MEDICINE AND HEALING IN THE ANCIENT MEDITERRANEAN WORLD

MEDICINE AND HEALING IN THE ANCIENT MEDITERRANEAN WORLD

including the Proceedings of the International Conference with the same title, organised in the framework of the Research Project 'INTERREG IIIA: Greece–Cyprus 2000–2006, Joint Educational and Research Programmes in the History and Archaeology of Medicine, Palaeopathology and Palaeoradiation'

and

the 1st International CAPP Symposium 'New Approaches to Archaeological Human remains in Cyprus'

Edited by

Demetrios Michaelides

Oxbow Books
Oxford & Philadelphia

Published in the United Kingdom in 2014 by
OXBOW BOOKS
10 Hythe Bridge Street, Oxford OX1 2EW

and in the United States by
OXBOW BOOKS
908 Darby Road, Havertown, PA 19083

Hardcover Edition: ISBN 978-1-78297-235-8
Digital Edition: ISBN 978-1-78297-236-5

A CIP record for this book is available from the British Library

Library of Congress Cataloging-in-Publication Data

Medicine in the Ancient Mediterranean World (Conference) (2008 : Nicosia, Cyprus), author.
Medicine and healing in the ancient Mediterranean world : including the proceedings of the international conference with the same title, organised in the framework of the Research Project INTERREG IIIA : Greece/Cyprus 2000/2006, Joint Educational and Research Programmes in the History and Archaeology of Medicine, Palaeopathology, and Palaeoradiation, and the 1st International CAPP Symposium "New Approaches to Archaeological Human Remains in Cyprus" / edited by Demetrios Michaelides.
p. ; cm.
Includes bibliographical references.
ISBN 978-1-78297-235-8
I. Michaelides, Demetres, editor. II. International CAPP Symposium "New Approaches to Archaeological Human Remains in Cyprus" (1st : 2008 : Nicosia, Cyprus), author. III. Biomedical Sciences in Archaeology (Conference) (1st : 2008 : Erakleion, Greece), author. IV. Title.
[DNLM: 1. History of Medicine--Mediterranean Region--Congresses. 2. Archaeology--Mediterranean Region--Congresses. 3. History, Ancient--Mediterranean Region--Congresses. 4. History, Medieval--Mediterranean Region--Congresses. WZ 70 GM35]
R135
610.938--dc23

2014014310

Printed in the United Kingdom by Berforts Information Press Ltd, Eynsham, Oxfordshire

For a complete list of Oxbow titles, please contact:

UNITED KINGDOM
Oxbow Books
Telephone (01865) 241249, Fax (01865) 794449
Email: oxbow@oxbowbooks.com
www.oxbowbooks.com

UNITED STATES OF AMERICA
Oxbow Books
Telephone (800) 791-9354, Fax (610) 853-9146
Email: queries@casemateacademic.com
www.casemateacademic.com/oxbow

Oxbow Books is part of the Casemate Group

Front cover: Mosaic of Saint Demetrios and an angel (before the 7th century AD). Basilica of Saint Demetrios, Thessaloniki (photo: 9th Ephoreia of Byzantine Antiquities).
Marble tombstone of the Athenian physician Jason (2nd century AD), Athens (photo: British Museum)

Back cover: Rodon (rose), illumination from mid-14th century manuscript (Padua, Biblioteca del Seminario, 194, f.134 r)
Roman limestone ex-voto of pair of eyes, of unknown origin, in the Cyprus Museum, Nicosia (photo: A. Koutas)
Wearing the plantago as a necklace to cure the headache (Codex Vindobonensis 93, f. 10 v).

Contents

1st International CAPP Symposium 'New Approaches to Archaeological Human remains in Cyprus'

Preface

In 1984, mechanical excavators working on the construction of Annabelle Hotel in Paphos chanced upon a large family tomb consisting of several rock-cut chambers arranged around an atrium. One of these contained a number of burials including that of a Roman surgeon of the late 2nd/early 3rd century AD, easily identifiable as such by the rich *instrumentarium* buried with him.[1] The study of the unusual and beautiful surgical instruments found there led me into the world of ancient Medicine, where I have stayed ever since.

In October 1995, on the occasion of the 'European Cultural Month' in Nicosia, the Archaeological Research Unit of the University of Cyprus, together with the Department of Mathematics and Statistics, and the Department of Computer Sciences, organised a very successful seminar entitled *The University of Cyprus and Medicine*, which was accompanied by a photographic exhibition on *Medicine and Hygiene in Ancient Cyprus*.

Another exhibition was organised by the Cultural Centre of the Laiki Group in 2006, covering different aspects of Medicine in Cyprus, from antiquity to the 20th century. The exhibition was accompanied by a substantial volume (in Greek) on the History of Medicine in Cyprus, to which I contributed the chapter dedicated to the ancient period.[2] Many of the panels with photographs and texts used for this exhibition were given to the Archaeological Research Unit through the kindness of Mrs Marina Vryonidou then of the Cultural Centre of the Laiki Group to be used during the conference *Medicine in the Ancient Mediterranean World*, which I had then begun to organise.

Already in 2005, Dr Constantinos Trompoukis, from the Laboratory for the History of Medicine and Medical Ethics of the University of Crete, had approached me with a proposal to put together an application for funding, though INTERREG III: Greece-Cyprus 2000-2006, for a Research Project entitled 'Joint Educational and Research Programmes in the History of Archaeology of Medicine, Palaeopathology and Palaeoradiation'. The application was successful and the programme started running in 2006. The international conferences *Biomedical Sciences in Archaeology* and *Medicine in the Ancient Mediterranean World* were part of this programme. The first was organised at Hersonissos, Crete, 24–26 September 2008, by Constantinos Trompoukis and the Laboratory for the History of Medicine and Medical Ethics of the University of Crete, with the assistance of the Archaeological Research Unit of the University of Cyprus. The roles were reversed for the second conference, which followed immediately afterwards, 27–29 September 2008. It took place in Nicosia, at the Archaeological Research Unit of the University of Cyprus.

For the organisation of the Cypriot conference, I was assisted by my colleagues Vasiliki Kassianidou and George Papasavvas, as well as the then PhD students Giorgos Papantoniou and Dimitrios Vitas, whom I was able to employ through the project. To all of them, as well as Dr Anthi Kaldeli and my then secretary Mrs Irida Chrysafi, I extend my thanks for all the assistance they offered during the preparation the conference. I am also grateful to the then undergraduate students Georgia Shiaelou and Nike Kyriakou; the post-graduate students Andreas Christou and Skevi Sykopetritou; and the PhD candidate Skevi Christodoulou, for the precious support they provided during the conference.

The aim of the conference was to cover as many aspects as possible of Medicine in the Mediterranean world during Antiquity and early Byzantine times. This is why I was happy to incorporate in it the 1st Symposium of the Cyprus Ancient Population Project (CAPP), which was put together by Dr Kirsi Lorentz. Another aim was to attract internationally established specialists on the history of medicine, as well as researchers in the early stages of their career.

The grouping of the contributions in the present volume follows that of the conference. A comparison between the programme of the conference and the list of contributions, however, reveals several differences. A number of colleagues had to cancel their participation to the conference at the last minute but sent their papers to be read by someone else. Others did not. Of the colleagues that made a presentation some sent their papers for publication others decided not to. Also, I had agreed to publish articles by several colleagues who right from the start informed me that, although they could not come to the conference, they wished to be included in the publication that would result from it.

Thus the present volume is not strictly speaking a volume of proceedings since, although it includes the largest part of the Nicosia conference (as well as the papers of the 1st Symposium of the Cyprus Ancient Population Project), it also includes a number of other contributions. I am most grateful to Professors Robert Arnott and Charalambos Bakirtzis for their invaluable input during the preparation of the present volume, and to Drs Alison South and Ian

Todd for assistance with the editing of the papers. As always, I am most thankful to the University of Cyprus for its support, financial and otherwise.

Demetrios Michaelides
Archaeological Research Unit
University of Cyprus
6 November 2013

Notes

1 D. Michaelides, 'A Roman Surgeon's Tomb from Nea Paphos', Part 1; and G. V. Foster, K. Kanada and D. Michaelides, 'A Roman Surgeon's Tomb, Part II: Ancient Medicines: By-products of Copper Mining in Cyprus', *Report of the Department of Antiquities, Cyprus* 1984, 315–32 and 1988, 229–34 respectively.

2 *Η Ιατρική στην Κύπρο, από την Αρχαιότητα μέχρι την Ανεξαρτησία*, Nicosia 2006.

Conference Programme

SATURDAY 27 SEPTEMBER 2008

08:30 – 09.00 Welcoming Remarks

Session 1: Medicine and Archaeology

Chairperson: Demetrios Michaelides

09:00–09:35 A. A. Diamandopoulos
Medicine and Archaeology

09:35–09:55 G. Karamitrou-Mendesidi and K. Moschakis
The Development of Medicine in Upper Macedonia during Antiquity

09:55–10:30 Coffee Break

Session 2: Media

Chairperson: Euphrosyne Rizopoulou-Egoumenidou

10:30–11:05 G. Cobolet
The Medical and Dental Academic Library of Paris (BIUM)

11:05 11:25 M. B. Ramos de Viesca, C. Viesca Treviño, S. Rodriguez Tierradentro and Itzel del Carmen Cruz Gaona
An Example of the Use of Multimedia Techniques for the Teaching of the History of Medicine

11:25–11:45 G. Sidiropoulos
City and Monument. Virtual Visualisation in the Classical World (The Case Study of Pergamon and its Asclepieion)

Session 3: The Aegean

Chairperson: Giorgos Papasavvas

11:45–12:20 R. Arnott
Healers and Medicines in Mycenaean Greek Texts

12:20–12:40 C. Morris and A. Peatfield
Health and Healing on Cretan Bronze Age Peak Sanctuaries

12:40–13:00 T. Sukhishvili
Medical Knowledge on the Evidence of Homeric Epic

13:00–14:30 Lunch Break

Session 4: Medical Authors/Schools of Medicine

Chairperson: Stella Demesticha

14:30–15:05 D. D. Lipourlis
Tracing the Origins of the Hippocratic Oath

15:05–15:25 A. Papachrysostomou and G. Gazis
Echoing Hippocrates: Aspects of Genre Intertextuality in the 5th Century BC

15:25–15:45 E. M. Kalokairinou
Ancient Medicine and Philosophy: A Philosopher's Perspective

15:45–16:05 N. A. E. Kalospyros
The Threshold of Pain. The Literary Embodiment of Pain and its Cognates in the Hippocratic Corpus

16:05–16:30 Coffee Break

16:30–16:50 F. Megaloudi
Knowledge and Practices of Andrology in the Hippocratic Medicine

16:50–17:10 D. Bacalexi
Le Traité de Galien De Pulsibus ad Tirones*: Pratique Médicale et Représentation du Corps Humain*

17:10–17:30 D. Koutroumpas and G. Papadopoulos
Galen of Pergamon's 'Art of Medicine': an Epitome of Medicine and its Different Fields

17:30–17:50 P. van der Eijk
Jones and After — Episodes in the Historiography of Malaria in the Classical World

17:50–18:10 A. Gautherie
Medical Dialogue in the Books on Dietetics in Celsus' De medicina

18:10–18:30 L. Cilliers
The Contribution of the 4th Century North African Physician, Helvius Vindicianus

SUNDAY, 28 SEPTEMBER 2008

Session 5: Surgery

Chairperson: Ourania Kouka

08:30–09:05 R. Jackson
Back to Basics: Surgeons' Knives in the Roman World

09:05–09:40 A. Musajo Somma
Alexander's Wounds as a Paradigm for War Surgery

09:40–10:15 S. Geroulanos
Surgery in Byzantium

10:15–10:35 M. Papadakis, E. Sfakiotakis, M. Fragakis, C. Trompoukis, M. Fragaki, M. Leivadara and A. Manios
Plastic Surgery of the Face in Byzantine Times

10:35–11:00 Coffee Break

Session 6: Medicaments and Cures

Chairperson: Vasiliki Kassianidou

11:00–11:35 G. Zanchin
The Headache Remedies of the Pseudo-Apuleius. A Modern Reappraisal

11:35–12:10 A. Touwaide
Formulas for Medicaments in Ancient Medicine: a First Approach

12:10–12:30 E. Photos-Jones and A. J. Hall
Alum, Astringency, Lemnian Earth and the Earths of the Aegean: an Archaeological Perspective

12:30–12:50 C. Tziraki-Segal and O. Y. Margalit
'Custom Designing your Offspring': Imagination and Progeny in Greco-Roman and Jewish Sources

12:50–13:10 Itzel del Carmen Cruz Gaona, S. Rodriguez Tierradentro, M. B. Ramos de Viesca and C. Viesca Treviño
Women and Contraception in the Ancient World

13:10–13:30 S. Gonzáles Soutelo
Spas in the Roman Age: Characteristics and Use of establishments with Mineral-Medicinal Water

13:30–15:00 Lunch Break

Session 7: Skeletal remains

Chairpersons: Kirsi O. Lorentz and Sherry C. Fox

15:00–15:20 A. L. Santos, F. Cortesão Silva, J. Márquez Pérez and J. Rosa
Care and Survival of a Child with Cranial Trauma at Augusta Emerita (Spain)

1st International CAPP Symposium 'New Approaches to Archaeological Human Remains in Cyprus'

15:20–15:30 Kirsi O. Lorentz
The Cyprus Ancient Populations Project (CAPP)

15:30–15:50 F. Le Mort, E. Crubezy, S. Duchesne, L. Haye, S. Lenorzer, S. Harter-Lailheugue, F. Bouchet, J.-D. Vigne and J. Guilaine
Health Status and Funerary Practices of the First Farmers of Cyprus: Inferences from Shillourokambos

15:50–16:10 Z. Parras
My Side of the Mountain: Initial Colonisation and Biological Regionalism on Cyprus through the Neolithic and Chalcolithic

16:10–16:30 K. O. Lorentz
Ante-Mortem Tooth Loss in Chalcolithic Populations of Cyprus. Comparisons between Cemetery and Settlement

16:30–17:00 Coffee Break

17:00–17:20 M. Gamble and K. O. Lorentz
A Preliminary look at the Health Status of Chalcolithic Populations: Inferences from Linear Enamel Hypoplasia

17:20–17:40 N. K. Harper
Spatial Patterning and Kinship within Kourion's Amathous Gate Cemetery

17:40–18:00 S. C. Fox, I. Moutafi, E. A. Prevedorou and D. Pilides
Trauma Patterns in Early Christian Cyprus

MONDAY, 29 SEPTEMBER 2008

Session 8: Asklepios and Incubation

Chairperson: Eleni Kalokairinou

09:00–09:20 J. Harrison
The Development of the Practice of Incubation in the Ancient World

09:20–09:40 I. Israelowich
The Authority of Physicians as Dream Interpreters in the Pergamene Asclepieion

09:40–10:00 G. Petridou
Asclepius the Physician. Asclepius the God Soter (Saviour): Epiphanies as Diagnostic and Therapeutic Tools

10:00–10:30 Coffee Break

Session 9: Byzantium

Chairperson: Maria Parani

10:30–11:05 C. Bakirtzis
The Hospital of St. Demetrios: Iconographic Issues

11:05–11:25 Father V. Trompoukis
Information of Medical Interest in Canon Law Texts

11:25–11:45 D. Papaioannou
Diseases as described in the Lives of Saints and their Cure

Session 10: Byzantine, Arab and Medieval Sources

Chairperson: Chris Schabel

11:45–12:05 C. Tsiamis, E. Poulakou-Rebelakou and G. Androutsos
The Role of the Egyptian Sea and Land Routes in the Justinian plague: the Case of Pelusium

12:05–12:25 M. Katouzian-Safadi
Du diagnostic différentiel aux thérapies prudentes: le traité de la rougeole et de la variole de Râzî

12:25–12:45 M.-M. Weker
The Ancient Background of Witelo's Theory of vision

Contributors to this volume

George Androutsos
History of Medicine
Athens Medical School
University of Athens
Athens
Greece
Email: lyon48@otenet.gr

Robert Arnott
Green Templeton College
University of Oxford
UK
Email: Robert.Arnott@medsci.ox.ac.uk

Dina Bacalexi
CNRS Centre Jean-Pépin (UPR_76)
L'Année Philologique
7 rue Guy-Môquet
F-94801 Villejuif Cedex
France
Email: bacalexi@vjf.cnrs.fr

Charalambos Bakirtzis
Anastasios G. Leventis Foundation
P.O. Box 2543
40, Gladstonos Street
1095 Nicosia
Cyprus
Email: charalambosb@yahoo.gr

Jean-Marc Bonmatin
Centre de Biophysique Moléculaire – CNRS
Rue Charles Sadron
45 071 Orléans Cedex 02
France
Email: bonmatin@cnrs-orleans.fr

Popi Chrysostomou
Cyprus Missing Persons Forensic Laboratory
Nicosia
Cyprus
Email: kaliopi05@gmail.com

Louise Cilliers
Department of Classics
University of the Free State
P.O. Box 339
Bloemfontein 9301
South Africa
Email: louise.cilliers@mweb.co.za

Guy Cobolet
Bibliothèque Interuniversitaire de Santé
12 rue de l'Ecole de Médecine
75006 Paris
France
Email: guy.cobolet@biusante.parisdescartes.fr

Filipa Cortesão Silva
Department of Life Sciences and CIAS
University of Coimbra
Apartado 3046
P-3001-401 Coimbra
Portugal
Email: filipacortesao@hotmail.com

Athanasios Diamandopoulos
St Andrew's State Hospital
1, Tertsidou Street
Patras
Greece
Email: tdiamandopoulos@yahoo.com

Sherry C. Fox
Wiener Laboratory
American School of Classical Studies at Athens
54, Souidias Street
Athens GR106-76
Greece
Email: sfox@ascsa.edu.gr

MARIA FRAGAKI
Department of Surgical Oncology
University General Hospital
Heraklion
Greece

MARIOS FRAGAKIS
Department of Dentistry
University General Hospital
Heraklion
Greece

MICHELLE GAMBLE
School of Historical Studies
Armstrong Building
Newcastle University
Newcastle-upon-Tyne NE1 7RU
UK
Email: michelle.gamble@ncl.ac.uk

AURÉLIEN GAUTHERIE
23 rue de Kembs
67100 – Strasbourg
France
Email: agautherie@yahoo.fr

GEORGIOS GAZIS
27, Matrozou Street
141 21 Neo Irakleio
Athens
Greece

STEFANOS GEROULANOS
University of Zurich
President, International Hippocratic Foundation
4, Papastratou Street
Kifissia
Athens 145 62
Greece
Email: stgeroulanos@gmail.com

SILVIA GONZÁLES SOUTELO
Universidade di Santiago de Compostela
Facultade de Xeografía e Historia
Universidade de Vigo
Campus Universitario As Lagoas, s/n
32004 Ourense
Spain
Email: silviatui2004@yahoo.es

ALLAN J. HALL
Department of Archaeology
University of Glasgow
Glasgow G12 QQ
Scotland
UK
Email: allan.hall@me.com

JULIETTE HARRISSON
Institute of Archaeology and Antiquity
University of Birmingham
Birmingham B15 2TT
UK
Email: Juliette.Harrisson@staff.newman.ac.uk

IDO ISRAELOWICH
Department of Classics and History
Tel Aviv University
Tel Aviv
Israel
Email: ido0572@post.tau.ac.il

RALPH JACKSON
Curator of Romano-British Collections
Department of Prehistory and Europe
British Museum
Great Russell Street
London WC1B 3DG
UK
Email: rjackson@thebritishmuseum.ac.uk

ELENI M. KALOKAIRINOU
Aristotle University of Thessaloniki
Department of Philosophy and Education
University Campus
541 24 Thessaloniki
Greece
E-mail: elenikal132@yahoo.gr

NICHOLAS A. E. KALOSPYROS
Department of Philosophy and History of Science
The National and Kapodistrian University of Athens
Athens
Greece
Email: nkalospy@phs.uoa.gr

Georgia Karamitrou-Mendesidi
30th Ephorate of Prehistoric and Classical Antiquities
Archaeological Museum of Aiani
P.O. Box 500 04
Aiani Kozanis
Greece

Mehrnaz Katouzian-Safadi
CNRS- Laboratoire SPHERE - CHSPAM - UMR 7219
Université Denis Diderot
75205 CEDEX 13 Paris
France
Email: katouzian.safadi@orange.fr

Demetrios C. Koutroumpas
Post-Doctoral Researcher
School of DentistryNational Kapodistrian University of Athens
Dem. Liouni 8
Keratea 19001
Greece
Email: dkoutrou@gmail.com

Moschoula Leivadara
Department of Surgical Oncology
University General Hospital
Heraklion
Greece

Demetrios Lypourlis
Arch. Oikonomide 1
54636 Thessaloniki
Greece
Email: dlipourlis@yahoo.gr

Kirsi O. Lorentz
Science and Technology in Archaeology Research Centre
The Cyprus Institute
Guy Ourisson Bldg. Athalassa Campus
P.O. Box 27456
1645 Nicosia
Cyprus
Email: k.o.lorentz@cyi.ac.cy

Efterpi Lyberopoulou
Intensive Care Unit
Onassis Cardiac Surgery Center
Syngrou 354
Athens 176-74
Greece
Email: efterpi.lyberopoulou@gmail.com

Andreas Manios
Department of Surgical Oncology
Univertsity General Hospital
Heraklion
Greece

Ohr Y. Margalit
Levinsky College of Education
Tel Aviv
Israel
Email: ohr.margalit@gmail.com

Juana Márquez Pérez
Consorcio Ciudad Histórico-Artística y Arqueológica de Mérida
C/ Reyes Huertas, 4
Mérida-Badajoz 06800
Spain
Email: juana@consorciomerida.org

Demetrios Michaelides
Archaeological Research Unit
University of Cyprus
Kallipoleos 75
Nicosia 1678
Cyprus
Email: d.michaelides@ucy.ac.cy/
dmichael@spidernet.com.cy

Christine Morris
Department of Classics and Centre for Mediterranean and Near Eastern Studies
Trinity College Dublin
Dublin 2
Ireland
Email: cmorris@tcd.ie

Kostas Moschakis
30th Ephorate of Prehistoric and Classical Antiquities
Archaeological Museum of Aiani
P.O.B. 500 04
Aiani Kozanis
Greece
Email: con.mosch@yahoo.gr

Ioanna Moutafi
Department of Archaeology
University of Sheffield
Sheffield
UK

ALFREDO MUSAJO SOMMA
Departimento ACTI
Università degli Studi di Bari
Via Calefati, 190
70122 Bari
Italy
Email: musajosomma@libero.it

CHARALAMBOS V. PANARETOS
204-206, Corinthou Street
Patras 26221
Greece
Email: panaretos.ch@gmail.com

ATHINA PAPACHRYSOSTOMOU
Open University of Greece
3, Valtetsiou Street
152 31 Kato Chalandri
Athens
Greece
Email: athina.papachrysostomou@uclmail.net

MARIOS PAPADAKIS
Department of Surgical Oncology
University General Hospital
Heraklion, Voutes 71110
Greece
Email: marios_papadakis@yahoo.gr

GIORGOS PAPADOPOULOS
School of Medicine
National Capodistrian University of Athens
Athens
Greece

DIMITRA PAPAIOANNOU
8th Ephorate of Byzantine Antiquities
Gorgopotamou 18
45221 Ioannina
Greece
Email: dipapaioannou@culture.gr

ZISSIS PARAS
2528 Kingsberry Cres.
Mississauga
Ontario L5B 2K5
Canada
Email: zparras@hotmail.com

ALAN PEATFIELD
School of Archaeology
University College Dublin
Dublin 4
Ireland
Email: alan.peatfield@ucd.ie

GEORGIA PETRIDOU
Department of Classics and Ancient History
University of Exeter
Amory Building
Rennes Drive
EX4 4RJ Exeter
Devon
UK
Email: G.Petridou@ex.ac.uk

EUPHEMIA PHOTOS-JONES
Analytical Services for Art and Archaeology (Ltd)
and
Department of Archaeology
University of Glasgow
Glasgow G12 QQ
Scotland
UK
Email: effie@sasaa.co.uk

DESPINA PILIDES
Department of Antiquities
Ministry of Communications and Works
Nicosia
Cyprus
Email: despo_pilides@hotmail.com

EFFIE POULAKOU-REBELAKOU
History of Medicine
Athens Medical School
University of Athens
Greece
Email: efpoulrebel@med.uoa.gr

ELENI ANNA PREVEDOROU
School of Human Evolution and Social Change
Arizona State University
Tempe, Arizona
USA

JOÃO ROSA
Department of Pediatrics
Hospital de Faro – E.P.E.
Rua Leão Penedo
8000-386 Faro
Portugal
Email: rosa.joao@gmail.com

ANA LUISA SANTOS
Department of Life Sciences and CIAS
University of Coimbra
Apartado 3046
P-3001-401 Coimbra
Portugal
Email: alsantos@antrop.uc.pt

Evangelos Sfakiotakis
Department of Plastic Surgery
Thriassio General Hospital
Magoula
Athens
Greece

Tamar Sukhishvili
Faculty of Humanities and Cultural Studies
Ilia Chavchavadze State University
0186 Tbilisi
Georgia
Email: tasukhi@yahoo.com

Alain Touwaide
Smithsonian Institution
Washington, DC
USA
Email: atouwaide@hotmail.com

Constantinos Trompoukis
Department of History of Medicine and Medical Ethics
University of Crete
Heraklion
Greece
Email: trompoukis@med.uoc.gr

Father Vasileios Chr. Trompoukis
40, Krystalli Street
Arta 47100
Greece
Email: vtrompoukis@hol.gr

Costas Tsiamis
History of Medicine
Medical School
University of Athens
Athens
Greece
Email: ctsiamis@med.uoa.gr

Chariklia Tziraki-Segal
Hebrew University
Ein Kerem
Israel
Email: tziraki@gmail.com

Philip Van der Eijk
Humbolt University
Berlin
Germany
Email: philip.van.der.eijk@staff.hu-berlin.de

Yiannis Violaris
Department of Antiquities
Ministry of Communications and Works
Limassol
Cyprus
Email: violarisyian@yahoo.gr

Maria-Magdalena Weker
Institute of Philosophy
Cardinal Stefan Wyszynski University
Warsaw
Poland
Email: m.weker@uksw.edu.pl

Giorgio Zanchin
Headache Centre
Department of Neurosciences
Padua University Medical School
Via Giustiniani 5
I 35128 Padova
Italy
Email: giorgio.zanchin@unipd.it

Part I

Medicine and Archaeology

1. Medicine and Archaeology

Athanasios A. Diamandopoulos

Defining the relationship between the history of medicine and archaeology is a chapter of the more general effort to define the relationship between history and archaeology. History has been roughly defined as a usually chronological record of events, as of the life or development of a people or institution, often including an explanation of or commentary on these events. Archaeology has been roughly defined as the systematic study of past human life and culture by the recovery and examination of remaining material evidence, such as graves, buildings, tools and pottery. Based on the above introduction, we can put forward the hypothesis that the archaeology of medicine makes the history of medicine more precise as it offers definite materials to be studied objectively, in contrast to texts that are usually more subjective. We will test this hypothesis in the course of this article.

Defining the relationship between the history of medicine and archaeology is a chapter in the more general effort to define the relationship between history and archaeology. History has been roughly defined as a usually chronological record of events, as of the life or development of a people or institution, often including an explanation of or commentary on these events. Traditionally, it is the study of the past using mainly documentary sources created by or about the society under scrutiny. Inevitably such investigations concentrated on societies where writing had been adopted.

Most of human history, however, is not described by any written records. Writing did not exist anywhere in the world until about 5000 years ago, and only spread among a relatively small number of technologically advanced civilisations. These civilisations are, not coincidentally, the best-known; they have been open to the inquiry of historians for centuries, while archaeology has appeared only recently. Even within a civilisation that is literate at some levels, many important human practices are not officially recorded. Any knowledge of the formative early years of human civilisation – the development of agriculture, cult practices of folk religion, the rise of the first cities – must come from archaeology.

Archaeology has been roughly defined as the systematic study of past human life and culture through the recovery and examination of remaining material evidence, such as graves, buildings, tools and pottery (*Britannica*). Hence, it would seem that, from a methodological point of view, history is concerned with events as they are documented in writing, while archaeology deals with materials of any form, even from illiterate societies. We should not, however, forget that written records tend to reflect the biases of the literate classes, and cannot be trusted as a sole source. The material record is nearer to a fair representation of society, although it is subject to its own inaccuracies, such as sampling bias and differential preservation. Several subfields of anthropology supplement the findings of archaeology, especially cultural anthropology (which studies behavioural, symbolic, as well as material dimensions of culture) and physical anthropology (which includes the study of human evolution and osteology). Other disciplines also supplement archaeology, such as palaeontology (the study of prehistoric life), including palaeozoology and palaeobotany, geography, geology, art history and classical studies.

There is considerable overlap between the objects of study of history and archaeology. Although written documents are the realm of history, some inscribed material lies in the field of archaeology. Epigrams on marble stelai, Egyptian papyri, illuminated medieval codices, words written on ceramics or coins are some such examples. On the other hand, legends, songs, poems and epic cycles, transmitted orally from generation to generation in illiterate societies, are studied by historians and not by archaeologists. Hybrid case-reports close to our interests abound. For example, when writing the history of a hospital, we are dealing with actual materials (the building, its contents, its landscape) but we are also studying the relevant written documents (its archives, the biographies of famous doctors or patients who worked or were treated there etc.).

Based on the foregoing introduction, we can put forward the hypothesis that the archaeology of medicine makes the history of medicine more precise as it offers definite materials to be studied objectively, in contrast to texts that are usually more subjective. We will test this hypothesis in the present paper. For the time being, I will mention that, just reviewing this year's published world literature, I noticed that there are some dozens of journals and books dealing with archaeology in medicine – a theme that has apparently caused great interest.

The next question was to find out how seriously the members of the International Society for the History of Medicine (ISHM) are interested in the topic; a kind of market research to decide if it was worth investing time and effort in writing this paper. As study material, I used the titles of the articles published in *Vesalius* and the proceedings of the ISHM congresses, as these are reported on the society's website (http://www.biusante.parisdescartes.fr/ishm/eng/acc_adh.htm). Overall, only 3.58% of all articles are of remote archaeological interest (Fig. 1.1). The percentage starts from the high of 100% in the section on prehistory (as was expected as there are no written sources of that period), to a low 1.64% in the varia section. The finding was disappointing and it might have discouraged any speculator from investing in the enterprise. However, I felt that our role is not to sell an idea but to promote it. Thus, the idea of monothematic meetings was first introduced after my election as President of ISHM in Bari four years ago, in order to investigate the relationship between medicine and the four elements. In order to avoid the risk of being seen as didactic in this swan-song of mine as president, I will refer briefly to the titles of my previous lectures at the opening ceremonies of this Society.

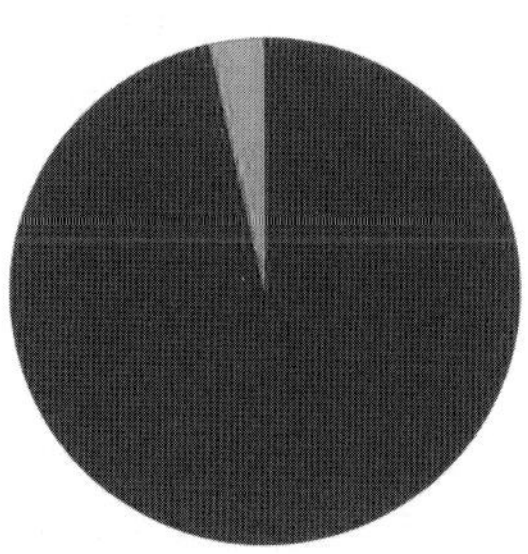

Fig. 1.1 Percentage of archaeo-medical to historico-medical subjects in ISHM Publications (A. Diamandopoulos)

At the 2005 meeting in Patras I spoke about 'Aqua and the Temple', promoting our interest in a natural element, something different from the human race, the usual subject of the history of medicine. In the 2006 Budapest congress I spoke about the fallacy of the statement 'The world is small', and tried to explain why the world is really vast and it just seems small because we try to minimise it according to our intellectual limits and preconceived ideas. But the world is not small, nor is it solid. We face two different worlds, contradicting each other and neither of them represents an erroneous image by claiming to be a representative sample of the whole. My aim then was to expand our studies in different parts of 'Old Europe'. In the 2007 Tuscany meeting the title of my lecture was 'When the air was impure', pointing to the moral obligations of our profession throughout history. And here I support the cooperation between historians and archaeologists for a further understanding of the history of medicine. The general goal of all these lectures was, and still is, to expand the set limits of our Society in order to face the challenges of new ideas, new academic environments and new cultural trends. The fact that we love the past should not fossilise us. Evolution is the key factor of survival. And in order for the ISHM to survive it has to push its frontiers beyond its traditional occupations, its fickle politics and its strongly Westernised orientation.

I will describe the benefits to the history of medicine from involving archaeology as one of its tools. The main archaeological objects useful to the history of medicine are human, animal and plant remains, medical instruments, pharmaceutical apparati, and ruins of buildings linked with medicine. These may include hospitals, health practitioners' residences, medical schools, tombstones and other funerary architectural fragments, as well as water supplies and drainage systems. The study of all the above will furnish the historian of medicine with an abundance of definite material to understand and sometimes revive the past of our profession. This is the main difference between history and archaeology in general, and in their use for the history of medicine in particular. But the benefits of this cooperation can be twofold. They also offer information for the archaeologists so that they can understand the reason for many calamities, and explain the use of several artefacts. When the professionals of both fields avoid asking hard questions about medicine and its practice and artefacts in the past, errors of interpretation are common. *It is not the unanswered but the unasked questions that undermine discourse and give an unbalanced slant to an entire field.*

Before proceeding to a brief presentation of examples from the archaeological record, a word of caution is in order about the dangers of an over-enthusiastic approach. Firstly, we should remember that archaeology *per se* has only recently acquired the prestige of a science. The exact origins of archaeology as a discipline are uncertain. Excavations of ancient monuments and the collection of antiquities have been taking place for thousands of years. It was only in the 19th century, however, that the systematic study of the past through its physical remains began to be carried out in a manner recognisable to modern students of archaeology. Prior to this, excavation had tended to be haphazard; the importance of concepts such as stratification and context was completely overlooked. Nowadays, an array of scientific methods supplements archaeological research, including nuclear technology, satellite photography, lithology, DNA analysis and thermography, to name but a few. Thus, we should be very careful to avoid being influenced in our studies by such pseudo-archaeological reports in the media like *The Mummy* or *Raiders of the Lost Ark*.

Secondly, when discussing archaeological medical material, we should devote more than a superficial glimpse to the technological aspects of the area and era to which the object belonged. Usually, we underestimate the advances of technology in the remote or more recent past when we discuss the history of medicine. The several improvements in metallurgy cannot be set apart from the evolution of scalpels and thus the improvement of surgery. Similarly, discoveries in the field of glassmaking are bound up with improvements in pharmaceutical vials, eye spectacles and x-ray screens. Analytic and synthetic chemistry are the cradle of many pharmaceutical products. The examples are many but the core of this point is that historians of medicine should be very careful when discussing any of the above medical applications while ignoring improvements in technology. The latter is not a keystone only of the present or the future, as is usually assumed, but it has been with us for millennia. A passage from Aeschylus' tragedy *Prometheus Bound* devoted to the ways that the Titan Prometheus helped mankind is revealing of the ancient Greeks' idea of medicine combined with technology:

> '[...] they had eyes but could not see, and ears but could not hear. ... They did not know how to build houses with bricks and facing the sun, nor to work with wood. They lived in sunless caves the way ants live in the ground ... They worked without useful calculations, until I showed them the risings and settings of stars ... I taught them numbers, the greatest stratagem, and writing, the mother of memory. I yoked beasts for them ... and I harnessed horses to chariots and taught them to heed the rein ... And it was nobody else who gave humans ships, sail-driven wagons that the sea buffets. ... The greatest was this: when they fell ill, they had no defence – no balm, no ointment, no elixir – and lacking medicine, they wasted away, until I showed them pharmacy so they could fend off various diseases. ...' (Aeschylus, *Prometheus Bound*, transl. H. W. Smyth, Cambridge MA, 1926, 477–506)

Keeping these prerequisites in mind, let us briefly review a few indicative examples of archaeological discoveries useful to the historian of medicine. These include ruins of buildings, skeletal remains, written texts, and metal and clay artefacts. For the sake of brevity, I choose only examples from the locations associated with recent and forthcoming activities of the ISHM: A) Greece (3rd meeting, 2005; B) Italy (4th meeting, 2007; C) Mexico (42nd congress, 2008; D) Cyprus (5th meeting, 2009); and E) Egypt (43rd congress, 2010).

A. Greece

For an example of textual evidence, I cite a votive marble stele from the temple of Asklepios in Epidauros. Unearthed by an archaeological excavation in 1882, it dates from the 4th century BC (See, Παυσανίας, Ελλάδος Περιήγησης [Κορινθιακά], vol. 2, Athens 1976, 27–34, p. 207). On it are incised dedicatory epigrams by patients who were cured there by divine intervention during incubation. These epigrams offer valuable information about the kind of diseases treated there and the cultural background of the grateful patients. However, even in antiquity some sceptics were scornful of the latter, saying: 'They would have been more numerous if those who were lost offered them than those who were saved' (Diogenes Laertius, *Lives of Eminent Philosophers*, VI, 59, referred to in Bergdolt 2008, 48).

From the field of osteology, I present a female skull, excavated at the Clazomenean colony at Abdera in Thrace (Agelarakis 2006). This woman's remains, which date to the second half of the 7th century BC, provide the earliest evidence of cranial surgery in Greece. The woman suffered a skull fracture on the back of her head, probably from a missile hurled from a sling by Thracians attacking the settlement. She underwent surgery and survived, living for another two decades. Even three centuries before Hippocrates' work *On Head Wounds* we notice that the doctor involved in treating the patient used exactly the same technique as recommended by the Father of Medicine, who wrote:

> 'It is necessary, if the wound is at the sutures and the weapon penetrated and lodged into the bone, to pay attention for recognizing the kind of injury sustained by the bone. Because ... he who received the weapon at the sutures will suffer far greater impact at the cranial bone than the one who did not receive it at the sutures. And most of those require trepanation, but you must not trepan the sutures themselves ... you are required to scrape the surface of the cranial bone with a rasp in depth and length, according to the position of the wound, and then cross-wise to be able to see the hidden breakages and crushes ... because scraping exposes the harm well, even if those injuries ... were not otherwise revealed' (trans. in Agelarakis 2006)

Faced with a compressed fracture with radiating fissure fractures and fearing damage to the dura mater, the surgeon scraped the bone in length, width and depth, removing fragments and eliminating the fissures through scraping and not trepanation. He would then have tended to any adjacent injured tissues. He probably used a type of rasp similar to the one found amongst a set of 4th-century surgical instruments at Abdera itself.

The last example from Greece comes from Patras: it is a Roman funerary stele for an oculist, as is clearly incised upon it. It proves beyond doubt that separate medical specialities were practised there about 2000 years ago.

B. Italy

From the written domain, I present two copies of Greek medical texts, housed in the Vatican Library. One is written in Greek and is a 10th or 11th century copy of Galen's *De usu partium* (2nd century AD), while the other is a Latin translation of Aristotle's *Libri naturales*, made by William of Moerbeke and others in northern Italy, during the late 13th or early 14th century (Beullens and Bossier 2000). These are but a negligible sample of a treasure of antique medical books in Italian libraries. Through them, the ancient medical knowledge spread in the West during the Middle Ages, but mainly during the Renaissance. Old books such as these are a disputed land between the historian and the archaeologist.

Ancient DNA research is a new way of investigating the history of disease. Dr Robert Sallares, of the Institute of Science and Technology of the University of Manchester has analysed DNA extracted from the bones of an infant that was buried at Lugnano in Umbria more than 1,500 years ago. This DNA revealed signs of infection with the parasite *Plasmodium falciparum*, which, according to British researchers, is the earliest genetic evidence that *malaria tropica* plagued the classical civilisations of Rome and Greece (Sallares and Gomzi 2001).

Italy hosts a treasure of monumental buildings linked to the history of medicine, but I will mention only one: Santa Maria della Scala, the monastery-hospital building in Siena, dating from the 10th century that was still used as a hospital until the middle of the 20th century. The patients' wards, murals and instruments housed there offer an abundance of information for the practice of medicine in a religious establishment from the early Renaissance onward (see http://www.newadvent/org Catholic Encyclopedia/hospitals).

C. Mexico

From Mexico I mention just two Maya clay figurines relevant to the history of medicine. One shows a man with plastic dwarfism; the other represents a group of laparotomised persons, possibly as part of a sacrificial religious rite (Miller 1985 and Gill n.d., respectively).

D. Cyprus

A very ancient artefact related to the history of medicine is a bronze object found at Kition, dating to the 13th century BC. It was considered by the excavator, V. Karageorghis, as an early representation of a kidney (Karageorghis and Masson 1971), but its purpose is disputed. It was either a votive offering to the temple by a grateful patient, or a device for teaching anatomy novices. The incisions on its outer surface are assumed to be similar to those found on Etruscan liver replicas. I published an article on the discovery (Marketos, Eftychiadis and Diamandopoulos 1993), and later an elaborate form of this object was used as the logo of the Association for the History of Nephrology, and even later it was depicted on the front cover of my book on the History of Greek Nephology (Diamandopoulos 2000). Closer to the ISHM is the logo of a forthcoming meeting for the history of medicine. This is an array of clay hot-water bottles found in Paphos (Michaelidou-Nicolaou, 1988; Nicolaou, 1989; Michaelides 2006, 26–7, figs 25–34), some of which are incorporated in the logo of the Vth Meeting of the International Society for the History of Medicine that took place in Cyprus in 2008.

E. Egypt

The best known medical text from Ancient Egypt is the Ebers papyrus, of *c.* 1550 BC, now in the University of Lepzig (www.scribd.com/doc/71736659/Ebers-Papyrus). One passage (Formula No. 618 [78, 10–11]) deals with the medical use of cannabis. It is a remedy for a toe-nail (or finger), and its ingredients include honey, ochre, smsm-t (hemp) and other substances.

From the world of art I present two painted works: one is the funerary stele of the priest Rom, of 1350 BC, now in the Carlsberg Museum in Copenhagen (Daniel and Robbins 1997, 5–22). It depicts a person with a limp leg and dropped foot, reputably due to poliomyelitis. The second is a funerary statue of the 4th or early 5th Dynasty, with a very realistic depiction of the dwarf Seneb, overseer of the palace dwarfs, with his family (Junker 1941).

***

Another quite different factor for employing archaeology in the study of the history of medicine, apart from its usefulness, is its intrinsic aesthetic value and its appealing sense of mystery. Famous doctors and historians of medicine of the past have been also amateur archaeologists. Heinrich Schliemann, the famous excavator of Troy in Asia Minor and Mycenae in the Peloponnese, Greece, who unearthed the Bronze Age remains associated with the Homeric legends, was a close friend of Rudolf Virchow, the famous

German pathologist, who was also the founder of the German Society for Anthropology, Ethnology and Prehistory. Schliemann in his first season at Troy worked alone with his wife Sophia. In 1879 he was assisted by Emile Burnouf, a classical archaeologist, and by Rudolf Virchow himself. The Gennadius Library in Athens acquired the letters from Virchow to Schliemann, documenting the pathologist's strong interest in archaeology (Kennell 2007).

Throughout his long life Sigmund Freud, the famous psychiatrist, had only one hobby: the collection of antiquities, which he began in 1896, when he really could not afford it. He had a hoard of Mycenaean and Cypriote antiquities, out of admiration for Heinrich Schliemann (D'Agata 1994). 'His waiting room, consulting room and study were filled almost to overflowing with beautiful, rare and interesting objects', wrote Ernest Jones, Freud's best known biographer. 'Egyptian, Etruscan, Greek and Roman pieces predominated, but there were others from farther afield'. Freud derived what he himself called 'unsurpassable comfort' from his glimpses of the world of ancient culture (Jones 1957, 317). In a remarkable passage written in 1909, Freud describes clearly the similarities between the unconscious and the archaeological artefact:

> 'I then made some short observations upon the psychological differences between the conscious and the unconscious, and upon the fact that everything conscious was subject to a process of wearing-away, while what was unconscious was relatively unchangeable; and I illustrated my remarks by pointing to the antique objects standing about my room. They were in fact, I said, only objects found in a tomb, and their burial had been their preservation: the destruction of Pompeii was only beginning now that it had been dug up' (Jones 197, 317)

The next example concerns the great benefactor of the history of medicine, Henry Wellcome and his medical officer Dr Ray, emphasising the fascination that this subject was having on the founder of Burroughs Wellcome & Company, one of the first giant pharmaceutical companies.

The last benefit for the historians of medicine from studying archaeology is the avoidance of cliché statements about the role of health and the feeling of wellbeing at different given periods. We are well aware of the definition of health by the Alma Ata declaration in 1978:

> 'The Conference strongly reaffirms that health, which is a state of complete physical, mental and social wellbeing, and not merely the absence of disease or infirmity, is a fundamental human right and that the attainment of the highest possible level of health is a most important world-wide social goal whose realization requires the action of many other social and economic sectors in addition to the health sector' (*World Health Organisation* 1978)

Thus, the image of a healthy man we recall from such a declaration coincides with the ancient Greek ideal about human beauty and harmony. But in other eras the feeling of mental and social wellbeing was very different from what we commonly think of as bordering the unhealthy. In a mural of the Hippokrateion Hospital chapel in Athens, depicting the pious Maria of Egypt, we recognise the withered flesh of the perpetually fasting Maria, who otherwise obtained a desirable high level of mental and social wellbeing by answering the divine call (Popović 1988). Lastly, an effigy of Buddha depicts, by modern standards, an unacceptably obese god, who, however, smiles happily immersed in his divine nirvana. So, different works of art propagandising mutually exclusive forms of physical, mental and social wellbeing challenge our firmly set ideas on health.

A paper about the relationship between the history of medicine and archaeology cannot be complete without a reference to the role of museums in the history of medicine. Medical museums are the institutionalised indicators of scientific interest and academic research spirit. Their foundations were laid upon the formation of scientific museums at the end of the 19th century, and medical sections were also incorporated in science and war museums. Today, many such museums, hygiene, health, medicine technology, and medical history museums, have been founded (Erbay 2004). While stating as strongly as possible the huge status-gap between the aforementioned colleagues and myself, I dare to add my own addiction to archaeology, which prompted me to arrange the closing ceremony of the 2005 ISHM meeting in Patras, in the ruins of the ancient Roman Baths in Kyllene, in western Greece – a fitting end to a gathering devoted to the relationship between water and medicine.

Bibliography

Agelarakis, A. 2006: 'Artful Surgery: Greek archaeologists discover evidence of a skilled surgeon who practiced centuries before Hippocrates', *Archaeology* 59/2, 26–9.

Beullens, P. and Bossier, F. (eds) 2000: *De Historia Animalium: Translatio Guilelmi De Morbeka (Aristoteles Latinus,* 17), Leiden, Boston and Cologne.

Bergdolt, K. 2008: *Wellbeing, A Cultural History of Healthy Living*, transl. by J. Dewhurst, Cambridge, UK and Malden, MA, USA.

Britannica: <http://concise.britannica.com/ebc/: Archaeology

D'Agata, A. L. 1994: 'Sigmund Freud and Aegean archaeology. Mycenaean and Cypriote material from his collection of antiquities', *Studi Micenei ed Egeo-Anatolici* 34, 7–41.

Diamandopoulos: Διαμαντόπουλος, A. A., 2000: *Ιστορία της Ελληνικής Νεφρολογίας. Πρώτος Τόμος "δι'ὕδατος"*, Athens.

El-Shahawy, A.: 2005, *The Egyptian Museum in Cairo: A Walk Through the Alleys of Ancient Egypt*, Cairo.

Erbay, F. 2004: 'The role of medical museums in the education of medicine', 99–101 in A. Musajo-Somma (ed.), *Proceedings of the 39th International Congress on the history of medicine. Bari-Metaponto, 5–10 September 2004,* vol. 2, Bari.

Gill, N. S. n.d.: 'Human sacrifice and the Maya appeasing the ancient gods', see ancienthistory.about.com/od/deathafterlife/qt/012709Maya Scrf.htm.

Jones, E. 1957: *Time, Life and Work of Sigmund Freud*, Vol. III, New York.

Junker, H. 1941: *Gîza V: Die Mastaba des Snb (Seneb) und die umliegenden Gräber* (Akademie der Wissenschaften in Wien: Philosophisch-historische Klasse, Denkschriften 71.2), Wien – Leipzig.

Karageorghis, V. and Masson, É. 1971: 'Un bronze votif inscrit (modèle de foie ou de rein?) trouvé à Kition en 1970', *Studi Ciprioti e Rapporti di Scavo* I, 237–48.

Kennell, S. 2007: 'Schliemann and his papers: a tale from the Gennadeion archives', *Hesperia* 76, 785–817.

Marketos, S. G., Eftychiadis, A. G. and Diamandopoulos, A. 1993: 'Acute renal failure according to ancient Greek and Byzantine medical writers', *Journal of the Royal Society of Medicine* May 1993; 86/5, 290–3.

Michaelides: Μιχαηλίδης, Δ. 2006: 'Ιατροί και Ιατρική στην Αρχαία Κύπρο', 12–68 in *Ιατρική στην Κύπρο, από την Αρχαιότητα μέχρι την Ανεξαρτησία*, Nicosia.

Michaelidou-Nicolaou: Μιχαηλίδου-Νικολάου, Ι. 1988: 'Ευρήματα που έχουν σχέση με Ασκληπιείο ή θεραπευτήριο στην Πάφο. Το Ασκληπιείο της Πάφου', 278–81 in *Πρακτικά του XII Διεθνούς Συνεδρίου Κλασικής Αρχαιολογίας. Αθήνα, 4–10 Σεπτεμβρίου 1983,* τόμ. Δ΄, Athens.

Miller, M. E. 1985: 'The dwarf motif in classic Maya art', 141-53 in E. P. Benson (ed.), *Fourth Palenque Round Table, 1980*, San Francisco.

Nicolaou, I. 1989 : 'Les bouillottes therapeutiques de Paphos et leurs paralleles hors de Chypre, *Bulletin de Correspondance hellénique* 113, 301–18.

Popović, Monk Justin 1998: 'Sermon: Pius Maria of Egypt', in *Pashalne Besede*, Beograd.

Robbins, F. C. and Daniel, T. M. (eds) 1997: 'A history of poliomyelitis', 5-22 in F. C. Robbins and T. M. Daniel (eds), *Polio*, Rochester, N.Y.

Sallares, R. and Gomzi, S. 2001: 'Biomolecular archaeology of malaria', *Ancient Biomolecules* 3, 195–213.

World Health Organisation 1978: *Primary Health Care. Report of the International Conference on Primary Health Care, Alma-Ata, USS.* Geneva.

2. Η Ιατρική στην Αιανή και την Άνω Μακεδονία κατά την Αρχαιότητα

Γεωργία Καραμήτρου-Μεντεσίδη και Κώστας Μοσχάκης

English summary

Present-day Western Macedonia, a region bounded by mountain ranges of varying size and traversed by the River Haliakmon, belonged to the mountainous Upper Macedonia of antiquity, which extended beyond the borders of modern Greece and included the River Erigon, Lakes Achris (Ochrid) and Prespa and the lands bounded by the Dautica, Babuna and Dren Mountains to the north (Fig. 2.1).

Upper Macedonia, with the kingdoms of Elimeia, Tymphaea, Eordaea, Orestis, Lyncestis, Pelagonia and Derriopus, as well as other 'tribes from the interior' did not become socially and culturally isolated and weakened, as was, unfortunately, formerly claimed by researchers working only with a scant supply of archaeological and historical evidence. This fact has been demonstrated by the early dating, wealth, quality and character of the finds yielded by systematic research at Aiani and elsewhere (Fig. 2.2), which has made it necessary to re-examine earlier archaeological finds from a new perspective.

Our research for this paper concerns the four prefectures of present-day Western Macedonia and does not extend to the parts of ancient Macedonia which are today outside the borders of Greece. We have established the fact that all areas have remarkable finds, but most examples come from Elimeia, with a total of 23, while Eordaea follows with ten, Tymphaea with three, and Orestis and Lyncestis with two. Of all the 23 finds from Elimeia, 19 come from its capital Aiani and its surrounding area (Fig. 2.3). The categories, according to the material, are the following:

A. Sculptures of Asclepios and Hygieia

From Platania village comes a torso of an Asclepios marble statuette (Fig. 2.5), surviving in three parts. Beside its left foot there is part of a small column with a representation of a snake and a cane. It is certain that in the area where the statuette was found there was an Asclepios sanctuary, which is now completely destroyed. From Diporo village comes a relief votive stele with a representation of Asclepios along with an inscription: *Ἀσκληπιῷ εὐχὴν* (Fig. 2.6), and from Leukovrisi village, a relief stele with a representation of Hygieia and an inscription: *[ὁ (ἡ) δεῖνα Ἀσκ]ληπι[ὸν] καὶ τὴν Ὑγείαν* (Fig. 2.7). From Aiani we have an arched stele depicting two women. One of them holds a *phiale* towards a snake, which coils on her left hand. It is certainly a representation of Hygieia (Fig. 2.8). From the city of Kozani comes a female statuette (probably Hygieia) with a snake on her left side coiling towards her breast (Fig. 2.9).

B. Relief votive stelai with representations of medical instruments

A relief votive stele found in the village of Agalaioi (Fig. 2.10) represents a cupping vessel for bloodletting (Greek: *sikya*, Latin: *cucurbitula*). In Kelli, a gravestone with a representation of several people was found (Fig. 2.11). On the stele a female doctor among her assistant and servants can be identified. Bloodletting cups, a small cup and scissors (Greek: *pshalis*, Latin: *forfex*) are also depicted. A wooden open probe case, in the centre of the representation, includes a complete set of instruments: probes (*spathomele*), scalpels, sharp hooks/obstetrical hooks (*agkistron*) and also a small probe/curette (*cyathiscomele*).

C. Inscriptions referring to doctors

From the island of Agios Achilleios, in the Lake of Small Prespa, comes a grave altar with an inscription that mentions doctor K. Ioulios Neiketes (Fig. 2.12).

A grave stone was found in the village of Kato Kleines with a multi-person representation and a long inscription that mentions doctor Theodoros.

D. Representations of body parts on votive stelai

Representations of body parts on votive stelai form a large category. These stelai are considered as thank-offerings to gods, for the healing of specific parts of the body. In other cases they are used as an invocation to a god, for perception and understanding. Three stelai come from Aiani representing ears, one from Xirolimni (Fig. 2.13) and one from Karyochori (Fig. 2.14). From Velvento comes a stele with a representation of eyes, dedicated by Theodotos to the gods (Fig. 2.15).

E. Inscriptions with the name Asklepiades

The god-bearing name Asklepiades is written on a sarcophagus from the village of Kentron, as well as a bronze seal (today lost) from Aiani, and on a votive stele to Apollo Mesoriskos, from Xirolimni.

F. Vessels

A series of very interesting utensils of unusual manufacture come from Aiani (Fig. 2.16), while there is also one example from Eordaea. The fact that they are made from different materials is of great interest. Two of them are made of bronze, two of an alloy of copper and lead, and one of clay.

G. Instruments

Cosmetic or medical/pharmaceutical use is attributed to bronze ear spoons and also spoons made of bone. There are many examples from Aiani (Fig. 2.17) and Eordaea.

Observations and Conclusions

The archaeological finds connected to Asclepios and the practice of medicine continue to increase as research continues in Upper Macedonia. Aiani and Kozani prefectures are the best researched areas in Western Macedonia, with the most finds. In the other prefectures the majority of the finds connected to Asclepios and medicine are gravestones and votive stelai, most of them being random finds.

Aiani has, up to now, the earlier finds from the Classical and Hellenistic periods. In the broader region of Western Macedonia artefacts that have been found date to the Roman period. But as the archaeological research and excavations become more systematic and extensive, we hope that in the future the number of relevant finds will increase.

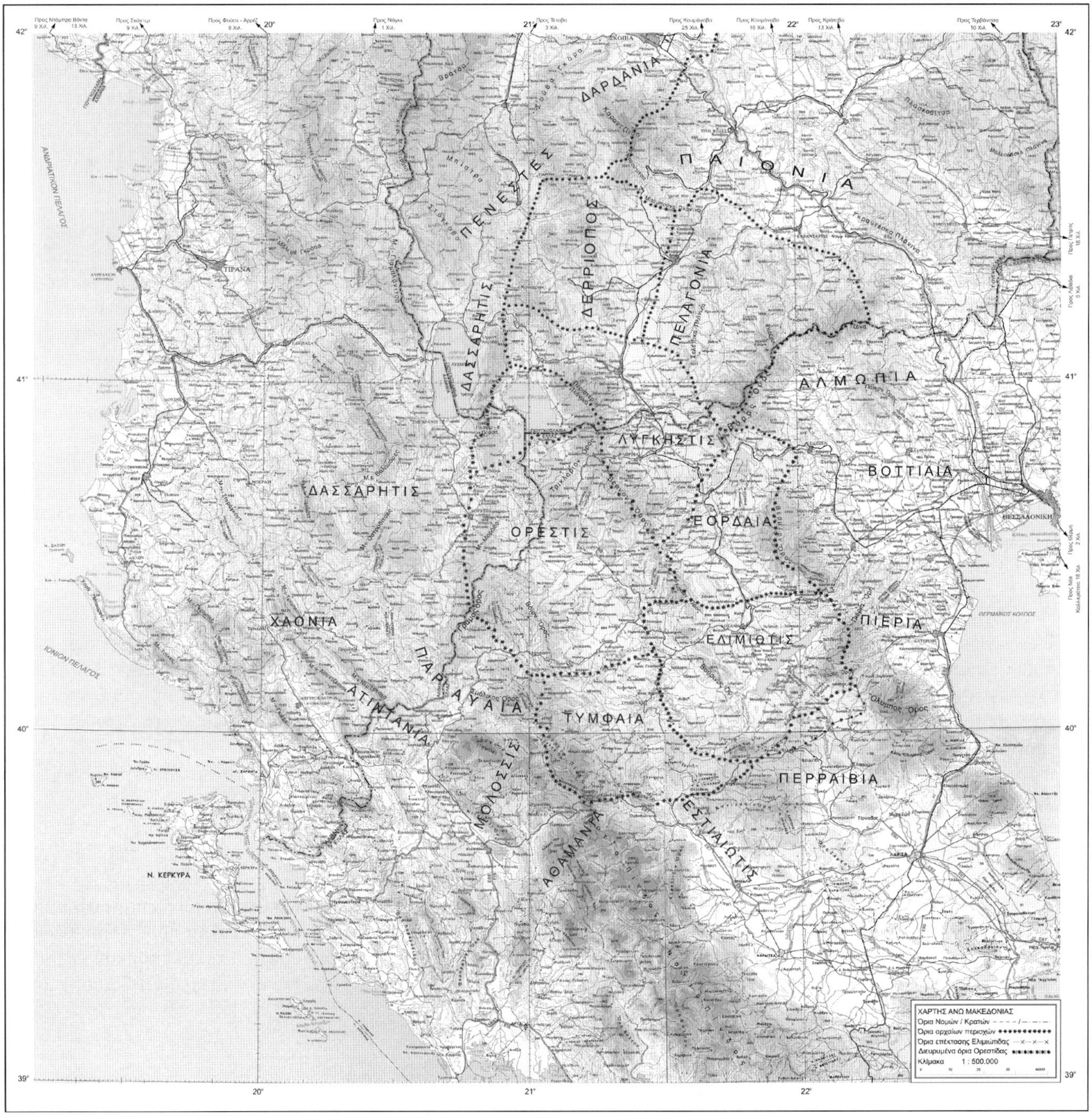

Εικ. 2.1. Χάρτης Άνω Μακεδονίας

Εισαγωγή

Άνω Μακεδονία

Η σημερινή Δυτική Μακεδονία, χώρα που ορίζεται από μικρούς και μεγάλους ορεινούς όγκους και διατρέχεται από τον ποταμό Αλιάκμονα, ανήκει στην Άνω – ορεινή – Μακεδονία των αρχαίων, η οποία εκτεινόταν πέρα από τα σύγχρονα ελληνικά σύνορα και περιλάμβανε τον ποταμό Εριγώνα, τις λίμνες Αχρίδα και Πρέσπες και τις περιοχές μέχρι τα όρη Dautika, Babuna, Dren στα βόρεια (Εικ. 2.1).

Κατά τη διάρκεια της 2ης χιλιετίας π.Χ. η Άνω Μακεδονία υπήρξε ορμητήριο, αφετηρία και σταθμός της πορείας του "πολυπλάνητου" έθνους των βορειοδυτικών ελληνικών φύλων, τα οποία ονομάστηκαν μακεδονικά στο βορρά και δωρικά στο νότο, κατά τον Ηρόδοτο (Ι, 56 και VIII, 43). Σύμφωνα με τον Ησίοδο (8ος αι. π.Χ., από Στέφανο Βυζάντιο

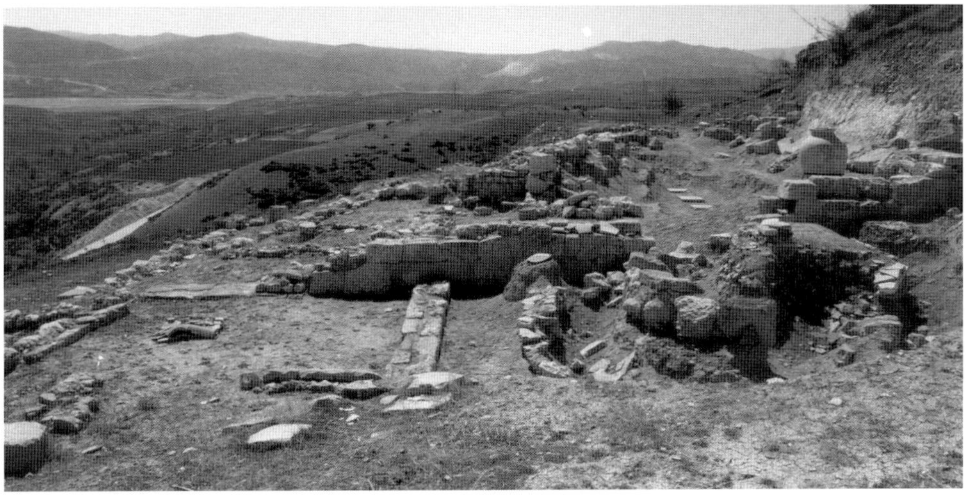

Εικ. 2.2. Άποψη από την αρχαία πόλη της Αιανής

στη λέξη 'Μακεδονία'), ο Μακεδών ήταν αδελφός του Μάγνητα, γιοι και οι δυο του Δία και της Θυίας, κόρης του Δευκαλίωνα και αδελφής του Έλληνα. Κατά τον Ελλάνικο (από Στέφανο Βυζάντιο στη λέξη 'Μακεδονία'), συγγραφέα του 5ου π.Χ. αι., ο Μακεδών ήταν γιος του Αιόλου και εγγονός του Έλληνα. Η σημασία των αρχαίων αυτών πηγών, που δεν εξαντλούνται στις παραπάνω, έγκειται στο ότι μας δείχνουν με ποιον τρόπο οι νότιοι Έλληνες αντιλαμβάνονταν, ήδη από τα ομηρικά χρόνια, την ενότητα του ελληνικού έθνους, στο οποίο ανήκαν και οι Μακεδόνες – ας μη ξεχνάμε άλλωστε ότι οι θεοί κατοικούσαν στον Όλυμπο.

Από τη σύγχρονη ιστορική έρευνα εντάσσονται στην Άνω Μακεδονία η Ελιμιώτις με την Τυμφαία, η Λυγκηστίς, η Ορεστίς, η Εορδαία, η Πελαγονία με τη Δερρίοπο, η Ατιντανία και η Δασσαρήτις. Ομοφωνία μελετητών υπάρχει για τις περισσότερες από αυτές, ενώ οι ανένταχτες περιοχές στα δυτικά-βορειοδυτικά, κυρίως, της Άνω Μακεδονίας και γύρω από την Αχρίδα μπορούν να συμπεριληφθούν στα "ἄλλα ἔθνη ἐπάνωθεν" του Θουκυδίδη (2.99) αν ήταν μακεδονικές και όχι ηπειρωτικές. Οπωσδήποτε, τμήμα της θεωρούμενης Δασσαρήτιδας, όπως και της Ατιντανίας, ανήκε στην Ήπειρο, ενώ η περιοχή γύρω από τη Λυχνίτιδα-Αχρίδα μπορεί να ενταχθεί στην Άνω Μακεδονία (Καραμήτρου-Μεντεσίδη 1999α). Από τις περιοχές της Άνω Μακεδονίας θα αναφερθούμε ιδιαίτερα στην Αιανή (Νομός Κοζάνης) διότι αποτελεί έναν από τους κύριους χώρους της έρευνάς μας.

Η Αιανή, της οποίας η ετυμολογική συσχέτιση με το επίρρημα *ἀεί*, *αἰεί* (= πάντοτε) φαίνεται πιθανή, υπήρξε «πόλις Μακεδονίας», σύμφωνα με τον ιδρυτικό μύθο, που διέσωσε ο Στέφανος Βυζάντιος (στη λέξη 'Αιανή'), και κτίστηκε από τον Αιανό, γιο του βασιλιά Ελύμου. Ήταν πρωτεύουσα του βασιλείου της Ελίμειας ή Ελιμιώτιδας, ενός από τα ισχυρότερα της Άνω Μακεδονίας και είχε βασιλείς που αναφέρονται από τον Θουκυδίδη (σχολ. στον Θουκυδίδη, 1.57.3, Gomme 1945–1981, τόμ. I, 203, 212, 218, Θουκ. 1.57. 1.61) και τον Ξενοφώντα (*Ελληνικά*, 5.2.38): Αρριδαίος (σύγχρονος του Αλεξάνδρου Α΄ των Αιγών και γυναικάδελφος), τρεις βασιλείς με το όνομα Δέρδας, βασιλόπαις Μαχάτας (το όνομά του αναφέρεται πιθανόν σε αργυρό αγγείο του τάφου του Φιλίππου), Φίλα (πρώτη σύζυγος του Φιλίππου Β': Αθήναιος 13.557C και 10.336C), ενώ, κατά μία άποψη, η μητέρα του Φιλίππου Ευρυδίκη καταγόταν από τον ελιμιωτικό βασιλικό οίκο (Αριστοτέλης, *Πολιτικά*, 58.11).

Η ανασκαφική έρευνα στους αρχαιολογικούς χώρους της Αιανής και γενικότερα η φροντίδα για όλο τον Νομό Κοζάνης συστηματοποιήθηκε στα μέσα της δεκαετίας του 1980 και συνεχίζεται χωρίς διακοπή. Από την αρχή διαπιστώθηκε ότι η σημασία της Αιανής έγκειται στην πρωιμότητα και διαχρονικότητα των ευρημάτων της, μνημείων λαμπρού πολιτισμού από τα προϊστορικά έως τα ρωμαϊκά και βυζαντινά χρόνια. Αποκαλύφθηκαν κατοικίες και οικοδομήματα με δημόσιο χαρακτήρα, που διαμορφώνουν την εικόνα μιας πόλης με οικιστική οργάνωση και πολιτική ανάπτυξη από τα υστεροαρχαϊκά και κλασικά χρόνια (αρχές 5ου–4ος αι. π.Χ., ενώ και ο 6ος αι. π.Χ. αντιπροσωπεύεται με κεραμεική), γεγονός που τεκμηριώνει την άποψή μας ότι υπήρχαν ακμαίες και οργανωμένες πόλεις στην Άνω Μακεδονία πολύ πριν από την ενοποίηση του μακεδονικού ελληνισμού από τον Φίλιππο Β' (359–336 π.Χ.), στον οποίο οι ιστορικοί απέδιδαν την ίδρυση των πρώτων πόλεων-αστικών κέντρων. Συγχρόνως η αποκάλυψη εκτός της αρχαίας πόλης μνημειακών κτιστών τάφων αλλά και απλών λακκοειδών του 6ου και 5ου αι. π.Χ. με πλούσια κτερίσματα, φώτισε δύο αιώνες πρώιμης ιστορίας των Μακεδόνων. Συμπερασματικά μπορούμε να πούμε ότι στην Αιανή αποτυπώνεται η διαχρονία του μακεδονικού ελληνισμού (Καραμήτρου-Μεντεσίδη 2001γ, 2008) (Εικ. 2.2).

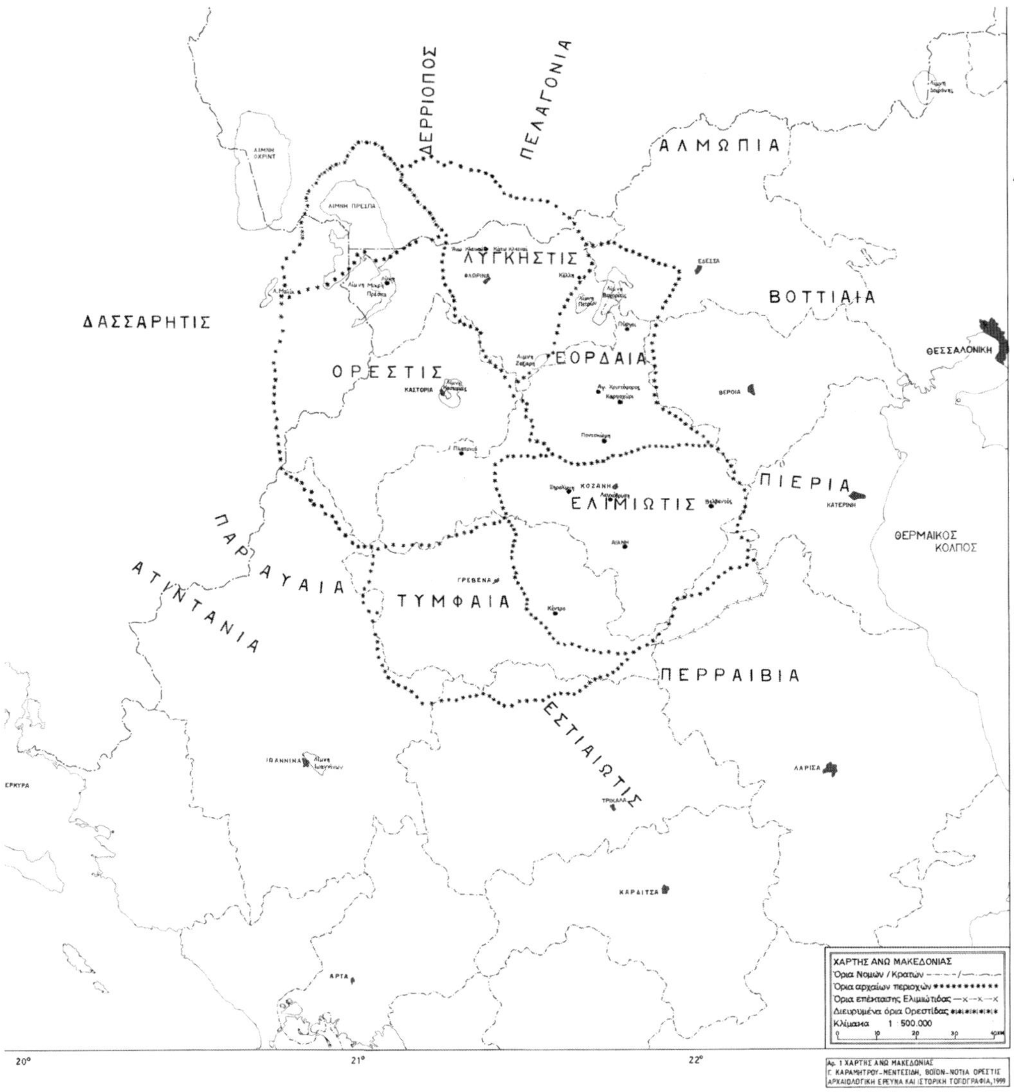

Εικ. 2.3. Θέσεις προέλευσης υλικού έρευνας

Το υλικό της έρευνας

Η έρευνά μας για το υλικό αυτής της εργασίας αφορά και στους τέσσερις νομούς της σύγχρονης Δυτικής Μακεδονίας και, εκτός από μικρές αναφορές, δεν επεκτάθηκε στα τμήματα των περιοχών της αρχαίας Άνω Μακεδονίας, τα οποία σήμερα βρίσκονται εκτός ελληνικών συνόρων. Διαπιστώσαμε ότι με ευρήματα σχετικά αντιπροσωπεύονται όλες οι περιοχές, αλλά τα περισσότερα παραδείγματα προέρχονται από την Ελίμεια, συνολικά 23, ακολουθούν η Εορδαία με δέκα, η Ορεστίδα και η Λυγκηστίδα με δύο, η Τυμφαία με τρία. Από τα 23 παραδείγματα της Ελίμειας τα 19 αφορούν στην πρωτεύουσά της Αιανή και την περιοχή της (Εικ. 2.3). Οι κατηγορίες, ανάλογα με το υλικό, είναι οι παρακάτω.

Α. Γλυπτά με Ασκληπιό και Υγεία

Τα αγαλμάτια και ανάγλυφα Ασκληπιού και Υγείας που παρουσιάζονται εδώ προέρχονται όλα από τον Νομό Κοζάνης.

1) Τμήμα Αγάλματος Ασκληπιού, Αιανή, αρ. Κατ. 263 (Εικ. 2.4)

Τμήμα αγάλματος Ασκληπιού, βρέθηκε και παραδόθηκε από θέση κοντά στην Μεγάλη Ράχη, όπου βρίσκεται η πόλη της αρχαίας Αιανής. Σώζεται σε ύψος 0.29 μ (Καραμήτρου-Μεντεσίδη 1982).

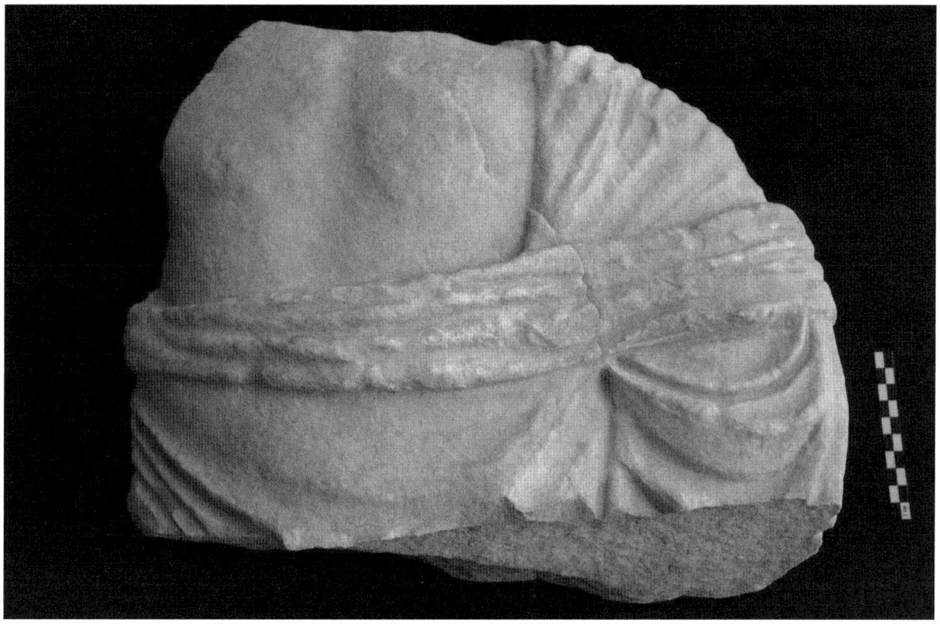

Εικ. 2.4. Τμήμα Αγάλματος Ασκληπιού, Αιανή, αρ. Κατ. 263

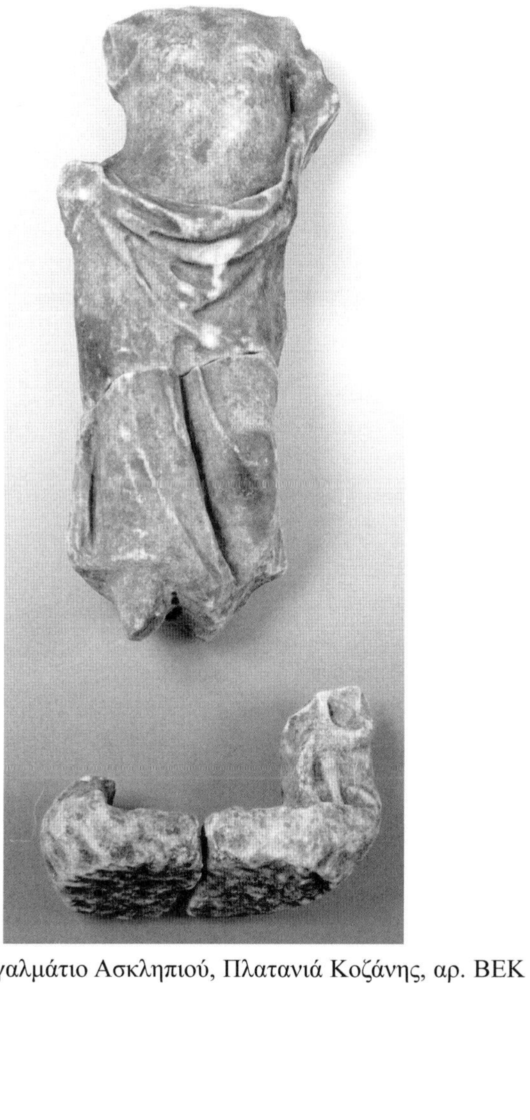

Εικ. 2.5. Αγαλμάτιο Ασκληπιού, Πλατανιά Κοζάνης, αρ. ΒΕΚ 3300

***2) Αγαλμάτιο Ασκληπιού, Πλατανιά Κοζάνης, αρ. ΒΕΚ[1] 3300* (Εικ. 2.5)**

Ύπαρξη ιερού μαρτυρεί με βεβαιότητα το εύρημα που παραδόθηκε και προέρχεται από τη θέση Ανάνα Πλατανιάς (Καραμήτρου-Μεντεσίδη 1999α, 227). Πρόκειται για κορμό μαρμάρινου αγαλματίου αντρικής μορφής, υστεροελληνιστικών χρόνων, σε τέσσερα κομμάτια, την ελλειψοειδή βάση του και το τμήμα πλίνθου με βάθυνση για την ένθεσή του. Η μορφή είναι ντυμένη με ιμάτιο που αφήνει γυμνό το δεξιό ώμο. Το τμήμα κιονίσκου, το οποίο σώζεται δίπλα στο αριστερό πόδι με τμήμα φιδιού και ράβδου, τη χαρακτηρίζει ως Ασκληπιό.[2]

***3) Τμήμα ενεπίγραφης ανάγλυφης στήλης, Δίπορο Γρεβενών, ΓΡΕΒ. 2392* (Εικ. 2.6)**

Ύπαρξη ιερού του Ασκληπιού, πιθανότατα, δηλώνει και το τμήμα μαρμάρινης αναθηματικής στήλης, από την οποία σώζεται το κάτω μέρος (αδημοσίευτη). Βρέθηκε κατά τις εργασίες διαπλάτυνσης αγροτικού δρόμου στον προαύλιο χώρο της εκκλησίας του Αγίου Νικολάου στο Δίπορο Γρεβενών. Ο Ασκληπιός παριστάνεται όρθιος με το δεξί του πόδι να προβάλλει και τείνει το δεξί του χέρι κρατώντας αυγό σε φίδι,[3] το οποίο ελίσσεται σε κορμό δένδρου ή βακτηρία.[4] Η παράσταση είναι ιδιαίτερα προβληματική εξαιτίας της κακής απόδοσης του ανάγλυφου. Καταλήγουμε ότι πιθανότατα υπάρχει και παράσταση βακτηρίας, η οποία κρύβεται από το δέντρο και μέρος της μόνο εμφανίζεται σε δεύτερο επίπεδο. Χρονολογείται στον 2ο αι. μ.Χ.

Στο κάτω πλαίσιο της στήλης υπάρχει επιγραφή: *Ἀσκληπιῷ εὐχήν.*

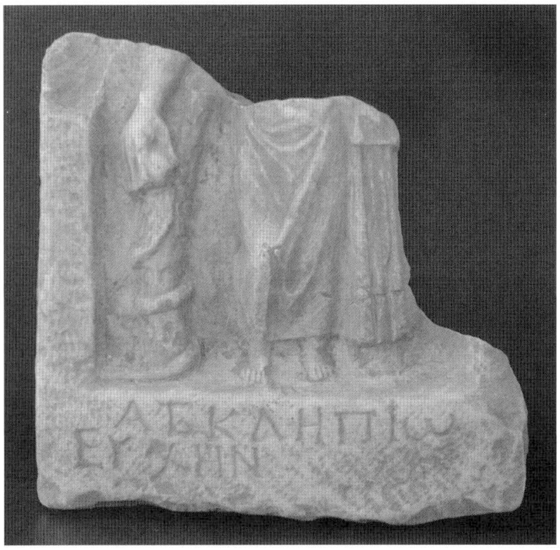

Εικ. 2.6. Τμήμα ενεπίγραφης ανάγλυφης στήλης, Δίπορο Γρεβενών, ΓΡΕΒ. 2392

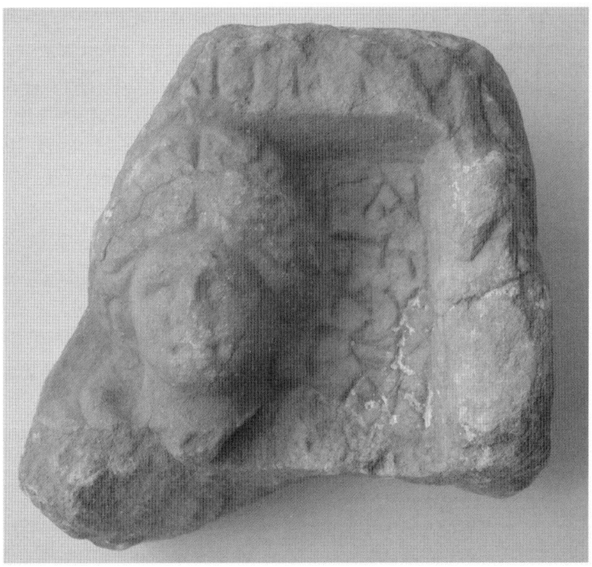

Εικ. 2.7. Τμήμα ενεπίγραφης ανάγλυφης στήλης, Λευκόβρυση Κοζάνης, αρ. ΒΕΚ 19

4) Τμήμα ενεπίγραφης ανάγλυφης στήλης, Λευκόβρυση Κοζάνης, αρ. ΒΕΚ 19 (Εικ. 2.7)

Σώζεται μόνο το δεξιό άνω τμήμα της μαρμάρινης αναθηματικής στήλης. Σε ορθογώνιο βάθυσμα υπάρχει παράσταση, στην οποία διακρίνεται κατενώπιον με ελαφρά κλίση προς τα αριστερά κεφαλή γυναικείας μορφής, προφανώς Υγείας.[5] Φέρει επιγραφή στην επάνω οριζόντια ταινία-πλαίσιο και στο έδαφος του βαθύσματος, δεξιά από την κεφαλή (Ριζάκης και Τουράτσογλου 1985, 24–5, αρ. 8). Χρονολογείται στον 2° αι. μ.Χ.

Επιγραφή: *[ὁ (ἡ) δεῖνα Ἀσκ]ληπι[ὸν] καὶ τὴν Ὑγείαν.*

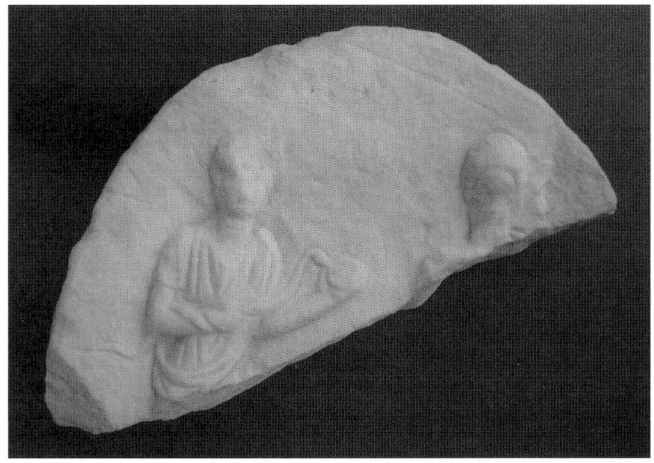

Εικ. 2.8. Τμήμα αναθηματικής στήλης, Αιανή, αρ. Κατ. 13

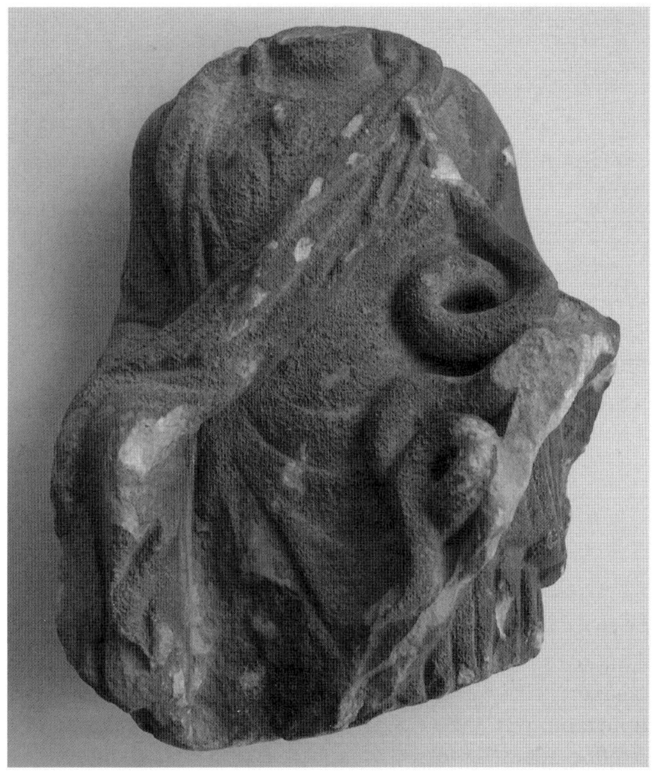

Εικ. 2.9. Αγαλμάτιο Υγείας, Κοζάνη, αρ. ΒΕΚ 53

5) Τμήμα ανάγλυφης αναθηματικής στήλης, Αιανή, αρ. Κατ. 13 (Εικ. 2.8)

Το πάνω μέρος μαρμάρινης αψιδωτής στήλης με παράσταση δύο γυναικών, από τις οποίες η μία τείνει φιάλη με το αριστερό της χέρι σε φίδι που περιελίσσεται στο δεξί της χέρι, και προφανώς πρόκειται για παράσταση της Υγείας (Σιαμπανόπουλος 1974, 192). Χρονολογείται στον $2^{o}/3^{o}$ αι. μ.Χ.

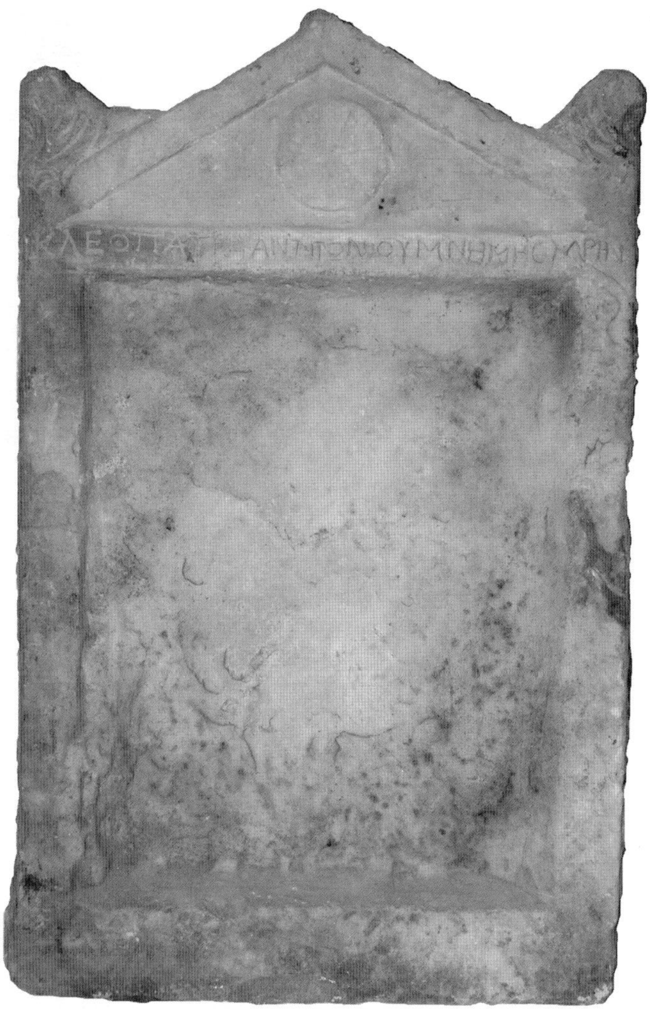

Εικ. 2.10. Επιτύμβια στήλη, Αγαλαίοι Γρεβενών

6) Αγαλμάτιο Υγείας, Κοζάνη, αρ. ΒΕΚ 53 (Εικ. 2.9)

Τμήμα ακέφαλου αγαλματίου ιματιοφόρου γυναίκας που σώζεται από τη βάση του λαιμού μέχρι τα γόνατα. Στην αριστερή της πλευρά φίδι που ελίσσεται ανεβαίνει στο στήθος της (Καραμήτρου-Μεντεσίδη 1993, 78 Εικ. 43). Χρονολογείται στον $2^{ο}$–$3^{ο}$ αι. μ.Χ.

Β. Ανάγλυφες επιτύμβιες στήλες με παραστάσεις ιατρικών εργαλείων

1) Επιτύμβια στήλη, Αγαλαίοι Γρεβενών (Εικ. 2.10)

Μαρμάρινη αετωματική επιτύμβια στήλη από το χωριό Αγαλαίοι, στον νάρθηκα της εκκλησίας του Αγίου Δημητρίου (Ριζάκης και Τουράτσογλου 1985, 65, αρ. 55). Σε ορθογώνιο βάθυσμα υπάρχει ανάγλυφη παράσταση, ιδιαίτερα φθαρμένη. Σώζονται τα πόδια και τα περιγράμματα άνδρα, παιδιού και γυναίκας, κατενώπιον με ιμάτιο. Στην αριστερή κατακόρυφη παραστάδα-πλαίσιο του βαθύσματος σώζεται παράσταση σικύας (βεντούζας).[6] Χρονολογείται στο β΄ μισό του $2^{ου}$ αι. μ.Χ.

Επιγραφή: *Κλεοπάτρα Ἀντιγόνου μνήμης χάριν.*

2) Επιτύμβια στήλη με παράσταση γιατρού, εργαλειοθήκης και άλλων ιατρικών εργαλείων, Κέλλη Φλώρινας, αρ. Κατ. ΠΤΟΛ 79 (Εικ. 2.11)

Πρόκειται για τυχαίο εύρημα από την περιοχή της Κέλλης Φλώρινας που παραδόθηκε στο Ανθρωπολογικό-Παλαιοντολογικό Μουσείο της Πτολεμαΐδας (Μοσχάκης 2004, 2009). Στο πρώτο διάχωρο της στήλης η κυρίαρχη μορφή είναι της τιμώμενης νεκρής, δηλαδή της γιατρού. Στην άλλη πλευρά απεικονίζεται νεαρός με κοντό χιτώνα και ένδυμα από το οποίο εξέχει κύλινδρος. Η ανυπομονησία στη στάση, η νεότητα, καθώς και ο κύλινδρος, μας επιτρέπουν την υπόθεση ότι πρόκειται για μαθητή και ίσως τον γιο της γιατρού, ο οποίος μετά τον θάνατό της μητέρας του παρουσιάζεται έτοιμος να συνεχίσει το έργο της.

Το κεντρικό τμήμα της παράστασης καταλαμβάνουν τα αντικείμενα του ιατρείου, εκτός από μία σικύα (βεντούζα), η οποία κρέμεται δίπλα στον μαθητή. Στηριγμένη και ανοικτή πάνω σε χαμηλό τραπέζι ή κρεβάτι βρίσκεται η εργαλειοθήκη. Η θήκη (ξύλινη ή μετάλλινη) είναι απαραίτητη για την αποθήκευση των εργαλείων ενός γιατρού και κυρίως για την μεταφορά τους, όπου και όποτε αυτό είναι αναγκαίο.[7]

Στο πάνω μέρος της κεντρικής παράστασης διακρίνεται μία ακόμη σικύα, κρεμασμένη όπως και η προηγούμενη. Οι σικύες είναι συνήθως γυάλινες ή από χαλκό και χρησιμοποιούνται ήδη από τα κλασικά χρόνια, όπως φαίνεται από παραστάσεις σε αγγεία και στήλες. Στα ρωμαϊκά χρόνια είναι σε ευρεία χρήση και βρίσκονται σε πολλούς τάφους γιατρών.[8] Δίπλα στη σικύα υπάρχει ψαλίδι,[9] που απεικονίζεται, όπως και τα υπόλοιπα αντικείμενα, ιδιαίτερα μεγάλο και ο λόγος είναι κατανοητός. Τη χρήση αυτού του εργαλείου στην ιατρική περιγράφει ο Ορειβάσιος στο έργο του *Ἰατρικαὶ Συλλογαί* (45, 18,16,1–2). Παρόμοια ψαλίδια είναι γνωστά από παραστάσεις σε στήλες, καθώς και από ανασκαφικά ευρήματα, ιδιαίτερα στην Ιταλία και τη Γερμανία. Τέλος δίπλα στην εργαλειοθήκη έχουμε και την απεικόνιση μικρού αγγείου με στενό λαιμό. Παρόμοια αγγεία είναι συνήθως χάλκινα ή γυάλινα και μερικές φορές πήλινα. Όπως φαίνεται περιείχαν τις αναγκαίες φαρμακευτικές ουσίες.

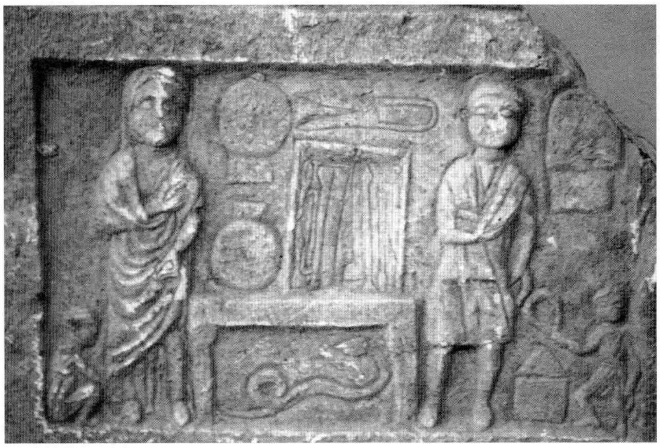

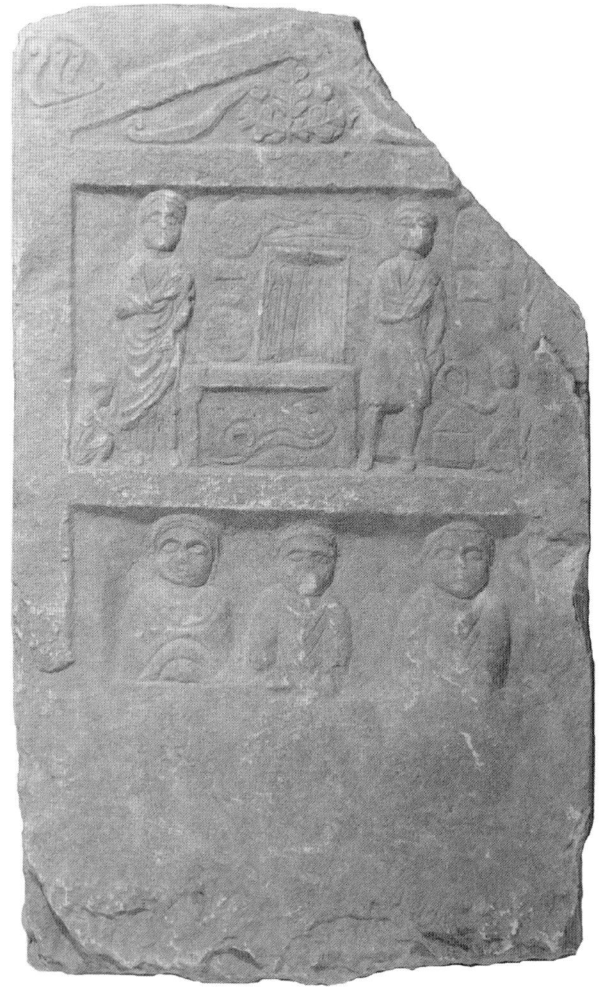

Εικ. 2.11. Επιτύμβια στήλη, Κέλλη Φλώρινας, αρ. Κατ. ΠΤΟΛ 79

Το περιεχόμενο της εργαλειοθήκης

Στο εσωτερικό της εργαλειοθήκης απεικονίζονται τα εργαλεία που συμπληρώνουν τη συλλογή του γιατρού. Δυστυχώς η ποιότητα της απόδοσης του αναγλύφου είναι πολύ κακή με αποτέλεσμα η αναγνώριση κάποιων να παραμένει προβληματική. Πρώτο έχουμε ένα νυστέρι (μάχαιρα ή σμίλη), ένα από τα αρχαιότερα εργαλεία, του οποίου ελάχιστα η χρήση του έχει διαφοροποιηθεί (Γαληνός, *Περὶ ἀνατομικῶν ἐγχειρήσεων* 2, 248, 2). Είναι γνωστό ότι ήδη από την αρχαιότητα είχαν εξελιχθεί πολλές μορφές του νυστεριού και στις απεικονίσεις εμφανίζεται σε πολλούς διαφορετικούς τύπους. Δίπλα στο νυστέρι απεικονίζονται δύο άγκιστρα (hamus acutus), που αποδίδονται με κοντά κυλινδρικά κακοδουλεμένα στελέχη που απολήγουν το ένα σε κλειστό και το άλλο σε λιγότερο καμπύλο άγκιστρο. Ανάλογα με την μορφή του το άγκιστρο είναι εργαλείο με πολλές χρήσεις στη χειρουργική (Ορειβάσιος, 45, 18,16,1–2), σε τραύματα, για εξαγωγή αμυγδαλών ή ακόμη και για επεμβάσεις στο πτερύγιο του ματιού. Ακολουθεί δεύτερο νυστέρι διαφορετικό από το προηγούμενο, και απεικονίζεται με πεπλατυσμένο στέλεχος που απολήγει σε λεπίδα. Δεν είναι ευδιάκριτη η δεύτερη απόληξη του εργαλείου, η οποία πιθανότατα χρησιμοποιούνταν επίσης ως εργαλείο, αφού δεν μοιάζει με λαβή. Η πρώτη σειρά τελειώνει με απεικόνιση κυλινδρικής εργαλειοθήκης (specillotheca).[10] Πρόκειται για μία δεύτερη, μικρή εργαλειοθήκη, η οποία είναι συνήθως χάλκινη ή οστέινη, όπου τοποθετούνταν τα μικρότερα εργαλεία, όπως οι μήλες και οι χειρουργικές βελόνες.

Στο δεύτερο τμήμα της εργαλειοθήκης η σειρά ξεκινά με ένα ακόμη νυστέρι, που είναι το τρίτο της συλλογής. Η λεπίδα του είναι κυκλική, όπως και στο πρώτο νυστέρι, και το στέλεχος μάλλον πεπλατυσμένο. Δεν είναι ευδιάκριτο αν απολήγει σε λαβή ή το άκρο του διαμορφώνεται σε εργαλείο, επίσης. Ακολουθεί μία οξεία μήλη με σπάτουλα, η οποία είναι διπλό εργαλείο και χρησιμοποιείται από τις δύο πλευρές. Το στέλεχός της είναι πλατύ και απολήγει στη μία του πλευρά σε φλογόσχημο οξυκόρυφο άκρο και στην άλλη του πλευρά σε πεπλατυσμένη σπάτουλα. Το όγδοο εργαλείο είναι μία μήλη.[11] Η κακή απόδοση δεν βοηθά στην αναγνώριση του εργαλείου, καθώς δεν διακρίνεται αν η άνω απόληξή του χρησιμεύει ως λαβή ή ως ένα δεύτερο εργαλείο. Ανήκει σε μία μεγάλη κατηγορία εργαλείων με διάφορους τύπους. Διευκόλυνε κυρίως στην εξέταση του ασθενή, αλλά χρησίμευε και στις εγχειρίσεις και άλλες επεμβάσεις. Το τελευταίο, ένατο στη σειρά, εργαλείο που απεικονίζεται δεν διακρίνεται με ευκρίνεια, καθώς η απόδοσή του είναι ιδιαίτερα κακή.

Τελειώνουμε με μια μικρή αναφορά στο φίδι, το οποίο γεμίζει το κενό ανάμεσα στα πόδια του τραπεζιού. Το φίδι, πολύ γνωστό θέμα στα επιτύμβια μνημεία του ελληνικού κόσμου, συνδέεται με χθόνιες θεότητες και θεωρείται ότι συνοδεύει μαζί με το άλογο τον αφηρωισμένο νεκρό. Είναι επίσης συνδεδεμένο με τον Ασκληπιό, όπως και η βακτηρία, ενώ εμφανίζεται και σε παραστάσεις της Υγείας. Ακόμη και σε παραστάσεις ίασης ασθενών, χωρίς απαραίτητα άμεση την παρουσία του Ασκληπιού, υπάρχουν απεικονίσεις φιδιού, όπου η παρουσία του υπονοεί επίκληση και ανταπόκριση του θεού. Άλλωστε είναι πιθανή η λατρεία

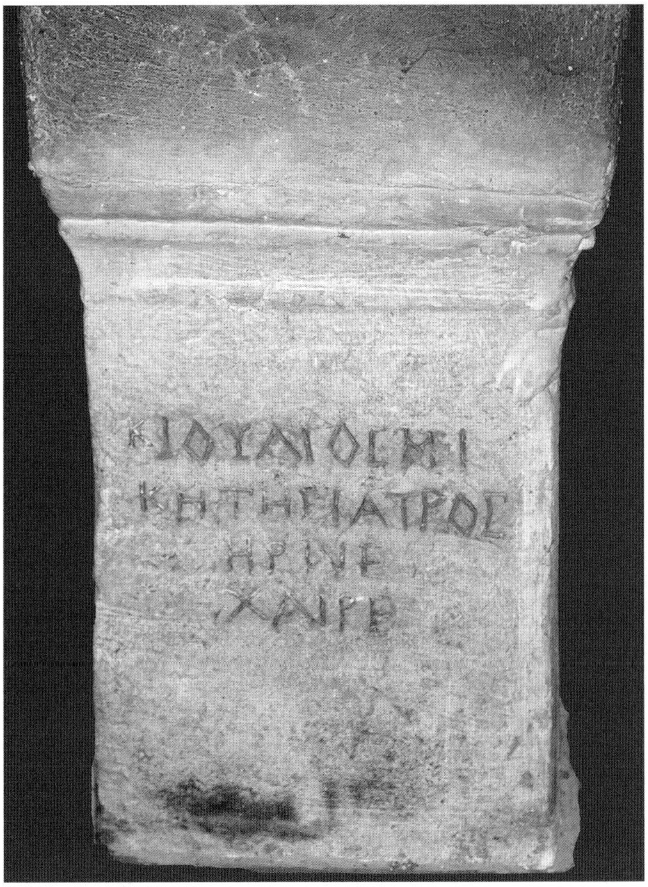

Εικ. 2.12. Βωμός με επιγραφή, Άγιος Αχίλλειος Φλώρινας

του Ασκληπιού και με την μορφή φιδιού. Στην περίπτωση της στήλης που εξετάζουμε ίσως η παρουσία του φιδιού να είναι διττή, καθώς συνεχίζεται μία ελληνική παράδοση αιώνων, ενώ ταυτόχρονα σχετίζεται με το επάγγελμα του νεκρού και εμμέσως με τις ιδιότητες του Ασκληπιού.

Γ. Επιγραφές με αναφορά σε γιατρούς

1) Βωμός με επιγραφή, Άγιος Αχίλλειος Φλώρινας (Εικ. 2.12)

Μαρμάρινος επιτύμβιος «μακεδονικός» βωμός με συμφυή βάση και επίθημα. Μεταφέρθηκε στην Πύλη, όπου χρησιμοποιείται ως βάση της αγίας τράπεζας του ναού του Αγίου Γεωργίου. Σώζεται επιγραφή στην κύρια όψη (Ριζάκης και Τουράτσογλου 1985, 151–2, αρ. 165). Χρονολογείται στις αρχές του $3^{ου}$ αι. μ.Χ.

Επιγραφή: *Κ. Ἰούλιος Νει-/κήτης ἰατρὸς/ ἥρως / χαῖρε.*

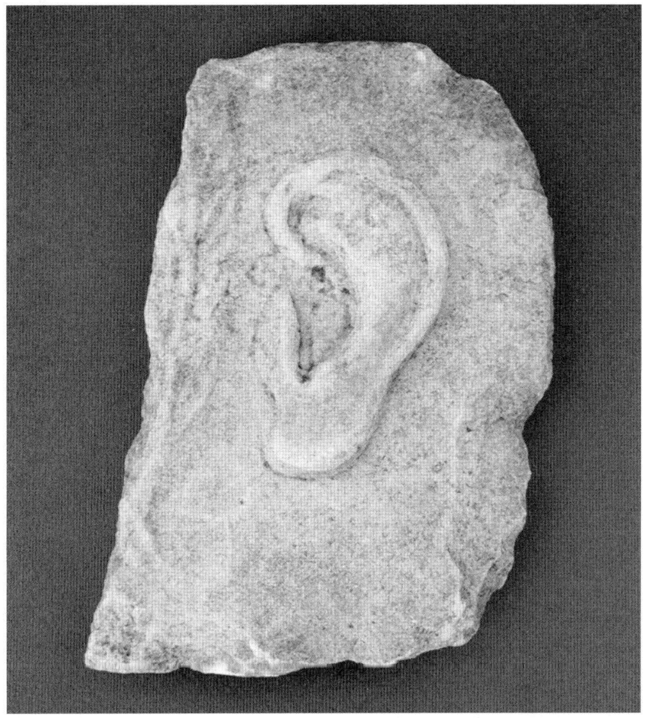

Εικ. 2.13. Μαρμάρινο αναθηματικό ανάγλυφο, Ξηρολίμνη, αρ. ΒΕΚ 6551

2) Επιτύμβια στήλη, Κάτω Κλεινές Φλώρινας (Μουσείο Θεσσαλονίκης, αρ. Κατ. 201)

Μαρμάρινη παραλληλεπίπεδη επιτύμβια στήλη με ανάγλυφη παράσταση κατενώπιον πέντε όρθιων μορφών: Στρατιωτικός με θώρακα, ασπίδα και δόρυ (Άρης;), καλυπτροφόρος και ιματιοφόρος γυναίκα, Ηρακλής με λεοντή και ρόπαλο, ιματιοφόρος άνδρας και γενειοφόρος με τρίαινα (;) στο αριστερό χέρι (Ποσειδών;). Σώζεται πολύστιχη επιγραφή κάτω από την παράσταση, που διακόπτεται από γυναικεία ανάγλυφη προτομή (Ριζάκης και Τουράτσογλου 1985, 144–5, αρ. 157). Χρονολογείται στα τέλη του $2^{ου}$–αρχές του $3^{ου}$ αι. μ.Χ.

Επιγραφή (στίχοι 6–9):
[..]όμοῦ ____ θέτο σῆμ' ἐπὶ τύ[μβῳ]
[...]ριδίκῃ ____ τε θυγατρὶ ἐῇ φρεσὶ
[..] ΑΕΙΔΥΙΗ ____ γαμβρῷ τε ἰητρῷ [Θ-]
εοδῶρῳ σοφῷ ἀνδρὶ vac.

Σημειώνουμε ότι η χρήση του ιωνικού τύπου *Ἰητρὸς* είναι συνηθισμένη στα επιγράμματα. Η στήλη του γιατρού Θεόδωρου δεν έχει μελετηθεί, επαρκώς, μολονότι σώζει πολύ ενδιαφέρουσα πολυπρόσωπη παράσταση θεοτήτων και στην επιγραφή της διαφαίνεται λατρεία του Μεγάλου Αλεξάνδρου.

Ο Γαληνός και ο Αρχιγένης, που έζησαν μετά τα μέσα του $2^{ου}$ αι. μ.Χ., καθώς και ο Αέτιος και ο Αλέξανδρος ο

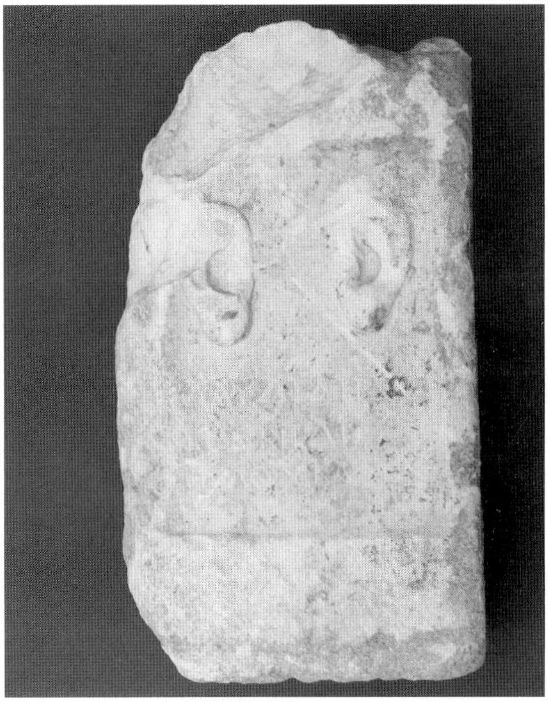

Εικ. 2.14. Αναθηματική στήλη, Καρυοχώρι Εορδαίας, αρ. ΒΕΚ 3347

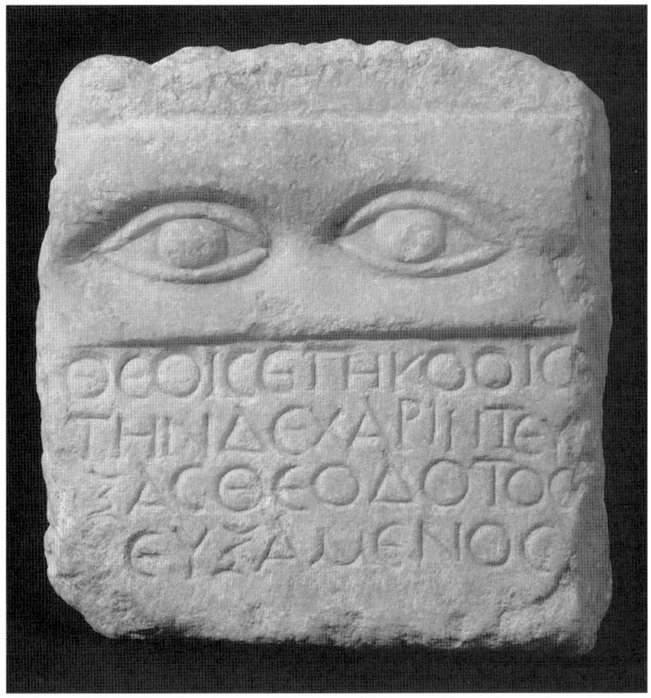

Εικ. 2.15. Ανάγλυφη ενεπίγραφη αναθηματική στήλη, Βελβεντό, αρ. ΚΑΒΕ 62

Τραλλιανός (6ος αι.), διέσωσαν τμήματα από το έργο του ιατρού και φαρμακολόγου Θεόδωρου του Μακεδόνα. Θεωρείται ιδρυτής πνευματικής σχολής, αλλά για τη ζωή του δεν σώθηκε καμιά πληροφορία, παρά μόνο τμήματα των συγγραμμάτων του (Γεωργακόπουλος 1998, 218). Αν και η υπόθεση είναι γοητευτική δεν μπορούμε με βεβαιότητα να υποστηρίξουμε την άποψη της ταύτισης του Θεόδωρου των πηγών με τον Θεόδωρο της επιγραφής των Κάτω Κλεινών, που χρονολογείται στα τέλη του 2ου αι. μ.Χ., όπως αναφέραμε.

Δ. Παραστάσεις ανθρώπινων μελών σε αναθηματικές στήλες

1) Μαρμάρινο αναθηματικό ανάγλυφο, Αιανή, αρ. Κατ. 192

Προέρχεται από την Ράχη Τσέικα της Αιανής (Πέτσας 1961–2, 216 πίν. 257δ, Σιαμπανόπουλος 1974, 145–6). Φέρει παράσταση δεξιού αυτιού, πιθανόν ως ιαθέν μέλος. Χρονολογείται στον 2ο–3ο αι. μ.Χ.

2) Μαρμάρινο αναθηματικό ανάγλυφο, Αιανή, αρ. Κατ. 193

Φέρει παράσταση δεξιού αυτιού, πιθανόν ως ιαθέν μέλος (Σιαμπανόπουλος 1974, 145–56). Χρονολογείται στον 2ο–3ο αι. μ.Χ.

3) Μαρμάρινο αναθηματικό ανάγλυφο, Ξηρολίμνη, αρ. ΒΕΚ 6551 (Εικ. 2.13)

Φέρει παράσταση αυτιού ως ιαθέν μέλος (Καραμήτρου-Μεντεσίδη 1999β, 340 εικ. 4). Αποτελεί ανασκαφικό εύρημα από τον χώρο του ιερού Απόλλωνα με τα επίθετα Νόμιος και Μεσωρίσκος, καθώς και της Αρτέμιδος, του Διονύσου και ενδεχομένως και άλλων σύνναων θεών.[12] Χρονολογείται στον 2ο αι. μ.Χ.

4) Ανάγλυφη αναθηματική στήλη, Αιανή, αρ. Κατ. 36

Φέρει παράσταση αυτιών σε ρηχό βάθυσμα και επιγραφή. Βρέθηκε στην περιοχή της θέσης Παλιούρι Αιανής (Σιαμπανόπουλος 1974, 148· Ριζάκης και Τουράτσογλου 1985, 38–9, αρ. 23). Χρονολογείται στον 2ο–3ο αι. π.Χ.

Επιγραφή: *Πετρωνία Που-/πλίου ευχήν.*

5) Αναθηματική στήλη με παράσταση αυτιών, Καρυοχώρι Εορδαίας, αρ. ΒΕΚ 3347 (Εικ. 2.14)

Στήλη αναθηματική στην Αρτέμιδα Λοχία με παράσταση

δύο αυτιών. Η στήλη προέρχεται από εντοπισμένη από το 1992 θέση ιερού ρωμαϊκών χρόνων, όπως διαπιστώσαμε από τα αρχιτεκτονικά μέλη, τα οποία εμφανίστηκαν από ισοπέδωση που επιχειρήθηκε (Καραμήτρου-Μεντεσίδη 2001β, 622).

Επιγραφή: *[Κ]λαυδία Ἡδόνα /[Ἀ]ρτέμιδι /Λοχία.*

6) Ανάγλυφη ενεπίγραφη αναθηματική στήλη, Βελβεντό, αρ. ΚΑΒΕ 62 (Εικ. 2.15)

Μαρμάρινη αναθηματική στήλη σε δεύτερη χρήση από το εσωτερικό της εκκλησίας των Αγίων Αποστόλων. Φέρει παράσταση δύο ανθρώπινων ματιών και αφιερώνεται από τον Θεόδοτο, στους θεούς επηκόους (Ριζάκης και Τουράτσογλου 1985, 39, αρ. 23α, Καραμήτρου-Μεντεσίδη 1994, 48–9). Χρονολογείται στον 2ο–3ο αι. μ.Χ.

Επιγραφή: *Θεοῖς ἐπηκόοις /τήνδε χάριν τεύ-/ξας Θεόδοτος/ vac. εὐξάμενος.*

Συμπερασματικά για τις παραπάνω παραστάσεις αυτιών μπορούμε να παρατηρήσουμε ότι στην κατηγορία αυτών, στα οποία τα αυτιά ερμηνεύονται ως ιαθέντα μέλη και όχι ως παράσταση που δηλώνει το *«ευήκοο»* από μέρους των θεών, ανήκουν τα τρία ανάγλυφα (δύο της Αιανής, αρ. 1 και 2, και ένα της Ξηρολίμνης, αρ. 3), όπου παριστάνεται με βεβαιότητα ένα αυτί. Στην στήλη από το Καρυοχώρι (αρ. 5) έχουμε παράσταση «ευήκοων ώτων» και ίσως το ίδιο συμβαίνει και με το ανάγλυφο της Αιανής (αρ. 4), που φέρει παράσταση δύο αυτιών.

Τέλος, το ανάγλυφο από το Βελβεντό (αρ. 6) «μιλά» από μόνο του, αφού παριστάνει ιαθέντα μάτια.[13]

Ε. Επιγραφές με το όνομα Ασκληπιάδης

1) Σαρκοφάγος, Κέντρον Γρεβενών

Μεγάλη μαρμάρινη παραλληλεπίπεδη μονολιθική σαρκοφάγος, ελλιπής σε μερικά σημεία, χωρίς το κάλυμμά της. Φέρει ανάγλυφες παραστάσεις σε δύο από τις τέσσερις πλευρές. Στη μια στενή πλευρά φέρει παράσταση Βελλερεφόντη σε Πήγασο εναντίον Χίμαιρας και πάνω από αυτόν ιπτάμενης σφίγγας. Στη μακριά πλευρά δύο σκηνές κυνηγιού, αριστερά κάπρου και δεξιά ελαφιού. Στο κάτω μέρος της αριστερής παραστάδας φέρει ανάγλυφη παράσταση παιδιού. Τέσσερις επιγραφές σώζονται στη μακριά πλευρά (Ριζάκης και Τουράτσογλου 1985, 69–70, αρ. 60). Φυλάσσεται στην Αρχαιολογική Συλλογή Κοζάνης. Χρονολογείται στον 3ο αι. μ.Χ.

Επιγραφή: α) *[Ζῶν Ἀσκ]ληπιάδης ληνὸν θέτο τήνδε ἑαυτῷ /---ην μελετῶν ἐρχομένου θανάτου.*

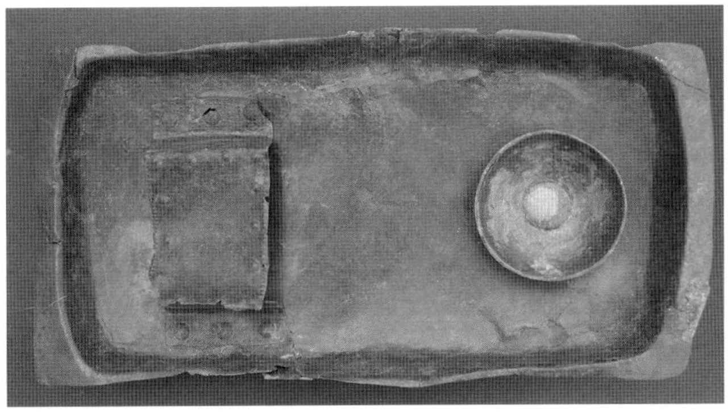

Εικ. 2.16. Χάλκινο σκεύος, αρ. κατ. 12350, Νεκρόπολη αρχαίας Αιανής

2) Χάλκινη σφραγίδα, Αιανή

Χάλκινη σφραγίδα, η οποία βρέθηκε στην περιοχή της Αιανής πιθανόν το 1912, βρίσκονταν στη κατοχή κατοίκου της Αιανής αλλά αργότερα χάθηκε (Ριζάκης και Τουράτσογλου 1985, 76, αρ. 69). Έφερε την επιγραφή *Ασκληπιάδης* και χρονολογείται στον 3ο (;) αι. π.Χ.

3) Αναθηματική στήλη στον Απόλλωνα Μεσωρίσκο, Ξηρολίμνη, αρ. ΒΕΚ 6569

Αναθηματική στήλη στον Απόλλωνα Μεσωρίσκο.[14] Σώζεται τμήμα του δεξιού πέρατος του κορμού, με την αρχή του πλαισίου της παράστασης σε βαθύτερο επίπεδο και τμήμα του κανόνα, πάνω στον οποίο σώζεται δεξιό πέρας δίστιχης επιγραφής (Καραμήτρου-Μεντεσίδη 2001α, 64–5). Χρονολογείται στο δεύτερο μισό του 2ου αι. μ.Χ.

Επιγραφή: *[Ἀπόλλωνι Μεσ]ωρίσκῳ/[ὁ δεῖνα Ἀσκλ]ηπιάδου.*

Σύμφωνα με την έρευνα το συγκεκριμένο θεοφόρο όνομα Ασκληπιάδης δινόταν σε θεραπευτές που εργάζονταν σε Ασκληπιεία και ιερά καθώς οι γιατροί θεωρούνταν απόγονοι του Ασκληπιού (Pollak 2005, 46).

ΣΤ. Σκεύη

Μεγάλο ενδιαφέρον παρουσιάζει σειρά ιδιόμορφων στην κατασκευή σκευών, τα οποία προέρχονται από την Αιανή και ένα από την Εορδαία. Ενδιαφέρον παρουσιάζει, επίσης, η διαφορά του υλικού κατασκευής τους: δύο από αυτά είναι χάλκινα, δύο από κράμα χαλκού και μολύβδου και ένα πήλινο (Καραμήτρου-Μεντεσίδη 2007, 42–3).

1. Χάλκινο σκεύος, Νεκρόπολη αρχαίας Αιανής, αρ. Κατ. 12350 (Εικ. 2.16)

Χάλκινο αγγείο αβαθές με εξωστρεφές κάθετο στο σώμα

περιχείλωμα, τονισμένο στις στενές πλευρές. Στο εσωτερικό του, κατά μήκος της μίας στενής πλευράς, προσηλώθηκε ταινιωτή ορθογώνια λαβή. Κάτω από αυτό είχε εισχωρήσει χάλκινη φιαλίσκη. Από τα συνευρήματα εντάσσεται στο β΄ μισό του 4^{ου} αι. π.Χ. (Καραμήτρου-Μεντεσίδη 2007).

2. Χάλκινο-μολύβδινο σκεύος, Ανατολικό Νεκροταφείο της Αρχαίας Αιανής, αρ. Κατ. 17460

Το σκεύος προέρχεται από την ανδρική ταφή 192, όπως συμπεραίνουμε από τη σιδερένια αιχμή δόρατος και την επίσης σιδερένια στλεγγίδα, μολονότι η τελευταία εντοπίζεται και σε ταφές γυναικών και παιδιών. Είναι κατασκευασμένο από κράμα χαλκού και μόλυβδου, ως ορθογώνια ρηχή φιάλη με επίπεδο χείλος (το μήκος του 0,27 και το πλάτος 0,12 μ.). Στη μια πλευρά του εσωτερικού υπάρχει ένα σχετικά πλατύ χάλκινο έλασμα, το οποίο κάμπτεται σε ορθή γωνία και τα άκρα του κολλούσαν στον πυθμένα δημιουργώντας ένα είδος λαβής. Στην άλλη πλευρά βρέθηκε μια χάλκινη φιαλίσκη (αρ. Κατ. 17441), διαμέτρου 0,11 μ. (Καραμήτρου-Μεντεσίδη 2007).

3. Χάλκινο-μολύβδινο σκεύος, Ανατολικό Νεκροταφείο Αιανής, αρ. Κατ. 1367

Πρόκειται για παρόμοιο με το παραπάνω αγγείο και από το ίδιο υλικό, το οποίο όμως προέρχεται πιθανότατα από γυναικεία ταφή (ταφή 8α), κρίνοντας από τις τέσσερις χάλκινες τοξωτές πόρπες (αρ. Κατ. 1361–1364) του β΄ μισού του 4^{ου} αι. π.Χ. Στην ίδια ταφή και από το ίδιο υλικό υπήρχαν κυλινδρικός καδίσκος (αρ. Κατ. 1365) και τρίποδας (αρ. Κατ. 1366) (Καραμήτρου-Μεντεσίδη 2007).

4. Πήλινο σκεύος, Ανατολικό Νεκροταφείο Αιανής, αρ. Κατ. 17443

Άβαφο πήλινο χειροποίητο αγγείο, εντοπίστηκε στην διαταραγμένη ταφή 183, το οποίο μπορούμε να θεωρήσουμε ότι αποδίδει στον πηλό ορθογώνιο μεταλλικό σκεύος. Παρατηρούμε ότι στην πήλινη μορφή του το αγγείο είναι χειροποίητο με βαθύ κυλινδρικό σώμα.[15] Στη μια άκρη του εσωτερικού υπάρχει η σχετικά πλατιά «λαβή», ενώ εξωτερικά το σώμα είναι κυρτό και καμπύλο έως τη βάση (Καραμήτρου-Μεντεσίδη 2007).

5. Χάλκινο σκεύος, Άγιος Χριστόφορος Εορδαίας

Από την περιοχή της Εορδαίας και τον Άγιο Χριστόφορο προέρχεται παρόμοιο με τα παραπάνω χάλκινο σκεύος. Έχει περισυλλεγεί από διάλυση τάφου στη θέση Ζούνολο. Από τα υπόλοιπα ευρήματα μπορεί να ενταχθεί στα μέσα του 4^{ου} αι. π.Χ. (Καραμήτρου-Μεντεσίδη 2001β, 624 εικ. 14· 2007).

Τα αγγεία αυτά, άγνωστα σε μας από αλλού, ερμηνεύουμε ως αγγεία μείξης διαφόρων υλικών με χρήση ιατρική ή καλλυντική, με τοποθέτηση φαρμακευτικών ή άλλων ουσιών και λιγότερο ως ιδιόμορφα τελετουργικά αγγεία. Πιθανότατα, μάλιστα, μπορούμε να αποδώσουμε διπλή χρήση, ιατρική και ως αγγείο καλλωπισμού, όπως συμβαίνει και με πολλά μικρά και λεπτά εργαλεία. Αν η ερμηνεία μας είναι ορθή οδηγούμαστε πιθανόν στο συμπέρασμα ότι ο άντρας της ταφής 192 ήταν γιατρός στο επάγγελμα.[16]

Ζ. Εργαλεία

Χρήση καλλυντική ή ιατρική-φαρμακευτική αποδίδεται σε χάλκινα ωτογλύφανα, όπως ονομάζονται ή μικρές μήλες (Krug 1997, 98), σε διάφορες σπάτουλες (Krug 1997, 97), καθώς και σε οστέινα κοχλιάρια.

Τα ωτογλύφανα, αντικείμενα με επίμηκες στέλεχος, συνήθως κυκλικής διατομής, που απολήγουν σε πεπλατυσμένα πέρατα σαν μικροσκοπικά κουταλάκια, αποκαλύπτονται συχνά σε ταφές και οικιστικά κατάλοιπα. Τα στελέχη αυτών των εργαλείων διακοσμούνται με κυκλικές εγχαράξεις ή κυκλικές ανάγλυφες ταινίες. Από την Αιανή έχουμε τρία χαρακτηριστικά παραδείγματα χάλκινων ωτογλύφανων, το πρώτο (αρ. Κατ. 1345), από τη Νεκρόπολη της αρχαίας πόλης στη θέση Λειβάδια, το δεύτερο (αρ. Κατ. 5661), από το Ανατολικό Νεκροταφείο και το τρίτο (αρ. Κατ. 17090) (Εικ. 2.17), παραδόθηκε από ιδιώτη προερχόμενο από την ευρύτερη περιοχή της νεκρόπολης της θέσης Λειβάδια. Από το ρωμαϊκό νεκροταφείο της Ποντοκώμης προέρχεται αργυρό ωτογλύφανο (ΕΡΔ 411) από τον χτιστό τάφο 42 (Καραμήτρου-Μεντεσίδη 2000, 618–23).

Για το διπλό οστέινο κοχλιάριο (αρ. Κατ. 344), που βρέθηκε μέσα σε γυάλινο αγγείο (αρ. Κατ. 342), και προέρχεται από ρωμαϊκό χτιστό τάφο της θέσης Ράχη Τσέικα Αιανής, μπορούμε με μεγαλύτερη πιθανότητα να υποστηρίξουμε ότι είχε φαρμακευτική χρήση. Από τον χτιστό τάφο 42 της Ποντοκώμης προέρχονται δύο κοχλιάρια από ήλεκτρο (αρ. Κατ. 413 και 418) και από ταφές του ίδιου νεκροταφείου δύο οστέινα, ταφή 79 (αρ. Κατ. 533) και από την ταφή 97 (αρ. Κατ. 584) (Καραμήτρου-Μεντεσίδη 2000, 622, εικ. 24).

Από την αρχαία πόλη της Αιανής, προέρχεται μία χάλκινη σπάτουλα (αρ. Κατ. 1763). Μεγαλύτερες σπάτουλες με αδιευκρίνιστη χρήση προέρχονται επίσης τόσο από την αρχαία πόλη της Αιανής όσο και την αρχαία Νεκρόπολη (αρ. Κατ. 455 και 5696). Τέλος από την Μαυροπηγή Εορδαίας προέρχεται μια δεύτερη χάλκινη σπάτουλα.

Αδιευκρίνιστη παραμένει προς το παρόν η χρήση δύο σιδερένιων εργαλείων που απολήγουν σε τριπλά άγκιστρα από τη μία τους πλευρά και σπάτουλα από την άλλη (αρ. Κατ. 9316 από τη θέση Βέρβερη Αιανής και το αρ. Κατ. 13390 από την αρχαία Νεκρόπολη της Αιανής). Χαρακτηριστικό τους είναι η έντονη καμπύλωση του μεσαίου από τα τρία άγκιστρα. Σύμφωνα με την A. Krug (1997, 88), παρόμοια εργαλεία χρησιμοποιούνται για την

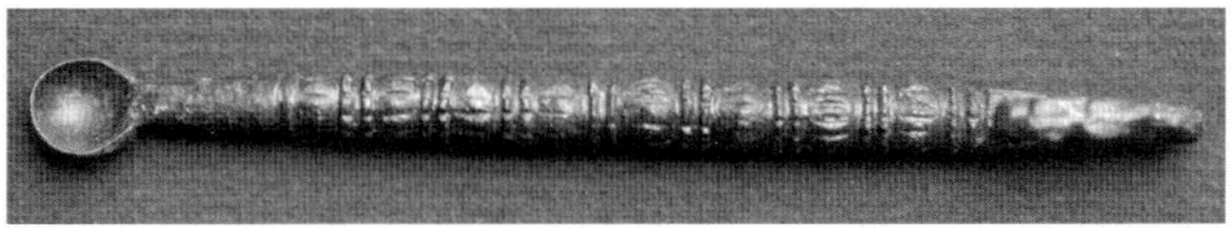

Εικ. 2.17. Χάλκινο ωτογλύφανο ή μήλη από την αρχαία πόλη της Αιανής, αρ. Κατ. 17090

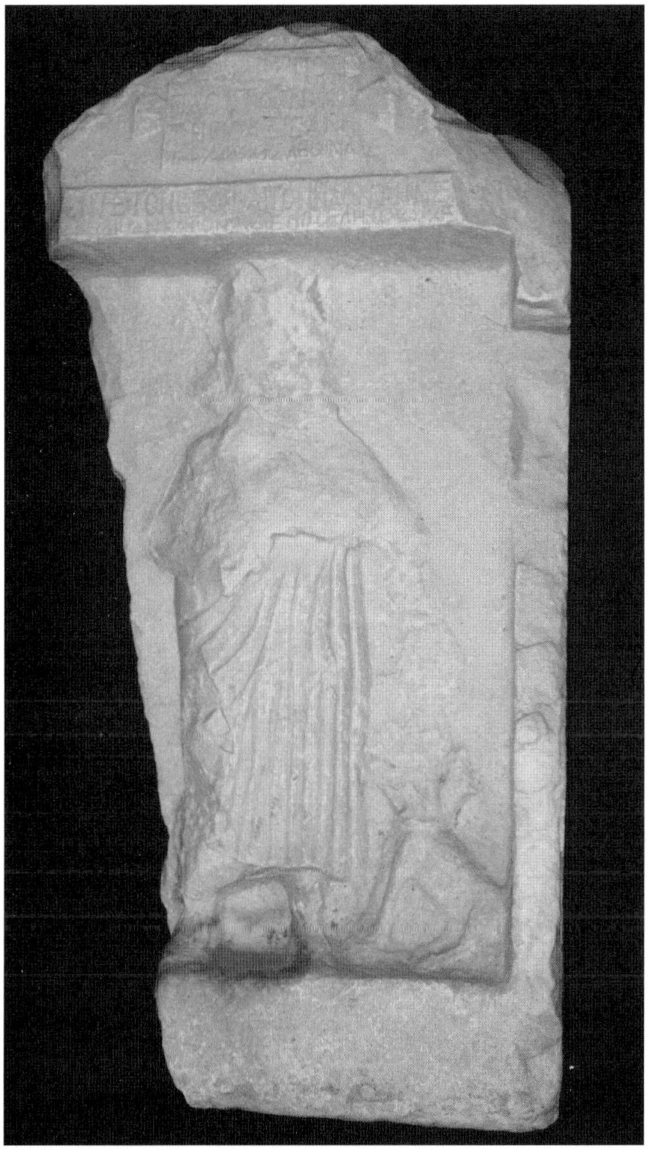

Εικ. 2.18. Αναθηματική στήλη, Αιανή, αρ. Κατ. 3

ακινητοποίηση στα χείλη τραυμάτων ή σε τμήματα ιστών. Στην περίπτωση των εργαλείων της Αιανής ενδέχεται να έχουμε μία πρώιμη χρήση αυτών των εργαλείων.

H. Varia

1) Αναθηματική Στήλη με παράσταση Πλούτωνα, Αιανή, αρ. Κατ. 3 (Εικ. 2.18)

Μαρμάρινη αναθηματική ανάγλυφη στήλη με τριγωνική απόληξη, ελλιπής στο αριστερό τμήμα και απολεπισμένη δεξιά. Μέσα σε ιδιαίτερα βαθύ πεδίο παράσταση κερασφόρου (;) Πλούτωνα κατενώπιον, με μακρύ χιτώνα, που κρατά στο αριστερό του χέρι από αλυσίδα, τον τρικέφαλο Κέρβερο, το δεξί του χέρι είναι διπλωμένο στο στήθος (Ριζάκης και Τουράτσογλου 1985, 31, αρ. 15). Χρονολογείται περί τα τέλη του 2ου μ.Χ αι.

Επιγραφή:

1α) *Θεῷ Δεσπότῃ/ Πλούτωνι καὶ/ τῇ πόλει Ἐανῇ/ Τ. Φλαύιος Λεωνᾶς*

1β) *ἰδὼν αὐτ]όν τε τὸν θεὸν καὶ τὸν ναὸν τὴν στ[ήλην ἀνέ-]/*
θηκα ἐκ τ]ῶν ἰδίων κατ' ὄναρ δι' ἐπιμελητοῦ Ἀρχε[λάου;]

Σύμφωνα με τους Ριζάκη και Τουράτσογλου (Ριζάκης και Τουράτσογλου 1999, 952), από το κείμενο της επιγραφής συνάγεται ότι στο χώρο υπήρχε ναός με λατρευτικό άγαλμα και προφανώς και *εγκοιμητήριον*. Οι ίδιοι τεκμηριώνουν την υπόθεση αναφέροντας ότι στα ρωμαϊκά χρόνια πολλά Πλουτώνια είχαν μεταβληθεί σε ένα είδος ιατρο-θεραπευτικών μαντείων υποκαθιστώντας κατά κάποιο τρόπο τα Ασκληπιεία.

Συμπεράσματα

Τα παραδείγματα αυξάνουν ανάλογα με το πόσο η έρευνα εξελίσσεται σε κάθε χώρο της Άνω Μακεδονίας. Η Αιανή, και ο Νομός Κοζάνης γενικότερα, αποτελούν τους καλύτερα ερευνημένους χώρους της Δυτικής Μακεδονίας και είναι φυσικό να αντιπροσωπεύονται με περισσότερα δείγματα. Στην πλειοψηφία τους τα παραδείγματα από τους άλλους Νομούς αφορούν σε επιτύμβιες και αναθηματικές στήλες, ως τυχαία ευρήματα.

Η Αιανή διασώζει μέχρι σήμερα τα πρωιμότερα παραδείγματα (κλασικά-ελληνιστικά χρόνια). Για την υπόλοιπη Δυτική Μακεδονία, όμως, σχεδόν όλα τα παραδείγματα χρονολογούνται στους ρωμαϊκούς χρόνους και τούτο οφείλεται ενδεχομένως στην περιορισμένη έρευνα. Άλλωστε στην Καμενίτσα, κοντά στην Κορυτσά, σήμερα στην Αλβανία, που συμπεριλαμβανόταν στην αρχαία Ορεστίδα, έχει διαπιστωθεί κρανιοτομή για θεραπευτικούς λόγους σε τάφο του 7ου–6ου αι. π.Χ. από τύμβο της Εποχής Σιδήρου.

Σημειώσεις

1 Στον κατάλογο χρησιμοποιούνται οι ακόλουθες συντομογραφίες:
Αρ. Κατ. (Αιανή): Αριθμός Καταλόγου καταγραφών Αρχαιολογικού Μουσείου Αιανής·
Αρ. Κατ. (Θεσσαλονίκη): Αριθμός καταγραφής Αρχαιολογικού Μουσείου Θεσσαλονίκης·
ΒΕΚ: Βιβλίο Εισαγωγής Αρχαιολογικού Μουσείου Κοζάνης·
ΓΡΕ: Κατάλογος Αρχαιοτήτων Γρεβενών·
ΕΡΔ: Κατάλογος Αρχαιοτήτων Εορδαίας·
ΚΑΒΕ: Κατάλογος αντικειμένων Βελβεντού·
ΠΤΟΛ: Κατάλογος Αρχαιολογικής Συλλογής Ανθρωπολογικού-Παλαιοντολογικού Μουσείου Πτολεμαΐδας.

2 Το ύψος του είναι 0,41 το πλάτος 0,15 και το πάχος του 0,105 μ. Για παραστάσεις Ασκληπιού σημειώνουμε ενδεικτικά μόνο, τα γλυπτά από το Ιερό του Απόλλωνα Μαλεάτα και του Ασκληπιού από την Επίδαυρο (Κατάκη 2002).

3 Οι παραστάσεις, στις οποίες ο Ασκληπιός τείνει αυγό προς το φίδι είναι σπάνιες: βλ.Grimm 1989.

4 Το σωζόμενο ύψος του είναι 0,25 και το πλάτος 0,27 μ.

5 Οι παραστάσεις της Υγείας με φίδι είναι πολλές στον αρχαίο ελληνικό κόσμο, αναφέρουμε εδώ το αγαλμάτιο Υγείας με φίδι που ελίσσεται πάνω της από το Εθνικό Αρχαιολογικό Μουσείο (Ρωμιοπούλου 1997, 271) και το ανάγλυφο από το Δίον (Παντερμαλής 1997, 336–7). Πολλές φορές συνοδεύει τον Ασκληπιό, ενδεικτικά αναφέρουμε το ανάγλυφο από την Θεσσαλονίκη (Βουτυράς 1993, 253).

6 Συνήθως απεικονίζονται δύο σικύες στα ανάγλυφα και ενδεικτικά αναφέρουμε αυτό από το Ασκληπιείο της Αθήνας (Σβορῶνος 1903, 343 πίν. 47).

7 Πολύ γνωστή είναι η μαρμάρινη βάση με παράσταση ανάγλυφης εργαλειοθήκης από το Ασκληπιείο της Αθήνας (Νότια κλιτύς Ακρόπολης), η οποία βρίσκεται στο Εθνικό Αρχαιολογικό Μουσείο (Σβορῶνος 1903, 323 πίν. 47· Svoronos 1908, 247).

8 Ίσως η πρωιμότερη απεικόνιση σικύας σε ανάγλυφο είναι αυτή στη στήλη καθιστού γενειοφόρου γιατρού, η οποία βρίσκεται στο Μουσείο Τέχνης της Βασιλείας (Krug 1985, 33 εικ. 4). Πιθανότατα απεικόνιση σικύας έχουμε και σε ένα από τα αμφίγλυφα του Τηλέμαχου ιδρυτή του Ασκληπιείου της Αθήνας (Beschi 1982, 31–43, σχ. 41). Στη αγγειογραφία σικύες-βεντούζες απεικονίζονται και σε αρύβαλλο του ζωγράφου της Κλινικής, που χρονολογείται στο 480-470 π.Χ. (Beazley 1984, 813). Τέλος αξίζει να αναφερθεί ότι σικύα αναφέρεται σε επιγραφή με κατάλογο από το Ασκληπιείο του Πειραιά (*Inscriptiones Graecae* II/III2 47). Για τη χρήση της σικύας (cucurbitula) στα ρωμαϊκά χρόνια και για την απεικόνιση της σε αγγεία και στήλες, καθώς και για σικύες που προέρχονται από τάφους γιατρών από πολλές περιοχές του ρωμαϊκού κόσμου (Ελλάδα, Ιταλία, Ισπανία, κεντρική Ευρώπη, Βαλκανική, Μικρά Ασία και της Αιγύπτου: Matthäus 1989· Künzl 1982). Στη Μακεδονία μία χάλκινη σικύα βρέθηκε σε τάφο γιατρού στον Μακρύγιαλο Πιερίας (Χρυσοστόμου 2002, 105 εικ. 5).

9 Στο ρωμαϊκό ανάγλυφο του Kom Ombo της Αιγύπτου (Stettler 1982, 48), απεικονίζεται όμοιο ψαλίδι μαζί με άλλα πολλά εργαλεία, επίσης παρόμοιο απεικονίζεται σε στήλη κατασκευαστή και πωλητή εργαλείων από την Όστια (Matthäus 1989, 80 Εικ. 38). Τέλος όμοιο ψαλίδι προέρχεται μαζί με πολλά άλλα εργαλεία από την Πομπηία (Καμπάνης 2002, 58 Εικ. 20).

10 Συνήθως οι εργαλειοθήκες αυτές είναι χάλκινες στα ρωμαϊκά χρόνια, χωρίς όμως να αποκλείεται και η κατασκευή τους από άλλο υλικό. Αυτή που βρέθηκε στον Μακρύγιαλο Πιερίας είναι οστέινη με χάλκινο πώμα. Δεν αναφέρεται στη δημοσίευση αν περιείχε στο εσωτερικό της μικρά εργαλεία (Χρυσοστόμου 2002, 105, εικ. 6). Θήκη με ένα μόνο εργαλείο στο εσωτερικό της (κυαθυσκομήλη) βρέθηκε και στην Αμφίπολη, σε τάφο γιατρού πιθανότατα (Αμοιρίδου και Μαλαμίδου 2008, 78 εικ. 5).

11 Οι μήλες γενικά εμφανίζονται σε πολλούς τύπους και με πολλές χρήσεις (Krug 1997, 96–8).

12 Από το ιερό του Απόλλωνα προέρχονται συνολικά 8 επιγραφές (Καραμήτρου-Μεντεσίδη 2001α, 58–68 εικ. 5–12).

13 Αναλυτικά για τις παραστάσεις ιαθέντων μελών και «ευήκοων» ώτων: Forsén 1996, 13–9. Ο Δ. Λυπουρλής σημειώνει επίσης ότι με την πράξη αυτή τα θεραπευμένα μέλη έμπαιναν κάτω από την προστασία του θεού, ο οποίος τα προστάτευε και από μία μελλοντική αρρώστια (Λυπουρλής 2008, 80–1).

14 Για το επίθετο Μεσωρίσκος πιθανότερη θεωρούμε την ερμηνεία που το συνδέει με τη θέση του ιερού στο μέσο των ορέων Βερμίου και Ασκίου. Για την ανασκαφή και τα ευρήματα (Καραμήτρου-Μεντεσίδη 1999α, 212–5· 1999β, 337–45· 2000, 607–10 και Καραμήτρου-Μεντεσίδη και Μπουλακάκης 2004).

15 Οι διαστάσεις είναι βάθος 0,065 μ. και στην πάνω επιφάνεια, μήκος 0,14, πλάτος 0,101, πάχος χείλους στις στενές πλευρές 0,022 και στις μακρές 0,01 μ.

16 Τάφος γιατρού βρέθηκε στο Κίτρος Πιερίας και χρονολογείται στο β΄ μισό του 4ου αι. π.Χ. (Χρυσοστόμου 2002, 105), τάφος γιατρού ρωμαϊκών χρόνων βρέθηκε στην Αμφίπολη (Αμοιρίδου-Μαλαμίδου 1998, 78).

Βιβλιογραφία

Αμοιρίδου, Ν. και Μαλαμίδου, Δ. 1998: «Ανασκαφική έρευνα στο ρωμαϊκό νεκροταφείο της Αμφίπολης», *Αρχαιολογικό Έργο στη Μακεδονία και Θράκη* 12, 77–83.

Beazley, J. D. 1984: *Attic Red-figure Vase Painters 2*, New York.

Beschi, L. 1982: 'Il relievo di Telemachos ricompletato', *Αρχαιολογικά Ανάλεκτα εξ Αθηνών* XV, 31–43.

Βουτυράς, Ε. 1993: «Η λατρεία του Ασκληπιού στην Αρχαία Μακεδονία», *Αρχαία Μακεδονία V*, τόμος 1, 251–65.

Γεωργακόπουλος, Κ. 1998: *Αρχαίοι Έλληνες Ιατροί*, Αθήνα.

Forsén, B. 1996: *Griechische Gliederweihungen. Eine Untersuchung zu ihrer Typologie und ihrer religions- und sozialgeschichtlichen Bedeutung* (Papers and Monographs of the Finnish Institute at Athens IV).

Gomme, A. W. 1945–1981, *A Historical Commentary on Thucydides*, 5 vols, Oxford.

Grimm, G. 1989: "Alexander the False Prophet and his god Asclepius-Glycon – Remarks concerning the Representation of Asclepius with an Egg ('type Nea Paphos – Alexandria –

Trier)", 168–81 στο V. Tatton-Brown (ed.), *Cyprus and the East Mediterranean in the Iron Age. Proceedings of the 7th British Museum Classical Colloquium, April 1988,* London.

Καμπάνης, Π. 2002: *Συλλογή Γ. Τσολοζίδη, Ιατρικά και χειρουργικά εργαλεία της ύστερης αρχαιότητας,* Θεσσαλονίκη.

Καραμήτρου-Μεντεσίδη, Γ. 1992: «Νομός Κοζάνης», *Αρχαιολογικό Δελτίο* 37, 305.

Καραμήτρου-Μεντεσίδη, Γ. 1993: *Κοζάνη, Πόλις Ελιμιώτιδος, Αρχαιολογικός Οδηγός,* Θεσσαλονίκη.

Καραμήτρου-Μεντεσίδη, Γ. 1994: «Αρχαιότητες του Βελβεντού. Τα πρώτα ιστορικά συμπεράσματα», *Βελβεντό, Χθές, Σήμερα, Αύριο, Πρακτικά του Συνεδρίου 1993,* Θεσσαλονίκη.

Καραμήτρου-Μεντεσίδη, Γ. 1999α: *Βόιον-Νότια Ορεστίς, Αρχαιολογική Έρευνα και Ιστορική Τοπογραφία,* Θεσσαλονίκη.

Καραμήτρου-Μεντεσίδη, Γ. 1999β: «Νομός Κοζάνης 1999: Ανασκαφές εν οδοίς και παροδίως», *Αρχαιολογικό Έργο στη Μακεδονία και Θράκη* 13, 337–68.

Καραμήτρου-Μεντεσίδη Γ. 2000: «Νομός Κοζάνης 2000: Ανασκαφές εν οδοίς και παροδίως», *Αρχαιολογικό Έργο στη Μακεδονία και Θράκη* 14, 607–40.

Καραμήτρου-Μεντεσίδη Γ. 2001α: «Νομός Κοζάνης: νεώτερα επιγραφικά ευρήματα», 49–78 στο Τουλουμάκος, Ι. (επιμ.), *Α΄ Πανελλήνιο Συνέδριο Επιγραφικής (Πρακτικά), Στην μνήμη Δημητρίου Κανατσούλη, Θεσσαλονίκη 22–23 Οκτωβρίου 1999,* Θεσσαλονίκη.

Καραμήτρου-Μεντεσίδη Γ. 2001β: «Εορδαία: Δήμος Αγίας Παρασκευής», *Αρχαιολογικό Έργο στη Μακεδονία και Θράκη* 15, 611–30.

Καραμήτρου-Μεντεσίδη, Γ. 2001γ: *Αιανή, Αρχαιολογικός οδηγός, Ταμείο Αρχαιολογικών Πόρων και Απαλλοτριώσεων,* Αθήνα 1996 (1η έκδοση), 2001 (2η έκδοση).

Καραμήτρου-Μεντεσίδη, Γ. 2007: «Αιανή 2007. Η έρευνα στο Ανατολικό Νεκροταφείο», *Αρχαιολογικό Έργο στη Μακεδονία και Θράκη* 21, 2007, 37–46.

Καραμήτρου-Μεντεσίδη, Γ. 2008: *Η Αιανή και η συμβολή της στη διαμόρφωση της νέας ιστορικής φυσιογνωμίας της Άνω Μακεδονίας* (Μακεδονική Λαϊκή Βιβλιοθήκη, 43, Δημοσιεύματα της Εταιρείας Μακεδονικών Σπουδών), Θεσσαλονίκη.

Καραμήτρου-Μεντεσίδη, Γ. και Μπουλακάκης, Γ. 2004: «Θεσσαλικά Νομίσματα στην Αιανή και την Ελιμιώτιδα», 291–310 στο *Γ΄ Επιστημονική Συνάντηση, Το Νόμισμα στο Θεσσαλικό Χώρο, Οβολός 7, Οι Φίλοι του Νομισματικού Μουσείου, Βόλος, 24–27 Μαΐου 2001,* Αθήνα.

Κατάκης, Σ. 2002: *Επίδαυρος, Τα γλυπτά των ρωμαϊκών χρόνων από το Ιερό του Απόλλωνος Μαλεάτα και του Ασκληπιού,* Αθήνα.

Krug, A. 1985: *Heilkunst und Heilkult. Medizin in der Antike,* München.

Krug, A. 1997: *Αρχαία Ιατρική* (ελληνική μετάφραση Ε. Μανακίδου και Θ . Σαρτζή), Αθήνα.

Künzl, E. 1982: 'Ventosae cucurbitae romanae, Zu einem angeblich antiken Schropfkopftypus', *Germania* 60, 513–32.

Λυπουρλής, Δ. 2008: *Ιατρική στην Αρχαία Ελλάδα,* Θεσσαλονίκη.

Matthäus, H. 1989: *Der Arzt in römischer Zeit, medizinische Instrumente und Arzneien. Archäologische Hinterlassenschaft im Siedlungen und Gräber* (Limes-museum, Aalen 43), Stuttgart.

Μοσχάκης, Κ. 2004: «Επιτύμβια στήλη γιατρού από την Κέλλη», *Εταιρία* τεύχος 38–9, 6–13.

Μοσχάκης, Κ. 2009: «Η ανάπτυξη της Ιατρικής στην Άνω Μακεδονία κατά τους ρωμαϊκούς χρόνους. Παράσταση ιατρού και συλλογής εργαλείων σε επιτύμβια στήλη από την περιοχή της Φλώρινας», 23–34 στο Ε. Χριστοπούλου-Αλετρά (επιμ.), *3ο Συνέδριο Πανελλήνιας Εταιρείας Ιστορίας της Ιατρικής, «ΥΓΙΕΙΝΑ ΠΑΡΑΓΓΕΛΜΑΤΑ». Η ιστορία της Δημόσιας Υγείας και της Υγιεινής από την Αρχαιότητα μέχρι σήμερα», Θεσσαλονίκη 1–2 Δεκεμβρίου 2006,* Αθήνα 2009.

Παντερμαλής, Δ. 1997: «Λατρείες και Ιερά του Δίου Πιερίας», *Αρχαία Μακεδονία* ΙΙ, 336–7.

Πέτσας Φ. 1961–2: «Αρχαιότητες και Μνημεία Δυτικής Μακεδονίας», *Αρχαιολογικό Δελτίο* 17, 1961/2, *Χρονικά* Β2, 213–26.

Pollak, K. 2005: *Η Ιατρική στην Αρχαιότητα* (ελληνική μετάφραση Α. Μαυρουδής), Αθήνα.

Ριζάκης, Θ. και Τουράτσογλου, Γ. 1985: *Επιγραφές Άνω Μακεδονίας (Ελίμεια, Εορδαία, Νότια Λυγκηστίς, Ορεστίς),* Τόμος Α΄, Αθήνα.

Ριζάκης, Αθ. και Τουράτσογλου, Ι. 1999: «Λατρείες στην Άνω Μακεδονία. Παράδοση και νεωτερισμοί», 949–65 στο *Αρχαία Μακεδονία, Έκτο Διεθνές Συμπόσιο,* Θεσσαλονίκη.

Ρωμιοπούλου, Κ. 1997: *Ελληνορωμαϊκά γλυπτά του Εθνικού Αρχαιολογικού Μουσείου,* Αθήνα.

Σβορῶνος Ν. 1903: *Τὸ ἐν Ἀθήναις ἐθνικὸν Μουσεῖον,* Αθήνα.

Svoronos, N. 1908: *Das Athener Nationalmuseum I,* Athen.

Σιαμπανόπουλος, Κ. 1974: *Αιανή, Ιστορία-Τοπογραφία-Αρχαιολογία,* Θεσσαλονίκη.

Stettler, A. 1982: 'Der instrumentenschrank von Kom Ombo', *Antike Welt* 13, 48–53.

Χρυσοστόμου, Π. 2002, «Συμβολές στην Ιστορία της Ιατρικής στην Αρχαία Μακεδονία», *Ευλιμένη* 3, 99–116.

3. Ancient Greek Votives, Vases and Stelae Depicting Medical Diseases

Stefanos Geroulanos

Illustrations of medical themes such as illnesses, trauma, bleeding or therapeutic issues are on the whole seldom depicted on vases, gravestones or votive offerings. However, during the last two decades these topics have been the subject of major research and much new knowledge has been added to Hollaender's classic work of 1912.

Illustrations of medical themes such as illnesses, trauma, bleeding or therapeutic issues are on the whole seldom depicted on vases, gravestones or votive offerings. However, during the last two decades these topics have been the subject of major research by M. Grmek and D. Gourevitch (1998) and the author (with R. Bridler: 1994; 1998), and much new knowledge has been added to Hollaender's classic work of 1912. Grmek and Gourevitch have focused mainly on illnesses, the author on trauma and its healing; while major work has also been done by the archaeologist Veronique Dasen on dwarfism, multiple births and phocomelia.

Through these two works (Grmek and Gourevitch 1998; Geroulanos and Bridler 1994; 1998) 412 illustrations of medical themes have been published; 27 of which are published in both. At least another 100 votive offerings and vases depicting medical subjects are in the collection of the author but are unpublished.

This icono-diagnostic investigation has compared more than eighty ancient medical illustrations with depictions of the same illness in today's medical handbooks. It provides clear evidence that the antique illustrations were made to document the underlying disease, either for medical purposes, or as an exact representation of what the god was asked to cure; and they were definitely not done unintentionally. However, the illustration of all of them in a paper is not possible and the following few examples must suffice.

1. As far as we are able to prove, the earliest European illustration of a disease is a Minoan depiction of a lymphoedema. Grmek and Gourevitch (1998, 293) speak of elephantiasis[1] of the left leg of a female subject. It was found at Traostalos and dates back to around 1800 BC (Davaras 1976, 246, fig. 85) (Fig. 3.1). Filariasis that could be the cause was well known in ancient Egypt but less so in Greece; however a congenital cause of the lymphoedema cannot be excluded. Another possibility could be a venous thrombosis with swelling of the leg; however, the colour of the two legs, that has partially survived, shows no difference.
2. The oldest depiction of a traumatism is depicted on a fresco of Thera (Santorini), which dates back to 1500 BC. It shows a pretty young girl, who has stopped dancing and sits on a stone. She is very concerned about the bleeding wound of her left big toe (Geroulanos and Bridler 1998, cover).
3. Two cases of phocomelia have been published by Dasen (1997, 5) probably originating from Selinus in Sicily and going back to the 7th or 6th century BC. One (Fig. 3.2) looks more or less identical with the Russian Nicolas Kobelkopf, who was born in Siberia in the middle of the 19th century AD (Witkowski 1920, 143, fig. 47). The only difference is that the ancient person depicted has one arm, in contrast to the Russian Nicolas, who has no extremities at all. Similar cases were observed in the 1960s after ingestion of the sedative-hypnotic drug Contergan, the so-called thalidomide embryopathy. Depending on the day the drug was taken, no ears (34–38th day), no arms (40–44th day), or no

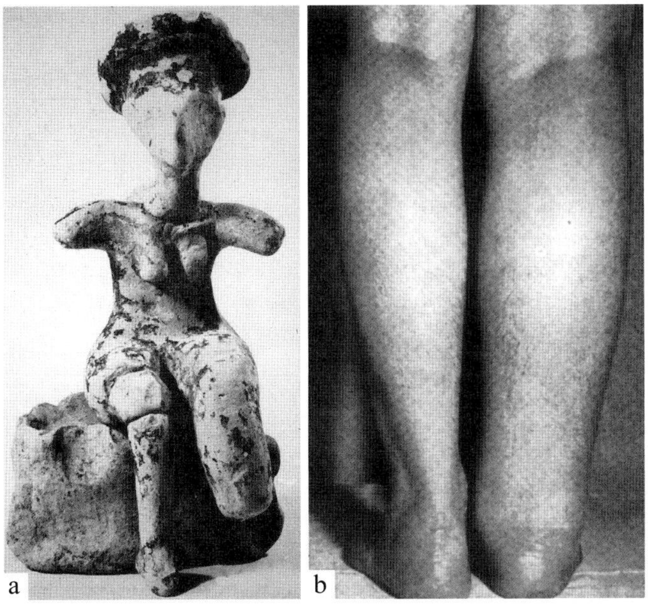

Fig. 3.1. a. Minoan votive offering from Traostalos dating to 1800 BC, showing massive lymphoedema of the left leg (elephantiasis?), Archaeological Museum, Heraklion (photo: National Archaeological Museum, Athens); b. Recent appearance of a lymphoedema of the right leg (photo: Urs Brunner)

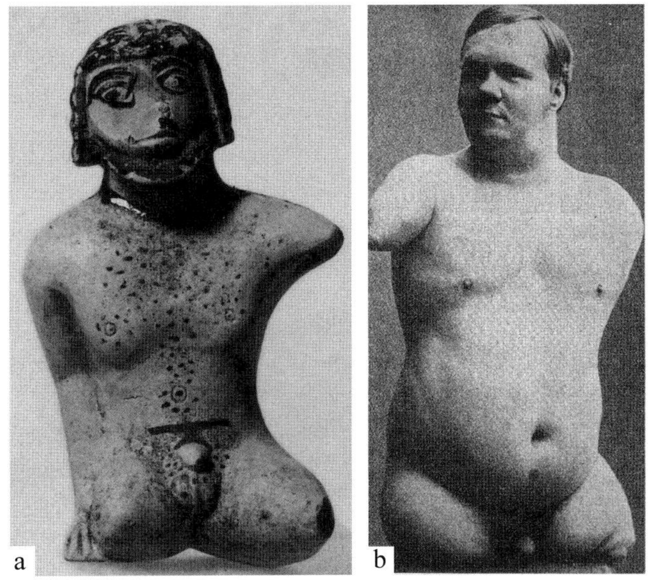

Fig. 3.2. a. Corinthian ex-voto of the 6th or 7th century BC, depicting phocomelia: Musée d'Art et d'Histoire, inv. HR79, Geneva (photo: Veronique Dasen); b. Photograph of Nicolas Kobelkopf, born in the 19th century in Siberia with complete amelia of all four extremities (photo: Witkowski 1920, 140, fig. 47)

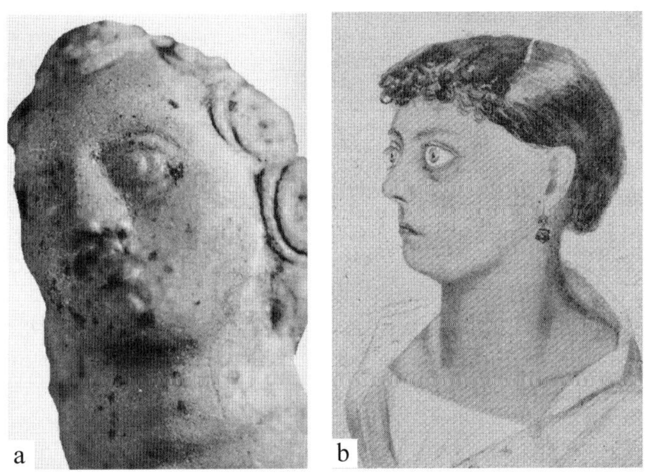

Fig. 3.3. a. Terracotta head from Troy, exhibiting swelling of the goitre accompanied by bilateral exophthalmos, Basedow syndrome, Musée du Louvre, Paris (photo: Louvre Museum, D 556); b. Exophthalmic goitre (from a drawing in St Bartholomew's Hospital Museum, London, cited by Riddle 1914, 789)

legs (43–46th day) were developed. If the drug was taken daily between the 34th and 46th day, complete phocomelia (amelia) was observed.

4 Several depictions of dwarfs have been published by Dasen (1988, 253–76). They can be compared to the achondroplastic dwarfs who are living around us and frequently make their living in circuses.

5 Acromegaly, Morbus Cushing and Morbus Basedow with exophthalmus and swelling of the goitre are some examples of the endocrine disorders occasionally depicted, as in a 1st century BC terracotta head from Troy (Besques 1971–72, vol. III, 94) (Fig. 3.3).

6 Several other votive offerings depict illnesses, traumatisms, tumours, blindness or enucleation of the eyes. The most common are diverse forms of strabismus, as in the ex-voto of Aurelia Artemisia from Ephesus (3rd century AD), with left-sided strabismus convergens (Antikensammlung Inv. 35: Hornbostel 1978, 215) (Fig. 3.4).

7 Even a Claude Bernard-Horner syndrome can clearly be identified on a Roman portrait of an unknown man, in the Chateau d'Erbach (Besques 1971–72, III, 94) (Fig. 3.5). As Grmek and Gourevitch (1998, 275, fig. 219) observe, the artist has beautifully depicted not only the drooping of the eye-lid (blepharoptosis) but also the asymmetry of the pupils (miosis), the sinking of the eye (enophthalmus) and the very infrequent hemi-atrophy of the face. The aetiology is either congenital (autosomal dominant) or acquired due to an injury of the ciliospinal centre in the spinal cord or the cervical sympathetic nervous system (the stellate ganglion). In this portrait, congenital aetiology seems more probable, as the hemi-atrophy of the face is more common in this form.

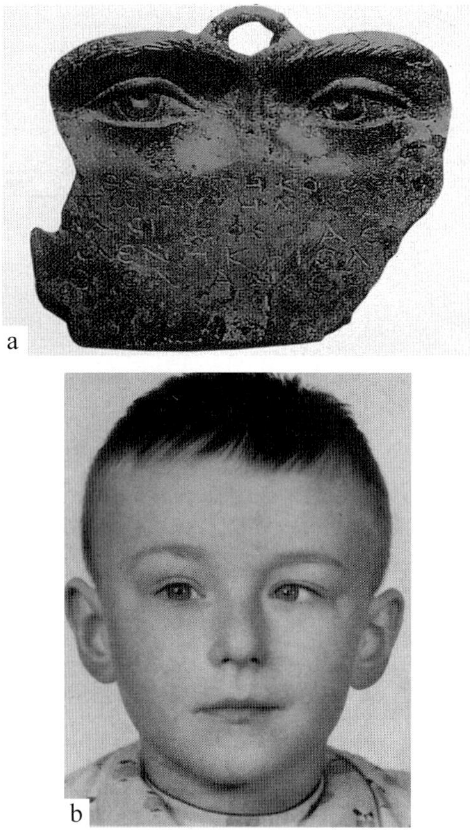

Fig. 3.4. a. Ex-voto with dedication of Aurelia Artemisia from Ephesus (3rd century AD), with left-sided strabismus convergens, Museum für Kunst und Gewerbe, Hamburg (photo: Hornbostel 1978, 215); b. Recent photograph of a child with left sided squinting (photo: author's archive)

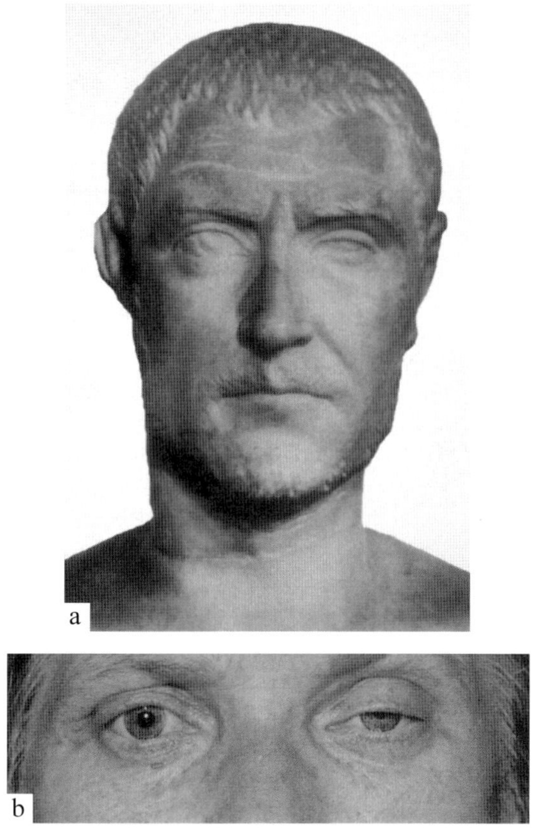

Fig. 3.5. a. Roman statue of a man, now in the Chateau d'Erbach, with Claude Bernard-Horner syndrome: blepharoptosis, miosis and pseudoatrophy of the left part of the face (photo: Fittschen 1977, pl. 41, figs 1–4); b. Modern photograph of a woman with Claude Bernard-Horner Syndrome (photo: author's archive)

8 The loss of hair in circumscriptive areas (alopecia areata) is most probably the correct diagnosis of the head, considered to be Greek, found at the temple of Minerva medica in the Quirinale in Rome, now kept in the Antiquarium Communale (Hollaender 1912, 304, fig. 196) (Fig. 3.6a). The curly hair that has been placed on the head forms such accurate circumscriptive areas without hair that it is impossible that it could have fallen away in such a manner just by chance. Sambon (1895, 147), who was the first to describe this head, is also sure that the circumscriptive areas were done on purpose. The comparative photograph from the Family Encyclopaedia of Medicine (Riddle 1914) beautifully illustrates the similarity (Fig. 3.6b). The cause of the illness is still not clear; however, antiseptic ointments and/or cortisone seem to be helpful, thus making an infection probable. Antimicrosomal antibodies and antibodies to thyreoglobulin, gastric parietal cells and adrenal cells may be present. The prognosis is poor if alopecia is extensive and involving other parts of the body, but alopecia confined to a few areas is often reversed in a

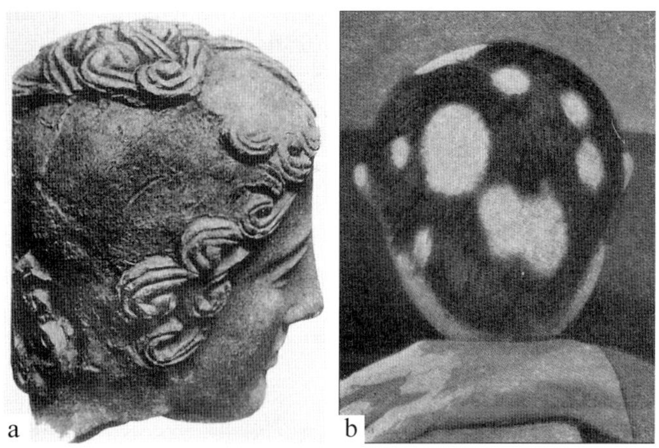

Fig. 3.6. a. Ancient head depicting alopecia areata, in the Antiquarium Communale in Rome (photo: Antiquarium, cited by Hollaender 1912, 304, fig. 196); b. Modern case of alopecia areata (photo: Riddle 1914, 65)

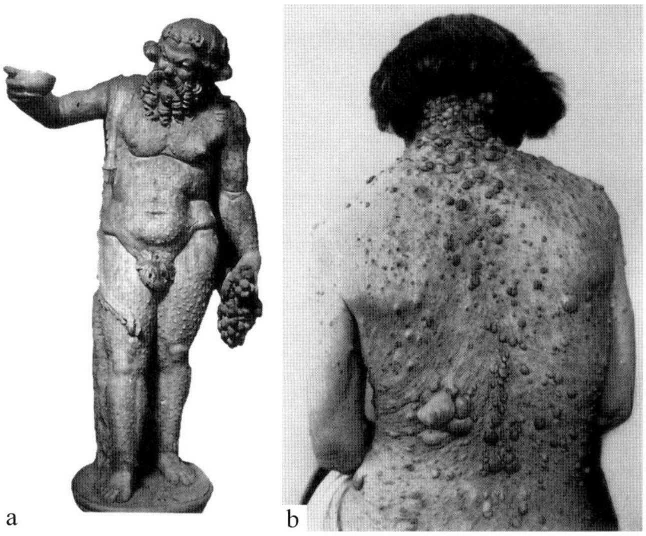

a b

Fig. 3.7. a. Statuette of Silenus in the, Villa Albani, Rome (Hollaender 1912, 309, fig. 203); b. Modern case of neuro-fibromatosis Recklinghausen (photo: unknown)

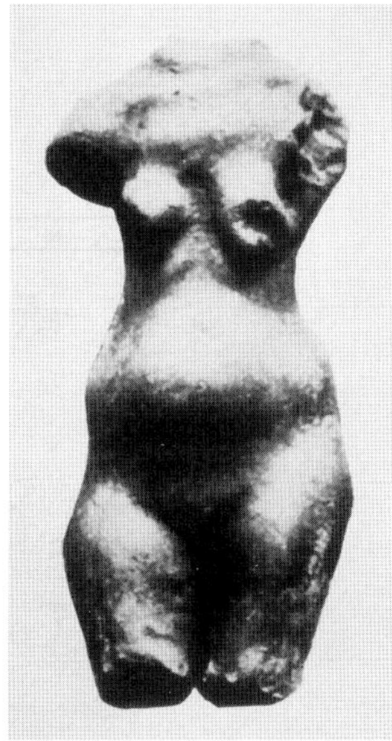

Fig. 3.8. Female statuette from Smyrna with an exulcerated breast tumour left; Note also the enlargement of the left mamma; Meyer-Steineg Collection, Jena (photo: Meyer-Steineg Collection, cited by Hollaender 1912, 301, fig. 194).

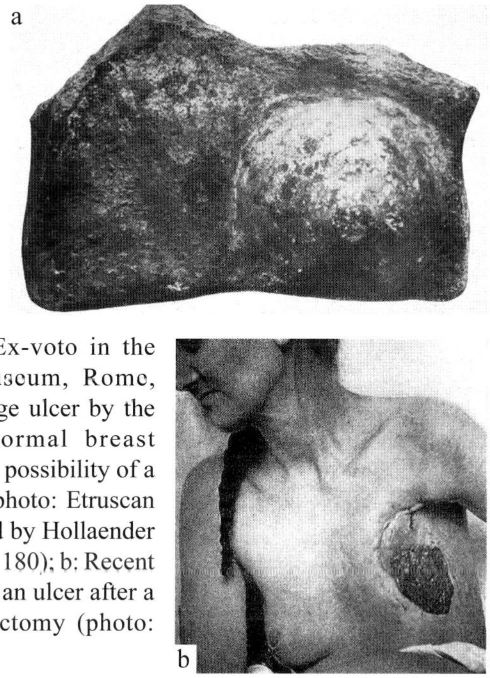

a b

Fig. 3.9. a. Ex-voto in the Etruscan Museum, Rome, showing a large ulcer by the side of a normal breast suggesting the possibility of a mastectomy (photo: Etruscan Museum, cited by Hollaender 1912, 288, fig. 180); b: Recent photograph of an ulcer after a radical mastectomy (photo: unknown)

few months, even without treatment. Recurrences are common (Berkow, Beers and Burs 1999, 814): a perfect disease for asking help from the temple.

9 Extremely interesting is also a statuette in the Villa Albani in Rome (Fig. 3.7a) published by Hollaender in 1912 (309, fig. 203). Grmek and Gourevitch (1998, 344, fig. 273) think that the way the satyr's skin is rendered is due to artistic license. However, the photograph of a patient with neurofibromatosis Recklinghausen shows major similarities (Fig. 3.7b) and at least it leaves the question open. The resemblance of the two cannot be neglected. There is, however, a question mark as the skin of both feet of the villa Albani satyr and the paragenital region are tumour free.

10 The trunk of the human body as depicted on ancient artefacts also shows many afflictions. Clearly depicted are Siamese twins (Thoracopagus), hermaphroditism, torticolis, one-sided breast atrophy, gynecomastia, rachitis (rickets), scoliosis, kyphosis, kyphoscoliosis, opisthotonus, tetanus and many others. Obesity, steatopygia, cachexia and hydrops are also clearly depicted on ex votos or statuettes (Hollaender 1912, 298–9; Grmek and Gourevitch 1998, 197).

11 Breast cancer was probably not as common as it is today, but early descriptions go back to 1600 BC in Egypt, where a male is described with a malignant tumour of the breast (case 45 in 'The Edwin Smith Papyrus': see Beasted 1930). In the case shown in a female statuette from Smyrna, in the Meyer-Steineg Collection, Jena (Hollaender 1912, 301, fig. 190) (Fig. 3.8), the left breast of the woman is enlarged and exulcerated; while on an ex-voto in the Etruscan Museum, Rome (Hollaender 1912, 288, fig. 180) (Fig. 3.9a), a large ulcer by the side of a normal breast suggests the possibility of a mastectomy. The operation is known to have been performed already in the 5th century BC, despite the fact that Hippocrates did not recommend it as a regular treatment. A recent photograph of an ulcer after a radical mastectomy (Fig. 3.9b) illustrates the similarity, although the technique of a mastectomy was in antiquity much simpler and explains the localisation of the wound in the ex-voto.

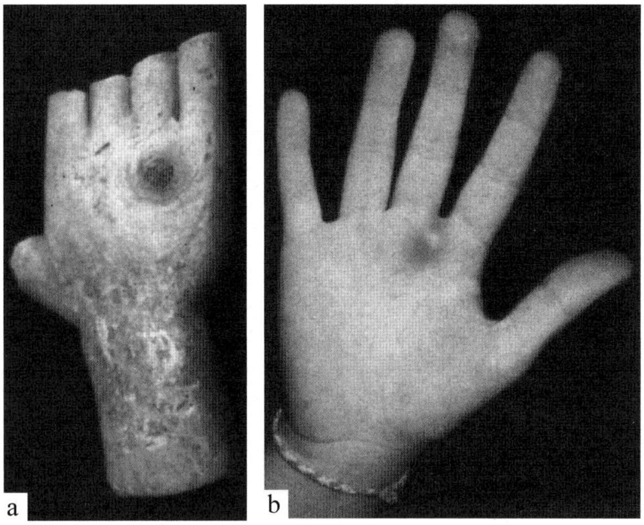

Fig. 3.10. a. Clay ex-voto depicting a hand with an abscess, found in the Asklepieion of Corinth, 480–325 BC, Archaeological Museum of Corinth (photo: author); b. Recent photo of a hand abscess (photo: unknown)

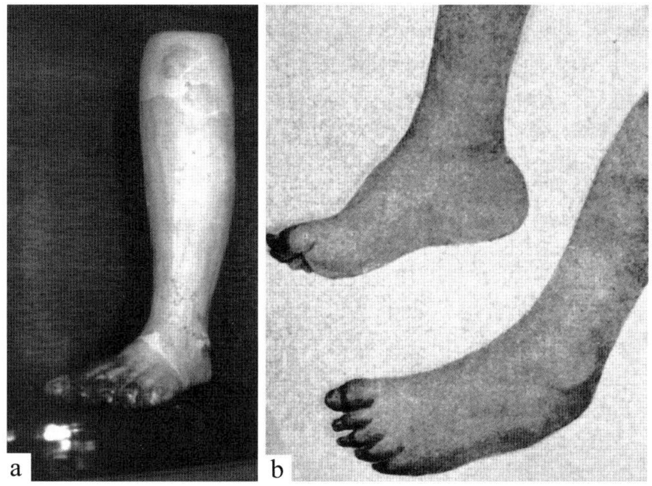

Fig. 3.11. a. Clay ex-voto depicting a gangrene of the foot; note the necrotic toes of the left foot. From the Asklepieion of Corinth, 480–325 BC, Archaeological Museum of Corinth (photo: author); b. Symmetrical gangrene of both feet (from a drawing at St Bartholomew's Hospital Museum, cited by Riddle 1914, 964)

12 Umbilical, inguinal and scrotal hernias, hydrocele and varicocele are also subjects depicted on votives. The same is true for phimosis, hypospadias and priapism. Even a double penis and a rectal prolapse are depicted (Grmek and Gourevitch 1998, 187–90).

13 In artefacts depicting the upper extremities we can recognise a congenital atrophy of an arm (Grmek and Gourevitch 1998, 304, figs 239 and 240), several luxations, a hand abscess, as on a clay ex-voto from the Asklepieion of Corinth, (Fig. 3.10) or a paronychia (Hollaender 1912, 305–9).

14 In the lower extremities an exarticulation of the left coxa (Wagoner 1929, 599) and luxations of other joints, congenital anomalies of the feet, like club foot, malformations of the feet of Hephaistos (Bazopoulou-Kyrkanidou 1997, 144), or even tetra or hexadactyly (Penso 1984, 257, fig. 132) are clearly diagnosed on a number of artefacts. Varices of the lower leg (Hollaender, 1912, 291, fig. 182), one-sided atrophies of the foot (poliomyelitis?) or gangrene, e.g. a clay ex-voto from the Asklepieion of Corinth (Fig. 3.11), are some of the diseases or injuries of the extremities depicted on votives and can clearly be identified today.

15 More than 50 stelae have been found depicting the knee bent at approximately 120° (Hollaender 1912, 295–6, figs 184–5). Are these blockades due to meniscus lesions? The meaning of the stelae is not always clear. However an injury that is so common today must also have been observed in Antiquity. Probably the patients were coming to the Asklepieia to ask for a deblocking of the knee.

Looking at all these diseases and injuries we can conclude that:

a The first medical illustration in Europe goes back as far as 1800 BC;

b Most of the artists who have depicted or painted them had extensive knowledge of external and internal anatomy;

c A large percentage of the votive offerings and the gravestones found were coloured. Unfortunately this colouring has very often been lost, making the exact diagnosis sometimes very difficult or even impossible.

Icono-diagnosis is a method that greatly helps to define diseases. The collaboration of archaeologists with physicians and other specialists helps us to understand the past much better.

Note

1 Furthermore, during the conference Robert Arnott expressed the opinion that it is the thinner of the two legs that shows the pathology.

Bibliography

Bazopoulou-Kyrkanidou, E. 1997: 'What makes Hephaestus lame?', *American Journal of Medical Genetics* 72, 144–55.

Berkow, R., Beers, M. H. and Burs, M. 1999: *The Merck Manual of Diagnosis and Therapy. Centennial Edition*, Whitehouse Station, NJ.

Besques, S, 1971–2: *Musée Nationale du Louvre. Catalogue raisonné des figurines et reliefs en terre cuite grecs, étrusques et romains*, vol. III, Paris.

Dasen, V. 1988: 'Dwarfism in ancient Egypt and Classical Antiquity. Iconography and medical history', *Medical History* 32, 253–76.

Dasen, V. 1997: 'Autour de l'estropié du Musée d'art et d'histoire de Genève. Une représentation archaique grecque d'hémimélie?' *Gesnerus* 54, 5–22.

Davaras, C. 1976: *Guide to Cretan Antiquities*, Park Ridge, NJ.

Fittschen, K. 1977: *Katalog der antiken Skulpturen in Schloss Erbach*, Berlin.

Geroulanos S. and Bridler R. 1994: *Trauma; Wundentstehung und Wundpflege im antiken Griechenland*, Mainz am Rhein.

Geroulanos S. and Bridler R. 1998: Γερουλάνος, Σ. και Bridler, R. 1998*: ΤΡΑΥΜΑ; Πρόκληση και Φροντίδα του Τραύματος στην Αρχαία Ελλάδα,* Athens.

Grmek, M. and Gourevitch, D. 1998: *Les Maladies dans l'Art Antique*, Paris.

Hollaender, E. 1912: *Plastik und Medizin*, Stuttgart.

Hornbostel, W. 1978: 'Kunst der Antike', *Jahrbuch der Hamburger Kunstsammlungen* 23, 215–6. Museum fur Kunst und Gewerbe, Antike Abtlg. Inv.

Penso, G. 1984: *La médecine romaine. L'art d'Esculape dans la Rome antique*, Paris.

Riddle, H. 1914: *The Family Encyclopaedia of Medicine*, London.

Sambon, L. 1895: 'Donaria of medical interest in the Oppenheimer Collection of Etruscan and Roman antiquities', *British Medical Journal* 2, 146–50 and 216–9.

Wagoner, G. W. 1929: 'An Etruscan bronze statuette depicting a posterior dislocation of the hip'. *Annals of Medical History* 1, 599.

Witkowski, G. J. 1920: *Curiosa de médicine*, Paris.

4. The Anatomical Ex-votos of Hellenistic and Roman Cyprus

Demetrios Michaelides

The aim of one of the projects initiated under the programme 'Greece-Cyprus: Joint Educational and Research Programmes Greece-Cyprus in the History and Archaeology of Medicine, Palaeopathology and Palaeoradiation' (INTERREG IIIA 2006–2008) *is to catalogue all surviving examples of medical ex-votos of Cypriot origin that can be traced, as well as to record all information regarding them. The present paper will give a short, general overview of the evidence regarding the anatomical ex-votos of the Hellenistic and Roman periods.*

Cyprus has a particularly interesting series of ancient ex-votos that fall into two main categories. The first consists of terracotta and, less frequently, stone figurines representing either the preparations for childbirth or the actual moment of parturition (Vandenabeele 1988, 31; Hermary1989, 442–3, nos 913–15; Vandervondelen 1977; Karageorghis 1998, 65–6, 78–9). The second consists of limestone ex-votos in the shape of organs or parts of the human body. One of the projects initiated during the programme *'Greece-Cyprus: Joint Educational and Research Programmes Greece-Cyprus in the History and Archaeology of Medicine, Palaeopathology and Palaeoradiation' (INTERREG IIIA 2006–2008)* aims to collect the evidence for and prepare as complete a catalogue as possible of the known examples of both these categories (for a general account of both types, see Michaelides 2006, 44–9; see also Mitropoulou 1985 for eye ex-votos). The present paper will deal briefly with the second group only.

The Cypriot anatomical ex-votos are made of limestone and are sculpted either in the round or in high relief, in the shape of organs or parts of the human body. In a much less frequent variety the anatomical details (normally a face) are painted on a flat stone plaque. Some of these ex-votos are fairly crude but there are also several groups which exhibit amazing anatomical detail. More rarely, there is extra detail applied in paint, or even an inscription, making the nature of the ailment more explicit. Most, but not all, have holes for hanging.

It is difficult to know if these objects were dedicated to a god by the sick person or members of his or her family entreating a cure, or whether they are offerings thanking the deity for the cure of a trauma, an illness or an infirmity. In any case, this is irrelevant for the purposes of this paper.

Some isolated discoveries aside, most of these ex-votos were found buried in large groups, in *bothroi* associated with sanctuaries, dating to the Hellenistic and Roman periods. The general type is, of course, well-known in Greece, Italy, Etruria in particular, and elsewhere (see, amongst others, Forsén 1996). Unfortunately, most of the Cypriot ex-votos were found during the 19th century and were neither properly excavated nor well published. Furthermore, soon after their discovery they were dispersed in different collections and museums of Europe and the USA, while a great number of them seem to have disappeared since.

Before examining the evidence, we have to eliminate some other ex-voto dedications with anatomical representations, which, although fairly similar in appearance to the group we are going to examine, are of a very different nature. For example, the raised hands sometimes represented on some plaques are not the ailing limbs of a dedicant but a gesture of prayer.[1] Similarly feet or foot imprints are intended as a reminder to a god, often Serapes or Isis, that the faithful visited his or her sanctuary and prayed therein.[2] We must also eliminate ex-voto-like marble objects with breasts in relief, which are, in fact, weights.[3]

It is worth pointing out, although as yet no satisfactory explanation can be given, that all the ex-votos with known

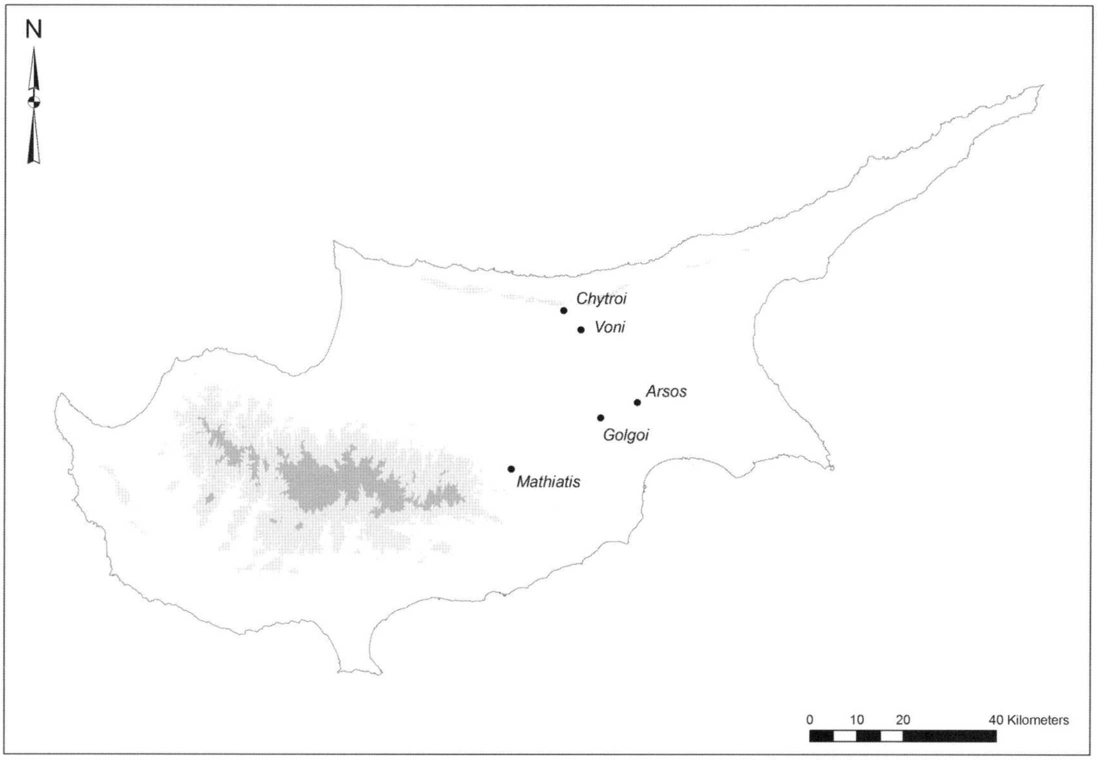

Fig. 4.1. Map of Cyprus with location of sanctuaries discussed (Athos Agapiou)

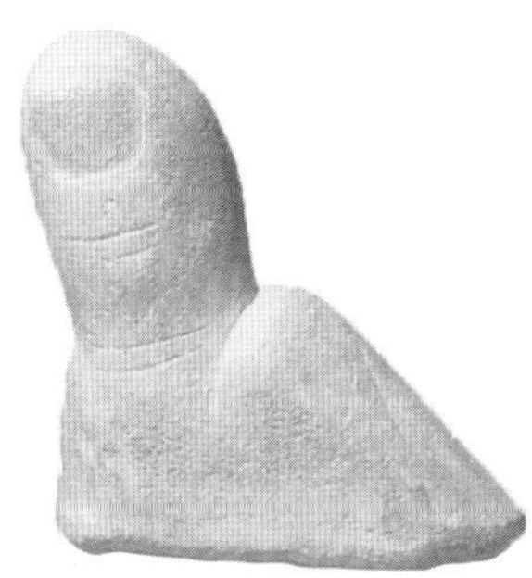

Fig. 4.2. Ex-voto of a toe from Golgoi, Metropolitan Museum, New York (Karageorghis 2000, fig. 419)

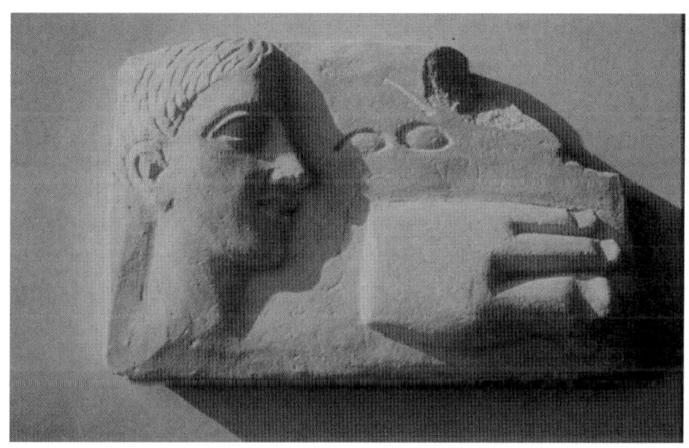

Fig. 4.3. Composite ex-voto from Golgoi now in the Louvre, Paris (Hermary 1989, fig. 934)

provenance come from inland sites (Fig. 4.1[4]): Arsos (see below), Chytroi (Karageorghis 1975), Golgoi (see below), Mathiates (Hadjisavvas 1984, figs 166–7) and Voni (Ohnefalsch-Richter 1893, pl. xl. 6–7). Chytroi, although fairly close to the northern coast (as the crow flies), is separated from it by the Pentadaktylos mountain range and belongs to the Mesaoria plane.

The largest group was excavated in 1870 by L. Palma di Cesnola at the locality *Ayios Photios* of Atheainou, ancient Golgoi. Most of these ex-votos are now in the Metropolitan Museum of Art, New York, and the Pitt Rivers Museum, Oxford (Doell 1873, 54; Cesnola 1877, 157–8; Cesnola 1885, vol. I: 3, pl. cxxii: 910, pl. cxxix: 924–36; Myres 1914, 280, nos 1675–87, pp 539–40, nos 1881–2; Masson 1997; Karageorghis 2000, 258–9, nos 417–20). Little is known about the conditions of their discovery except that the objects appeared to have been placed all together as if in front of an altar or a deity with healing powers. The types represented include faces, one or a pair of eyes, pairs of and single ears, noses, lips, a single and pairs of breasts, male genitals, thumbs, hands, toes (Fig. 4.2) and feet. There is also a composite relief, which seems to belong to this group,

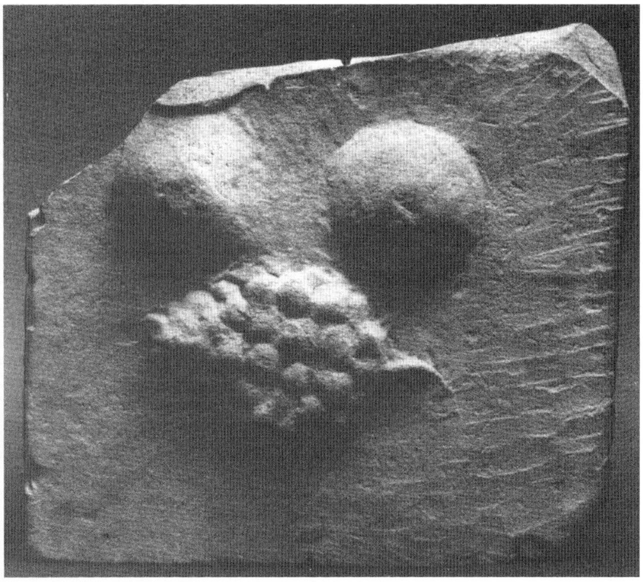

Fig. 4.4. Ex-voto with a pair of breasts and a bunch of grapes from Golgoi, Metropolitan Museum, New York (Masson 1997, pl. viii)

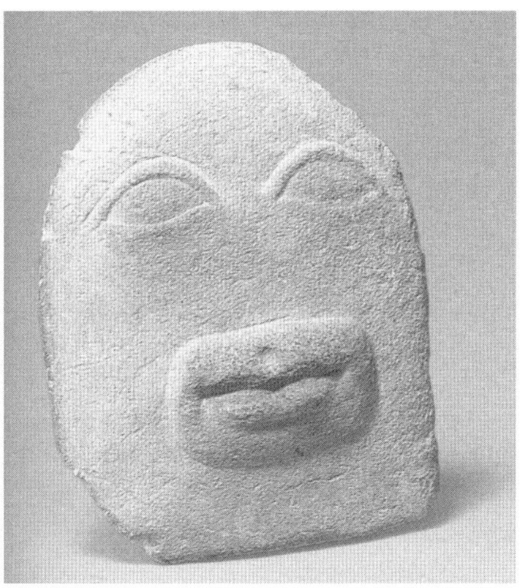

Fig. 4.5. Face with swollen lips and no nose from Golgoi now in the Metropolitan Museum, New York (Karageorghis 2000, fig. 417)

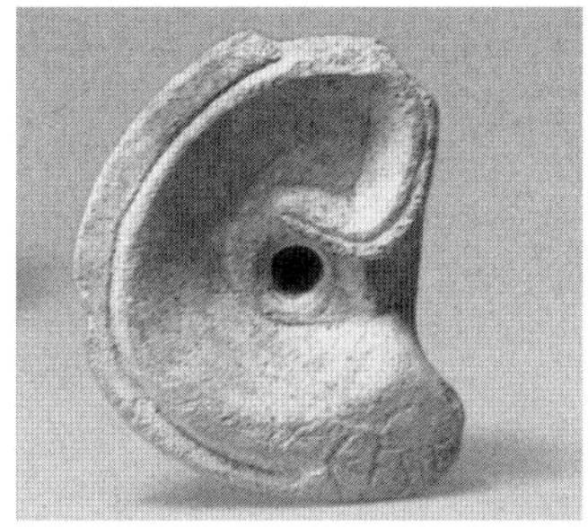

Fig. 4.6. Ex-voto of an ear with syllabic inscription from Golgoi now in the Metropolitan Museum, New York (Karageorghis 2000, fig. 418)

Fig. 4.7. Ex-voto dedicated to *Theos Hypsistos* by Chariton, from Golgoi now in the Louvre, Paris (Maria Parani)

depicting a head in profile, a pair of eyes and a foot with only three toes (Fig. 4.3). Of special interest is a plaque with a pair of breasts under which there is a bunch of grapes, a common symbol of fertility (Fig. 4.4). Also, a face without nose, the swollen lips of which are marked with red colour, is surely an indication of a medical condition (Fig. 4.5). Even more interesting are two ears in the round inscribed in syllabic Greek. One is difficult to make out, the other reads «τῶ (ἀ)πώτω ἠ(μί)», meaning 'I belong to the one without ears', underlining the fact that the dedicant had hearing problems (Fig. 4.6) (Masson 1997, 28–9). The syllabic inscription and some other factors have led scholars to attribute this group of offerings to the early Hellenistic period, perhaps the 4th or 3rd century BC, which makes it by far the earliest collection of anatomical ex-votos known in Cyprus; and the only one dating to before the Roman period.

Another very interesting group was found in the 1890s, again at Golgoi but at a different location from that of Cesnola. These ex-votos date to the Imperial period, probably to the 2nd century AD, and they are now in the Louvre (Perdrizet 1896; Masson 1971; Hermary 1989, nos 935, 940–942; Masson 1990, 33; and Masson 1997). They include three flat, tile-like plaques on which some of the main outlines of the features are traced by an incision but all details and inscriptions are applied in black paint. According to Perdrizet (1896, 362) more plaques with suspension holes were found but they had lost all traces of whatever was painted on them, and it is impossible to be certain that they were of medical nature. Of the three in the Louvre, two show a pair of large eyes with thick eyebrows, under which one has the inscription: Θεῷ Ὑψίστῳ εὐξάμενος

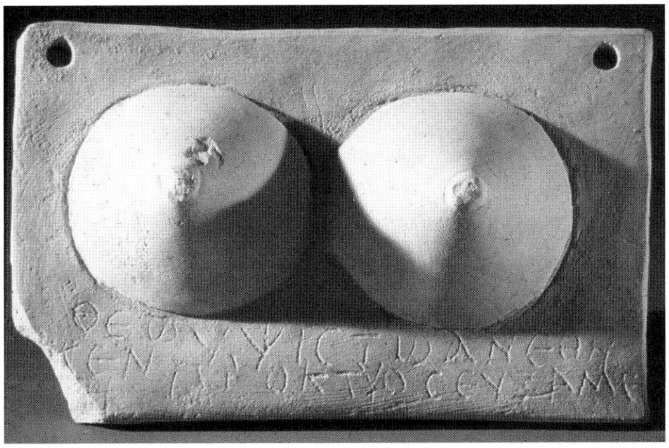

Fig. 4.8. Ex-voto of a pair of breasts dedicated to *Theos Hypsistos* by Proktyos, from Golgoi, now in the Louvre, Paris (Archaeological Research Unit, University of Cyprus)

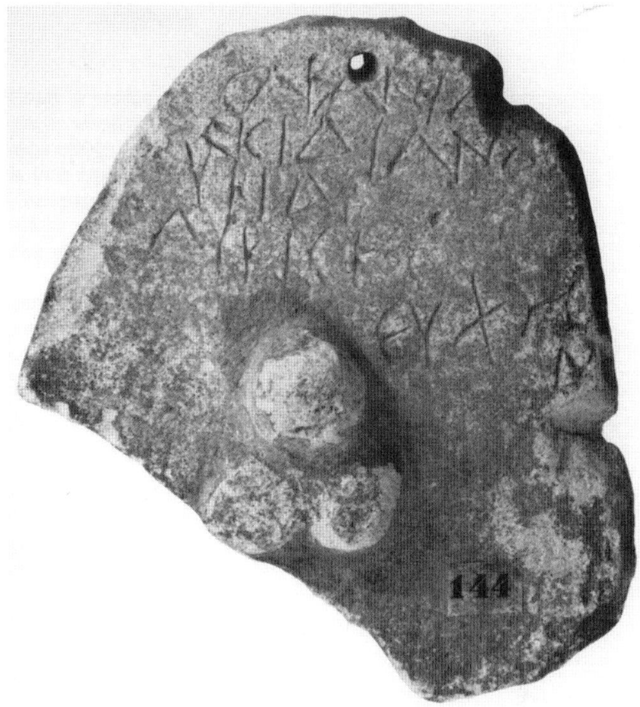

Fig. 4.9. Ex-voto of male genitals dedicated by Lykiskos to Isis, Serapis and Anubis, from Arsos now in the Louvre, Paris (Hermary 1990, pl. 1:2)

Χαρίτων ἀπέδωκεν (Fig. 4.7); the other: Θεῷ Ὑψίστῳ ἀνέθηκεν εὐξάμενος Μᾶρκος...ς (?). The third example is difficult to make out (a nose?) but the inscription reads Θεῷ Ὑψ[ίστῳ] Ἀφροδείσις ἀνέθηκεν εὐξάμενος. The *Theos Hypsistos,* the 'Highest of Gods', often stands for Jehovah but the name could also be associated with Zeus (Derda and Ajtar 1987), Apollo or Serapes (see Aupert and Masson 1979, 378–83, for a general discussion). What is certain is that the form in which he is mentioned here, as well as elsewhere (see, for example, the ex-voto from Athens mentioned below), is that of a healing god. Interestingly, all three of these plaques were dedicated by men, while, according to Derda and Ajtar (1987), the dedicants to Zeus Hypsistos were mostly women. A fourth ex-voto from this group is, indeed, dedicated by a woman: It is a rectangular plaque with a pair of breasts in relief, just below which there is the inscription Θεῷ Ὑψίστῳ ἀνέθηκεν Πρόκτυος εὐξαμέ[ν]η (Fig. 4.8). Of great interest is the fact that a practically identical ex-voto was found in the Agora of Athens (Forsén 1996, 66, no. 8.11, fig. 59). The plaque is very similar, but made of marble, with a pair of breasts in relief and the inscription Διονυσία Ὑψίστῳ εὐχήν. The similarity is certainly not accidental and opens up questions of provenance or at least of prototypes for some of these ex-votos – issues that need to be investigated further.

A rich and interesting group of ex-votos from nearby Arsos was brought back to France by the de Vogüé, Waddington and Duthoit mission in 1862 (Masson 1980, Hermary 1989, 449–53, nos 925–33, 936–9; Hermary 1990). Melchior de Vogüé writing about the ex-votos from Arsos mentioned: '*... J'ai formé une collection ou toutes les parties du corps humain sont représentées. Plusieurs de ces singuliers monuments portent l'inscription suivante*: Ἴσιδι, Σεράπιδι, Ἀνούβιδι εὐχήν' (Masson 1980, 273). Edmond Duthoit in a letter of 27 March 1862 mentioned: '*des centaines de parties sexuelles mâles et femelles en pierre avec des inscriptions dédicatoires*' (Hermary 1989, 449). This is almost certainly an exaggeration but we can assume that the ex-votos were fairly numerous and included a lot of male and female genitals. However, only a small number of these ex-votos, mostly of rather crude execution, have been located so far. They include a plaque with a single eye, and one with three eyes; one breast, male and female(?) genitals, arms and feet. The inscriptions on two plaques with male genitals in relief confirm the information given by de Vogüé. One reads: Ἴσιδι, Σεράπιδι, Ἀνούβιδι Λυκίσκος εὐχήν (Fig. 4.9); the other: Πασικράτης ἀνέθηκεν Ἴσιδι, Σεράπιδι, Ἀνούβι. The possibility that the temple in which these ex-votos were found was dedicated to Serapis, Isis and Anubis is further supported by the inscription on a small column found together with them: [Ἴσ]ιδ[ι, Σερ]άπιδι, [Ἀ]νούβιδι εὐχήν. All three gods, of Egyptian origin, are well known, Isis in particular, for their role in medicine and cure.

Another collection, about which very little is known, includes ex-votos in the round, in relief and of the painted plaque-type (Pieridou 1966). They can be attributed to the Roman period and some of them are of a generally higher quality than most Cypriot examples. Of unknown provenance, they entered the Cyprus Museum in 1951, and include the usual types: one face (painted), a pair of eyes (Fig. 4.10), one ear, one breast, two male genitals (Fig. 4.11), one arm

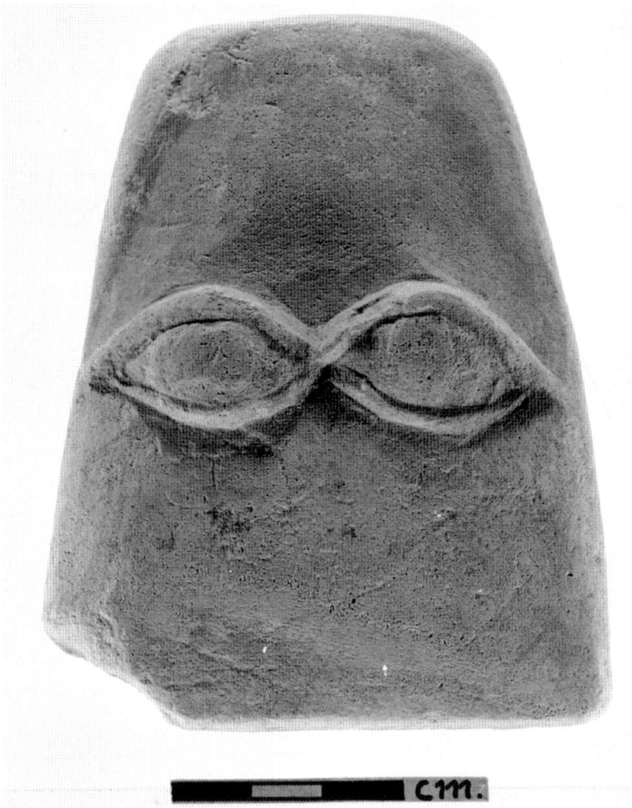

Fig. 4.10. Ex-voto of pair of eyes, of unknown origin, in the Cyprus Museum, Nicosia (A. Koutas)

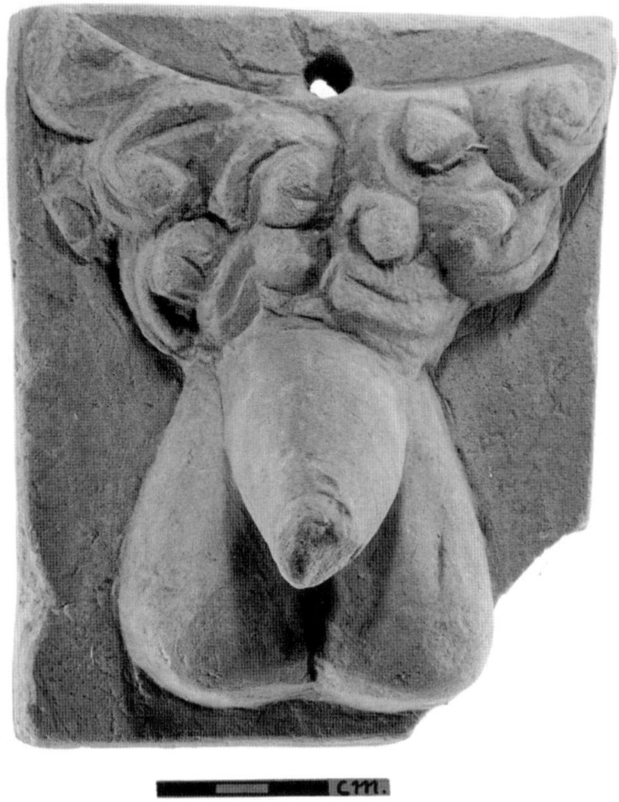

Fig. 4.11. Ex-voto of male genitals, of unknown origin, in the Cyprus Museum, Nicosia (A. Koutas)

(Fig. 4.12) and one foot (Fig. 4.13). Two are of special interest: One of the representations of male genitals has a considerable swelling of the pubic area marked with a red dot which must surely be indicative of a problem (Fig. 4.14). Similarly, the lack of the left eyebrow and, above all, the difference between the two eyes on a painted plaque ex-voto must also be indicative of the dedicant's complaint (Fig. 4.15). In fact, the differently sized pupils are reminiscent of cases of unilateral Argyll Robertson pupil.

These groups of ex-votos, and many more isolated examples now dispersed in museums and private collections in Cyprus and overseas, give us a picture of the concerns and health problems of the ancient Cypriots – and they represent a tradition that is still alive on the island: very similar anatomical ex-votos, but now made of beeswax, are commonly hang in front of icons in churches, with exactly the same purpose.

Naturally, it is necessary to collect the maximum of examples before any statistics can be made or conclusions drawn. Even with only part of the sample, however, we can see some trends that must certainly reflect the general situation. For example, it is very surprising that there is a total absence of internal organs, such as intestines and the uterus, which are commonly found elsewhere. Even if some

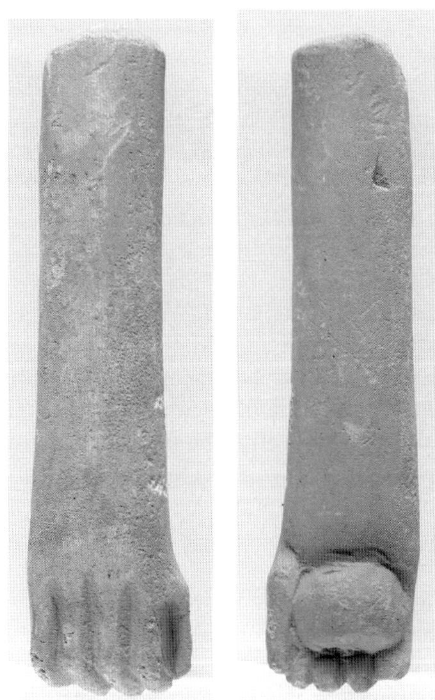

Fig. 4.12. Ex-voto of an arm, of unknown origin, in the Cyprus Museum, Nicosia (A. Koutas)

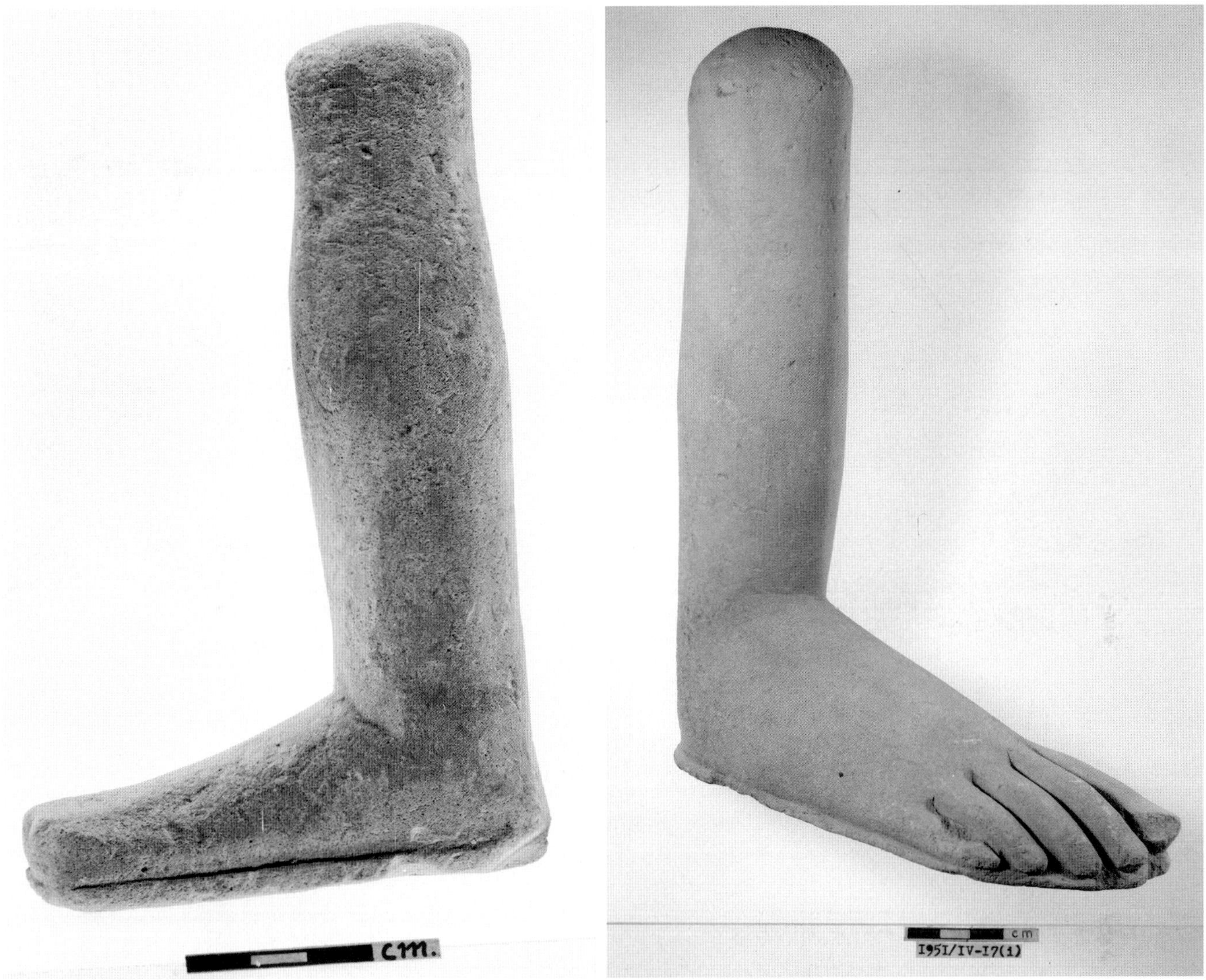

Fig. 4.13. Ex-voto of a foot, of unknown origin, in the Cyprus Museum, Nicosia (A. Koutas)

examples do eventually turn up, they will always be a minute percentage of the whole. The large number of examples of limbs or fingers and toes is not surprising since these are very vulnerable parts of the body – especially in a society engaged in agriculture and manual labour. If we are to judge by the known ex-votos, eye complaints must have been widespread in ancient Cyprus. Single or pairs of breasts are common and at least some of them must be related to lactation problems. However, the marked absence of female genitals, despite Edmond Duthoit's claim (see above) is very surprising – unless with female 'parties sexuelles' he meant representations of breasts. In fact, only one item from Arsos (Fig. 4.16) amongst the ex-votos collected so far can probably be interpreted as representing female genitals. By contrast, the large number of male genitals is rather puzzling – unless, in some cases, the phallus plays its common role as a generic symbol of fertility and well-being, rather than being an anatomical ex-voto.

Many of these ex-votos have been published briefly. The programme through which they are being re-examined is trying to locate as many examples as possible in museums around the world, in an attempt to reconstruct the original groups and, hopefully, locate new ones. With more and/or larger groups of offerings it is hoped that it will be possible to identify the different workshops that produced them and compare their work with that of workshops from outside Cyprus. This will also enlighten the question of whether some of the Cypriot ex-votos follow prototypes from outside the island. Petrographic analysis will certainly contribute valuable information in this direction, and it is hoped that it will be possible to analyse at least some examples. It is also hoped that through the reconstruction of original groups

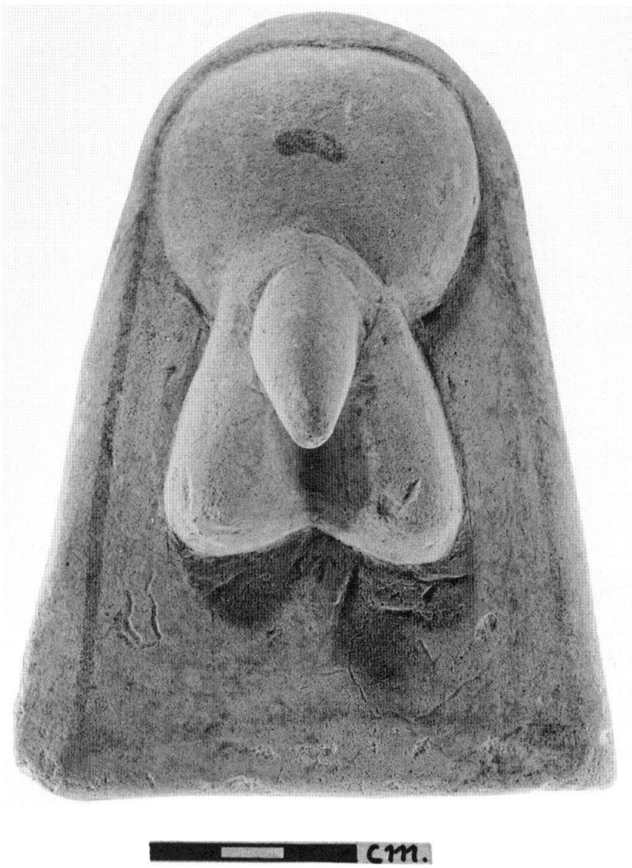

Fig. 4.14. Ex-voto of male genitals, of unknown origin, in the Cyprus Museum, Nicosia (A. Koutas)

Fig. 4.15. Ex-voto of face without an eyebrow and a dilated pupil, of unknown origin, in the Cyprus Museum, Nicosia (A. Koutas)

it might be possible to understand if the god worshipped in a given sanctuary specialised in the healing of one or more particular ailments. Examining the ex-votos as one large group will certainly reveal the main health concerns of the inhabitants of Hellenistic and Roman Cyprus.

Notes

1 E.g. an inscribed marble plaque from Enkomi, now in Alexandria: Voskos 2002, 100–1, 312–3, fig. 10.

2 See an example in the Paphos District Museum: Michaelides 1991, pl. L.

3 I know of one example from Cyprus, found in a tomb at *Pervoli tou Englezou* of Polis, which the excavator, Eutychia Zachariou, was kind enough to show me. For this type of weight, see Forsén 1996, 9–13; and for an illustrated Roman example from Athens, see Poupaki 2000, 116, no. 105.

4 I would like to thank Athos Agapiou for preparing Figure 4.1.

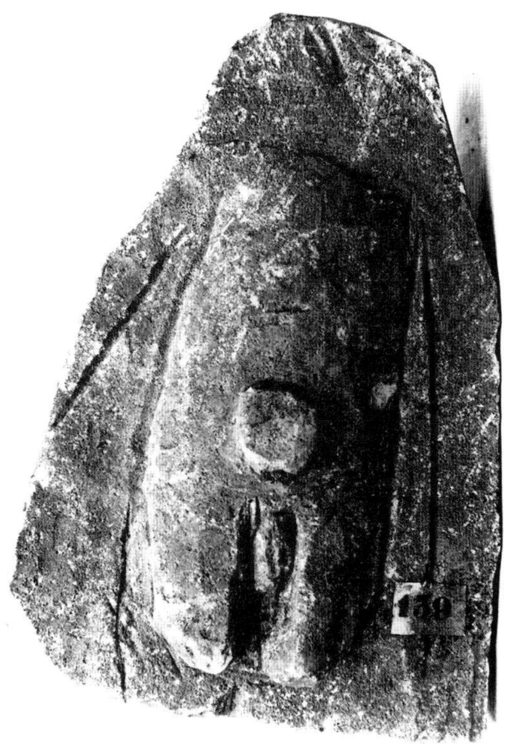

Fig. 4.16. Ex-voto with a representation of female genitals (?), from Arsos (Hermary 1989, fig. 937)

Bibliography

Aupert, P. and Masson, O. 1979: 'Inscriptions d' Amathonte I', *Bulletin de Correspondance hellénique* 103, 361–89.

Cesnola, L. Palma di. 1877: *Cyprus its Ancient Cities, Tombs and Temples,* London.

Cesnola, L. Palma di. 1885: *A Descriptive Atlas of the Collection of Cypriote Antiquities in the Metropolitan Museum of Art, New York,* I:3, Boston.

Derda, T. and Ajtar, A. 1987: 'An Athenian dedicatory inscription to Zeus Hypsistos reconsidered', *Zeitschrift für Papyrologie and Epigrafik* 70, 163–4.

Doell, J. 1873: *Die Sammlung Cesnola* (Mémoires de l'Académie Impériale des Sciences de St. Petersbourg VIIe sér. XIX, no. 4), Saint Petersburg.

Forsén, B. 1996: *Griechische Gliederweifungen* (Papers and Monographs of the Finnish Institute at Athens vol. IV), Helsinki.

Hadjisavvas, S. 1984: in V. Karageorghis 'Chronique des fouilles à Chypre en 1983', *Bulletin de Correspondance hellénique* 108, 964–5.

Hermary, A. 1989: *Musée du Louvre, Département des antiquités orientales. Catalogue des antiquités de Chypre. Sculpture,* Paris.

Hermary, A. 1990: 'Cinq ex-voto d'Arsos retrouvés au Musée du Louvre', *Cahier du Centre d'Études chypriotes* 14, 45–8.

Karageorghis, V. 1976: *Annual Report of the Director of the Department of Antiquities for the year 1975*, 41, figs 74–5.

Karageorghis, V. 1998: *The Coroplastic Art of Ancient Cyprus,* V. *The Cypro-Archaic period. Small female figurines* A. *Handmade/ Wheelmade Figurines,* Nicosia.

Karageorghis, V. 2000: *Ancient Art from Cyprus. The Cesnola Collection in The Metropolitan Museum of Art,* New York.

Masson, O. 1971: '*Kypriaka IX. Recherches sur les antiquités de Golgoi* ', *Bulletin de Correspondance hellénique* 104, 331–2.

Masson, O. 1980: 'Notes sur un sanctuaire d'Arsos', *Bulletin de Correspondance hellénique* 104, 273–5.

Masson, O. 1990: 'Paul Perdrizet à Chypre en 1896', *Cahier du Centre d'Études chypriotes* 13, 27–41.

Masson, O. 1997: 'Les ex-voto trouvés par L. Palma di Cesnola à Golgoi en 1870', 25–9 in M. Amandry, H. Cassimatis, A. Caubet and A. Hermary (éds), *Mélanges Olivier Masson, Cahier du Centre d'Études chypriotes* 27.

Michaelides, D. 1991: 'Paphiaca II: a) A stone "Footprint" from Nea Paphos', *Report of the Department of Antiquities, Cyprus,* 191–2.

Michaelides: Μιχαηλίδης, Δ. 2006: 'Ιατροί και Ιατρική στην Αρχαία Κύπρο', in *Η Ιατρική στην Κύπρο, από την Αρχαιότητα μέχρι την Ανεξαρτησία,* Λευκωσία, 12–68.

Mitropoulou 1985: Μητροπούλου, Ε.: 'Ὁ Ὀφθαλμὸς ὡς ἀνάθημα στὴν Κύπρο', 403–13 in Θ. Παπαδόπουλλος και Σ. Α. Χατζηστυλλής, *Πρακτικά του Δεύτερου Διεθνούς Κυπρολογικού Συνεδρίου (Λευκωσία, 20–25 Απριλίου 1982), Τόμος Α΄,* Λευκωσία.

Myres, J. L. 1914: *The Metropolitan Museum of Art. A Handbook of the Cesnola Collection of Antiquities from Cyprus,* New York.

Ohnefalsch-Richter, M. 1893: *Kypros. Die Bibel und Homer: Beiträge zur Cultur-, Kunst- u. Religionsgeschichte des Orients im Alterthume*, Berlin.

Perdrizet, P. 1896: 'Un sanctuaire de dieu guérisseur à Golgoi', *Bulletin de Correspondance hellénique* 20, 361–3.

Pieridou 1966: Πιερίδου, Α.: 'Αναθηματικοί «πίνακες» προς θεούς-ιατρούς εις Κύπρον', *Κυπριακαί Σπουδαί* 30, 35–8.

Poupaki 2000: Πουπάκη, Ε.: στο Λ. Παρλαμά και Ν. Χρ. Σταμπολίδης (επιμ.), *Η πόλη κάτω από την πόλη. Ευρήματα από τις ανασκαφές του Μητροπολιτικού Σιδηροδρόμου των Αθηνών,* Αθήνα.

Vandenabeele, F. 1988: 'Kourotrophoi in the Cypriote terracotta production from the Early Bronze Age to the Archaic Period', *Report of the Department of Antiquities, Cyprus* 1988/2, 31–2.

Vandervondelen, M. 1997: 'L'accouchement à Chypre dans l'Antiquité. Etudes de Sculptures', 271–88 in E. De Smet, H. Melaerts, C. Saerens (eds), *In Honorem Aloysi Gerlo* (Studia Varia Bruxellensia IV), Leuven.

Voskos 2002: Βοσκός, Α. Ι.: *Αρχαία Κυπριακή Γραμματεία 3: Πεζογραφία,* Λευκωσία.

Part II

Media

5. Providing Online Access to Graeco-Roman Medicine: BIUM's Electronic Corpus of Ancient Physicians

Guy Cobolet

The paper presents the services offered by the Bibliothèque Interuniversitaire de Médecine and particularly the digital open-access collection Medic@.

The Bibliothèque Interuniversitaire de Médecine (BIUM, Paris, http://www.biusante.parisdescartes.fr/) is basically an academic medical library dedicated to health professionals and researchers. However, its holdings, dating back to the end of the 14th century, make it a major repository for the history of Western medicine, together with a few others (e.g. the US National Library of Medicine, Wellcome Institute). Since 2000, it has been developing a digital open-access collection, Medic@ (http://www.biusante.parisdescartes.fr/histmed/medica.htm), that covers a wide spectrum of topics, a part of which focuses on Ancient Medicine.

1. Medic@ digital library

Initiated in the autumn of 2000, Medic@ digital library is the digitisation project of the BIUM Department for the History of Medicine. It is a complement of other information products developed by the Department (images databank, bio-bibliographic database of physicians, virtual exhibits, 'ask a librarian' service, etc.). As of September 2008, the digital library offered online 5,200 electronic documents (1.4 M pages).

The project has been developed according to the following guidelines:

Goals:

- provide Web access to electronic resources dealing with the history of medicine and dentistry, in a field (health) where online publications are used daily.
- reach a new audience in France and abroad.
- promote the BIUM's old and rare collections, as well as its information services.
- enhance the BIUM's visibility.
- make the BIUM a reservoir of primary resources, and not just a distributor of secondary information.
- set up a French-speaking portal in a domain where English-speaking websites predominate.

Targets:

- researchers interested in the history of medicine, dentistry and health.

Medic@ aims primarily to serve specialists, and to provide the documents and tools they need and use. However great or small their numbers may be, Medic@ is designed to reach these communities, the specialists who are users and who teach students. These communities are international, and are located mainly in Europe and in North America.

- people interested in the history of medicine, dentistry and health. Some are members of learned societies; some have already used the BIUM's services.
- the general and lay public, who use search engines such as Google, Yahoo or others to seek information.
- students (post doctoral, graduate, undergraduate, high-school) who may need information (texts, images) for academic purposes.

Content:

Medic@ includes several series dedicated to medical specialties, epidemics and diseases, famous scientists, reference sources (dictionaries, dissertations, catalogues), 19th century journals, and promotes multidisciplinary topics that broaden the perspectives of the field and place medical practice within a larger context (scientific, social and artistic).

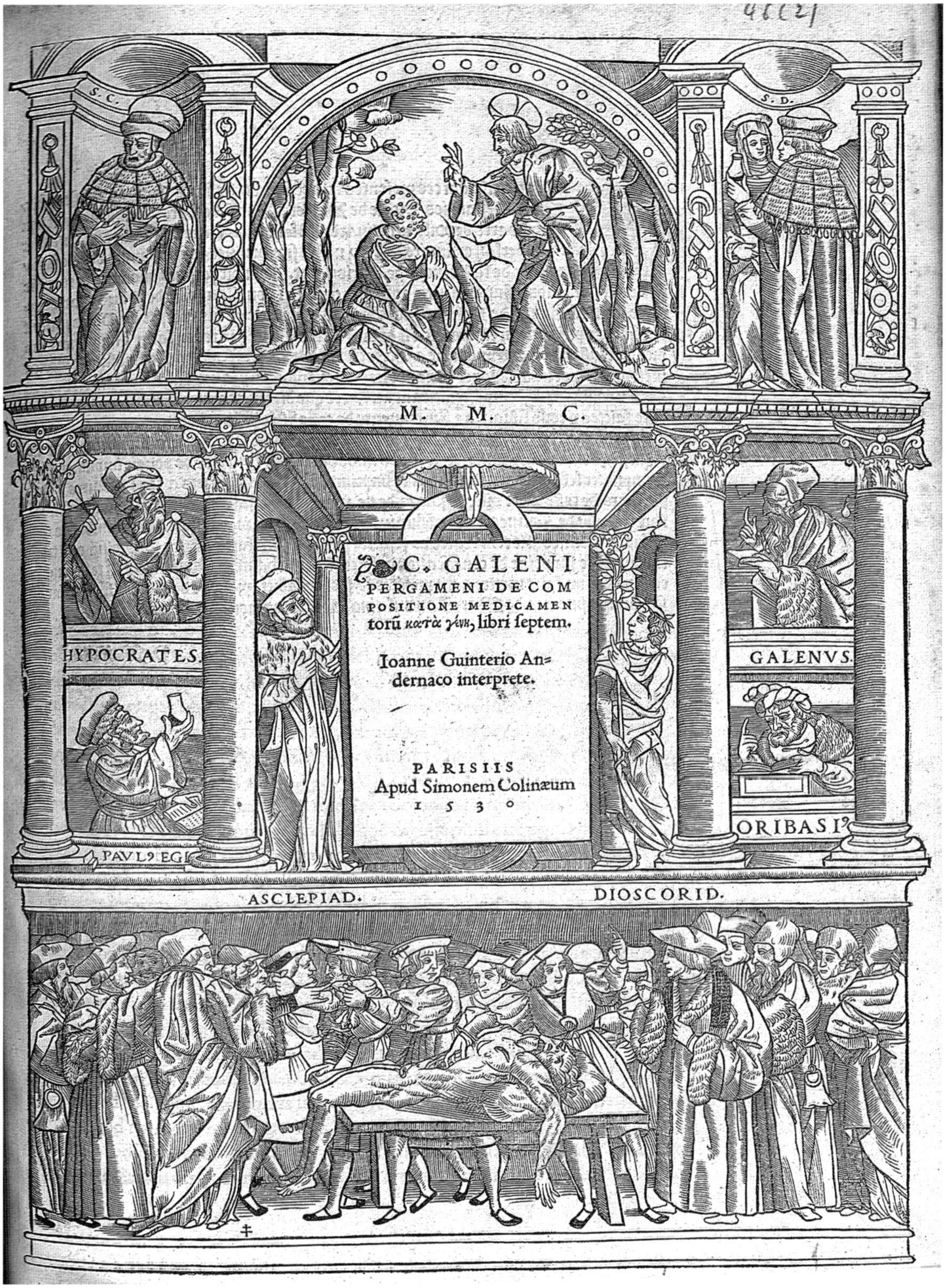

Fig. 5.1. Galen: C. Galeni *De compositione medicamentorum kata genē libri septem*. Parisiis, Apud Simonem Colinaeum, 1530. http://www2.biusante.parisdescartes.fr/livanc/?cote=00046x02&p=1&do=page

2. The Electronic Corpus of Ancient Physicians

The project started in 2001, with the active collaboration of several philologists of the University of Paris IV-Sorbonne (Marie-Laure Monfort, Véronique Boudon, Jacques Jouanna) who helped to select a panel of Hippocratic editions. Then, it was enriched by the addition of many authors: Galen, Soranos of Ephesus, Aetius, Oribasius, Alexander of Tralles, Apollonius of Citium, Aretaeus of Cappadocia, Celsus, Dioscorides, Erotianus, Nicander of Colophon, Paulus of Aegina, Nicholas of Damascus, Philostratos, Pliny, Priscianus, Rufus of Ephesus, *et al.*

The corpus presently comprises almost 500 volumes and over 100,000 image-mode pages, and includes both BIUM's holdings (the majority) and those of Gallica (that are harvested via Bibliothèque nationale de France's OAI-PMH[1] repository). Every material is searchable, readable and downloadable in many ways (page, chapter or full PDF).

The scanned materials cover a long period of printing and editorial activity: the best editions from the Renaissance up to the 19th century. So one can access the Latin princeps edition of Galen's works published in Venice by Diomedes Bonardus in 1490, the princeps Greek edition of the same published by Aldus Manutius in 1525, and Hippocrates' works by Émile Littré as well (Paris, 1839–1861).

Among the various series provided by Medic@, the corpus is actually one of the most popular, along with a few other series (anatomy, botany and catalogues of medical instruments, which all offer plenty of illustrations and plates): many of its titles are listed among the top 100 downloaded materials, showing that the aimed target has been reached – worldwide (researchers, students, philologists, historians and paleopathologists specialised in ancient medicine).

In the near future, we plan to enlarge the set by adding some neglected editions and minor authors, and by taking into account hippiatry (Vegetius, Pelagonius, for example) that was so close to human medicine in ancient times.

This digitisation project is a part of a larger entity that aims at the building of a specialised portal dedicated to Graeco-Roman Medicine, which already includes several other pieces:

- an online newsletter, "Medicina : Bulletin de médecine ancienne / Ancient Medicine Newsletter", that provides information on congresses, researchers, other scanned materials and a bibliographic database (http://www2.biusante.parisdescartes.fr/medicina/debut.htm);
- the organisation of meetings ('Lire les médecins grecs à la Renaissance', Paris, 2003; 'Femmes en médecine', Paris, 2006; 'L'édition René Chartier des œuvres d'Hippocrate et de Galien', Paris, 2010);
- the publication of some reprints (major sources): Littré's edition of Hippocrates, Kühn's edition of Galen (available at http://www.deboccard.com/).

Conclusion

The Electronic Corpus of Ancient Physicians is basically a tool made by and for researchers, and provides philologists and historians with free digital information and modern technologies in order to help them access the core literature they daily need. Still under construction, it has a worldwide audience and a good feedback, that encourage the BIUM to continue as a research library capable not only of providing access to information but also of producing and offering new tools specially designed for the academic community, when requested.

Note

1 Open Archives Initiative's Protocol for Metadata Harvesting.

Part III

The Aegean

6. Healers and Medicines in the Mycenaean Greek Texts

Robert Arnott

The Mycenaean Linear B tablets were records of the day-to-day management of an agricultural palace-based centralised regional economy. Two of the tablets, PY Eq 146 and PY Vn 1314, found at Pylos, tell us something about the practice of medicine and the status and work of healers or physicians in the Mycenaean world and a series of tablets, mostly from Mycenae, identify the use of spices which are for medicinal uses. I also examine the additional evidence that exists for Mycenaean healers and medicines to see if it corroborates anything that is found in the texts.

Introduction

In 1931, the medical historians Blaxland Stubbs and Bligh wrote optimistically: 'If it were possible to interpret the Minoan texts we should doubtless find matters of medical interest which would throw light on later Greek developments …' (Blaxland, Stubbs and Bligh 1931, 40). Unfortunately, following the decipherment of Linear B in 1952, as an early form of Greek, we were to be disappointed. The Late Bronze Age Aegean possesses nothing remotely comparable to the Egyptian or Near Eastern medical texts. All the Mycenaeans had were temporary records of the day-to-day management of what was a largely rural economy, such as land tenure, the distribution of labour and production. The tablets only survive because of the fires that caused the destruction of the buildings in which they were stored. There are no literary or historical texts.[1]

Outside archaeology and the study of human skeletal remains, the little we are able to learn from these texts about healers and their medicines in the Mycenaean world is largely derived from two individual tablets, PY Eq 146 and PY Vn 1314, both found in the Mycenaean palace at Pylos in Messenia in south-west Greece, dating to its destruction in approximately 1200 BC and some additional tablets, mainly from Mycenae, such as the MY Ge series, that point to the nature of the medicines they used.

Tablet PY Eq 146

This tablet was found during the earliest excavation season at Pylos in 1939, on a southwest facing bench in the west corner of Archive Room 7, subsequently numbered PY Eq 146, dating to a period likely to be made in the period immediately before the final destruction of the palace at the end of the Late Helladic IIIB period, in approximately 1200 BC (Blegen and Rawson 1966, 99; Palaima 2003, 163–4). It forms part of the E series of tablets, which mostly relates to land tenure and the annual distribution of seed grain. It is expressed in this way in order to indicate the size of land holdings by a series of individuals, most likely to be palace officials, craftsmen or servants and offers a glimpse of their status in society (Ventris and Chadwick 1973, 232–79).

Tablet PY Eq 146 (Arnott 1999c, 274) is a clay rectangular or page-shaped tablet (dimensions H. 18.9 cm, W. 9.5 cm, Th. *c.* 2.2 cm), attributed by Palaima to the Scribe 74/Hand 1 (the Master-Scribe), as were all the tablets in the same series found at the site, PY Eq 36[+]887, 213, 1451, 1452 (Palaima 1988b, 37–9, 204); these latter two perhaps also part of PY Eq 36 (Bennett and Olivier 1973, 134). Some fragments have been subsequently joined (Melena 1992–3, 310; 1994–5, 95), but the text is unaffected. The first two tablets in the series have roughly the same size and are rectangular, or 'page-shaped' as PY Eq 146 (Palaima 1988b, 204). The tablet is now transliterated as follows:

PY Eq 146 (S74-H1)

.1 o-da-a$_2$⌊ ⌋ te-re-ta, e-[
.2 ko-ro, to-so-de, pe-mo [[GRA]] GRA [
.3 o-da-a$_2$, po-ro-te-u, e-ke, to-so-de, pe-mo GRA 1
.4 o-da-a$_2$, re-pi-ri-jo, e-ke, to-so-de, pe-mo GRA 1
.5 o-da-a$_2$, a-de-me-we, e-ke, to-so-de pe-mo GRA 1 V 3
.6 *vacat*
.7 *vacat*
.8 *vacat*
.9 o-da-]a$_2$, [..]me-no, i-ja-te, o-na-to,
.10 e-]ke, to-so-de⌊ ⌋pe-mo GRA 1
.11 o-da-a$_2$, a-si-wi-jo, i-qo-na-to-mo,
.12 o-na-to, e-ke[to-]so-de pe-mo GRA T 7
.13 *vacat*
.14 *vacat.*
.15 *vacat*
.16 to-so-de pe-]mo GRA T 3

Notes
.2 *-de* over erasure, possibly [[*pe*]]; [[GRA]] only half erased, possibly [[GRA T]]; trace at right possibly T[, but after space for numbers
.3 *e-ke* over erasure
.4 *re-pi-* over erasure; *-so-* over erasure
.9 Now thought likely to be [..] ro-me-no
.16 3 in upper register, possibly incomplete

This tablet is of particular interest, not necessarily for its record of land tenure, important as that is, but for its unique reference to the word *i-ja-te*, which points to a Mycenaean healer or physician and his land holdings. He appears on line .9, continued on line .10, which can now be translated as:

.9 o-da-]a$_2$, [..]ro-me-no, i-ja-te, o-na-to,
And thus, [..]ro-*meno*, physician, holds a portion of beneficial land
.10 e-]ke, to-so-de⌊ ⌋pe-mo GRA 1
and so much seed grain GRAIN (= 96 litres)

Ventris and Chadwick were the first to identify from the tablet the phonetic resemblance of the word *i-ja-te* to the ἰατήρ, which also occurs in later Greek and Cypriot texts (but was subsequently replaced by Attic ἰατρός), as a healer or physician named *[..]-meno* (or -μενος) (Ventris and Chadwick 1973, 123, 547) or possibly *[..] ro-meno* (or -ρομενος), although regrettably the tablet does not place him in an occupational context. This translation has been subsequently supported by a number of other Linear B scholars, including Palmer and Morpurgo Davies (Palmer 1963, 422; Morpurgo Davies 1979, 99) and remains to date unchallenged.[2]

Research into Mycenaean land tenure and the distribution of rations has interpreted these lines as meaning that our healer or physician held a lease of land and was issued with one annual measure or ration of seed grain, in return for certain services rendered. This is standard for the E-series of tablets, especially the En and Ep land tenure series, which make it clear that the principal landholders, such as this healer or physician, are *te-re-ta* and that they sub-leased land to smallholders. Many of these *te-re-ta* at Pylos receiving similar rations are uniquely also royal craftsmen, namely a *ke-ra-me-u* (king's potter) and a *ka-na-pe-u* (king's fuller or clothes dresser) or sometimes associated with the cult of the goddess Potnia with the title of *do-e-ro* and *do-e-ra* or servant, such as *i-je-re-u* or priest, *i-je-re-ja* or priestess, *i-je-ro-wo-ko* or sacrificing priest, *ka-ra-wi-po-ro* or key bearer, perhaps another religious office, possibly a priestess (Palaima 1997). There are also interesting parallels to specialist craftsmen in the contemporary Hittite kingdom or ^{GIŠ}TUKUL-men, who also performed services for the royal and religious institutions and were rewarded with land grants (Beal 1988). However, unlike Mycenaean Greece, it does not include references to craftsmen-healers.[3]

The E series tablets from Pylos specifically record various amounts of seed-grain, but as Hooker pointed out, these texts are chiefly concerned with transactions involving parcels of land; the distribution of seed-grain being an indication of the size of land held, with the productivity and yield of the land being of greater importance than its actual linear size. The word *pe-mo* (sometimes *pe-ma*) that precedes the ideogram for wheat in PY Eq 146 means seed-grain and therefore each entry for wheat is likely to the amount of seed-grain required to sow a plot of land (Hooker 1980, 133–4). This is based on the revised calculations of Ventris and Chadwick, where one unit of ration equals 96 litres of seed-grain is equivalent to 1.92 hectares, not 120 as originally understood (Ventris and Chadwick 1973, 393–4) and suggests that this land may not only have been of the right size to maintain his immediate family but perhaps also to cultivate medicinal plants that were not gathered in the wild.

The i-ja-te: a physician and healer

It is unlikely that our healer had any special status over and above that of a craftsman. This tablet, as an indicator of the landholding of our *i-ja-te*, suggests that it is modest and is on the scale of the other *te-re-ta*, in this case, craftsmen and lower officials referred to in the E-series, including others referred to on PY Eq 146. Other officials, *te-o-jo*, *do-e-ro* and *do-ea-ra*, held much smaller parcels of land, perhaps garden holdings, which would produce welcome additions to the food stocks of their families or social units. It is regretful that the tablets do not record the location or quality of our healer's land. We are, however, fortunate to have both a personal name and a brief occupational reference and an indication that our *i-ja-te* was the sole landholder and did not share it with others, other than his tenants.

There is no supporting pictorial evidence from the prehistoric Aegean of medical practice, but the place of an *i-ja-te* on the tablet may be an indication of the existence of a healer in his social and economic, but not in his occupational context. It is not yet possible to determine whether he was a palace healer and a royal servant or not. If he was, he would usually enjoy the designation *wa-na-ka-te-ro* or 'royal' (Palaima 1997). However, the size of his landholding and that the master scribe (Hand 1) of PY Eq 146 fluctuates in using the designation *wa-na-ke-te-ro*, may suggest that he served the palace in some manner. As Palaima has pointed out, '... land tenure was a system of reciprocally obligatory compensation, support or reward of individuals for various levels of service to the palatial centres or within religious districts and sanctuaries' (Palaima 2003, 166).

It is possible, of course, that the *i-ja-te* owed his rations and allegiance not to the king or wanax, but to a religious centre or sanctuary. If that were the case, however, he should have had the designation *do-e-ro* or *do-e-ra* which, like the royal designation, is also missing. However, known palace servants and craftsmen at Pylos, for example the king's fuller or cloth dresser, *ka-na-pe-u*, the king's potter *ke-ra-me-wo* and who held the royal designation, held land of almost similar land holdings.

Considering that the economic and social resources of the palaces were much greater than any other, it is only natural to assume that some healers are likely to have been dependent upon the palace in return for rations or land. If our healer did serve the palace, then this would mirror exactly what was happening in other contemporary Late Bronze Age societies at this time. The cuneiform records of Babylonian and to a lesser extent Hittite medical practice, like the Linear B tablets, are records of palace-based activities, with the work of the Sumerian ^{LÚ}A.ZU, or the Akkadian *asû* and *āšipu* (Ritter 1965; Arnott 2002), largely confined to the elite. In ancient Egypt, the term *swnw*, which is usually translated as physician, probably had other meanings, and 'one who treats the ailments of the upper classes' has been suggested by one scholar as being nearer to an understanding of their role (Weeks 1995, 1789).

The existence of a healer serving a much earlier mainland ruling family is also reflected in the skeletal evidence and helps to indicate the existence of the social variation in the provision of medical practice in that period. From the very end of the Middle Helladic Period there is the skeleton of an adult female, found in Grave Γ of Grave Circle B at Mycenae (58 My.), dated to *c.* 1550 BC, and a member of one of the elite families, as confirmed by the quality of the grave goods found with her. She had a perfectly healed midshaft three-part fracture to her right humerus without overriding of the ends or shortening of the bone (Angel 1972, 380–1, 389), probably resulting from a traumatic injury; it could not have healed naturally in this way. Many of the occupants of nearby contemporary and slightly earlier lower-status cemeteries in the Argolid, such as those at Asine and Lerna, often present fractures with faulty union, often in abnormal positions, with consequent permanent dysfunction, which had clearly not received any medical attention (Arnott 1996). Accordingly, in this grave there are the remains of someone of status who will have had access to better medical treatment. Perhaps by the very end of the Late Bronze Age in Pylos, the provision of medical assistance to a wider population was in evidence.

In the Late Bronze Age the material culture points to the practice of a great many crafts, but they need not always have been the work of individual specialists. Whether our healer worked exclusively in medicine we may never know, but the physical condition and lifestyle of those who lived in or under the immediate control of the palaces would have been such as to provide sufficient full-time work. In Homer, the ἰατήρ, the battlefield surgeon in this case, was considered a craftsman, equal to such important figures such as weapon makers or armourers (Tzavella-Evjen 1981, 185; Salazar 2001, 136–7). In Homer's *Odyssey* (xvii.383–4), physicians are δημιοεργοὶ together with carpenters, soothsayers and bards. In the *Iliad* (xi.507), physicians, like good craftsmen, were eagerly sought after, and 'worth many people'. Assuming a craftsman status for our *i-ja-te*, a physician or healer; we are again reminded of his status as similar to other craftsmen that of the *ke-ra-me-u* or king's potter and a *ka-na-pe-u*, or king's fuller or clothes dresser, with his position in society, tied to the *wanax* or a religious sanctuary.

Tablet PY Vn 1314

There is a second tablet PY Vn 1314, also from the palace at Pylos that is of special interest in medical terms. This unique tablet and obscure Mycenaean text, found in 1957 in Room 99 is completely unconnected with the others found nearby and also dates to the destruction of the palace at the end of the Late Helladic IIIB period, in approximately 1200 BC. This tablet, formerly known as PY Un 1314, has been re-classified as PY Vn 1314, following the work by Bennett (Bennett 1992, 120) and the deletion of the ideogram. The original translation (Janko 1981) has been re-examined by Bennett (Bennett 1992, 120; Bendall 2003, 222–23), who has introduced a variation in the text, but the basic translation remains the same.

PY Vn 1314		(H Cii) Room 99
.1	a-wa-ra-ka-na-o , pa-ma-ko	
.2	jo-qi , wo-to-mo , pe-re 1	
.3A	, do-we-na-qe , KA 20	KA possibly 100
.3B	a wa ra ka na o pi ka , ka-ja , pa-ra-we	

Translated as:

.1	A medicine (pharmakon) of Awarakanao (a healer?)
.2	which Wotomo brings
.3A	made of wood (?), 20 or 100 units
.3B	for Awarakanao (tame-) mallows... (2 WORDS UNKNOWN)

As to the contents, Janko originally translated it to show that tree-mallow or common mallow, *e-pi-ka* or ebiskos or hibiscus (ἡ ἐβίσκος), thought to be *Malva silvestris* L. or *Lavatera arborea* L. was brought to the palace for the sake of its medicinal properties. Also known from the archaeological record, it is anti-inflammatory, soothing, refreshing, and its emollient properties are attributed to the common mallow. Mallow extract has a high mucilage content that, when in contact with water, swells and forms a soft, soothing, protective gel. The dried peeled root of the mallow or althaea is a commonly known remedy for gastro-intestinal disturbances and inflammations, particularly to the mouth.

This tablet also includes the word *pa-ma-ko* (or φάρμακα), which Ventris and Chadwick suggest are likely to be a record of drugs or medical supplies presumably for a healer or physician (Ventris and Chadwick 1973, 568), possibly called *awarakanao*. There is some evidence to suggest continuity into the 1st millennium BC of Mycenaean practices in the understanding and use of particular drugs and it is in Homer that one first understands the concept of the word *farmakon* and it would be wrong to believe that what Homer says about φάρμακα is simply magical (Scarborough 1991, 139).

Of course, it may be possible to look at this tablet in another way, as it may contain a reference to another healer, this time in an occupational context. Whilst Janko (1981, 32–3) has identified the word *pa-ma-ko,* that is usually translated as φάρμακον, this word may be that for a healer who has the name of *awarakanao* and that the preparation based on *e-pi-ka* mentioned in the text was brought to him by *wotomo* for one of his patients, but this does not change the context.

Medicines

From the study of a number of the tablets from the Mycenaean palace records of Knossos, Pylos and Mycenae, and largely based on the work of Hein, it is possible to detect the existence of a number of plants (Table 6.1) some of which have known medicinal properties; but their context within the tablets does not directly concern medicine (Hein 1961). The pharmacological properties of these plants are confirmed by Flückiger and Hanbury (1879) and most are also mentioned in the work of the 1st century AD herbalist Dioscorides Pedanius, *De Materia Medica* (Gunther 1934;

Table 6.1. Plants with medicinal properties found in the Linear B tablets

Tablet	Text	Name
MY Ge 604	*se-ri-no*	**Celery** (*Apium graveolens* L.)
PY Un 267 MY Ge 605 MY Ge 605 KN Ga 674 PY Au 616 KN Ga 415 KN Ga 418+	*ko-ri-a$_2$-da-na* *ko-ri-ja-da-na** *ko-ri-jo-da-na** *ko-ri-ja-do-no* *ko-ri-ja-do-no**	**Coriander** (seed) (*Coriandrum sativum* L.)
MY Ge 602+ MY Ge 603+ MY Ge 604+ MY Ge 605+605a+607[+]fr	*ku-mi-no*	**Cumin** (*Cuminum cyminum* L.)
KN Ga 454 KN Ga 465 KN Ga 517+ KN Ga 519 KN Ga 8005 PY Un 249 PY Un 267 PY An 616 PY Fr 1201 PY Fr 1203	*ku-pa-ro* *ku-pa-ro ** *ku-ra-ro* (?)*	**Cyperus grass** (*Cyperus rotundus* L. or *C. esculentus* L.)
MY Ge 602+	*ma-ra-tu-wo*	**Fennel** (*Foeniculum vulgare* Mill.)
KN F 841 KN Gv 862 KN Gv 864 PY Er 880	*su-za*	**Figs** (*Ficus carica* L.)
KN 594 KN L 5927 KN L 8159	*ri-ta*	**Flax** (*Linum usitatissimum* L.)
KN F 935+955 MY Ge 602+ MY Ge 603+ MY Ge 606	*ko-no* *ko-i-no**	**Ginger grass** (*Cymbopogon schoenanthus* L.)
KN Od 2026 KN Od 8202 PY Un 249	*wi-ri-za*	**Iris root** (*Iris germanica* L. or *I. cretica* L.)
MY Ge 604	*ka-da-mi-ja*	**Kardamia/Cress** (*Nasturtium officinale* L. or *Lepidium sativum* L.)
MY Ge 602+	*mi-ta*	**Mint** (*Mentha viridis* L.)
KN E 842	*ki-da-ro*	**Onions** (*Allium cepa* L.)
MY Ge 605	*ka-ra-ko*	**Pennyroyal** (*Mentha pulegium* L.)
PY Fr 1203 PY Fr 1204+	*wo-do-we*	**Rose** (*Rosa centifolia* L.)
MY Ge 602+ MY Ge 608	*ka-na-ko e-ru-ta-ra* *ka-na-ko re-u-ka*	**Safflower** (*Carthamus tinctorius* L.) Safflower seeds
KN X 974+5742	*ko-ro-ki-no*	**Saffron** (*Crocus sativus* ssp., *C. oreocreticus* L. or *C. cartwrightiensis* L.)
PY Fr 1202 PY Fr 1220+	*pa-ko-we* (Scented with sage)	**Sage** (*Salvia triloba* L. fils)
MY Ge 602 MY Ge 603+ MY Ge 604+ MY Ge 605+605a+607[+]fr MY Ge 606	*sa-sa-ma*	**Sesame** (*Sesamum indicum* L.)
KN Ga 1530 KN X 1385	*ki-ta-no*	**Terebinth** (*Pistacia terebinthus* L. or *P. atlantica* L.)
PY Vn 1314	*ep-i-ka*	**Tree-mallow or ebiskos** (*Malva silvestris* or *Lavatera arborea* L).

* variant spelling

Beck 2005). Although these plants are the likely ingredients of remedies, regrettably there is no mention of prescriptions or the final products and their uses and it is only possible to conjecture about their use, and about what precise ailments any remedies may have been used to treat. Ventris and Chadwick assumed that these plants were foods or spices, and many are at Pylos mentioned in connection with the perfumed oil industry (Ventris and Chadwick 1973, 219–31; Shelmerdine 1985), but they could equally as well have had medicinal uses and Milani has translated *a-ke-a*$_2$ found on tablet PY Vn 130 from Pylos as a 'remedy' contained within a wine-jar or other form of vessel (Milani 1986, 34). Wylock believes that a number of plants in the MY Ge series tablets from Mycenae, a centre of trade in herbs and spices, were medicinal (Wylock 1972), in light of the small amounts referred to, and that they were not being used in the kitchen or industrially. However, the records of spices in the MY Ge tablets from Mycenae are taxation records of the standard type found at other palace centres and record the delivery of spices to the palace. Whilst the unity of the consignments is related to their origin that may not apply to their final use and medicinal purposes cannot be ruled out. It is thought they may have been gathered by herb-gatherers, as the consignments suggest that they were gathered from various locations possibly locally, and not cultivated or imported (Killen 1983).

It is also worth noting at this point that the seeds of at least five of the spices identified from the MY Ge series tablets from Mycenae have specific medicinal, especially anti-flatulent properties: pennyroyal, coriander, cumin, celery and fennel. With the diet of the Mycenaean palaces rich in pulses, figs and coarse meal, then these and other members of the family of *umbelliferae* not mentioned in the tablets, but known from organic residue analysis, such as dill and aniseed, would have been valued as treatment for gastrointestinal disorders. However, if the plants mentioned in the Linear B tablets are generally for non-medicinal uses, for example, for perfumed oils, then plants with exclusive medicinal use will not be mentioned because of their small-scale use within the palaces, or because they were used by healers outside the palaces.

By the late 13th century BC, the Mycenaeans had developed a highly organised palace-controlled perfumed oil industry (Shelmerdine 1986), and it is possible that some plants were either imported, or especially cultivated in palace gardens as components of a palace-based industry on a smaller scale, manufacturing remedies, perhaps under the supervision of the palace healer. There is no evidence at present, however, for the medical application of various perfumed oils manufactured in the Aegean in industrial quantities, an important function of similar oils in the Near East in the 2nd millennium BC, but their use as external remedies cannot be discounted.

Naturally, some popular therapeutics would, of course, have been made-up from local ingredients and used domestically. Both Shaw and Walberg believe that the discovery in excavations of flower-pots, clay and faience vessels with an aperture at the base, clearly indicates some cultivation of flowers or other plants in the Aegean, some of which may have had medicinal use (Shaw 1993, 661 n.14; Walberg 1992). Despite the hierarchical control that the Linear B tablets document in most areas of production and (internal) distribution, there are likely to have been factors of export and exchange that may have been practiced on a more individualistic basis, in exchange for raw materials, luxury products and other goods, such as medicines. From the variety of pottery forms in use in the prehistoric Aegean, both open and closed shapes, it is possible that any number could have been used for the making, storing or transport of medicines. For example, many of the pottery vessels and other objects used in the Mycenaean perfumed oil industry could easily have also been used pharmaceutically.

Healers in the Late Bronze Age Aegean

The experience of healers in the Late Bronze Age (Arnott 1996; 1997) would have been based upon observable physical causes, much of it trauma, and they probably knew much about wounds caused by weapons (Arnott 1999a), tools or accidents, and treated them accordingly. However, the causes of strokes or epilepsy, for example, would have been quite mysterious and frightening and healers may have regarded these patients as being possessed by a spirit or demon. Whether the healers were able to go much beyond the sacrifices, spells and incantations of their time, and give a natural explanation to a disease is not known, but in any case, they would have practised with the *materia medica* at their disposal and performing surgery, tending the wounds and setting bones.

An important role for the Mycenaean healer must have been to provide medical services to the warrior elites and those that served them. Weapons that pierced the body would have been extracted, haemorrhages stopped by bandaging, wounds washed and picked clean of debris, and cranial injury treated by cranial trepanation (Arnott 1997). One of the most difficult problems facing them would have been the removal of arrowhead barbs, the curse of battlefield surgery in the ancient world and they would have enlarged the wound with a knife to extract the arrow, or perhaps pushed it through, after removing the flight. Perhaps some of the instruments used in these procedures were similar to those found in Chamber Tomb K (in a pit used as an ossuary or bone depository), of the Palamidi-Pronoia cemetery at Nauplion in 1971, dated to the Late Helladic IIB period (*c.* 1450–1400 BC) (Protonotariou-Deilaki 1973, 92–3; Arnott 1997, 271–5), although some of the nearby graves can be dated both earlier and later, from Late Helladic IB through to Late Helladic IIIB (Protonotariou-Deilaki 1973, 90–2). These instruments, made from bronze, together with a grinding stone and grinder (mortar and pestle) for the preparation of remedies, would have belonged to a healer and have been buried with him. The close similarity of these instruments to many of those listed in a medical text from Ugarit (Ras Shamra) (KTU 4.285) and of the same date, is of interest. The Ugarit tablet includes references to forceps, scalpels, lancets and a whetstone (Stieglitz 1981).

How healers were trained in preparing remedies, the setting of bones and the treatment of all forms of trauma will probably never be known. This is not unique; Palaima has pointed out that we know nothing about when young boys are likely to have been apprenticed as tablet makers and scribes, or anything about their system of training; nor are there any documents intended for scribal reference or training (Palaima 2003, 154). Perhaps both professions passed from father to son, or through an apprenticeship relationship, but for healers it is likely mostly to have been acquired through practice and through observing lesions on the living, mostly gained in combat, accident, or even punishment. It is reasonable to assume from much of the pathological evidence, that palace healers possessed some very basic anatomical knowledge, at least of the most vulnerable parts of the body, such as limbs, neck and head, which they would have been able to observe. A little could also have been learned from the butchering or the treatment of cattle and domestic animals. Details on a Minoan ivory and gold kouros found at Palaikastro in eastern Crete, dated to the Late Minoan IA period (*c.* 1600–1500 BC), show a remarkable knowledge of human surface anatomy (Musgrave 2000); Coulomb goes so far as to suggest that the Minoans may have acquired some of it through the dissection of cadavers (Coulomb 1979, 39 n.27). Probably little would have been known about the respiratory, cardiovascular and digestive systems, other than the effectiveness of a particular remedy used to treat a particular internal ailment.

The evidence, however, from cut marks on the inner surface of the ribs of children's bones found by Warren at Knossos shows that they were cut from the front of the body. This implies that the thoracic cavity had been skilfully opened and the heart and lungs removed before these cut marks were made. The brain had been similarly treated (Wall, Musgrave and Warren 1986, 373, 375, 386). It only remains to speculate as to whether they were able to teach their skills and give dietary advice, and whether they were capable of associating certain diseases and conditions with food eaten or with animal or plant origins. They must surely have recognised the basic aetiology, which might have occurred as the consequence of overexposure to heat or cold, overeating, eating contaminated food or drinking too much alcohol. That some diseases may have been communicable was possibly recognised, but there would have been no perception of how it originated. However, all illness would generally have been considered as intrusive, entering the body from outside.

The treatment of parasitic and digestive disease is fundamental to the origin of human medicine. Many illnesses would have been gastrointestinal, as would be expected in a society in which there was often contamination of water and food, inadequate food preservation, common use of kitchen utensils, and other factors that encourage intestinal disorders, such as food poisoning and gastroenteritis, leading to the passing of blood, rectal strictures, constipation and flatulence. Such problems would have been treated by a variety of means, including mixtures taken orally, suppositories and enemas. Many of the forms of treatment would have been based on herbal plants that are known from the Linear B tablets and before (Arnott 1996, 267–8; 2007).

All forms of medicine fulfil a social need and the amicable co-existence of religion and practical medicine is one aspect of pluralism in later Greek medicine that it is speculated may have originated in the Bronze Age. For both the earlier Minoans on Crete and the Mycenaeans, there would have been religious and in some cases magical healing for people to address their need for long-term relief or cures, perhaps internal or neurological ailments or mental illness. Priests or priestesses may have helped perform these cures, although it is likely to have been of a personal nature, similar to the healing cult of the earlier Minoan Peak Sanctuaries with its votives seeking cures or giving a thank offering for a cure (Arnott 1999b; Morris and Peatfield, this volume). The cause of disease and the operation of remedies would have been so closely linked to a religious belief in their efficacy that diseases would have been considered to be manifestations of the displeasure of deities or spirits, and their own prime purpose would be to appease the deity or exorcise the spirit from the body of the sick person. There would have been in use a number of religious and magical media, including spells and incantations. Our *i-ja-te*, whilst not directly referred to as *i-je-re-u*, or a priest, may even have had an association with a local sanctuary of some description. In the Late Bronze Age in Egypt and the Near East, the status of the doctor or physician was enhanced by the fact that they were exchangeable commodities. We know nothing as to whether the Aegean healers were similarly exchanged. A Mycenaean healing deity was certainly known in the Hittite capital (Arnott 2002, 45–6), but whether this involved Mycenaean healers working in Hattuša is unknown.

Other forms of non-palace medicine, such as community or folk medicine, would have combined elements of both the practical and the magical. As in other areas of life in the Aegean, outside the world of the palace, the population largely fended for themselves, and the tradition of self-help, independent of palace control, will always have existed. Domestic medicine would have provided one area of activity. Another example is midwifery, most likely practised, as in other ancient societies, by women probably with elements of magical practice so often associated with childbirth. On tablet PY Aa 815 from Pylos, amongst a list of women and their occupations, there appears the word *a-ke-ti-ra*$_2$ which Ventris and Chadwick originally interpreted as a nurse, foster-mother or midwife (Ventris and Chadwick 1973, 158, 418, 529); Hippocrates used the word, ἀκεστρίς for a midwife (Hippocrates *Medica, Carn.*, 19), but the context is that of textile workers, perhaps a spinner or weaver (Palmer 1963, 405–511). Milani believes that *a-ke-te-re* (a variant spelling of *a-ke-te*) found on tablet PY Jn 832 from Pylos, traditionally believed to be a tradesman may also refer to a nurse (Milani 1986, 35). Another interpretation may be ἀκεστήρ, as 'healer' but both are speculative.

Unlike other aspects of medical practice in the Aegean, there is specific archaeological evidence for childbirth and the work of midwives. There are the terracotta votive models of women depicting parturition found at the peak sanctuary of Mount Juktas on Crete, and a fragment from the peak sanctuary of Petsofas depicting a seated pregnant woman (Peatfield 1990, 122), placed by those seeking a trouble-free birth and some of the seated Mycenaean figurines may well represent parturient woman sitting on obstetric chairs, as this position, with legs dangling down over the edge, was formerly the natural position for childbirth (Householder 1974). The seated Mycenaean figurine found in a Late Helladic IIIA/B chamber tomb at Berbati in 1934 (Holmberg 1983, 43, fig. 27), has been thought to be such, although rather conventionalised. Similar figurines, of unknown provenance are in the Danish National Museum, Copenhagen and the Louvre in Paris possesses some from Mycenae (Holmberg 1983, 43 n. 11; Amandry 1986). As two of the seated figurines are each holding a small child, this may be an indication that they have just given birth. There is no archaeological and textual evidence for birth rituals such as practised, for example, by the Hittites (Beckman 1983; Pringle 1983).

Similar to what Nutton has proposed in his model of community medicine in Greek and Roman urban centres (Nutton 1992, 17), there would have been both in Minoan and Mycenaean towns and larger rural communities, healers outside the control of the palaces. They were probably both male and female, perhaps competing with each other, and amongst them would have been magicians and exorcists, faith-healers, bone-setters, root-cutters and 'wise-women' and would certainly not have been above conscious quackery and drug-fraud. The 'wise-woman' is also a feature of Hittite medicine whose specialisations within the family or community may have included those of midwife, nurse, wet-nurse or magico-ritual attendant. In the royal archives of Hattuša she is to be identified as the *Hašauwa*, meaning the 'one of birth giving'; she may also be the 'Old Woman' of the Hittite Old Kingdom tablets who performed a wide variety of purificatory and healing rituals (Pringle 1983, 132–4; Beckman 1993, 36–9). The term 'old' or 'wise' woman perhaps derives from rural usage, and was the exponent of the simplest form of patient care as well as magic.

Perhaps some wise-women and others were very experienced and proficient, existing at a level between the palace healers and domestic medicine and self-help and combining a mixture of folk-remedies and magic, some working with herbal medicine and performing primitive surgery. Some community practitioners were possibly barbers or smiths with particular skills, perhaps tooth-pulling, put to everyday use. Some may even have been peripatetic. This was certainly likely later in the Iron Age. We read from the *Odyssey* (xvii.381), that healers or physicians were amongst the few, along with singers and bards that were readily admitted to a home. However, in the rural communities, the population would have relied on self-help and fended for themselves, as many of the community healers may only have been a particular feature of Late Bronze Age urban towns.

Conclusion

If the word *i-ja-te* is to be identified as a healer or physician, then it is perhaps a little surprising that more evidence for this has not been forthcoming over the years, although it must be noted that the Linear B records are very uneven and perhaps further references may for reasons of serendipity, never appear. We are reminded that the scale of known documents is rather small, with only approximately 5,500 inscribed clay documents and approximately 160 painted vase inscriptions known from all the sites in the Mycenaean palatial period (approximately 1450–1200 BC) (Palaima 2003, 154; Driessen 2000, 21). Perhaps craftsman with other titles performed healing and practised medicine. The finding, however, in the future of a Linear B archive that lists the specific ingredients of medicines and links them to an *i-ja-te* or another craftsman which we may also interpret as a healer or physician, may provide some of the answers.

To move forward a few hundred years from the Mycenaeans, it must now be assumed that it is possible to conjecture that the eventual establishment in the mid-first millennium BC of the healing cults and the Hippocratic School of practice on Kos and elsewhere is likely to have drawn upon Mycenaean healing traditions. It cannot be possible that all the remedies described by the Hippocratic School originated exclusively then. It points to the Hippocratic healers systematising a traditional body of knowledge rather than asking fundamentally new questions.

Acknowledgements

I acknowledge Professor Demetrios Michaelides and his team from the University of Cyprus for their organisation of this conference and particularly Professor Michaelides for his subsequent collaboration. This paper would not be in its present form without the help and advice of Professor Thomas G. Palaima, to whom I am deeply grateful, although any omissions and solecisms are mine alone. I also wish to acknowledge the advice and help of the late Dr John Chadwick FBA, Professor John Killen FBA and Dr Lisa Bendall with aspects of this research and to Professor Vassos Karageorghis for his reference to the Idalion text from mid fifth century BC Cyprus. I am also very grateful to Frau Sabine Beckman for help with the identification of certain plants referred to in the text.

Notes

1 For a basic introduction to Linear B and its decipherment see Bennett 1984; 1985; Chadwick 1967; 1976; Duhoux and Davies 2008; Hooker 1979; 1980; Killen 1985; Palaima 1984; 1988a; 1988b; 2003; Ventris and Chadwick 1973. For a general overview of the current state of Linear B scholarship, see Palaima 2003.

2 There is also a very speculative suggestion of an earlier reference to a healer. From the palace at Phaistos (Palace Magazine 27) comes an earlier Linear A inscription (PH Zb 4) on a pithos (Heraklion Museum HM 1620) (Godart and Olivier 1982, 93, GORILA 4 S.93) dated to the Late Minoan IA period (*c.* 1550 BC), which has been very tentatively read by Owens and Trench as SI-MA • I-JA-TE and suggests that I-JA-TE is similar in meaning to the Linear B tablet PY Eq 146 (Owens and Trench 1996). If this is the case, it might point to a Cretan origin of the word *i-ja-te.* An alternative interpretation is 'of/from I-JA' (Younger 2008).

3 Evidence of the granting of land in exchange for medical services is also found much later in Cyprus in the mid-1st millennium BC, on the double-sided Idalion Tablet, now in the Bibliothèque National in Paris. The text refers to an agreement made by the King of Idalion and a physician named Onasilos and his brothers. The physician undertook to treat the wounded from the war against the Medes and the Phoenicians (478–440 BC) and in return the King and the city would pay Onasilos and his brothers a silver talent or to grant them state owned land on which they would not be required to pay taxes. If the land was reclaimed, they would be paid compensation. The tablet was deposited in the Temple of Athena, the patron of the city. See Karageorghis 1982, 159; Masson 1983, 235–44 (no. 217).

Bibliography

Amandry, P. 1986: 'Sièges mycéniens tripodes et trépied pythique', 167–84 in *Φίλια Ἔπη εἰς Γεώργιον Ἐ. Μυλωνᾶν*, Τόμος Α´, Athens.

Angel, J. L. 1972: 'Human skeletons from Grave Circles at Mycenae', 379–97 in G. E. Mylonas (ed.), *Ὁ Ταφικὸς κύκλος Β´ τῶν Μυκηνῶν*, Athens.

Arnott, R. 1996: 'Healing and medicine in the Aegean Bronze Age', *Journal of the Royal Society of Medicine* 89, 265–70.

Arnott, R. 1997: 'Surgical practice in the prehistoric Aegean', *Medizinhistorisches Journal* 32, 249–78.

Arnott, R. 1999a: 'War wounds and their treatment in the Aegean Bronze Age', 499–506 in R. Laffineur (ed.), *Polemos: le contexte guerrier en Egée à l'âge du bronze* (Aegaeum 19), Liège and Austin.

Arnott, R. 1999b: 'Healing cult in Minoan Crete', 1–6 in P. P. Betancourt, V. Karageorghis, R. Laffineur and W.-D. Niemeier (eds), *Meletemata: Studies in Aegean Archaeology Presented to Malcolm H. Wiener as he enters his 65th Year* (Aegaeum 20), Liège and Austin.

Arnott, R. 1999c: 'Healing and medicine', 262–79 in Y. Tzedakis and H. Martlew (eds), *Minoans and Mycenaeans: Flavours of their Time*, Exhibition Catalogue: National Archaeological Museum, July–December 1999, Athens.

Arnott, R. 2002: 'Disease and medicine in Hittite Asia Minor', 41–52 in R. Arnott (ed.), *The Archaeology of Medicine* (British Archaeological Reports International Series 1046), Oxford.

Arnott, R. 2007: 'Chrysokamino, occupational health and the earliest medicine on Crete', 108–20 in Y. Tzedakis, H. Martlew and M. K. Jones (eds), *Archaeology Meets Science: Biomolecular and Site Investigations in Bronze Age Greece,* Oxford.

Beal, R. H. 1988: 'The ^{GIŠ}TUKUL-Institution in Second Millennium Hatti', *Altorientalische Forschungen* 15, 289–92.

Beck, L. Y. (tr. and ed.) 2005: *De materia medica by Pedanius Dioscorides*, Hildesheim.

Beckman, G. M. 1983: *Hittite Birth Rituals*, 2nd ed. (Studien zu den Boğazköy-Texten 29). Wiesbaden.

Beckman, G. M. 1993: 'From cradle to grave: women's role in Hittite medicine and magic', *Journal of Ancient Civilisations* 8, 25–39.

Bendall, L. M. 2003: 'A reconstruction of the Northeastern building at Pylos: evidence for a Mycenaean redistributive center', *American Journal of Archaeology* 107, 181–231.

Bennett, E. L., Jr. 1992: 'A selection of Pylos tablet texts', 103–27 in J.-P. Olivier (ed.), *Mykenaïka: Actes du IXe Colloque international sur les textes mycéniens et égéens, Athènes, 2–6 octobre 1990,* Paris.

Bennett, E. L. and Olivier, J.-P. 1973: *The Pylos Texts Transcribed*, Vol. I: *Texts and Notes,* Rome.

Bennet, J. 1984: 'Text and context: levels of approach to the integration of archaeological and textual data in the Late Bronze Age Aegean', *Archaeological Review from Cambridge* 3, 63–75.

Bennet, J. 1985: 'The structure of the Linear B administration at Knossos', *American Journal of Archaeology* 89, 231–49.

Blaxland Stubbs, S. G. and Bligh, G. W. 1931: *Sixty Centuries of Health and Physick*, London.

Blegen, C. W. and Rawson, M. 1966: *The Palace of Nestor at Pylos in Western Messenia*, Vol. 1, Princeton.

Chadwick, J. 1967: *The Decipherment of Linear B*, 2nd edition, Cambridge.

Chadwick, J. 1976: *The Mycenaean World*, Cambridge.

Coulomb, J. 1979: 'Le "Prince aux lis" de Knosos reconsidéré', *Bulletin de Correspondance hellénique* 103, 29–50.

Driessen, J. 2000: *The Scribes of the Room of the Chariot Tablets at Knossos: Interdisciplinary Approach to the Study of a Linear B Deposit*, (Minos Supplement 15), Salamanca.

Duhoux, Y. and Davies, A. M. (eds) 2008: *A Companion to Linear B: Mycenaean Greek texts and their World*, Vol. I, Louvain-la-Neuve.

Flückiger, F. A. and Hanbury, D. 1879: *Pharmacographia. A*

History of the Principal Drugs of Vegetable Origin met with me in Great Britain and British India, London.

Godart, L. and Olivier, J.-P. 1982: *Recueil des Inscriptions en Linéaire A*, Vol. 4, *Autres Documents* (Études Crétoises, 21.4, GORILA 4), Paris.

Gunther, R. T (ed.) 1934: Dioscorides Pedanius, *De Materia Medica*, translated by J. Goodyear in 1655 [*The Greek Herbal of Dioscorides*], Oxford.

Hein, W.-H. 1961: 'Die Bedeutung der Entzifferung des Linear B für die Arzneimittel-geschichte', *Pharmazeutische Zeitung* 106, 1145–8.

Holmberg, E. J. 1983: *A Mycenaean Chamber Tomb near Berbati in Argolis*, Göteborg.

Hooker, J. T. 1979: *The Origin of the Linear B Script (*Minos Supplement 8*),* Salamanca.

Hooker, J. T. 1980: *Linear B: An Introduction*, Bristol.

Householder, M. S. 1974: 'A historical perspective on the obstetric chair', *Surgical Gynecology and Obstetrics* 139, 423–30.

Janko, R. 1981: 'Un 1314: herbal remedies at Pylos' *Minos* 17, 30–4.

Karageorghis, V. 1982: *Cyprus: from the Stone Age to the Romans*, London.

Killen, J. 1983: 'On the Mycenae Ge tablets', 216–33 in A. Heubeck and G. Neumann (eds), *Res Mycenaeae: Akten des VII. Internationalen Mykenologischen Colloquiums in Nürnberg vom 6.–20. April 1981*, Göttingen.

Killen, J. 1985: 'The Linear B tablets and the Mycenaean economy', 241–305 in A. M. Davies and Y. Duhoux (eds), *Linear B: A 1984 Survey: Proceedings of the Mycenaean Colloquium of the VIIIth Congress of the International Federation of the Societies of Classical Studies, Dublin, 27 August – 1 September 1984,* Louvain-La-Neuve.

Masson, O. 1983: *Les Inscriptions chypriotes syllabiques. Recueil critique et commenté* (École française d'Athènes, Études Chypriotes I), Paris.

Melena, J. 1992–3: 'Joins and quasi-joins of fragments in the Linear B tablets from Pylos', *Minos* 27–8, 307–24.

Melena, J. 1994–5: '28 joins and quasi-joins of fragments in the Linear B tablets from Pylos', *Minos* 29–30, 95–100.

Milani, C. 1986: 'Notizie sulla farmacopea micenea', 31–7 in C. Milani and O. Carruba (eds), *La farmacia nel mondo minoico-miceneo ed egeo-anatolico*, Chieti.

Morpurgo Davies, A. 1979: 'Terminology of power and terminology of work in Greek and Linear B', 87–108 in E. Risch and H. Mühlestein (eds), *Colloquium Mycenaeum: Actes du Sixième Colloque International sur les textes mycéniens et égéens, tenu à Chaumont sur Neuchâtel du 7 au 13 Septembre 1975*, Neuchâtel and Geneva.

Musgrave, J. H. 2000: 'The anatomy of a Minoan masterpiece', 97–101 in J. A. MacGillivray, J. M. Driessen and L. H. Sackett (eds), *The Palaikastro Kouros: a Minoan Chryselephantine Statuette and its Bronze Age Context* (British School at Athens Studies 6), London.

Nutton, V. 1992: 'Healers in the market place: towards a social history of Graeco-Roman medicine', 15–58 in A. Wear (ed.), *Medicine in Society*, Cambridge.

Owens, G. and Trench, G. 1996: 'A possible reading of Linear A PH Zb 4', *Kadmos* 25, 171–2.

Palaima, T. G. 1984: 'Scribal organization and palatial activity', 31–9 in C. Shelmerdine and T. G. Palaima (eds), *Pylos Comes Alive,* New York.

Palaima, T. G. 1988a: 'The development of the Mycenaean writing system', 269–342 in J.-P. Olivier and T. G. Palaima (eds), *Texts, Tablets and Scribes (*Minos Supplement 10*), Salamanca.*

Palaima, T. G. 1988b: *The Scribes of Pylos*, Rome.

Palaima, T. G. 1997: 'Potter and fuller: the Royal craftsmen', 407–12 in R. Laffineur and P. P. Betancourt (eds), *TEXNH Craftsmen, Craftswomen and Craftsmanship in the Aegean Bronze Age* (Aegaeum 16), Liège and Austin.

Palaima, T. G. 2003: 'Archives and scribes and information hierarchy in Mycenaean Greek Linear B records', 153–94 in M. Brosius (ed.), *Ancient Archives and Archival Traditions: Concepts of Record-keeping in the Ancient World*, Oxford.

Palmer, L. R. 1963: *On the Interpretation of Mycenaean Greek Texts*, Oxford.

Peatfield, A. A. D. 1990: 'Minoan peak sanctuaries: history and society', *Opuscula Atheniensia* 18, 117–31.

Pringle, J. 1983: 'Hittite birth ritual', 128–41 in A. Cameron and A. Kuhrt (eds), *Images of Women in Antiquity*, London.

Protonotariou-Deilaki: Πρωτονοταρίου-Δεϊλάκη, Ε.: 1973: 'Ἀρχαιότητες καὶ μνημεῖα Ἀργολίδος-Κορινθίας 1971–1972 – Ἀκροναυπλία', *Ἀρχαιολογικὸν Δελτίον*, 28 (Β΄:1 *Χρονικά*), 90–4.

Ritter, E. K. 1965: 'Magical-Expert (=Āšipu) and Physician (=Asû): notes on two complementary professions in Babylonian medicine', 299–321 in H. G. Güterbock and T. Jacobsen (eds), *Studies in Honor of Benno Landsberger on his Seventy-Fifth Birthday, April 21, 1965* (Oriental Institute of the University of Chicago Assyriological Studies 16), Chicago.

Salazar, C. F. 2001: *Treatment of War Wounds in Graeco-Roman Antiquity* (Studies in Ancient Medicine 21), Leiden.

Scarborough, J. 1991: 'The pharmacology of sacred plants, herbs and roots', 138–74 in C. A. Faraone and D. Obbink (eds), *Magika Hiera: Ancient Greek Magic and Religion*, Oxford.

Shaw, M. C. 1993: 'The Aegean garden', *American Journal of Archaeology* 97, 661–85.

Shelmerdine, C. 1985: *The Perfume Industry at Pylos* (Studies in Mediterranean Archaeology Pocket Book 34), Göteborg.

Stieglitz, R. B. 1981: 'A physician's equipment list from Ugarit', *Journal of Cuneiform Studies* 33, 52–5.

Tzavella-Evjen, H. 1981: 'Homeric medicine', 185–8 in R. Hägg (ed.), *The Greek Renaissance of the Eighth Century BC: Tradition and Innovation*, Stockholm.

Ventris M. and Chadwick, J. 1973: *Documents in Mycenaean Greek*, 2nd ed., Cambridge.

Walberg, G. 1992: 'Minoan floral iconography', 317–22 in R. Laffineur and J. L. Crowley (eds), *EIKΩN. Aegean Bronze Age Iconography: Shaping a Methodology* (Aegaeum 8), Liège.

Wall, S. M., Musgrave, J. H. and Warren, P. M. 1986: 'Human bones from a Late Minoan IB house at Knossos', *Annual of the British School at Athens* 81, 333–88.

Weeks, K. R. 1995: 'Medicine, surgery, and public health in Ancient Egypt', 1787–98 in J. M. Sasson (ed.), *Civilizations of the Ancient Near East*, Vol. III, New York.

Wylock, M. 1972: 'Les aromates dans les tablettes Ge de Mycenès', *Studi micenei ed egeo-anatolici* 15, 105–46.

Younger, J. 2008: *Linear A Lexicon*, http://people.ku.edu/~jyounger/LinearA/lexicon.html (Accessed 27 December 2008).

7. Health and Healing on Cretan Bronze Age Peak Sanctuaries

Christine Morris and Alan Peatfield

The peak sanctuaries of the Cretan Bronze Age are well-known for having a healing dimension. These ritual sites, of which around 25 are known, are characterised by both their location – on or near mountain peaks – and their distinctive finds of clay figurines of animals, humans, and detached anatomical models, termed 'votive limbs' within Aegean archaeology. By analogy with anatomical offerings elsewhere, these votive limbs quickly suggested to the earliest excavators, such as Myres at Petsophas in Eastern Crete and Evans at Jouktas above Knossos, that issues of health and healing were a significant element of Minoan peak sanctuary cult. Alternative interpretations of the finds – that they are parts of puppets, dolls or sacrificial dismembered body parts – are not supported by the evidence. Relatively few of the figurines can be recognised as explicitly representing illnesses, but the large category of votive limbs, including legs, arms, torsos with incised genitalia, and vertically split bodies, resonate with offerings familiar from later and more fully documented healing cults in the Mediterranean area. Indeed, the offering of anatomical models is a tradition which also finds expression in the contemporary metal tamata *and wax models found in Greek Orthodox churches. The Minoan votive limbs have, somewhat surprisingly, not been studied or published in any detail. In this paper we review the study of the anatomical offerings from peak sanctuaries, considering them within the wider context of the figurine assemblages. In addition, we will explore the evidence for the processes or mechanics of healing in relation to ritual action and embodied experience at the peak sanctuaries.*

When Sir John Myres excavated the mountain-peak sanctuary of Petsophas in east Crete in 1903, he found a class of finds that are often cited in discussions of Minoan religion, but which are actually little-studied and less understood (Myres 1902–3). These are the clay anatomical models or body parts, which Minoan archaeologists call 'votive limbs' following Myres' insightful interpretation that they are offerings concerned with healing (*ibid.*, 381). This group of finds, therefore, represents some of the earliest evidence for healing concerns within Greek archaeology. This material has mostly been discussed in relation to its votive role, rather than as evidence for health concerns. In this paper, therefore, we review some of the interpretative debate around these 'votive limbs' and offer some more considered ways in which their deeper value as archaeological evidence may begin to be drawn out.

Peak sanctuaries in context

Since the excavation of Petsophas, more than 25 peak sanctuaries have been identified (Fig. 7.1).[1] Their identification rests on conformity with two sets of characteristic features: location – a distinctive set of topographic features; and finds – a typical shared assemblage of artefacts (Peatfield 1983; 1990). In summary, the topographic features are:

1) Visibility: on or near mountain peaks, they appear to be the most prominent local high point, and they have good views of the surrounding valleys from which worshippers come;
2) Accessibility: they can be reached in less than two hours walk from the lowland settlements, and they are close to upland pastures and fields, familiar to the herders and farmers (Rutkowski 1972, 185; 1986, 94). As noted in earlier papers, they are not – in contrast to mountain

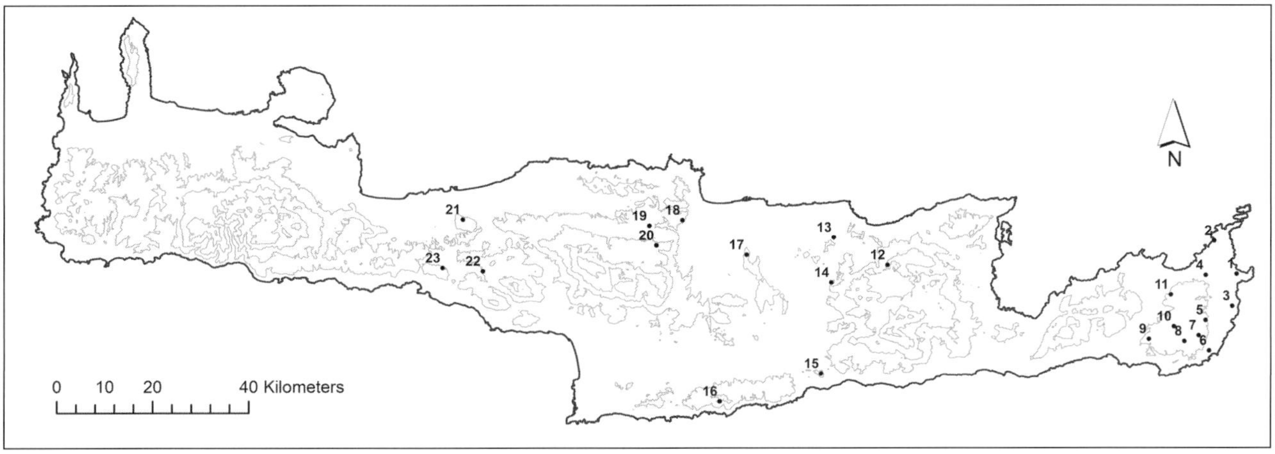

Fig. 7.1. Map showing the location of Minoan peak sanctuaries (map: Will Megarry)

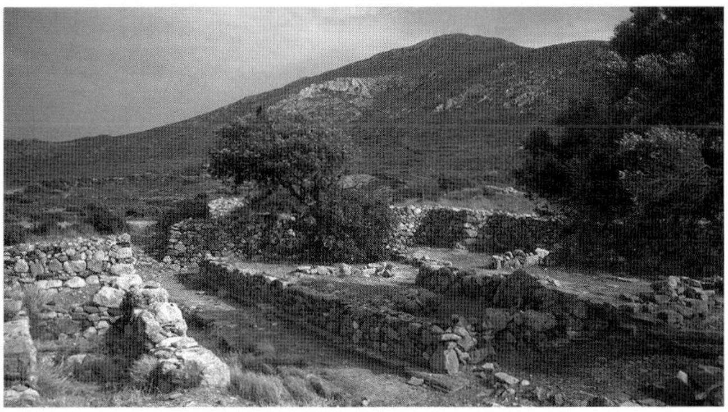

Fig. 7.2. View looking S.E. from Palaikastro towards the peak sanctuary of Petsophas (photo: Alan Peatfield)

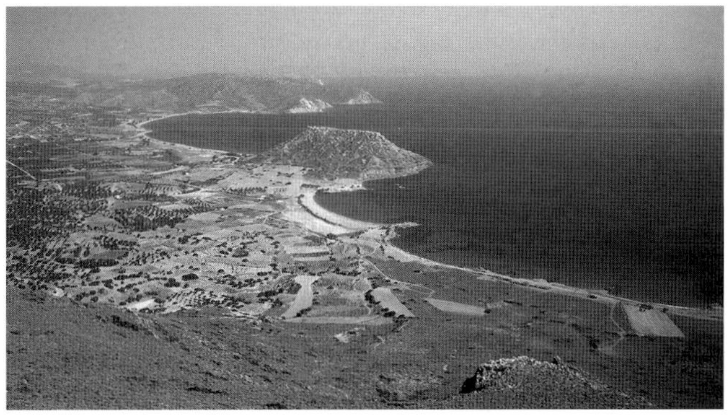

Fig. 7.3. View down from Petsophas to Palaikastro (photo: Alan Peatfield)

sanctuaries in many other cultures – sites of 'remote and arduous pilgrimage' (Peatfield 1990, 120; 1994, 23–5). Both of these features are well illustrated with the views between Petsofas and the town of Palaikastro (Figs 7.2–3; see also Nowicki 2007 for further examples);

3) They are also intervisible with other peak sanctuaries (Peatfield 1994, fig. 2.1).

These characteristics emphasise the local, popular nature of the sites as an expression of the Minoan sacred landscape.

The primary elements of the characteristic find assemblage are large numbers of clay figurines of three main types: animal figurines (mostly domestic – cattle, pigs, sheep, and goats); human figurines (male and female); and detached anatomical models, i.e. the votive limbs. Minoan clay figurines are, of course, found in a wide range of contexts other than peak sanctuaries, but it is not simply their presence, but their presence in *large quantities* that is particularly distinctive. Within the figurine assemblage the votive limbs stand out as unique to peak sanctuaries, making them of central importance to any discussion of the ritual roles of these sites.

Of these 25-plus sites, around 18 have been excavated, some fully, but many only superficially. Unfortunately, little of the material from these excavations has been published, which presents difficulties for the interpretation of peak sanctuaries. Petsophas is still the best known site, followed by Jouktas, extensively excavated and reported by Karetsou in the 1970s and 1980s, and Atsipadhes Korakias, excavated by us in 1989, and reported in various articles (Petsophas: Myres 1902–3; Rutkowski 1991; Jouktas: Karetsou 1974; 1975; 1976; 1977; 1980; 1981a; 1981b; 1984; Atsipadhes: Peatfield 1992; Morris and Peatfield 1995; Morris and Batten 2000).

In terms of distribution, peak sanctuaries are to be found over most of Crete, from Petsophas on the east coast, at least as far west as the Rethymnon district of west central Crete (Fig. 7.1). There is also a shared chronology. The available evidence suggests that the first peak sanctuaries were founded late in the Early Minoan/Prepalatial period, around 2200 BC, and spread all over the island, as a popular cult during the Middle Minoan/Protopalatial period. At least two peak sanctuaries – Atsipadhes and Traostalos – are also reported as having even earlier material from Final Neolithic/ Early Minoan I. In the case of Atsipadhes a case has been made for this being a deposit of ritual rather than domestic/ mundane character. This opens up the possibility that mountain locations were perceived of as having a ritual significance at a much earlier date, but given the limited nature of the evidence (material from only two sites, and the lack of continuity), it would be unwise to press the point further (Atsipadhes: Morris and Batten 2000; Traostalos: Chryssoulaki 2001, 63).

In the following Neopalatial period, from about 1650 BC, there is confirmed evidence of use at only eight of the 25 peak sanctuaries. These sites are closely associated with Neopalatial palaces and regional power centres, strongly suggesting an elite appropriation and centralisation of what had been a popular, vernacular cult (Peatfield 1987; 1990). These 'palatial' peak sanctuaries also have evidence of built structures, rarely more than simple stone enclosures, but still stratigraphically late additions to the sites. Only the Jouktas peak sanctuary, associated with the palace of Knossos, has a more complex, multi-roomed building. Poor, Protopalatial peak sanctuaries, such as Atsipadhes, have no evidence for structures.

This is a simplified summary of the archaeology of peak sanctuaries, but it serves to set the scene for our discussion of the anatomical models, the 'votive limbs', and the healing dimension of the peak sanctuaries.

Votive limbs from Minoan peak sanctuaries

As noted above, the first peak sanctuary excavators, Myres at Petsophas, followed by Arthur Evans excavating at Jouktas near Knossos, were quick to suggest that issues of health and healing were a significant element of peak sanctuary cult (Myres 1902–3, 381; Evans 1928, 153). The obvious analogies to draw with the votive limbs were the detached anatomical offerings from elsewhere in the material record, notably the offerings at classical Asklepios temples, and the medical votive offerings offered in Christian churches (Rouse 1902, 210–6, 239; de Waele 1933; van Straten 1981, 100–1, 148–9; Simon 1986, 364; Teske 1980; Dubisch 1995, 88–90).

Beyond such simple comparisons, little more has been made of these analogies, though they offer enormous potential both for developing a better understanding of the Minoan votive limbs and, on a broader scale, for a cross-cultural study of the phenomenon of making and using votive body parts in the context of healing. A comparative study of this kind could bring into sharper relief the distinctive features in each specific context and culture within a diachronic perspective: for example, choices of materials and artefact form, attitudes to the body and fragmentation, and to ritual practice and performance.

For the present, limited publication of the Minoan votive limbs is a hindrance to such research ambitions. Remarkably, the finds from Petsophas, published in 1903, still remain the best known collection of these Minoan anatomical offerings. There is, therefore, currently no corpus of finds which would enable detailed comparison either between the Minoan sites or with similar artefacts from later Greek traditions, or indeed from other potentially comparable traditions. To cite only a few examples, these wider traditions include the vast number of ancient Italic anatomical offerings in terracotta, notable for the representation of internal organs as well as external body parts (Fenelli 1975; Lesk 2002; Potter and Wells 1985; Turfa 1994; 2006), as well as the modern *milagros*, made from metal and from wax, best known from the Hispanic Catholic tradition (Vidal 1974; Egan 1991; Nolan and Nolan 1989, 71–8; Oktavec 1995; Francis 2007).

We are far then from being able to establish a corpus of the full range and distribution of this material. But through years of study of peak sanctuaries and their finds, including our own from the Atsipadhes excavation, we are in a position to present an informed review of the material. Firstly, with the excavator's perspective, it is important to be able to distinguish anatomical models from anatomical fragments, i.e., pieces broken off from fully made human figurines. This is sometimes difficult when a piece is worn, but it is

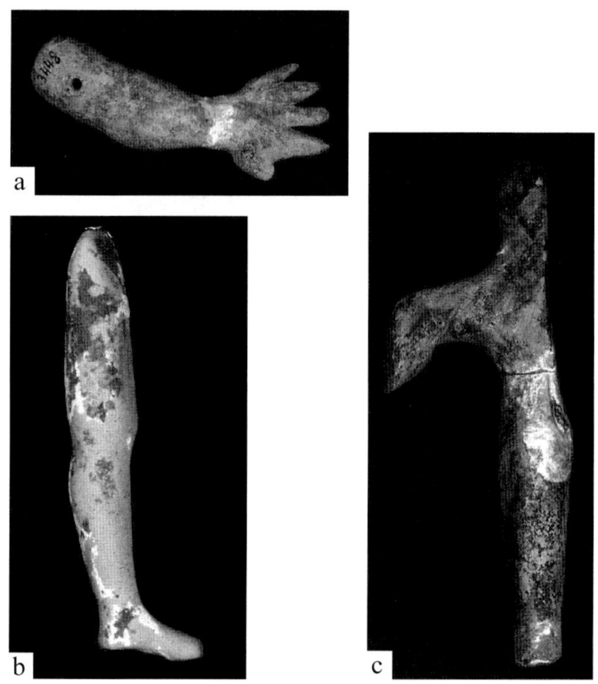

Fig. 7.4 a–c. Votive limbs from Petsophas: arm, leg and split torso (photo: Alan Peatfield)

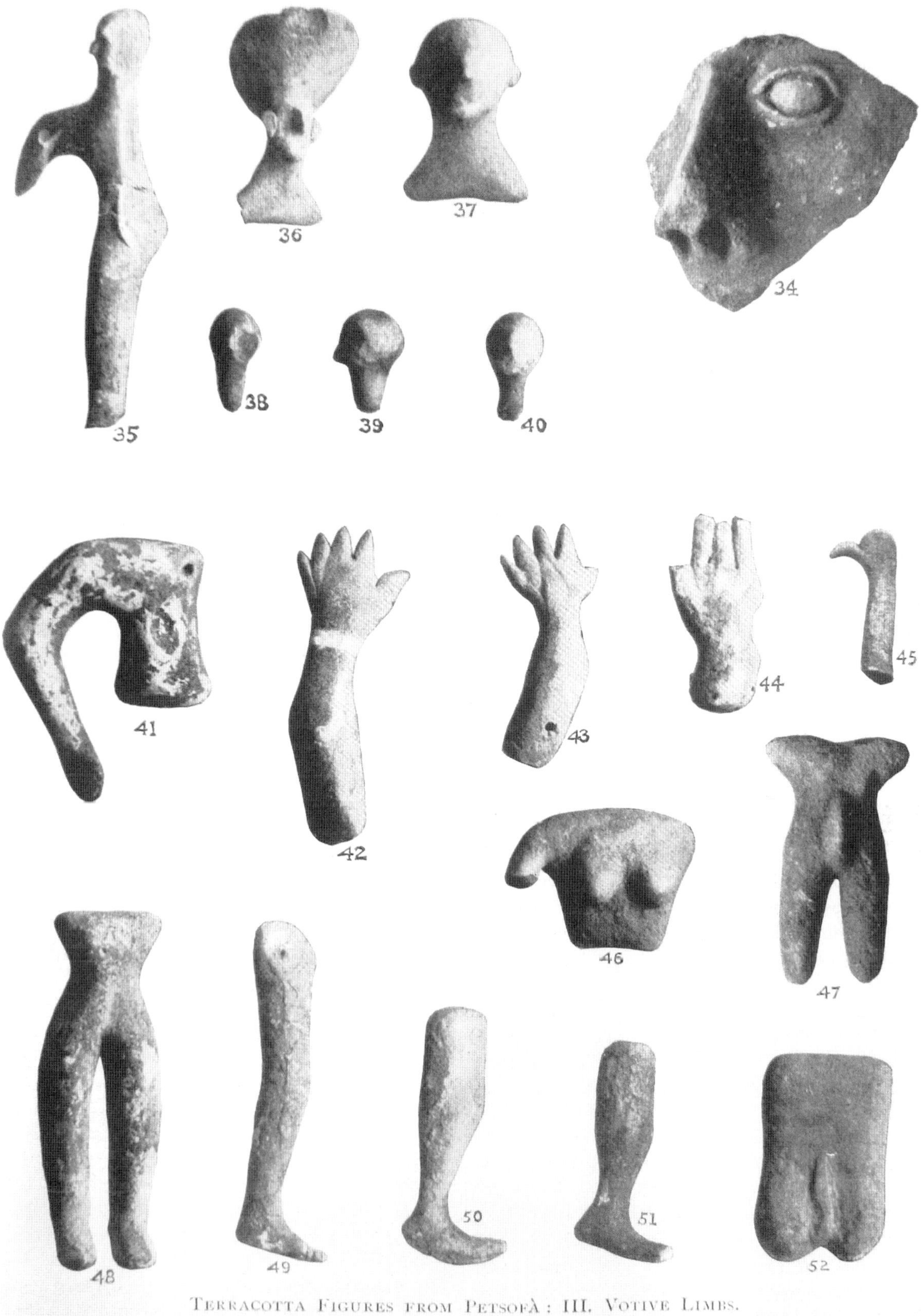

Fig. 7.5. Votive limbs from Petsophas as published by Myres (after Myres 1902–3, pl. xii)

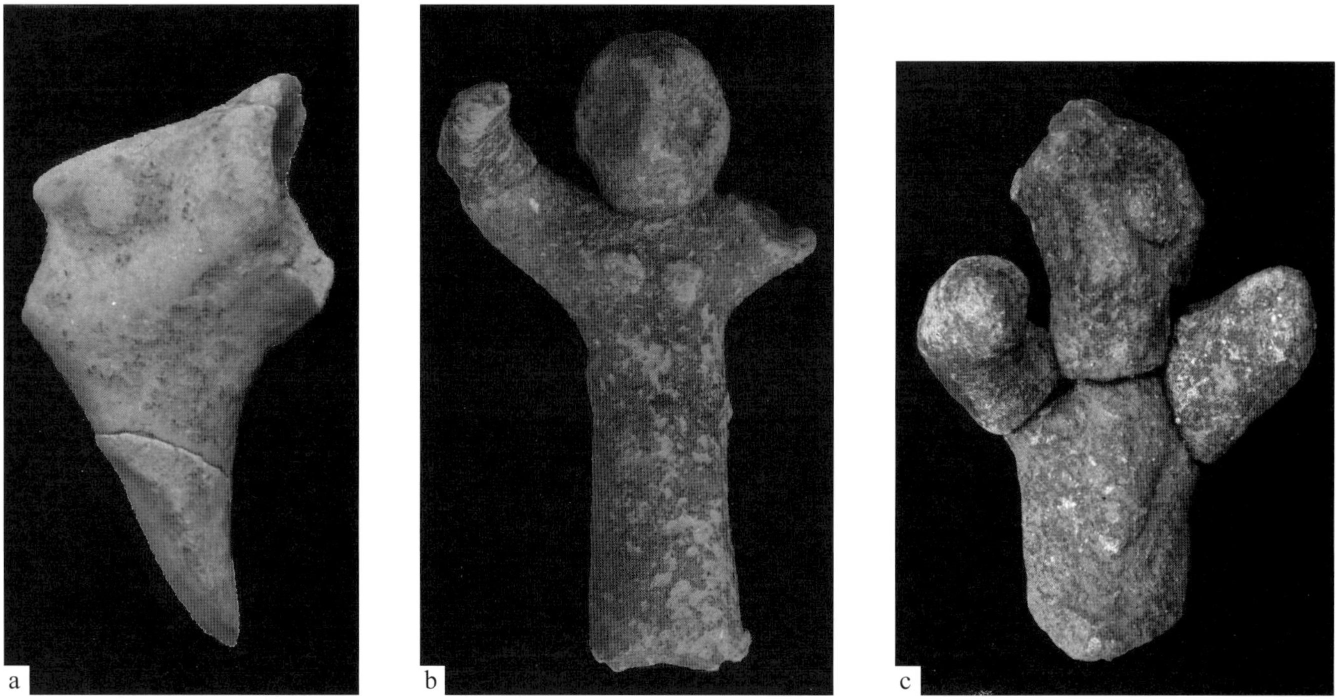

Fig. 7.6a–c. Clay figurine heads from Atsipadhes, showing various forms of shaping and pegging for attachment to the figurine body (photos: Alan Peatfield)

the presence of finished edges around the piece, rather than a broken edge, that indicates the model. Many, but not all of the Minoan votive limb models, also have one or more pierced holes at one end or the corners of the piece. This suggests that a period of suspension formed part of the use or 'life cycle' of these anatomical models. We shall return to this feature later. The range of modelled body parts is quite consistent. Most obvious are the true limbs: arms, hands, legs and feet. There are also torso models, particularly of the lower torso, and vertically-split half-bodies, head to foot (Fig. 7.4).

Heads are usually included in the lists of 'detached' limbs alongside the arms, legs and partial torsos; they are, for example, illustrated on a plate showing votive limbs in the Petsofas report (Fig. 7.5; Myres 1902–3, pl. xii, 36–40). Comparisons can readily be made with the terracotta votives from the Corinth Asklepieion, or with the extensive Italic votive deposits, where separate heads are clearly present in the votive assemblages, but we urge a note of caution here in relation to the Minoan material. In his report Myres notes correctly that the 'detached heads' are *separately* modelled, and he specifically describes the different construction forms these take: from 'mere peg' and tapering 'to a sort of wedge' through to more elaborate 'shouldered busts' (Myres 1902–3, 375). This is not necessarily because they were intended as detached body parts, but because this is how Minoan clay figurines are made, i.e. in several pieces joined together. At Atsipadhes, heads with a variety of construction forms, including sharply angled pegs and squared neck/shoulders, have been found to attach to torsos to form part of complete figurines (Fig. 7.6). Whereas a limb with a pierced hole and clearly finished edges can be assigned to the anatomical offering category with confidence, the situation regarding heads is more ambiguous, making this an area which would repay more careful study.[2]

Before discussing the evidence in more detail, we should comment briefly on alternative interpretations, since some scholars have doubted the association of the Minoan votive limbs with healing. Rutter, for example, has suggested that they could be body parts belonging to complete figurines or 'dolls' (Rutter n.d.). The arms and legs do bear some resemblance to the jointed or articulated limbs of 'dolls' known from Archaic and Classical Greece (Elderkin 1930). There are, however, no preserved Minoan torsos perforated and socketed in such a way that they would fit together with limbs. Moreover, it is important to draw attention to the fact that the peak sanctuary torsos are deliberately formed as *partial* body torsos emphasising a particular body feature, and *not* as complete torsos, thus making the doll or puppet hypothesis untenable.

In the early years of Minoan discovery, that great scholar of Greek religion, Martin Nilsson noted the absence of body parts such as eyes and breasts, which are well represented at later healing sanctuaries, and he puzzled over the half-bodies, 'cloven from crown to groin' (Nilsson 1950, 74). Nilsson tentatively suggested that the votive limbs were simulacra body-parts, associated with a sacrificial-like ritual, 'in which living animals, human puppets and miscellaneous objects were thrown into the fire' (*ibid.*, 75). He does admit, however, that this is a 'mere guess', and that he finds the body parts 'enigmatical'. Subsequent exploration of peak sanctuaries requires modification of the view that sacrificial bonfires were a consistent, central aspect of the cult, since evidence of burning is completely absent from some sites. Following Nilsson's line of argument, Dietrich later suggested that the body parts should be interpreted as a ritual of dismemberment, suggesting that the limbs were remnants of a kind of proto-Dionysiac human sacrifice, the 'savage worship performed for a great goddess, a worship which fell into disuse at a relatively early time' (Dietrich 1969, 269; 1974, 302). Most recently, dismemberment has again resurfaced as an interpretation for the votive limbs at Petsophas, with the suggestion that they should be linked to the dismembering of the body of the Egyptian god, Osiris (MacGillivray, Driessen and Sackett 2000). Among the many reasons for rejecting this 'Osiris hypothesis', we mention only the presence of *female* body parts amongst the finds from Petsophas (Rutkowski 1991, pl. xliv.4, 10; also on display in Ayios Nikolaos museum from Davaras' later excavation of the site).

The observation that the Minoan votive limbs appear less varied than the assemblages from later healing sanctuaries merits further comment. This presupposes that the Minoan offerings should exactly mirror the later votive assemblages or indeed that these are all closely similar to one another. As noted above, Nilsson found this problematic, and, in the absence of modelled eyes and breasts recorded in classical sanctuaries, wondered if 'the people of Petsofa suffered only in their legs, arms and heads' (Nilsson 1950, 74). With respect to the focus on limbs, study of Etruscan and also Roman terracotta anatomical offerings shows that limbs can indeed have a high visibility, since 'in rural or pre industrial populations, walking and working are of prime importance, and healing of hands and feet is commonly sought' (Turfa 2006, 105). It is easy also to overlook the point that the Minoan votive limbs are true figurines, that is, *miniature* offerings, whereas the comparable terracottas from the Asklepieion at Corinth or the numerous Italian sanctuaries are closer to life-size (Corinth: de Waele 1933; Italy: Lesk 2002; Turfa 2006). The pierced legs from Petsophas, for example, fall in the range of 8–11 cm in height (for comparison, complete standing figurines range around 11–17 cm). At this kind of scale, separately modelled elements such as eyes and breasts would be impractically tiny, and if we speculate for a moment that concerns for these parts of the body could be represented in the Minoan finds, then it might be as part of a head of torso (or even a complete figurine). This indeed seems to be the case with

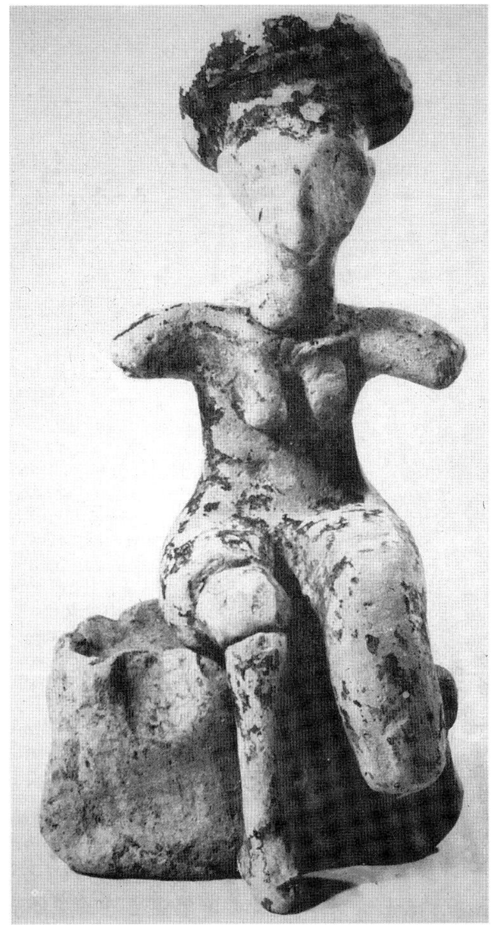

Fig. 7.7. Traostalos seated female figurine with swollen leg

the lower torso models that explicitly depict the female genitalia. Finally, it is important to emphasise again that our knowledge of the Minoan material is based on a limited amount of data, and that only fuller study and publication of additional sites will help to clarify whether there are other, as yet, unidentified body parts within the material,[3] and whether the votive limbs are more characteristic of some sites, regions or phases than others.

Representing ailments?

Returning therefore with confidence to the healing interpretation, we can review and explore the material evidence in more detail. First, there are some unusual or exceptional finds (not known to earlier writers such as Nilsson) which offer further strong support for the role of healing on peak sanctuaries. Although few in number, these finds clearly show illness or pathology. In other anatomical offering traditions explicit representation of ailments is also relatively rare. At Corinth, de Waele notes a leg with swollen

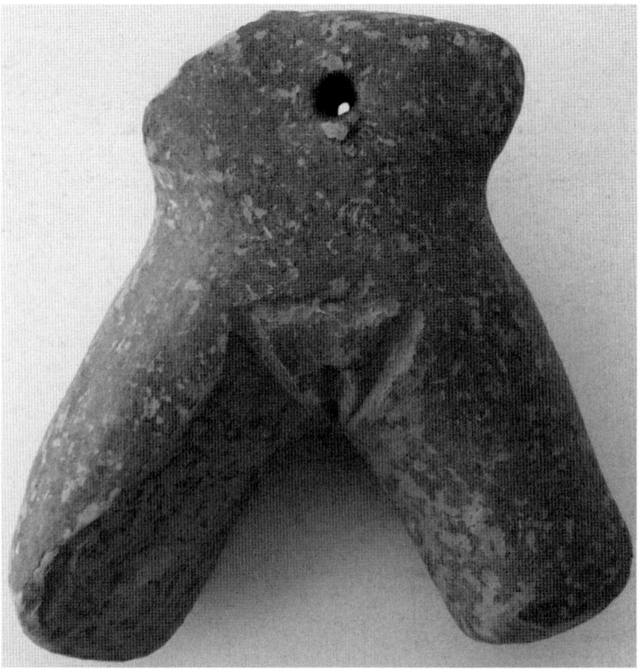

Fig. 7.8. Separately modelled female lower torso with vulva clearly shown (from Prinias) (photo: Alan Peatfield)

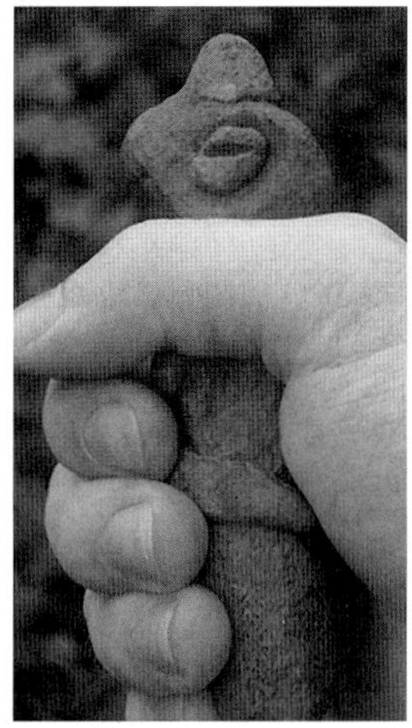

Fig. 7.9. Carrying a peak sanctuary figurine (from Atsipadhes) (photo: Christine Morris)

arteries, a hand with a tumour, and hands with bent fingers, perhaps arthitic (1933, 443–4), but these seem to be the exception alongside large numbers of anatomical models without pathologies. There are a number of possible reasons for this. If the offering is in thanks for healing (ex-voto) as opposed to an offering making a request for healing (both are widely attested), then a representation of a healthy body part might be expected. The manufacturing process for many of these offerings was, and is, one which favoured standardised or 'off-the-peg' offerings – whether the Corinthian mouldmade terracottas or metal reliefs such as Greek *tamata* or Hispanic *milagros* – which show the relevant body part but not the specific ailment. More simply, representation of the ailment may have been considered unnecessary or even inappropriate since the offering would most probably be made in a wider ritual context involving prayers and performance.

The Minoan figurines were handmade, and therefore the manufacturing tradition was more permeable both to individualisation and to stylistic variation. A good example of a highly individualised offering is the well-known, seated female figurine from Traostalos that has one heavily swollen leg (Fig. 7.7; Davaras 1976, 246, fig. 138). Normally, female figurines are shown wearing a bell-skirt – hence, the figurine maker has departed from convention in order deliberately to emphasise the legs. Attempts to interpret the pathology of the leg have included suggestions that the larger left leg shows elephantiasis or lymphedaema (Peatfield 1990, 122, fig. 10; Arnott 1999, 4). Robert Arnott has more recently proposed that it is the right leg that shows the pathology, 'possibly a necrosis' (Arnott forthcoming, pers. comm. April 2009).[4] These different diagnoses underline the difficulties in interpretation, but the unusual form of the figurine and the obvious differences in leg size make it clear that the intention is to show an ailment.

The current excavator at Traostalos reports another figurine, a male head which seems to show a 'protruding thyroid gland' (Chryssoulaki 2001, 62). Several of the Atsipadhes figurines also have unusual protruberances in the throat area created by an applied clay lozenge, but it is not clear to us whether this is an attempt to show an ailment or to represent a distinctive neck ornament, given that arm bands and bracelets are also added in clay. It has been observed too that some of the hand/arm models from Petsophas portray a distinct puffy or swollen quality, very different from the slender lines of arms attached to complete human figurines (Rutkowski 1991, pl. xlv, 14–15; Arnott 1999, 4). Similarly there is at least one arm model from Petsophas with an emphasised thumb. Also from Petsophas, there are several figurines which clearly portray pregnant women.

The quality of *selectively emphasising* anatomical features is one of the things which separates the votive limbs from the complete human figurines. The whole point of the votive limbs seems to be to emphasise certain body features. We have already observed enlarged leg, thumb, bellies, but this emphatic quality is nowhere more apparent than on the female lower torsos. These draw attention to the female genitalia by deeply incising the pubic triangle and vulva (Fig. 7.8; see also, Rutkowski 1991, pl. xliv, 4, 10; and numerous examples on display in Ayios Nikolaos Museum). Another example from Zou Prinias shows a deeply incised vulva, bordered by incised pubic hair (Davaras n.d., fig. 42).

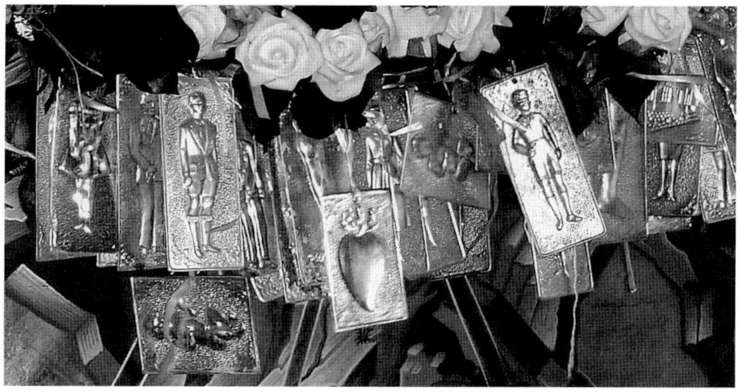

Fig. 7.10. Modern Greek *tamata*, including anatomical body parts, suspended in groups (photo: Alan Peatfield and Christine Morris)

Such explicit depictions of female genital nudity are remarkable, because nowhere else is it portrayed in Minoan art. There are also comparable male torsos, similarly pierced for suspension. This strongly suggests that all these representations are purposefully made to indicate, if not the symptoms, then certainly the location of concern or affliction. They show concern both with healing from illness and with health or protection for the body (for example, in pregnancy). In this way the Minoan models truly are similar to the Asklepios anatomical models, and to the modern *tamata*, which explicitly portray the relevant body parts. Within this context the 'enigmatical' half-bodies, split vertically, are also understandable, when one considers how strokes or similar disorders can paralyse entire sides of the body.

As noted above, another distinctive feature of the Minoan votive limbs is their small size. This contrasts with the later terracotta models which are substantially larger, often lifesize. The small size relates to the general portability of the peak sanctuary figurines (Fig. 7.9). Many, though not all, of the votive limbs have one or sometimes two perforations, suggesting that they were intended to be hung. Modern traditions illustrate this vividly, whether with the *tamata* in Greek Orthodox churches, typically strung around icons, or Spanish *milagros* arranged for display on walls (Fig. 7.10). The Classical Corinthian terracotta models were pierced for suspension and display on the temple walls (De Waele 1933, 443; Lang 1977), and this practice is also illustrated by a Boiotian vase where two legs and a hand hang on a wall behind a ritual scene (Rouse 1902, 221, fig. 33; Lang 1977, 18, fig. 16). According to Pausanias' description, votives at the Sikyon Asklepieion were also hung from the ceiling (2, 10, 3). Not all anatomical votives, however, were designed for hanging, a good example being the Italic terracottas which were not pierced (Lesk 2000; Turfa 2006).

In the Minoan case, suspension for display and as part of a ritual are likely, though in comparison to the later examples described above which occur within a built environment, such practices would have been constrained by the rocky nature of the peak sanctuaries, and the absence of buildings on many of them. The possibility that the anatomical offerings could also have been worn *on the body* prior to final deposition on the sites also deserves consideration. However, a more generalised life-use as protective charms or amulets would seem to be ruled out by the absence of these clay votive limbs from contexts other than peak sanctuaries. There may be some conceptual and functional overlap with the earlier amulets found in the Mesara tombs, particularly the foot amulets (Branigan 1970; Pini 1972; Watrous 1995). The meaning, however, is unlikely to be exactly the same as for the votive limbs, given the differences in materials, context and chronology.

When looking for evidence for illness and pathologies both on the anatomical body parts and on complete figurines, we stress the importance of being aware of the manufacturing process of the figurines and of their stylistic features. The figurines are usually modelled from several pieces of clay, which are joined more securely through the use of shaped clay pegs, for example at the neck or at the join between torso and skirt. Details of bodily form are rendered through modelling and simple pinching of the clay: rolled clay strips and pellets are used for eyes, ears, hair-locks, jewelry and belts, and details may also be pierced, impressed or painted.

Lopsided or assymetrical faces, and other lumpy or irregular features, have been interpreted by a number of scholars as evidence of specific pathologies. For example, medical specialists have suggested that a head fragment from Jouktas shows 'abnormality which may be showing a bilateral congenital facial cleft', though they note the view of the excavator, Alexandra Karetsou, that the features are due to the style of the figurine (Velegrakis *et al.* 1993, 880–1, fig. 4). The authors also suggest that the asymmetry of the face of a figurine fragment from the site of Piskokephalo[5] may be attributed to 'facial nerve weakness' (*ibid.*, 880–1, fig. 5). In this case the view of the excavator is not known. A fragmentary female figurine from Vrysinas in western Crete is described as having 'a pointed base for depositing at the sanctuary' and as having 'possible multiple pathologies' (Tzedakis and Martlew 1999, 263, fig. 263). The pointed base is the peg for attachment of the torso into the typical bell skirt worn by female figurines, and it also has the characteristic belt applied as a clay strip around the waist. While the figurine undoubtedly lacks elegance and has lopsided facial features, this is of itself not unusual within the stylistic range of peak sanctuary figurines. The divergent views of the excavator and the medical specialist concerning the Jouktas head fragment neatly illustrate the difficulties of interpretation and underline the importance of considering the manufacturing processes and stylistic range of the figurines in tandem with suggested pathologies.

In contrast to the well-known, elegant figurines which are repeatedly illustrated, many peak sanctuary figurines are lopsided, and others may seem barely human in their stylised forms to those not familiar with the material. Asymmetry of the face is quite common, and is in many cases the result of the way the head is formed from a rounded ball of clay with the eye sockets hollowed by the thumb and forefinger. In other, more fully documented, cultural contexts, anatomical offerings for healing more usually show a healthy representation of the relevant body part. This could provide an alternative model for thinking about the Minoan material – leaving explicit representation of illness in only some cases. The way forward here must be a closer collaboration between scholars with medical expertise and figurine specialists who are attuned to the formal characteristics and stylistic variants within the material. This, together with a clearer picture of the distribution and types of anatomical offerings across all the peak sanctuaries, will allow a deeper understanding of the healing dimension of Cretan Bronze Age religion.

Notes

1 This map reproduces the distribution of sites for which there is broad agreement in the literature. It is mostly the same as we have published elsewhere (Peatfield 1992), but with additions and omissions, based on more up-to-date reports. There are other sites suggested recently as peak sanctuaries (Nowicki, 2007), which we have not yet personally examined. More broadly, the theme of this paper precludes detailed discussion on topographic terminology and function.

2 Rutkowski, who restudied the Petsophas figurines, was also aware of the methodological difficulty of distinguishing between these two potential categories: 1) heads made as detached offerings; 2) heads which had become detached from complete figurines (Rutkowski 1991, 33).

3 Suggestions for other body parts include a liver or womb (Rutkowski 1991, 116), and possible embryos (Arnott 1999, 3).

4 We thank him for sharing this info with us (pers. comm. April 2009).

5 Piskokephalo is described as a peak sanctuary by Velegrakis *et al.* (1993) and elsewhere in the literature, but it does not display the combined topographic and finds features which are considered characteristic of these sites.

Bibliography

Arnott, R. 1999: 'Healing cult in Minoan Crete', 1–6 in P. P. Betancourt, V. Karageorghis, R. Laffineur and W.-D. Niemeier (eds), *Meletemata: Studies in Aegean Archaeology Presented to Malcolm H. Wiener as he enters his 65th Year* (Aegaeum 20), Liège, Austin.

Arnott, R. forthcoming, *Disease, Healing and Medicine in the Aegean Bronze Age*, Leiden.

Branigan, K. 1970: 'Minoan foot amulets and their Eastern counterparts', *Studi Micenei ed Egeo-Anatolici* 11, 7–23.

Chryssoulaki, S. 2001: 'The Traostalos peak sanctuary: aspects of spatial organization', 57–66 in R. Hägg and R. Laffineur (eds), *Potnia. Deities and Religion in the Aegean Bronze Age* (Aegaeum 22), Liège, Austin.

Davaras, C. 1976: *Guide to Cretan Antiquities*, Park Ridge, NJ.

Davaras, C. n.d.: *Hagios Nikolaos Museum*, Athens.

de Waele, F. J. 1933: 'The sanctuary of Asklepios and Hygieia at Corinth', *American Journal of Archaeology* 37, 417–51.

Dietrich, B. C. 1969: 'Peak cults and their place in Minoan religion', *Historia: Zeitschrift für Alte Geschichte* 18, 257–75.

Dietrich, B. C. 1974: *The Origins of Greek Religion*, Berlin.

Dubisch, J. 1995: *In a Different Place: Pilgrimage, Gender, and Politics at a Greek Island Shrine*, Princeton.

Egan, M. 1991: *Milagros. Votive Offerings from the Americas*, Santa Fe.

Elderkin, K. 1930: 'Jointed dolls in antiquity', *American Journal of Archaeology* 34, 455–79.

Evans, A. J. 1928: *The Palace of Minos at Knossos*, Vol. 1, London.

Fenelli, M. 1975: 'Contributo per lo studio del votivo anatomico: i votivi anatomici di Lavinio', *Archeologia Classica* 27, 206–52.

Francis, D. 2007: *Faith and Transformation: Votive Offerings and Amulets from the Alexander Girard Collection*, Santa Fe.

Karetsou, 1974: Καρέτσου, Α.: 'Το ιερό κορυφής του Γιούχτα', *Praktika tes en Athenais Archaiologikes Hetaireias*, 228–39.

Karetsou, 1975: Καρέτσου, Α.: 'Το ιερό κορυφής του Γιούχτα', *Praktika tes en Athenais Archaiologikes Hetaireias*, 330–42.

Karetsou, 1976: Καρέτσου, Α.: 'Το ιερό κορυφής του Γιούχτα', *Praktika tes en Athenais Archaiologikes Hetaireias*, 408–18.

Karetsou, 1977: Καρέτσου, Α.: 'Το ιερό κορυφής του Γιούχτα', *Praktika tes en Athenais Archaiologikes Hetaireias*, 419–20.

Karetsou, 1980: Καρέτσου, Α.: 'Το ιερό κορυφής του Γιούχτα', *Praktika tes en Athenais Archaiologikes Hetaireias*, 232–58.

Karetsou, 1981a: Καρέτσου, Α.: 'Το ιερό κορυφής του Γιούχτα', *Praktika tes en Athenais Archaiologikes Hetaireias*, 405–8.

Karetsou, A. 1981b: 'The peak sanctuary of Mt Juktas', 137–53 in R. Hägg and N. Marinatos (eds), *Sanctuaries and Cults in the Aegean Bronze Age, Proceedings of the First International Symposium at the Swedish Institute in Athens, 12–13 May 1980*, Stockholm.

Karetsou, 1984: Καρέτσου, Α.: 'Το ιερό κορυφής του Γιούχτα', *Praktika tes en Athenais Archaiologikes Hetaireias*, 600–14.

Lang, M. 1977: *Cure and Cult in Ancient Corinth: a Guide to the Asklepieion*, Princeton.

Lesk, A. L. 2002: 'The anatomical votive terracotta phenomenon in Central Italy: complexities of the Corinthian connection', 193–202 in G. Muskett, A. Koltsida and M. Georgiadis (eds), *SOMA 2001 Symposium on Mediterranean Archaeology*, Oxford.

MacGillivray, J. A., Driessen J. M. and Sackett, L. H. 2000: *The Palaikastro Kouros: A Minoan Chryselephantine Statuette and its Aegean Bronze Age Context*, British School at Athens, London.

Morris, C. E. and Batten, V. 2000: 'Final Neolithic pottery from the Atsipadhes Korakias peak sanctuary', *Proceedings of the 8th Cretological Conference, Iraklion 1996*, 373–82.

Morris, C. E. and Peatfield, A. A. D. 1995: 'Pottery from the peak sanctuary of Atsipadhes Korakias, Ay. Vasiliou, Rethymnon,' *Proceedings of the 7th International Cretological Congress, Rethymnon, August 1990*, 643–7.

Myres, J. L. 1902–3: 'Excavations at Palaikastro. II. The sanctuary-site of Petsofà', *Annual of the British School at Athens* 9, 356–87.

Nilsson, M. P. 1950 [1927]: *The Minoan-Mycenaean Religion and its Survival in Greek Religion*, Lund.

Nolan, M. L. and Nolan, S. 1989: *Christian Pilgrimage in Modern Western Europe*, Chapel Hill.

Nowicki, K. 2007: 'Some remarks on new peak sanctuaries in Crete: the topography of ritual areas and their relationship with settlements', *Jahrbuch des Deutschen Archäologischen Instituts* 122, 1–31.

Oktavec, E. 1995: *Answered Prayers: Miracles and Milagros along the Border*, Tuscon.

Peatfield, A. A. D. 1983: 'The topography of Minoan peak sanctuaries', *Annual of the British School at Athens* 78, 273–80.

Peatfield, A. A. D. 1987: 'Palace and peak: the political and religious relationship between palaces and peak sanctuaries', 89–93 in R. Hägg and N. Marinatos (eds), *The Function of the Minoan Palaces*, Stockholm.

Peatfield, A. A. D. 1990: 'Minoan peak sanctuaries: history and society', *Opuscula Atheniensia* 18, 117–31.

Peatfield, A. A. D. 1992: 'Rural ritual in Bronze Age Crete: the peak sanctuary at Atsipadhes', *Cambridge Archaeological Journal* 2:1, 59–87.

Peatfield, A. 1994: 'After the "Big Bang" – What? or Minoan symbols and shrines beyond Palatial collapse', 19–36 in S. E. Alcock and R. Osborne (eds), *Placing the Gods: Greek Sanctuaries in Space*, Oxford.

Pini, I. 1972: 'Weitere Bemerkung zu den minoischen Fuss-amuletten', *Studi Micenei ed Egeo-Anatolici* 15, 179–88.

Potter, T. W. and Wells, C. 1985: 'A Republican healing sanctuary at Ponte di Nona near Rome and the Classical tradition of votive medicine', *Journal of the British Archaeological Association* 138, 23–47.

Rouse, W. D. 1902: *Greek Votive Offerings*, Cambridge.

Rutkowski, B. 1972: *Cult Places in the Aegean World*, Warsaw.

Rutkowski, B. 1986: *The Cult Places of the Aegean*, New Haven.

Rutkowski, B. 1991: *Petsophas. A Cretan Peak Sanctuary*, Warsaw.

Rutter, J. n.d.: The Prehistoric Archaeology of the Aegean http://projectsx.dartmouth.edu/history/bronze_age/lessons/les/15.html (accessed July 15th 2009).

Simon, C. G. 1986: *The Archaic Votive Offerings and Cults of Ionia*. PhD thesis, University of California, Berkeley.

Teske, R. T. 1980: *Votive Offerings among Greek-Philadelphians: a Ritual Perspective*, Ayer, New Hampshire.

Turfa, J. M. 1994: 'Anatomical votives and Italian medical traditions', 224–40 in R. D. De Puma and J. P. Small (eds), *Murlo and the Etruscans: Art and Society in Ancient Etruria*, Madison.

Turfa, J. M. 2006: 'Votive offerings in Etruscan religion', 90–115 in N. T. De Grummond and E. Simon (eds), *The Religion of the Etruscans*, Austin.

Tzedakis, Y. and Martlew, H. (eds) 1999: *Minoans and Mycenaeans. Flavours of their Time*, Athens.

Van Straten, F. T. 1981: 'Gifts for the gods', 65–151 in H. S. Versnel (ed.), *Faith, Hope and Worship. Aspects of Religious Mentality in the Ancient World*, Leiden.

Velegrakis, G., Skoulakis, C., Bizakis, J., Segas, J. and Helidonis, E. 1993: 'Otorhinolaryngological diseases in the Minoan era', *Journal of Laryngology and Otology* 107, 879–82.

Vidal, T. 1974: *Los milagros en metal y en cera de Puerto Rico*, San Juan de Puerto Rico.

Watrous, L. V. 1995: 'Some observations on Minoan peak sanctuaries', 393–403 in R. Laffineur and W.-D. Niemeier (eds), *Politeia: Society and State in the Aegean Bronze Age* (Aegaeum 12), Liège, Austin.

8. Medical Knowledge on the Evidence of the *Iliad*

Tamar Sukhishvili

The paper focuses on the details of ancient medical knowledge and practice on the evidence of Homeric epic. Besides, it discusses Homeric epic as the earliest Greek literary source of the popular somatic vocabulary. The paper deals with the contextual uses of the somatic terms in the Iliad *with a special emphasis on the battle scenes. Homeric battle episodes contain valuable information on medical knowledge, including healing methods, detailed depictions of body parts/organs (as well as battle wounds), their functions, emotional motions of the body, etc. The poem provides important material for both the history of medicine and lexicology.*

The aim of the paper is to demonstrate the importance of Homeric anatomical (somatic) vocabulary for the history of ancient medicine and lexicology. Greek medical (anatomical) terminology standardised in Hippocratic writings and philosophic works and eventually providing a basis for the international anatomical terminology, emerged from the popular Greek vocabulary (Lloyd 1983, 149–68). Homeric epic is the earliest Greek literary source of the popular somatic terminology. The study of the rich anatomical vocabulary on the evidence of Homeric epic is noteworthy not only to get some information about ancient medical knowledge and practice but also to define lexical meanings and their motivations in the language. Thus, these poems provide important material for both the history of ancient medicine and lexicology. The study of somatic words concentrates mainly on two aspects: contemplating the uses of somatic words to collect information about the popular medical knowledge of the Homeric epoch in general, and revealing the values and functions of body parts and anatomical organs in daily life and human knowledge to demonstrate how these functions and meanings are reflected in phraseology.

The contextual uses of the somatic words in the *Iliad* are as follows: battles, daily scenes/ritual activities (with a special emphasis on the uses of somatic words during prayer, supplication and sacrifice), passages expressing gestures, emotions or some features of the characters, and passages depicting the acts of oath and curse (Gould 2001, 22–78; Pulleyn 1997, 56–70). Somatic words appear to be used very frequently in the battle scenes. These passages are especially interesting in respect of studying medical knowledge of those times. They prove that people had already gained quite important medical experience and accumulated knowledge about human anatomy, functions of the anatomical organs, about emotional motions of the body. The analysis of Homeric battle scenes shows the following results:

1. The battle passages present precise anatomical delineations: naturalistic scenes of inflicting/receiving wounds followed by detailed depiction of wounded body parts or organs, sometimes similar to the common anatomical descriptions referring to the location of a body part and specifying it afterwards by means of isolated words or subordinate clauses, with an appropriate nomination: struck upon the head above the ear – τὸν ῥ᾽ ἔβαλεν κεφαλὴν ὑπὲρ οὔατος ὀξέϊ χαλκῷ… (*Il.* 15.433); struck on the hip, where the thigh turns in the hip joint, that is called the cup, and crushed the cup-bone and broke the sinews:

> τῷ βάλεν Αἰνείαο κατ᾽ ἰσχίον, ἔνθα τε μηρὸς
> ἰσχίῳ ἐντρέφεται, κοτύλην δέ τέ μιν καλέουσι·
> θλάσσε δέ οἱ κοτύλην, πρὸς δ᾽ ἄμφω ῥῆξη τένοντε…
> (*Il.* 5.305–7).

Table 8.1

Somatic Name	*Location*
heart hJ kradivh	in the breast to; sth`qo~ (*Il.* 13.439)
breast to; sth`qo~	between shoulders oJ w\mo~ (*Il.* 5.41)
breast oJ mazov~	close to shoulder oJ w\mo~ (*Il.* 5.147)
spine oJ nw`to~	ties with shoulder oJ w\mo~ (*Il.* 5.147)
lung oJ pneuvmwn	behind the breast oJ mazov~ (*Il.* 4.528)
sinew of the head to; ijnivon th`~ kefalh`~S	behind tongue and teeth hJ glw`ssa, oJ ojdouv~ (*Il.* 5.74)
buttock oJ gloutov~	behind the bladder hJ kuvsti~ (*Il.* 5.66)

Sometimes there is a reference not only to the location of a body part/anatomical organ, but also to its functions, as discussed below in more detail.

2. Anatomical information disseminated throughout the poem gives us the possibility to develop a certain kind of micro-schemes of human anatomy. A small number of examples can be found in Table 8.1.

3. During the war serious damage to the following body parts causes death: temple ἡ κόρση (*Il.* 4.502), right breast τὸ στῆθος δεξίον (*Il.* 4.480), navel ὁ ὀμφαλός (*Il.* 4.525), neck ὁ αὐχήν (*Il.* 5.658, 10.456), liver τὸ ἧπαρ (*Il.* 11.579, 13.412, 17.349), windpipe ὁ ἀσφάραγος (*Il.* 13.388), carotid artery ἡ φλέψ that goes along the back (ὁ νῶτος, τὸ νῶτον) until it reaches the neck ὁ αὐχήν (*Il.* 13.546), joining (ὁ συνεοχμός) of head (ἡ κεφαλή) and neck (ὁ αὐχήν) on the topmost joint of the spine (ὁ ἀστράγαλος) (*Il.* 14.465–6), head above the ear ἡ κεφαλὴ ὑπὲρ οὔατος (*Il.* 15.433), etc.

4. The depictions of body parts/anatomical organs we encounter in the *Iliad* are in some instances similar to the passages from the medical treatises dealing with the reasons, nature and symptoms of the diseases. Homeric episodes usually include warning/advice as well as depictions of the somatic parts; warning: μάλιστα δὲ καίριόν ἐστιν, it is the fatal spot:

> (βάλε) ἄκρην κὰκ κορυφήν, ὅθι τε πρῶται τρίχες ἵππων κρανίῳ ἐμπεφύασι, μάλιστα δὲ καίριόν ἐστιν (*Il.* 8.83–4).

> …τὸν δ᾽ αὖ κορυθαίολος Ἕκτωρ
> αὐερύοντα παρ᾽ ὦμον, ὅθι κληῒς ἀποέργει
> αὐχένα τε στῆθός τε, μάλιστα δὲ καίριόν ἐστιν (*Il.* 8.324–6).

Moreover, in certain examples these warnings contain a strong reference to the vital importance of body parts:

> βέβληαι οὐδ᾽ ἅλιον βέλος ἔκφυγεν· ὡς ὄφελόν τοι
> νείατον ἐς κενεῶνα βαλὼν ἐκ θυμὸν ἑλέσθαι (*Il.* 11.380–1).

> ἀσπίδες ὅσσαι ἄρισαι ἐνὶ στρατῷ ἠδὲ μέγισται
> ἑσσάμενοι, κεφαλὰς δὲ παναίθῃσιν κορύθεσσι
> κρύψαντες (*Il.* 14.371–3).

5. There are also other passages to consider. Some episodes in the Iliad (books 4, 11, 15) speak of the healing practice with pain-killing drugs (mainly plants), i.e. cleaning of the battle wound, washing off blood with warm water and putting φάρμακον or chopped bitter root afterwards:

> ἀλλ᾽ ἐμὲ μὲν σὺ σάωσον ἄγων ἐπὶ νῆα μέλαιναν,
> μηροῦ δ᾽ ἔκταμ᾽ ὀϊστόν, ἀπ᾽ αὐτοῦ δ᾽ αἷμα κελαινὸν
> νίζ᾽ ὕδατι λιαρῷ, ἐπὶ δ᾽ ἤπια φάρμακα πάσσε… (*Il.* 11.828–30).

> ἔνθά μιν ἐκτανύσας ἐκ μηροῦ τάμνε μαχαίρῃ
> ὀξὺ βέλος περιπευκές, ἀπ᾽ αὐτοῦ δ᾽ αἷμα κελαινὸν
> νίζ᾽ ὕδατι λιαρῷ, ἐπὶ δὲ ῥίζαν βάλε πικρήν… (*Il.* 11.844–6).

These passages prove that the uses of plants marked out for their special qualities were the subject of intense interest from the earliest times. In a famous passage in the *Odyssey* (10.302), where Hermes gives Odysseus an antidote to those Circe used to turn men into beasts, he digs up a plant with a black root (Lloyd 1983, 119).

6. Apart from the battle episodes, the passages displaying somatic reflections (i.e. reflections on a physical level) of the emotions are of a special interest. Severe excitement (i.e. fear) usually stirs up these emotions, makes the heart tremble and increases the speed of palpitations. A person who suffers these emotions is stammering and pale with fear and the teeth chattered in his mouth: ὁ δ᾽ ἄρ᾽ ἔστη τάρβησέν τε βαμβαίνων – ἄραβος δὲ διὰ στόμα γίγνετ᾽ ὀδόντων – χλωρὸς ὑπαὶ δείους… (*Il.* 10.374–6), his limbs tremble beneath him – τρομέει δ᾽ ὑπὸ φαίδιμα γυῖα (*Il.* 10.95), ὑπὸ δ᾽ἔτρεμε γυῖα (*Il.* 10.390), his colour changes, χρὼς ἄλλυδις ἄλλῃ (*Il.* 13.279), the sweat flows down from his head and shoulders, κατὰ δὲ νότιος ῥέεν ἱδρὼς ὤμων καὶ κεφαλῆς (*Il.* 11.811–12), grief enfolds his eyes, κρατερόν ῥά ἑ πένθος ὀφθαλμοὺς ἐκάλυψε κασιγνήτοιο πεσόντος (*Il.* 11.249–50). Hence Homer paints a vivid portrait of an

anxious/nervous man. In the *Iliad,* 13 comparative characteristics of the two personages, brave and cowardly men, are based on natural somatic reflections:

τοῦ μέν γὰρ τε κακοῦ τρέπεται χρῶς ἄλλυδις ἄλλη,
οὐδὲ οἱ ἀτρέμας ἧσθαι ἐρητύετ' ἐν φρεσὶ θυμός,
ἀλλὰ μετοκλάζει καὶ ἐπ' ἀμφοτέρους πόδας ἵζει.
ἐν δέ τέ οἱ κραδίη μεγάλα στέρνοισι πατάσσει
κῆρας ὀϊομένῳ, πάταγος δέ τε γίγνετ' ὀδόντων·
τοῦ δ' ἀγαθοῦ οὔτ' ἄρ τρέπεται χρὼς οὔτέ τι λίην
ταρβεῖ, ἐπειδὰν πρῶτον ἐσίζηται λόχον ἀνδρῶν (*Il.* 13.279–85).

7. Another passage (the one concerning Hector's death) that seems obviously important considering ancient medical knowledge of Homeric times, drops a hint at an articulatory function of a windpipe/throat. In book 22 of the *Iliad,* Achilles kills Hector with a spear to his neck, but he acts in a very careful way, he tries not to harm his windpipe/throat (ὁ ἀσφάραγος) to the end that he might speak and leave his last words before he dies:

ἀντικρὺ δ' ἁπαλοῖο δι' αὐχένος ἤλυθ' ἀκωκή·
οὐδ' ἄρ' ἀπ' ἀσφαράγον μελίη τάμε χαλκοβάρεια,
ὄφρα τί μιν προτιείποι ἀμειβόμενος ἐπέεσσιν (*Il.* 22.327–9).

It might be proposed that people in the Homeric epoch were already aware of the information about voice apparatus and about the results of its possible damage, destroying the human articulatory function.

8. When studying somatic vocabulary in Homer we cannot avoid the blood motif, one of the most important motives in the *Iliad* that has long been the subject of investigations for scholars (Neal 2006, 15–33). There are many references to blood in Homer. In this instance the paper considers the definitions of the two terms, αἷμα and ἰχώρ in the *Iliad.* Αἷμα means 'blood' in general, and ἰχώρ is 'immortal blood', 'rotten blood', juice that flows in the veins of the gods (Liddell and Scott 1968, 846; Ebeling 1885, 49–50; Frisk 1960, 747; Snell 1991, 1266). Ἰχώρ is used only twice in the *Iliad* (*Il.* 5.340, 5.416). Blood flows from the wound of the goddess Aphrodite but that is not an ordinary blood, i.e. the mortal blood, that is immortal blood – ἄμβροτον αἷμα (this word combination is repeated only one more time in *Il.* 5.870 referring to the wound of the god Ares). In the first passage (*Il.* 5.340) the author of the *Iliad* tries to be precise in giving definition of the meaning of ἰχώρ, noting that it is not mortal blood – it is some specific juice that flows in the body of the gods. In the second passage (*Il.* 5.416) that actually follows the first one, mother Dione takes care of Aphrodite her daughter and cleans her wound, washing ἰχώρ flowing from it. The etymology of the word ἰχώρ is unknown (Boisacq 1950, 388). In the later texts, in the works of Plato, Aristotle and the Hippocratic writings, this word is synonymous with lymph or serum, though in Aeschilles' *Agamemnon* (1480) it is a synonym for blood, αἷμα (Kirk 1985, ad.5.340; Frisk 1960, 747). It is noteworthy how this word is reconstructed on the Indo-European level. The scholars Th. Gamkrelidze and V. Ivanov focus on the traces of lexical connections of the two linguistic areas of Greece and Asia Minor and provide a list of words presumably borrowed from the languages of Asia Minor by the Greek dialects. Ἰχώρ is also included in the list: Greek. Hom. ἰχώρ 'immortal blood of the gods', later 'blood': cf. Hitt. ešhar, išhar 'blood' (Gamkrelidze and Ivanov 1984, 902). Thus, the choice of the term ἰχώρ dealing with Asia Minor for denoting the immortal blood of Aphrodite, the goddess with non-Greek origin, might not be fortuitous.

The study of meanings of these words, αἷμα and ἰχώρ also leads us to the question concerning how to define the differences between man and god, i.e. between mortal and immortal. In the 'well-known passage elucidating immortal difference' (Neal 2006, 27) the answer to this question is based first of all upon the pure physiological level. In book 5 Homer depicts the gods as follows: they do not eat bread (σῖτος) and do not drink wine (οἶνος), hence they are bloodless – ἀναίμονες (*Il.* 5.340–2), and therefore, they are not humans (ἄμβροτοι), they are immortals (ἀθάνατοι):

οὐ γὰρ σῖτον ἔδουσ', οὐ πίνουσ' αἴθοπα οἶνον·
τούνεκ' ἀναίμονές εἰσι καὶ ἀθάνατοι καλέονται (*Il.* 5.341–2).

It might be suggested that the opposition mortal-immortal is based on the knowledge about physiological functions of blood, with an emphasis on the digestive function among them: mortal – eats – has blood, immortal – does not eat – does not have blood.

The investigation of the somatic words in Homeric epic reveals many important details that are valuable not only from the perspective of medical studies. The observation of the Greek somatic/anatomical terms, which eventually created a basis for medical terminology, gives us the reason for the proposition that the process of transformation (from popular nomenclature into technical/medical terminology) had already been started in the Homeric language (Benett 1978, 60–1). Hence, Homeric epic shows signs of terminological formations, i.e. reference to the body parts/organs by means of descriptive definition: οὐτάμεναι πρὸς στῆθος, ὅθι φρένες ἧπαρ ἔχουσι... strike in the breast where the midriff holds the liver... (*Od.* 9.301). A descriptive definition for a carotid artery also draws one's attention: the vein that runs along the back until it reaches the neck: ἀπὸ δὲ φλέβα πᾶσαν, ἥ τ' ἀνὰ νῶτα θέουσα διαμπερὲς αὐχέν' ἱκάνει... (*Il.* 13.546–7). And here are some more examples of the descriptive formations using the adjective πρυμνός, ή, όν denoting the lowest part, hindmost, undermost, endmost: πρυμνὸς ραχίων – upper part of an arm close to shoulder, πρυμνὴ γλῶσσα – the lowest part of a tongue, πρυμνὸς θέναρος – edge of a palm of a hand, etc. (Liddell and Scott 1968, 1543). The examples given above show that there are no special lexical units for denoting some body parts, i.e.

parts of the extremities, etc. and in this instance Homeric language successfully applies the descriptive method of word formation. However, anatomical terms are notably indeterminate or imprecise even in the medical texts (Lloyd 1983, 153–4). Apart from highlighting medical information provided in Homeric poems the study of Homeric anatomical terms regarding their lexical peculiarities and motivations also seems very important.

Bibliography

Benett, S. 1978: *Mind and Madness in Ancient Greece. The Classical Roots of Modern Psychiatry,* Ithaca and London.

Boisacq, É. 1950: *Dictionnaire étymologique de la Langue grecque. Étudiée dans ses rapports avec les autres langues indo-européennes,* 4ᵉ éd., Heidelberg.

Ebeling, H. (ed.) 1885: *Lexicon Homericvm*, Vol. I, Leipzig.

Frisk, H. 1960: *Griechisches etymologisches Wörterbuch*, Band I, Heidelberg.

Gamkrelidze, Th. and Ivanov, V. 1984: *Indo-European and Indo-Europeans. A Reconstruction and Historical Typological Analysis of a Protolanguage and a Proto-Culture,* (2 vols), Tbilisi.

Gould, J. 2001: *Myth, Ritual, Memory and Exchange. Essays in Greek Literature and Culture*, Oxford.

Kirk, G. S. (ed.) 1985: *The Iliad: A Commentary* (6 vols), vol. II, Cambridge.

Liddell, H. G., Scott, R. and Jones, H. S. (eds) 1968: *A Greek-English Lexicon*, Oxford.

Lloyd, G. E. R. 1983: *Science, Folklore and Ideology: Studies in the Life Sciences in Ancient Greece*, Cambridge.

Neal, T. 2006: 'Blood and hunger in the Iliad', *Classical Philology* 101, 15–33.

Pulleyn, S. 1997: *Prayer in Greek Religion*, Oxford.

Snell, B. 1979–91: *Lexikon des frühgriechischen Epos begründet von Bruno Snell*, Band 1 1979, Band 2 1991, Göttingen.

Part IV

Medical Authors / Schools of Medicine

9. Αναζητώντας Ίχνη του Ιπποκρατικού Όρκου

Δημήτριος Λυπουρλής

The authenticity of the Oath, which has been delivered to us in the context of the Corpus Hippocraticum, *has been debated by a large number of Hippocratists since the publication of the* Corpus *by É. Littré in the middle of the 19th century. The view expressed in 1943 by the pioneering Hippocratist L. Edelstein that this text is the work of a Pythagorean doctor of the second half of the 4th century BC, a totally revolutionary view for its time, has since found a substantial number of supporters. This view in itself implies the existence of an earlier/initial Hippocratic text, which was addressed to the doctors of the immediate circle of the great Coan. The paper presents part of the author's latest research in this field, which is based on a very interesting narration by Herodotus regarding a famous ancient doctor, Dekomedes of Croton in Magna Grecia.*

Δεν είναι ίσως άσκοπο να αρχίσω με μερικές γενικές πληροφορίες – μπορεί και να είναι χρήσιμες σε μερικούς από τους ακροατές μου.

Πληροφορία πρώτη: Με το όνομα του Κώου γιατρού Ιπποκράτη μάς παραδόθηκαν από την αρχαιότητα 60 περίπου έργα ιατρικού περιεχομένου. Στα έργα αυτά ως σύνολο αναφερόμαστε με τον όρο «Ιπποκρατική Συλλογή». Μπορούμε, ωστόσο, να είμαστε βέβαιοι ότι για διάφορους λόγους, που δεν είναι του παρόντος να τους αναφέρουμε, τα έργα αυτά δεν είναι δυνατό να προέρχονται όλα τους από τον «πατέρα της ιατρικής».

Πληροφορία δεύτερη: Ένα από τα έργα αυτά, το πιο μικρό από όλα τους, σίγουρα, πάντως, το πιο γνωστό από όλα, είναι ο *Όρκος*. «Το πιο μικρό», μαζί όμως και το πιο προβληματικό από όλα τα έργα της Συλλογής. Κάθε, πράγματι, φράση του κειμένου αυτού έγινε – χρόνια τώρα – αντικείμενο εξονυχιστικότατης διερεύνησης. Και το αποτέλεσμα; Γνώμες επί γνωμών. «So viele Kőpfe, so viele Meinungen», όπως είπε ένας μεγάλος Γερμανός φιλόλογος σε μιαν άλλη, ανάλογη περίσταση (Schadewaldt 1955).

Πληροφορία τρίτη: Το κύριο, βέβαια, ερώτημα είναι: Τι είναι βασικά ο *Όρκος*; Σχετίζεται πράγματι το κείμενο αυτό με τον Ιπποκράτη; Ένα πράγμα, πάντως, μπορεί να είναι απόλυτα σίγουρο: ότι το κείμενο αυτό είναι ασφαλώς η παλαιότερη, αλλά και η πιο σημαντική μαρτυρία ιατρικής ηθικής και δεοντολογίας, ένας ανεπανάληπτος οδηγός ιατρικής συμπεριφοράς.

Πληροφορία τέταρτη, ασφαλώς η σπουδαιότερη: Δύο είναι οι κύριες ερμηνευτικές γραμμές που ακολούθησε στις μέρες μας η σχετική με τον *Όρκο* έρευνα:

Σε ένα λαμπρό άρθρο του στα 1932 ο Karl Deichgräber παρουσίασε τις σκέψεις του για την *Ιατρική επαγγελματική ηθική του ιπποκρατικού όρκου*. Στην πραγματικότητα το άρθρο αυτό ήταν το εναρκτήριο μάθημα που ο Deichgräber έκανε στο πανεπιστήμιο του Βερολίνου στις 28 Απριλίου του 1931. Με μια μεθοδική μελέτη της δομής του *Όρκου* ο Γερμανός φιλόλογος οδηγήθηκε στην πίστη ότι το κείμενο αυτό πρέπει να ανήκει στα τέλη του 5^{ου} αι. π.Χ. Η πίστη αυτή προήλθε βασικά από δύο παρατηρήσεις: α) Για τον Έλληνα αυτής της εποχής, και μάλιστα για τον Έλληνα της Ιωνίας, είναι ιδιαίτερα χαρακτηριστική η προσήλωση στην ιδέα της *δικαιοσύνης*, της αρετής που όταν την έχει κανείς είναι σαν να έχει όλες μαζί τις αρετές (*«ἐν δὲ δικαιοσύνῃ συλλήβδην πᾶσ' ἀρετή ἐστιν»*), που φαίνεται όμως (η αρετή αυτή) με έναν ιδιαίτερο τρόπο στην *εγκράτεια* και στη *σωφροσύνη*: αυτήν τη δικαιοσύνη, με το ιδιαίτερο αυτό περιεχόμενό της, είναι που διεκδικεί, κατά τον Deichgräber, για τον εαυτό του και ο γιατρός του *Όρκου*. β) Η ηθική του *Όρκου* είναι, κατά τον Deichgräber, βασικά η απολλώνια ηθική, αφού η αγνότητα που θέλει για τον εαυτό του ο γιατρός είναι εκείνη ακριβώς που αποτελεί το ιδιαίτερο γνώρισμα του θεού Απόλλωνα· η έννοια «δίκαιος ιατρός» συμπίπτει, στην περίπτωση του *Όρκου*, με την έννοια «απολλώνιος γιατρός».

Τη δεύτερη ερμηνευτική γραμμή τη χάραξε ο πιο ρηξικέλευθος ιπποκρατιστής των νεότερων χρόνων, σύγχρονος του Deichgräber, ο Ludwig Edelstein, που με μια προσεκτικότατη ερμηνεία των επιμέρους προτάσεων του *Όρκου* και με μια αυστηρή ανάλυση της δομής του οδηγήθηκε στην πίστη ότι ο *Όρκος* έχει από την αρχή ως το τέλος του μια συνεπέστατη ενότητα και ότι η μορφή με την οποία τον έχουμε εμείς σήμερα είναι έργο ενός πυθαγόρειου γιατρού του δεύτερου μισού του 4ου αι. π.Χ. Δεν έχω, δυστυχώς, τον χρόνο, ούτε θα το θεωρούσα σκόπιμο να αναφέρω τα επιχειρήματα με τα οποία ο Edelstein στήριξε τη θεωρία του, βιάζομαι, ωστόσο, να δηλώσω ότι προσωπικά είμαι, από χρόνια τώρα, με το μέρος της δεύτερης αυτής ερμηνευτικής γραμμής. Είναι, τότε, φανερό ότι οι απαγορεύσεις που διαβάζουμε στον *Όρκο* είναι, κατά την ερμηνεία του Edelstein, υπαγορευμένες από μιαν ορισμένη φιλοσοφική διδασκαλία: στην πραγματικότητα ο γιατρός που δίνει στον όρκο του τις συγκεκριμένες υποσχέσεις ενεργεί με αυτόν τον τρόπο επειδή επιθυμεί να τηρήσει πιστά τους κανόνες που του ορίζει η φιλοσοφική διδασκαλία την οποία έχει ασπασθεί και στην οποία ανήκει.

(Μια παρενθετική σημείωση δεν είναι ίσως εδώ άσκοπη – ίσα ίσα για να υπενθυμίσουμε ότι τον αρχαίο αυτό όρκο τον συναντούμε και σε διάφορες άλλες, παραλλαγμένες μορφές, σε πεζό και ποιητικό λόγο, στους ελληνιστικούς και στους αυτοκρατορικούς χρόνους, στους Ρωμαίους και στους Χριστιανούς, στους Άραβες, στον Μεσαίωνα, στις δικές μας τέλος μέρες – και είναι πολύ φυσικό το ότι σε όλες αυτές τις μορφές συναντούμε στοιχεία που συνάδουν προς το ιδιαίτερο περιβάλλον μέσα στο οποίο ζει ο ορκιζόμενος γιατρός και σε συνάφεια προς το οποίο θα ασκήσει αύριο το ιατρικό του έργο.)

✢✢✢

Αν η άποψη του Ludwig Edelstein για την προέλευση του *Όρκου* είναι, όπως ο ίδιος – μαζί, βέβαια, με πολλούς άλλους – πιστεύω, η πιο σωστή, τότε ο *Όρκος*, το κείμενο που μας σώθηκε ως ένα από τα έργα της λεγόμενης «Ιπποκρατικής Συλλογής», προήλθε από κύκλους ολότελα διαφορετικούς από τους κύκλους των ιατρικών σχολών της Κω και της Κνίδου, που εκπροσωπούνται σ' αυτήν τη «Συλλογή». Μόνο με μια τέτοια παραδοχή μπορούν να λάβουν μια αξιόπιστη απάντηση ερωτήματα μπροστά στα οποία είχαν σταθεί αμήχανοι οι πριν από τον Edelstein μελετητές του *Όρκου*, αυτοί δηλαδή που πίστευαν ότι στον *Όρκο* καθρεφτίζεται η ιατρική του Ιπποκράτη και του κύκλου του· ερωτήματα π.χ. του τύπου «Πώς μπορεί να απαγορεύεται στον *Όρκο* η έκτρωση, τη στιγμή που αυτή ασκείται σε έργα της «Ιπποκρατικής Συλλογής;» ή «Γιατί ο γιατρός δεν πρέπει ποτέ να παίρνει στο χέρι του το μαχαίρι του χειρούργου, τη στιγμή που η «Ιπποκρατική Συλλογή» περιλαμβάνει τόσα χειρουργικά έργα και αφού τόσο συχνά γίνεται στα έργα που την αποτελούν λόγος για 'τομές'». Αν όμως λάβει κανείς υπόψη του ότι οι Πυθαγόρειοι αισθάνονταν αποστροφή για το ρέον αίμα και ότι θεωρούσαν την αφαίρεση της ζωής, με όποιον τρόπο και αν γινόταν, αθέμιτη, τότε η απάντηση σ' αυτού του είδους τα ερωτήματα δεν είναι και τόσο δύσκολη: Ο *Όρκος* ήταν για γιατρούς που είχαν τις ίδιες με τον συντάκτη του αντιλήψεις.

Μια τέτοια, βέβαια, διατύπωση θα πει ότι ο *Όρκος* είναι ένα καθαρά ιστορικό μνημείο, και αυτό πάλι με τη σειρά του θα πει ότι ο *Όρκος* γεννήθηκε από μια ιστορική πραγματικότητα, που πια δεν μπορεί με κανέναν τρόπο να επαναληφθεί ολόιδια. Όμως, από την άλλη, ο *Όρκος* σώθηκε στο πέρασμα των αιώνων, κάτι που, βέβαια, δεν θα είχε γίνει, αν το περιεχόμενό του δεν είχε αξία υπερχρονική. Πρέπει τάχα να μιλήσουμε, τότε, για μια αντίφαση; Σίγουρα όχι, αν δεχτούμε ότι ο *Όρκος* νίκησε τον χρόνο όχι τόσο λόγω της αξίας των επιμέρους προτάσεών του όσο λόγω της αξίας των βασικών, των θεμελιωδών αρχών από τις οποίες πήγασαν οι επιμέρους αυτές προτάσεις. Και ως τέτοιες μπορεί κανείς με απόλυτη σιγουριά να επισημάνει μέσα στο κείμενο αυτό τον σεβασμό προς τη ζωή, τον σεβασμό προς τον άρρωστο, τον σεβασμό προς την προσωπικότητα του αρρώστου, τον σεβασμό προς την επιστήμη και τους εργάτες της, την επιθυμία για διάκριση στην επιστήμη και στην κοινωνία μόνο με έντιμα και αξιοπρεπή μέσα, την άρνηση της εκμετάλλευσης των εύκολων περιστάσεων.

Νομίζω ότι μπορεί κανείς να είναι βέβαιος ότι σε τέτοιου είδους αρχές θα ήταν γερά θεμελιωμένος και ο παλαιότερος – που πρέπει αναμφίβολα να υπήρξε – καθαρά Ιπποκρατικός όρκος.

Για μια τέτοια υπόδειξη θέλησα να είναι ο λόγος μου στη σημερινή ανακοίνωσή μου. Τη βοήθεια μου την προσφέρει ο Ηρόδοτος, που στο τρίτο βιβλίο των *Ιστοριών* του μας μιλάει για έναν περίφημο, φαίνεται, στην αρχαιότητα γιατρό – περίφημο τουλάχιστο στον καθαρά επαγγελματικό τομέα –, τον Δημοκήδη από τον Κρότωνα της Μεγάλης Ελλάδας.

Δεν θα σας αναφέρω σήμερα εδώ όλες τις σχετικές με τον γιατρό αυτό πληροφορίες μας, που άσκησε με επιτυχία την τέχνη του στην Αίγινα, στην Αθήνα, στη Σάμο του Πολυκράτη προτού γίνει θεραπευτής του «Μεγάλου βασιλιά» της Περσίας, του γνωστού μας από τους Περσικούς πολέμους Δαρείου, κάτι που τον ανύψωσε τελικά σε ομοτράπεζό του. Δεν θα αναφερθώ σε όλες τις λεπτομέρειες, πρώτον γιατί, αν τις αναφέρω όλες, *«επιλείψει με»* ασφαλώς ο χρόνος, και δεύτερον γιατί δεν θα ήθελα να στερήσω από κανέναν σας την ευχαρίστηση να διαβάσει όλη τη σχετική διήγηση στο τρίτο, όπως σας είπα, βιβλίο των *Ιστοριών* του Ηροδότου (συγκεκριμένα στις παραγράφους 125 και 129–37).

Η λεπτομέρεια που λέω να μας απασχολήσει σήμερα εδώ σχετίζεται με μιαν αρρώστια της βασίλισσας Άτοσσας, της γυναίκας του βασιλιά (μας τη σκιαγράφησε, όπως θυμάστε, τόσο ωραία στους *Πέρσες* του ο Αισχύλος). Διηγείται λοιπόν ο Ηρόδοτος: «Η Άτοσσα, η κόρη του Κύρου και γυναίκα του Δαρείου, παρουσίασε ένα οίδημα στον μαστό της, που λίγο ύστερα έσπασε και απλωνόταν. Όσο το οίδημα ήταν μικρό, εκείνη το έκρυβε και από ντροπή δεν μιλούσε γι' αυτό σε κανέναν. Όταν όμως η κατάστασή της έγινε πολύ άσχημη, κάλεσε τον Δημοκήδη και του το έδειξε. Εκείνος της είπε ότι θα τη γιατρέψει και την έβαλε να ορκιστεί ότι και εκείνη, όμως, θα του κάνει όποια αντίχαρη της ζητήσει – και, φυσικά, της είπε, δεν επρόκειτο να της ζητήσει τίποτε από όσα φέρνουν ντροπή». Εύκολα, νομίζω, μπορεί κανείς να δεχτεί ότι η τελευταία φράση του Δημοκήδη – εντελώς, από κάποια άποψη, αφύσικη και άκομψη αυτή τη στιγμή στο στόμα του γιατρού της βασίλισσας – πρέπει να αποτελεί απήχηση της φράσης του *Όρκου* της «Ιπποκρατικής Συλλογής» «*Ἐς οἰκίας δὲ ὁκόσας ἂν ἐσίω, ἐσελεύσομαι ἐπ' ὠφελείῃ καμνόντων, ἐκτὸς ἐὼν πάσης ἀδικίης ἑκουσίης καὶ φθορίης, τῆς τε ἄλλης καὶ ἀφροδισίων ἔργων ἐπί τε γυναικείων σωμάτων καὶ ἀνδρῴων, ἐλευθέρων τε καὶ δούλων*» – μακριά, λοιπόν, θα μένω από κάθε πράξη αφροδισιακή πάνω σε σώματα γυναικεία ή αντρικά ελεύθερων ή σκλάβων.

Δεν πρέπει, κατά τη γνώμη μου, να υπάρχει καμιά αμφιβολία ότι την αφύσικη και άκομψη, όπως τη χαρακτηρίσαμε, φράση του γιατρού της βασίλισσας την έβαλε στο στόμα του ο ίδιος ο Ηρόδοτος που, ξέροντάς την από τον όρκο που έδιναν οι γιατροί της εποχής του, θέλησε με αυτήν να δηλώσει ότι ο γιατρός για τον οποίο ήταν ο λόγος του γνώριζε πολύ καλά και τηρούσε ευλαβικά τον βασικό αυτό κανόνα της ιατρικής δεοντολογίας.

Η εποχή όμως του Ηροδότου ήταν και του Ιπποκράτη η εποχή. Θα μπορούσε λοιπόν κανείς να υποστηρίξει – με πολλές ελπίδες ότι πετυχαίνει το σωστό – ότι πριν από την πυθαγορική, όπως πιστεύω και εγώ μαζί με τον Edelstein, μορφή του κειμένου του όρκου που έφτασε ως εμάς πρέπει να υπήρχε ένας άλλος όρκος, της εποχής του Ιπποκράτη αυτός, ή και παλαιότερος από τον μεγάλο γιατρό, που θα περιείχε και εκείνος την πρόταση που μας απασχολεί.

Αναφέρθηκα πρωτύτερα στις βασικές, τις θεμελιώδεις, όπως τις χαρακτήρισα, αρχές ιατρικής δεοντολογίας από τις οποίες πήγασαν, κατά τη γνώμη μου, οι συγκεκριμένες προτάσεις του *Όρκου* της «Ιπποκρατικής Συλλογής». Ως τελευταία ανάμεσά τους ανέφερα, όπως θα θυμάστε, την άρνηση κάθε εκμετάλλευσης των εύκολων περιστάσεων. Την αρχή αυτή αισθάνομαι ότι μπορώ, βασισμένος στη μαρτυρία του Ηροδότου, να θεωρήσω ότι την επισημάναμε και σε έναν όρκο παλαιότερο από τον *Όρκο* της «Ιπποκρατικής Συλλογής», που θα μπορούσε να είναι ο Ιπποκρατικός όρκος. Η έρευνα που συνεχίζω ελπίζω να οδηγήσει στην επισήμανση ότι στον παλαιότερο αυτό όρκο, τον όρκο των χρόνων του Ιπποκράτη, λειτουργούσαν και οι υπόλοιπες *θεμελιώδεις αρχές* ιατρικής δεοντολογίας που αναφέραμε – κάποιες όμως από τις συγκεκριμένες *προτάσεις* του *Όρκου* της λεγόμενης «Ιπποκρατικής Συλλογής» ασφαλώς δεν θα λειτουργούσαν στον παλαιότερο αυτό όρκο. Ας αρκεσθούμε, λοιπόν, σήμερα σ' αυτήν μόνο την επισήμανση, που ο ίδιος τη θεωρώ – εύλογα, ελπίζω, και κατά τη δική σας γνώμη – σημαντική.

Βιβλιογραφία

Deichgräber, K. 1932: 'Die ärztliche Standesethik des hippokratischen Eides', *Quellen und Studien zur Geschichte der Naturwissenschaften und der Medizin* 3, 1932, 29–49.

Edelstein, L. 1943: *The Hippocratic Oath: Text, Translation, and Interpretation*, Baltimore.

Schadewaldt, W. 1955: 'Furcht und Mitleid? Zur Deutung des Aristotelischen Tragödiensatzes', *Hermes* 83, 129–71 = pp. 246–88 in M. Luserke (ed.), *Die Aristotelische Katharsis. Dokumente ihrer Deutung im 19. und 20. Jahrhundert*, Hildesheim/New York 1991.

10. Echoing Hippocrates: Aspects of Genre Intertextuality in the 5th Century BC

Athina Papachrysostomou and Georgios Gazis

This paper identifies and traces aspects of the influence exercised by the Hippocratic corpus on the intellectual renaissance of the 5th century BC, and examines how this influence reveals itself through this era's literary works. Through a number of examples, we particularly highlight the specific aspects where the Hippocratic texts function as a stimulating impulse upon the developing arts and sciences of this period, e.g. upon historiography, philosophy and drama.

Introduction

Hippocrates of Cos proved to be a great and multifarious personality who continued exerting a vast influence over the ancient world even long after his death. It is assumed that he was born in the island of Cos around 460 BC. He came from the family of Asclepiades, a doctors' family, being their 19th descendant, according to the most reliable source. So he was a doctor, from a doctors' family and with a splendid background of eminent ancestors (Jouanna 1999, 14). The most renowned of them was Nevros who, participating in the first sacred war that was conducted by the Amphictyons against Krissa at the beginning of the 6th century, poisoned the potable water of that town, while his son was killed trying to climb up the walls. The oracle of Delphi honoured Nevros and with him the whole Asclepiades family for this contribution, by granting them the privilege of *promanteia* (the right of priority in oracular consultation).

With such a lineage, his initiation in medicine was expected to come from the side of his family, although several are the famous personages who claim to have been his instructors, such as Democritus and Gorgias. The strongest probability, however, lies in his father, Herakleides, being the first initiator in the secrets of medical art.

At an early age, Hippocrates left Cos for Thessaly, having already acquired a great deal of fame for his medicinal skills, and it was in Larissa where he was mostly active as a doctor, even if many of the cities of Thessaly are mentioned by the *Corpus Hippocraticum* as places where he cured his patients. From the books of the *Epidemics*, works that, according to Jouanna (1999, 388), were written in all probability by Hippocrates himself, we can deduce that he must also have visited northern Greece, because the place names that appear derive exclusively from this geographical region, the furthest limit of which reaches as far as Propontis. The evidence of his friendship with the Macedonian king Perdikkas argues for it.

Having travelled a great deal and with panhellenic recognition he died in Larissa between 375 and 351 BC. He had already left his indelible mark on the intellect of his time and this is further proved by the fact that he was declared a hero in later times and a cult was established in his name.

There are about 60 very interesting and diversified works attributed to Hippocrates. Today, it is ascertained that most of them could not have been written by Hippocrates himself, and there are many difficulties in identifying even those thought as most reliably to be his own work. In this article we will not concern ourselves with the identification or dating of the works included in the *Corpus Hippocraticum*. What we will attempt here will be to focus on the influence that this great doctor exerted with his art and his writings on the literary production of the 5th century. We are aware of the difficulties of this attempt, as well as of the possibility that many of our observations may be doubted. We are, however, convinced that an intertextual approach to the Hippocratic texts could contribute much in this direction and might above all elucidate the way in which medicine was viewed in Hippocrates' age, as well as the role that this science played in the creation of the Greek enlightenment.

Echoes of Hippocrates

When referring to the 5th century BC, we automatically evoke the golden age of Athens of Pericles, the Peloponnesian War and its documentation by Thucydides, the philosophical enquiries of Plato and the sophists, as well as the original creations of the major representatives of dramatic poetry. Faced with this prolific production of human intellect, it is hard to make time for the Hippocratic texts. The reasons why this happens are obvious since the *Corpus Hippocraticum* is not really a literary work, while its technical context keeps classicists away from ranking its study as a priority. However, it should not be overlooked that Hippocrates' contribution to medicine of the 5th century marked a revolutionary step in science, which may be regarded as equivalent to – or even greater than – the contribution of the Sophistic movement in philosophy.

The medical achievements of Hippocrates would by no means have passed the people of his time unnoticed, as they provided solutions to matters of survival and at the same time gave hope to patients who, about a century earlier, depended almost exclusively on gods and oracles. The latter was probably his greatest achievement; that is, he freed man from superstition and fear about his body and his physical nature. In the two major works attributed to Hippocrates which are related to this subject, *The Sacred Disease* and *Airs, Waters, Places*, any involvement of divine presence in human physiology is rejected by means of arguments that are based on reasoning and observation.

The aim of this paper is to detect traces of influence of the Hippocratic Corpus upon three major fields of intellectual production of the 5th century: historiography, philosophy and drama.

1. Historiography –Thucydides (by G. Gazis)

As has long been observed (Cochrane 1929, 14–9), the Hippocratic method exercised a considerable amount of influence on Thucydides' methodology. The latter refers to the real causes of the Peloponnesian war using the word πρόφασις, a term that appears identical in the Hippocratic texts which are relative to the causes of the diseases. Specifically, in Thucydides I.23 we read: τὴν μὲν γὰρ ἀληθεστάτην πρόφασιν, ἀφανεστάτην δὲ λόγῳ τοὺς Ἀθηναίους ἡγοῦμαι μεγάλους γιγνομένους καὶ φόβον παρέχοντας τοῖς Λακεδαιμονίοις ἀναγκάσαι ἐς τὸ πολεμεῖν.

There is an obvious similarity to the Hippocratic texts. In *Prognosticon*, after the mention of some symptoms, we read: κρίνεται δὲ ἐν ἡμέρῃ τε καὶ νυκτί, ἣν διὰ ταύτας τὰς προφάσιας τὸ πρόσωπον τοιοῦτον ᾖ (§1). Likewise, in the introduction to the *Sacred Disease*: περὶ μὲν τῆς ἱερῆς νούσου καλεομένης ὧδ' ἔχει· οὐδέν τί μοι δοκέει τῶν ἄλλων θειοτέρη εἶναι νούσων οὐδὲ ἱερωτέρη, ἀλλὰ φύσιν μὲν ἔχει καὶ αὕτη καὶ πρόφασιν (§1).

Similarly, when it comes to the description of the plague in Athens (II.48–50), Thucydides again echoes the Hippocratic reasoning. According to the historian, the purpose of this description is to alert the following generations to the possibility of the reappearance of the plague and to inform them about it. His accuracy in recognising and analysing the symptoms is extraordinary and resembles to a great extent the descriptions of diseases in the Hippocratic texts. It is almost impossible not to admit the analogies, as well as the obvious influence that medicine exercised on – at least – this particular passage. At this point, worth mentioning is the description of the plague that struck the Achaean camp in *Iliad* 1. Nothing in the Homeric passage relates the plague to concrete or natural causes, whereas doctors, like Machaon or Podaleirios, are not even mentioned. The Homeric plague comes as a result of the wrath of the gods, against which man can present little opposition. On the other hand, the plague described by Thucydides is a clearly natural phenomenon and can – theoretically – be combated. It might be objected here that poetry is seen through the same prism as historiography; however, it is not rare for social convictions and functions to be reflected in poetic writings.

If we were to examine the entire work of Thucydides, we would repeatedly encounter various examples that assert the historian's conscious thinking in medical terms. The aim alone of writing this history is inspired by the Hippocratic ideas; Thucydides writes not only in order to immortalise the incidents of his times, but also to benefit posterity by indicating the compound interrelations between acts and results and, in addition, based on empiric observation, to point out what must and what must not be done and when. The first work that crosses the reader's mind is *Air, Waters, Places* with its detailed descriptions of climate and its effect on the human organism, as well as the proposals about treating the consequences of this effect. Admittedly, Thucydides' history and *Air, Waters, Places* share a similar way of thinking; we are led towards feasible solutions through objective observation and data recording. Subjectivity is barred equally from both the science of medicine and the history of Thucydides.

2. *Philosophy – Plato (by G. Gazis)*

Examination may now turn to the parts of Plato's work in which the influence of Hippocrates is to be detected. As is widely known (Lypourlis 1991, 36), in the Platonic work there are two direct references to Hippocrates himself; the first appears in *Protagoras* 331b where Socrates, addressing a certain Hippocrates, says: Ὥσπερ ἂν εἰ ἐπενόεις παρὰ τὸν σαυτοῦ ὁμώνυμον ἐλθὼν Ἱπποκράτη τὸν Κῷον, τὸν τῶν Ἀσκληπιαδῶν.

The second and more extensive reference to Hippocrates is found in *Phaedrus* 270c, where, apart from the doctor's name, a theory relating to the body is also studied. What is additionally analysed is the degree to which this theory can be applied to the investigation of the nature of the soul. Thus, we can reasonably conclude that not only was Hippocrates a renowned personality, but he also played a leading role in science of his time. The citation of his name in *Phaedrus* reminds us of the degree to which the art of medicine had affected the philosophical currents of that period.

Furthermore, in *Phaedo* 86b Simmias argues in favour of the mortality of the soul and refers to the elements that compose the human body as follows: ὅτι τοιοῦτόν τι μάλιστα ὑπολαμβάνομεν τὴν ψυχὴν εἶναι, ὥσπερ ἐντεταμένου τοῦ σώματος ἡμῶν καὶ ξυνεχομένου ὑπὸ θερμοῦ καὶ ψυχροῦ καὶ ξηροῦ καὶ ὑγροῦ καὶ τοιούτων τινῶν. It is easy to detect the analogies between this Platonic passage and the Hippocratic work Περὶ Διαίτης, where the author analyses the components of the human body: τούτων δὲ προσκέεται ἑκατέρῳ τάδε· τῷ μὲν πυρὶ τὸ θερμὸν καὶ τὸ ξηρόν, τῷ δὲ ὕδατι τὸ ψυχρὸν καὶ τὸ ὑγρόν· ἔχει δὲ ἀπ' ἀλλήλων τὸ μὲν πῦρ ἀπὸ τοῦ ὕδατος τὸ ὑγρόν· ἔνι γὰρ ἐν πυρὶ ὑγρότης· τὸ δὲ ὕδωρ ἀπὸ τοῦ πυρὸς τὸ ξηρόν· ἔνι γὰρ ἐν ὕδατι ξηρόν.

Moreover, plenty of examples with doctors are to be found in Plato's *Lysis* (210a, 215d, 217a–b, 219a) and *Euthydemos* (280a, 289a, 291e). Through all the above references and also through a thorough study of Platonic works, it is possible to trace the impact of medicine in Plato's thought; hidden though it may be, this impact definitely exists. It is of course understandable that what is mentioned here is rather limited in comparison with the considerable amount of cases where the art of medicine appears through a variety of ways in Plato's texts. Despite the fact that these examples cannot ultimately prove the direct influence of Hippocrates on the Platonic work, we still think that they are the best evidence of the extent to which medicine had invaded the everyday life of classical Athens. When Socrates, in his simplifying examples, mentions along with the professions of a shoemaker, a farmer, an armourer etc., that of a doctor, we cannot resist assuming that medicine formed a basic and recognisable part of everyday life. We might even venture a step further and consider Hippocrates himself to have been one of the principle motivators of this evolution.

3. *Drama (by A. Papachrysostomou)*

Within the Homeric world the doctor figure is admittedly a highly respected one (cf. *Il.* 4.212 (referring to Machaon): ἰσόθεος φώς), but still a doctor's duties and responsibilities are limited to wrapping up in bandages an open trauma or applying soothing ointments on a wound (cf. *Il.* 4.218–9: αἷμ' ἐκμυζήσας ἐπ' ἄρ' ἤπια φάρμακα εἰδὼς / πάσσε).

Some three hundred years later the picture has utterly changed.[1] The science of medicine experiences a quantum leap — not only on the level of knowledge and skills acquired by doctors, but also in regard to the people's attitude, mentality and way of reception of this science. The 5th century, especially, saw an increased interest in medicine; by a 'trickle down' process this ground-breaking science became part of the fabric of the society, even to the point where playwrights writing for mass audiences could expect their public to know certain basic concepts. Indeed, the 5th century dramatists draw freely upon the contemporary medical vocabulary and knowledge, thus attesting to the fact that during the 5th century not only was the science of medicine thriving, but its achievements were also accessible to the masses.

The way in which Euripides in his tragedies describes the seizures suffered by both Orestes and Heracles is astonishing. In the plays *Iphigenia in Tauris*, *Orestes* and *Heracles* we read detailed enumerations of epileptic symptoms that are highly reminiscent of the Hippocratic texts. In these depictions of temporary mental insanity Euripides does not make up some random or imaginary symptoms; on the contrary, his reports are distinguished for their medical accuracy and correspond – in both content and vocabulary – to the Hippocratic treatise about *The Sacred Disease* (Περὶ ἱερῆς νούσου).

At this point, I consider useful a close, parallel reading of Euripides' plays and *The Sacred Disease*.[2] Let us start from the epilepsy seizure experienced by Orestes in *Iphigenia in Tauris*. Orestes suffers from convulsions (κάρα τε διετίναξ' ἄνω κάτω / ... ὠλένας τρέμων ἄκρας, vv 282–3), and hallucinations (τήνδε δ' οὐχ ὁρᾷς / Ἅιδου δράκαιναν ὥς με βούλεται κτανεῖν / δειναῖς ἐχίδναις;, vv 285–7), groans loudly (κἀνεστέναξεν ... / ... βοᾷ, vv 283–4), and finally collapses, while foam comes out of his mouth (στάζων ἀφρῷ γένειον, v. 308).

In the play *Orestes* further symptoms are recorded: sudden jumps in alarm out of bed (δεμνίων ἄπο / πηδᾷ δρομαῖος, πῶλος ὣς ὑπὸ ζυγοῦ, vv 44–5), loss of memory (πόθεν ποτ' ἦλθον δεῦρο; πῶς δ' ἀφικόμην; / ἀμνημονῶ γάρ, τῶν πρὶν ἀπολειφθεὶς φρενῶν, vv 215–16), loss of voice and physical weakness (ὅταν ἀνῇ νόσος / μανίας, ἄναρθρός εἰμι κἀσθενῶ μέλη, vv 227–8), eye-rolling (ὄμμα σὸν ταράσσεται, v. 253). Equally remarkable is the medical history recorded by Electra: she explains to the spectators that this is the sixth day since Clytemnestra's murder that Orestes has been experiencing these symptoms: ἕκτον δὲ δὴ τόδ' ἦμαρ (v. 39). The parallelism with the medical histories, numbered according to the day, recorded by the travelling doctor/author of the *Epidemics* is automatically drawn. Besides, Electra offers a rational explanation for the Erinyes as non-existent, but as mere hallucinations: ὁρᾷς γὰρ οὐδὲν ὧν δοκεῖς σάφ' εἰδέναι (v. 259) (Devereux 1970, 37).

The seizure that Heracles suffers, in Euripides' homonymous play,[3] is presented with symptoms, which we already encountered: convulsions (καὶ δὴ τινάσσει κρᾶτα βαλβίδων ἄπο, v. 867), loss of voice (σῖγα ... ἔστη σιωπῇ, vv 868, 930), eye-rolling (ἐν στροφαῖσιν ὀμμάτων ἐφθαρμένος, v. 932), foam dripping out of his mouth (ἀφρὸν κατέσταζ' εὐτρίχου γενειάδος, v. 934), and hallucinations (ἅρματ' οὐκ ἔχων ἔχειν / ἔφασκε δίφρου δ' εἰσέβαινεν ἄντυγας / κἄθεινε, κέντρον δῆθεν ὡς ἔχων, χερί, vv. 947–9). His frenzy proves fatal, since he ends up slaughtering his own children and wife. After coming to his senses, he has no recollection of what happened (οὐ γάρ τι βακχεύσας γε μέμνημαι φρένας, v. 1122).

These portrayals of madness suggest – more than anything else – that Euripides was well-acquainted with the science of medicine. The treatise about *The Sacred Disease* lists one by one the symptoms mentioned by the 5th century dramatist: convulsions (αἱ χεῖρες συσπῶνται ... ἀκρατεῖς γίνονται καὶ σπῶνται, §10), hallucinations (δείματα παρίσταται καὶ φόβοι καὶ παράνοιαι, §4), shouts (βοᾷ καὶ κέκραγεν, §18), foam from the mouth (ἀφρὸς ἐκ τοῦ στόματος ἐκρεῖ, §10), eye-rolling (οἱ ὀφθαλμοὶ διαστρέφονται, §10), loss of memory (ὑπ' αὐτοῦ δὲ τοῦ πάθεος καὶ ἐπιλήθεται, §18), loss of voice (ἄφωνος γίνεται καὶ πνίγεται, §10), panic jumpings from the bed (ἀναπηδήσιες ἐκ τῆς κλίνης, §4), and weakening of the limbs (ὁ δ' ἀὴρ ... τὴν κίνησιν τοῖσι μέλεσι παρέχει, ὥστε, ἐπειδὰν ἀποκλεισθῶσιν αἱ φλέβες τοῦ ἠέρος ὑπὸ τοῦ φλέγματος, ἄφωνον καθιστᾶσι καὶ ἄφρονα τὸν ἄνθρωπον, §10).

As the Hippocratic treatise explains, when the crisis is over and the flow of air is reinstated in the veins, the patient regains consciousness and returns to sanity (ὁκόταν σκεδασθῇ κατὰ τὰς φλέβας καὶ μιγῇ τῷ αἵματι ... ἐδέξαντο τὸν ἠέρα αἱ φλέβες καὶ ἐφρόνησαν, §10). Euripides does not omit this final detail, but presents both Orestes and Heracles experiencing the return to rationality (cf. *Or*. 277–9 and *HF* 1089–92 respectively). Devereux (1970, 37) characterises these and the following lines as a 'clinically flawless "supportive therapy" scene'.

This pattern of coming to one's senses receives further elaboration from Euripides in the stichomythia between Cadmus and Agave towards the end of *Bacchae* (vv 1263–1301) (Seaford 1996, 247–9). Agave, having just dismembered Pentheus, is still in a state of frenzy and totally disoriented. The stichomythia that follows could be acknowledged – and with good reason – as the first example of psychoanalysis and Freudian treatment in ancient literature; or, as Devereux puts it, as 'the first surviving account of an insight-and-recall oriented psychotherapy' (Devereux 1970, 35). Cadmus knows exactly what kind of questions to pose to Agave, and how to express them, so that she recovers from insanity. Indeed, as Cadmus asks Agave first about the outside world (vv 1264–7), next about her inner state (v. 1268), and finally about past events from her life, Agave gradually advances towards consciousness (γίγνομαι δέ πως / ἔννους, μετασταθεῖσα τῶν πάρος φρενῶν, vv 1269–70), shows signs of awareness (ἄρτι μανθάνω, v. 1296), and eventually acknowledges that she had been frenzied (ἀφροσύνης ἐμῆς, v. 1301) (for the entire process of psychotherapy, see Devereux 1970, 41–7).

Throughout Euripides' texts the poet clarifies that the crises suffered by both Orestes and Heracles are triggered not from a divine power but from some kind of physical malfunction (e.g. a mind abnormality); cf. *HF* vv 1091–3: ὡς <δ'> ἐν κλύδωνι καὶ φρενῶν ταράγματι / πέπτωκα δεινῷ καὶ πνοὰς θερμὰς πνέω / μετάρσι', οὐ βέβαια πνευμόνων ἄπο. As an antipode to Euripides' rational explanation stand Aeschylus' *Eumenides*, as well as Sophocles' *Ajax*. A brief study of these cases suggests itself here, for it will help us follow the gradual acknowledgment and adoption of medical knowledge by poetry.

Aeschylus in *Oresteia* (458 BC) treats the Erinyes as existent avenging divinities and not as a symptom of Orestes' madness (as Euripides does in the plays examined above). Clytemnestra's warning to Orestes in *Choephori* v. 924 (φύλαξαι μητρὸς ἐγκότους κύνας) already provides the Erinyes with real substance, while creating a feeling of expectation of their appearance at the same time. Indeed, towards the end of the play they appear on stage and start haunting Orestes. The play *Eumenides*, in particular, follows their transformation into benign goddesses and the establishment of their worship in Athens.

Written between 460 and 450 BC, *Ajax* is Sophocles' oldest surviving play. Therefore, it is not surprising that here the divine element – and particularly goddess Athena – is omnipresent, omniscient and omnipotent; in a way that strongly recalls the Homeric epics. From as early as the first lines of the prologue, Athena proudly announces that it was she who afflicted the terrible madness upon Aias; cf. (NB the emphatically positioned ἐγώ at the beginning of the lines) vv 51–2: ἐγώ σφ' ἀπείργω, δυσφόρους ἐπ' ὄμμασι / γνώμας βαλοῦσα, and 59–60: ἐγὼ δὲ φοιτῶντ' ἄνδρα μανιάσιν νόσοις / ὤτρυνον, εἰσέβαλλον εἰς ἕρκη κακά. Expectedly, Odysseus acknowledges the gods' powers (v. 86: γένοιτο μέντἂν πᾶν θεοῦ τεχνωμένου), and pities human fate (v. 126: εἴδωλ' ὅσοιπερ ζῶμεν ἢ κούφην σκιάν). Aias, in turn, attributes his insanity to Athena; cf. vv 401–3: ἀλλά μ' ἁ Διὸς / ἀλκίμα θεὸς / ὀλέθριον αἰκίζει. Until the end of the play there is a sense of predestined inevitability about Aias' fate. Besides, we should not fail to notice that Athena's portrait is painted with Homeric colours: not only does she take sides with mortals and capriciously chooses to support one (Odysseus) over another (Aias), but she also laughs at the latter's delusional state (v. 79).

Special reference also needs to be made to Philoctetes. In the *Iliad* no particular term or name is attributed to his illness; he is merely described as suffering from an evil ulcer: ἕλκεϊ μοχθίζοντα κακῷ (*Il*. 2.723). Nevertheless, in what survives from both Aeschylus' and Euripides' *Philoctetes* we come across a definite term, i.e. φαγέδαινα; cf. Aesch. fr. 253 Radt (φαγέδαινα<.>, ἥ μου σάρκας ἐσθίει ποδός), and Eur. fr. 792 Kannicht (φαγέδαινα <> ἥ μου σάρκα θοινᾶται ποδός). The term φαγέδαινα reoccurs regularly throughout the Hippocratic corpus, indicating a specific kind of ulcer; e.g. *A*ër. 10, *Ulc.* 10, *Epid.* 6.3.23, etc. (see further Jouanna 1999, 142–3). Nowadays, in modern dermatology the term 'phagedenic ulcer' describes 'a rapidly spreading ulcer attended by the formation of extensive sloughing' (*Online Medical Dictionary*, available from http://cancerweb.ncl.ac.uk/cgi-bin/omd). Despite the fact that in Sophocles' *Philoctetes* the very term φαγέδαινα does not occur, there are still numerous passages in this play where both the description of the disease and the symptoms experienced by Philoctetes correspond to the medical knowledge of that time. For example, it is observed that Philoctetes' malady is a πλάνης νόσος (v. 758–9), i.e. a disease that occurs at intervals. In the Hippocratic corpus both the adverb πεπλανημένως and the noun πλάνης are used as technical terms to denote the intermittent occurrence of a disease (mainly – but not exclusively – of fever); e.g. *Epid.* 1.3 (πυρετοῖσι φρικώδεσι σμικρὰ ἐφιδροῦντες, ἄλλοτε ἀλλοίως παροξυνόμενοι πεπλανημένως), *Epid.* 1.12 (πλανῆτες δὲ πυρετοί, καὶ τεταρταῖοι, καὶ πεμπταῖοι, καὶ ἑβδομαῖοι, καὶ ἐναταῖοι), etc.

The borders among the literary genres are constantly proven to be porous. Medical terminology infiltrates into late 5th century Comedy too. Towards the end of Aristophanes' *Peace* we come across an interesting line: τί δ' ἔστιν ὦ κακόδαιμον; οὔτι που λοφᾷς; (1211). What is astonishing here is that the verb λοφάω is an Aristophanic coinage that is modelled upon a whole series of verbs (better say, medical terms) that signify particular diseases; e.g. ποδαγράω ('suffer from gout'), στραγγουριάω ('suffer from strangury'), etc. The meaning in *Peace* 1211 is that the crest-maker is accused of suffering from an urge/manic obsession for manufacturing crests.[4] Not only does Aristophanes have some medical knowledge, but he also feels confident to coin a medical term and use it to advance his comic purposes (see also Olson 1998, 299). This is not an isolated case within the Aristophanic corpus; similar examples that reveal the poet's familiarity with the science of medicine are also to be found elsewhere, e.g. *Ra.* 814–17, *V.* 403, *Lys.* 464–5, 694, *Eq.* 41, etc.[5]

Conclusion

By focusing on a number of examples we have attempted to demonstrate the role that Hippocrates and medicine played in the intellectual renaissance of classical Athens (or, at least, the relation between the two phenomena). Of course, this has always been a multifaceted issue; here we simply dealt with some of its aspects — those we believe to be the most important.

In conclusion, we would like to underline how much the 5th century BC owes to Hippocrates. It is a truism that art and philosophy cannot bloom if the human body and mind are trapped in superstition and fear. It is logical that both innovative ideas and philosophical queries appear only when the human mind is freed from the unbearable threats of illness and death, which are perceived as results of divine vengeance. This, in combination with other contributing factors, is exactly what happened in Athens of the 5th century and Ionia of the 6th century BC. It should not be deemed as a coincidence that medicine and philosophy appear to follow a parallel path, without it always being easy to make out the real nature of their relation.

Finally, as evidence of the charm that medicine has always exerted on poetry, and generally on art, we would like to remind the reader of a passage from the *Argonautics* of Apollonius Rhodius. In Book III, vv 755–69 Apollonius describes the emotional situation of Medea on the night before she betrayed her father for the sake of Jason:

> πυκνὰ δέ οἱ κραδίη στηθέων ἔντοσθεν ἔθυιεν,
> ἠελίου ὥς τίς τε δόμοις ἐνιπάλλεται αἴγλη
> ὕδατος ἐξανιοῦσα, τὸ δὴ νέον ἠὲ λέβητι
> ἠέ που ἐν γαυλῷ κέχυται, ἡ δ' ἔνθα καὶ ἔνθα
> ὠκείῃ στροφάλιγγι τινάσσεται ἀίσσουσα·
> ὣς δὲ καὶ ἐν στήθεσσι κέαρ ἐλελίζετο κούρης.
> δάκρυ δ' ἀπ' ὀφθαλμῶν ἐλέῳ ῥέεν· ἔνδοθι δ' αἰεὶ
> τεῖρ' ὀδύνη σμύχουσα διὰ χροός ἀμφί τ' ἀραιὰς
> ἶνας καὶ κεφαλῆς ὑπὸ νείατον ἰνίον ἄχρις,
> ἔνθ' ἀλεγεινότατον δύνει ἄχος, ὁππότ' ἀνίας
> ἀκάματοι πραπίδεσσιν ἐνισκίμψωσιν Ἔρωτες.
> φῆ δέ οἱ ἄλλοτε μὲν θελκτήρια φάρμακα ταύρων
> δωσέμεν· ἄλλοτε δ' οὔ τι, καταφθίσθαι δὲ καὶ αὐτή·
> αὐτίκα δ' οὔτ' αὐτὴ θανέειν, οὐ φάρμακα δώσειν,
> ἀλλ' αὔτως εὔκηλος ἑὴν ὀτλησέμεν ἄτην.

> 'Over and over the heart within her breast fluttered wildly,
> as when a ray of sunlight bounds inside a house as it leaps
> from water freshly poured into a cauldron or perhaps
> into a bucket, and quivers and darts here and there
> from the rapid swirling –
> thus did the girl's heart tremble in her breast.
> Tears of pity poured from her eyes, and deep
> within a pain tortured her constantly as it smoldered
> through her body and along the delicate nerves and
> deep down beneath the nape of the neck,
> where the sharpest anguish penetrates whenever
> the tireless Loves inflict pains upon the spirit.
> At one moment she was determined to give him the drugs for charming
> the oxen; at another by no means to give them but to perish herself as well;
> then immediately neither to die herself nor to give the drugs,
> but to endure her calamity in silence just as she was doing.'
> (transl. W. H. Race)

It would be really hard to find a more harmonious blend of medical symptoms and poetry than this passage, which centuries later manages to overwhelm us with the elegance and the accuracy of its description.

Notes

1 Littré (1973, i. 3–65) meticulously traces the history of the science of medicine, as well as Hippocrates' sources of influence (e.g. in the form of predecessors).

2 The present fragment of Euripides' text, and also those following, do not imply that these literary creations could also be interpreted as clinical accounts. Our attempt is simply to highlight the subtle infiltration of concrete elements of clinical observation into poetry.

3 Heracles' madness and symptoms in Euripides' play are thoroughly studied by Holmes (2008). The article constitutes a brilliant case study of interaction between 5th-century medicine and tragedy.

4 Henderson 1998, 581, translates: 'What's the matter, poor fellow? Come down with a touch of plume-onia?'

5 Apostolides (1996) has collected – and commented upon – the majority of Aristophanic passages that bear a a relation to medicine.

Bibliography

Apostolides: Αποστολίδης, Π. 1996: Τα Ιατρικά του Αριστοφάνη, Αθήνα.

Barlow, S. A. (ed.) 1996: *Euripides: Heracles*, Warminster.

Cochrane, C. N. 1929: *Thucydides and the Science of History*, Oxford.

Cropp, M. J. (ed.) 2000: *Euripides: Iphigenia in Tauris*, Warminster.

Devereux, G. 1970: 'The psychotherapy scene in Euripides' *Bacchae*', *Journal of Hellenic Studies* 90, 35–48.

Dodds, E. R. (ed.) 1986: *Euripides: Bacchae,* Oxford.

Garvie, A. F. (ed.) 1986: *Aeschylus Choephori*, Oxford.

Henderson, J. (ed.) 1998: *Aristophanes. Clouds, Wasps, Peace*, Cambridge, MA.

Holmes, B. 2008: 'Euripides' Heracles in the Flesh', *Classical Antiquity* 27.2, 231–81.

Jones, W. H. S., Withington, E. T., Potter, P. and Smith, W. D. 1923–1995: *Hippocrates*, 8 vols, Cambridge, MA.

Jouanna, J. 1999: *Hippocrates* (English translation by M. B. DeBevoise), Baltimore.

Kannicht, R. 2004: *Tragicorum Graecorum Fragmenta Vol. 5: Euripides*, Göttingen.

Littré, É. (ed.) 1973–1989: Œuvres complètes d*'Hippocrate*, 10 vols, Amsterdam.

Lypourlis: Λυπουρλής, Δ. 1991: Δύο διαλέξεις και μια εισήγηση για τον Ιπποκράτη, Θεσσαλονίκη.

Olson, S. D. (ed.) 1998: *Aristophanes: Peace*, Oxford.

Radt, S. (ed.) 1985: *Tragicorum Graecorum fragmenta Vol. 3: Aeschylus*, Göttingen.

Seaford, R. (ed.) 1996: *Euripides: Bacchae*, Warminster.

Sidgwick, A. (ed.) 1902: *Aeschylus: Eumenides*, 3rd ed., Oxford.

Ussher, R. G. (ed.) 1990: *Sophocles: Philoctetes*, Warminster.

Willink, C. W. (ed.) 1986: *Euripides: Orestes*, Oxford.

11. Ancient Medicine and Philosophy: a Philosopher's Perspective

Eleni M. Kalokairinou

In this paper I explore the relations that ancient medicine had with philosophy. As I point out, since the Presocratic philosophers, Plato, Aristotle and the Hellenistic and Roman philosophical schools there has been a constant interaction between philosophy and medicine. The medical schools which developed in antiquity were all very good examples of the way in which the different philosophical trends influenced medicine at different periods. In this light I also examine Celsus' classical claim that Hippocrates of Cos was the man who separated medicine from philosophy and rendered it an independent branch of learning. The conclusion reached, therefore, is that, in spite of what has been argued by Celsus, ancient medicine was to a great extent formed by the philosophical tendencies that were prevailing at the time, while at the same time it attempted to define its own particular methods of research and practice and so become autonomous.

One of the recurrent questions of medicine, medical ethics and contemporary bioethics is whether medicine is 'art, science or practical wisdom' (Kuczewski and Polansky 2000, 31). The history of ancient medicine teaches us that in a way it is all three things at the same time, something which explains perhaps why it is so difficult to track down its relations to philosophy. Philosophy is both theoretical and practical, and it also involves practical wisdom, as Aristotle argued. Medicine is all three things too (Kuczewski and Polansky 2000, 31–56).

Medicine, a science which is closely related to man and to human nature, appears in a fairly progressive stage of human history and civilisation. In antiquity, when we talk about medicine, we usually refer to therapeutic practices, whereas the physician is not the scientist who possesses the specialised scientific knowledge he applies in action, but the practical healer who applies accepted practices for the healing of a wound or the cure of a disease. To be more precise, we should mention that these medical practices initially had a divine character. The ancient Greeks considered that diseases came from the gods, were supernatural, and that their cure, in whatever form, came from the gods too; however, they gradually realised that all diseases were both natural and divine and they sought for different means of cure. This is how the religious concept of medicine is slowly replaced by the philosophical one.

One of the most important problems of antiquity is the relation which exists between philosophy and medicine. As is to be expected, neither the philosophers nor the classicists nor the historians of ancient medicine agree on this. All of them recognise that philosophy and medicine are related in a rather complicated way in antiquity. Whereas some modern and contemporary classicists and philosophers claim that it was ancient Greek medicine which influenced ancient philosophical thought, according to others, it was the philosophers who provided the foundations of medical theory (Edelstein 1987, 399; Frede 1987, 225). It is worth mentioning at this point what Celsus writes in this connection:

> 'At first the science of healing was held to be part of philosophy, so that treatment of disease and contemplation of the nature of things began through the same authorities; clearly because healing was needed especially by those whose bodily strength had been weakened by restless thinking and night-watching. Hence we find that many who professed philosophy became expert in medicine, the most celebrated being Pythagoras, Empedocles and Democritus' (Celsus, *De medicina,* Proemium 6–7).

And he goes on:

> 'But it was, as some believe, a pupil of the last, Hippocrates of Cos, a man first and foremost worthy to be remembered, notable both for professional skill and for eloquence, who separated this branch of learning from the study of philosophy' (Celsus, *De medicina,* Proemium 7–8).

At one stroke therefore we realise that Celsus recognises the common origin of philosophy and medicine, while at the same time he underlines that it was Hippocrates who rendered medicine independent of philosophy. In the same way, the author of the treatise of the Hippocratic corpus entitled, *Decorum* or *Περὶ εὐσχημοσύνης* advises that philosophy be carried into medicine and medicine into philosophy. He writes:

> 'Wherefore resume each of the points mentioned, and transplant wisdom into medicine and medicine into wisdom. For a physician who is a lover of wisdom is the equal of a god. Between wisdom and medicine there is no gulf fixed; in fact medicine possesses all the qualities that make for wisdom. It has disinterestedness, shamefastness, modesty, reserve, sound opinion, judgment, quiet, pugnacity, purity, sententious speech, knowledge of the things good and necessary for life, selling of that which cleanses, freedom from superstition, pre-excellence divine' (Hippocrates, *Decorum,* vol. II, v, 1–13).

As is widely acknowledged by both philosophers and classicists, the relation between philosophy and medicine was very close and complicated. It is true that ancient philosophers showed a surprising amount of interest in medical questions. In particular, the first Milesian philosophers, Thales, Anaximander and Anaximenes, engaged more in physics and astronomy than in anthropology and medicine. However, with the Pythagoreans who settled in Italy, where there was a medical tradition, things changed. Alcmaeon of Croton, who was either a pythagorean or related to the pythagorean circle, was a philosopher-physician. Aristotle mentions him as a philosopher; however, Diogenes Laertius says that Alcmaeon wrote on medical issues (Aristotle, *Metaphysics* 986 a 23 – b 9 and Diogenes Laertius, *Lives of eminent philosophers* VIII 83). Alcmaeon rejects the ontological conception of disease which was prevailing in his time. On the contrary, he regards disease as a part of nature and, therefore, as subject to the same rules which govern the world. In an extant fragment from his work, *Περὶ φύσεως,* he argues that the balance (ἰσονομία) between a number of opposite forces of the body, i.e. hot–cold, moist–dry, sweet–bitter, etc., constitutes health, while the supremacy (μοναρχία) of any one of them over the others causes disease. Health, according to him, is the harmonious mixing (κρᾶσις) of all these forces (Diels and Kranz 1989, 24, B 4 [22]).

The influence of this medical theory was great. Because, as we shall see, through Empedocles' medical theory it was adopted by the Hippocratic corpus and in particular by the author of the treatise *On ancient medicine,* and constituted the theory of the four humours, widely known in the history of ancient medicine.

Empedocles was one of the leaders of the medical school of Italy, which was in disagreement with the Asclepiades of Cos and Cnidos (Diels and Kranz 1989, 31, A3). He was interested in finding out the beginning of beings. He put forward the theory that the cosmos consists of four different elements, i.e. fire, water, air and earth, which he called ῥιζώματα (Diels and Kranz 1989, 31, B 6, 7). On the analogies in which these different elements are mixed depend the different kinds of beings we end up with each time. The mixing of these four elements in different proportions explains how different beings are distinguished the one from the other and, furthermore, enables us to distinguish between individual human natures (Diels and Kranz 1989, 31, B 110). This is an important concept not only because, as Frede has pointed out, it has been adopted by the Hippocratic physicians who on the basis of it developed the idea of treatment and cure according to each individual patient, but mainly because it lays the foundations of what in contemporary medicine and bioethics has come to be known as 'genomics' (Frede 1987, 229). Moreover, according to Empedocles, there is no birth and destruction but only mixing and alternation of the four elements, which are subject to the two cosmic powers, the φιλότητα and the νεῖκος (Diels and Kranz 1989, 31, B 8, 16, 17, 18, 19, 26). But Empedocles' important contribution to medicine is that he attempted to develop a theory of human physiology by virtue of which to explain the most basic functions of the human organism (Diels and Kranz 1989, 31, B 100; Frede 1987, 229–30). It may be, as Frede argues, that Empedocles' physiology is not satisfactory; however, the credit goes to him for being the first philosopher–physician who considered such a physiological theory indispensable to the understanding of human beings (Frede 1987, 230).

Empedocles' teaching proved decisive for the subsequent development of medicine. Many of the philosophers who succeeded him attempted to elaborate more detailed accounts of human physiology. Among them, one should mention Anaxagoras, Diogenes of Apollonia, Democritus, Hippon of Samos, Philolaus of Croton and even Plato. Plato in his dialogue *Timaeus* is still under Empedocles' spell. After he has described how the world was created and 'Cosmos evolved out of Chaos', he then discusses the creation of man, he analyses the functions of the human body and the soul and, in the end, he offers an account of health and disease (Bury 1981, 5). He seems to hold Empedocles' theory of the four basic elements and to support the view that the world is compounded of them (Plato, *Timaeus,* 31–3). However, as the reader fairly soon realises, Plato is gradually moving away from this theory, since he conceives these four basic elements not as basic but as compound (Plato, *Timaeus*, 53–6). Plato's pupil, Aristotle, on the other hand, though he did not follow his father's profession, esteemed medicine highly, and taught it, together with biology and zoology, in the Lycaeum. Among his writings are included treatises which show his genuine interest in issues concerning man's physiology and pathology. Treatises like, *On the soul, On sense and sensible objects, On memory and recollection, On sleep and waking, On length and shortness of life, On respiration, On breath* etc. express Aristotle's explicit concern for medical and anthropological matters, which his philosophical training enabled him to discuss in a more thorough manner than a simple physician would have done. According to him, medicine and philosophy are two inextricably related disciplines, since neither the philosophers can avoid studying medicine in the end, nor the physicians can get their reasoning started unless they invoke the first principles of natural philosophy. As he writes:

> 'It is further the duty of the natural philosopher to study the first principles of disease and health; for neither health nor disease can be properties of things deprived of life. Hence one may say that most natural philosophers, and those physicians who take a scientific interest in their art, have this in common: the former end by studying medicine, and the latter base their medical theories on the principles of natural science' (Aristotle, *On sense and sensible objects* 436 a19–b1).

And he repeats:

> 'For those physicians who have subtle and inquiring minds have something to say about natural science, and claim to derive their principles therefrom, and the most accomplished of those who deal with natural science tend to conclude with medical principles' (Aristotle, *On respiration* 480 b27–31).

This is the state of things which was prevailing around the 4th century BC. Furthermore, this close relationship which exists between philosophy and medicine becomes more obvious in the treatises of the Corpus Hippocraticum. Thus, while in some treatises the author makes an attempt to explain the medical phenomena by arguing from certain hypotheses or axioms to the conclusions in the same way as philosophers do, in certain others he criticises this method. In particular, in the treatise *On Ancient Medicine,* the author first rejects the position of his opponents and then he puts forward his own thesis. He condemns the position of those who reduced medicine to one principle. As he writes:

> 'All who, on attempting to speak or to write on medicine, have assumed for themselves a postulate as a basis for their discussion – heat, cold, moisture, dryness, or anything else that they may fancy – who narrow down the causal principles of diseases and of death among men, and make it the same in all cases, postulating one thing or two, all these obviously blunder in many points even of their statements, but they are most open to censure because they blunder in what is an art, and one which all men use on the most important occasions, and give the greatest honours to the good craftsmen and practitioners in it' (Hippocrates, *On Ancient Medicine* vol. I, I, 1–11).

The author of the treatise rejects such a monistic thesis in medicine and then he broadens his criticism so as to include every form of philosophical medicine. He writes in the same treatise:

> 'Certain physicians and philosophers assert that nobody can know medicine who is ignorant what a man is; he who would treat patients properly must, they say, learn this. But the question they raise is one for philosophy; it is the province of those who, like Empedocles, have written on natural science, what man is from the beginning, how he came into being at the first, and from what elements he was originally constructed' (Hippocrates, *On Ancient Medicine* vol. I, XX, 1–8).

What these modern physicians claim is that medicine does not have its own method, it is not an independent science because in order to acquire knowledge of man, of his constitution and his existence presupposes or has recourse to cosmology. So the writer of the treatise proposes his thesis:

> 'But my view is, first, that all that philosophers or physicians have said or written on natural science no more pertains to medicine than to painting. I also hold that clear knowledge about natural science can be acquired from medicine and from no other source, and that one can attain this knowledge when medicine itself has been properly comprehended, but till then it is quite impossible' (Hippocrates, *On Ancient Medicine* vol. I, XX, 9–10).

The physician need not take recourse to philosophical views in order to show that man is composed of certain basic elements. All he needs is to study the body's reactions to certain foods, drinks or exercises and so to define the various kinds of human nature. If philosophy attempts to define the principles of human nature, then the object of medicine is to study the different kinds of human nature, that is human natures in plural, which are the result of the rational study of the relation which exists between diet and body. In this way, medicine is entirely distinguished from philosophy, it becomes an independent science, the science of man.

A similar attack against philosophical medicine is put forward by the author of the treatise *Nature of man.* He writes:

> 'He who is accustomed to hear speakers discuss the nature of man beyond its relations to medicine will not find the present account of any interest. For I do not say at all that a man is air, or fire, or water, or earth, or anything else that is not an obvious constituent of a man; such accounts I leave to those that care to give them' (Hippocrates, *Nature of man* vol. I, I, 1–8).

I have mentioned these quotations which include the polemic against philosophy at quite some length because I wish to make my point and, consequently, my contribution to this conference clear. The interpretation that is normally given to these particular references is the one which, as we saw, Celsus gives, namely that Hippocrates or the author of the treatises has succeeded in distinguishing medicine from philosophy. But this interpretation, as one would have thought, is too simplistic. However, if we look at the recent literature written whether by classicists or by philosophers, we realise that things are somewhat more complicated. Longrigg, for instance, admits that there are obvious philosophical influences in the Hippocratic Corpus (Longrigg 1993, 89–90). However, he is not so certain when it comes to deciding the origin of each of them. He points out that some of them may be the result of the influence of one particular philosopher, others may be traced back to the Presocratics, yet others do not come from a particular theory but from a number of philosophical theories and in this sense they are eclectic, while some others condemn the introduction of philosophy into medicine, but in their attempt to define their principles independently of philosophy, they end up in vagueness, ambiguity and confusion (Longrigg 1993, 90). Longrigg's claim gives us a good insight into the kind of position I am trying to defend. In other words, is Hippocrates attacking philosophy as such in the two above-mentioned treatises or is he attacking a particular philosophical theory? Can it be, for instance, that he is attacking a particular philosophical theory, the one that assumed one postulate as a basis for the discussion from which, by means of deductive reasoning, he attempted to reach conclusions regarding issues of health and disease? What reasons do we have to claim that this is most likely what has been attacked in these two treatises?

This is a fairly familiar issue in bibliography. G. E. R. Lloyd in his article asks a more or less similar question (Lloyd 1963, 108–26). Is the author of the treatise combating all the thinkers who attached undue weight to the effect that the traditional opposites had on bodily health or is he attacking a whole medical school rather than a particular individual?

I think it would be somewhat naïve to argue that what is attacked in these treatises is philosophy as such, as if medical theory could exist in a vacuum and independently of any philosophical account. I wish to argue that, on the contrary, what is attacked is a particular philosophical school, the school that argued from one postulate or ὑπόθεσις, whether monistic or not, to certain conclusions. This way of reasoning or arguing was known in the philosophical tradition as Rationalism. And even though it proved very successful in philosophical theorising, physicians thought that it was not sufficient for such a complicated science as medicine. They perhaps thought not so much that medicine did not need a theory of first principles as that it needed a philosophical theory more akin to its nature. And this is why they attacked it. By way of reminder, there is a constant influence, or, better, an interrelation or interchange between philosophy and medicine in antiquity (as there is an analogous interchange between the two nowadays). The Dogmatist physicians were influenced by Rationalism or the Rationalist philosophy. But this does not imply that all subsequent medical schools were not influenced by other philosophical schools. In a similar manner, the Empiricists argued that experience came first and medical theory second. One had to work through the observation and the study of the particular cases, acquire knowledge, and in this case medical knowledge, and on the basis of it formulate one's theory (Frede 1987, 236). But by arguing in this way they actually attacked the Dogmatists because, in their opinion, they did not have an alternative way of acquiring knowledge. In an analogous manner, the Methodists criticised both the Dogmatists and the Empiricists and tried to steer a middle course between the two. They argued that neither of them understood by which kind of method one comes to know the right form of treatment. In their opinion, the kind of knowledge the physician relies on is neither exclusively practical nor theoretical. The physician does not rely on experience, as the Empiricists do, in order to gain knowledge. Nor does he depend upon reason in order to derive conclusions from hidden and unobservable powers to observable ones, as the Dogmatists do. The Methodists rely on reason in order to reach medical knowledge in the sense that they infer from the observable symptoms of all diseases, which were nothing else but forms of constriction and dilation, the indicated methods of treatment and cure (Frede 1987, 237).

Paul Carrick neatly explains how the different medical schools in antiquity were influenced by the different philosophical schools (Carrick 2001, 40–1). Behind the manifest symptoms of a disease the Dogmatists assumed the existence of the hidden causes of it, which, to a great extent, determined the kind of treatment which was to be applied to the particular patient. Their views can be traced back to Hippocrates' theory of humours, to Plato's teleological conception of the creation of Cosmos and to Empedocles' theory of basic elements or ῥιζώματα (Carrick 2001, 40). The Empiricists do not agree with this kind of approach. Being influenced by the sceptic school, they dispute the Dogmatists' hypothesis that hidden causes may exist behind the observable symptoms of the disease. They emphasised the important role that observations played and the close study of the symptoms of each case for the acquisition of medical knowledge and, therefore, for the treatment of the disease. Although they acknowledge their debt to Aristotle, they do not share his concern for finding out the hidden causes of phenomena (Carrick 2001, 40–1). In a similar manner, the Methodists being influenced by the atomic philosophers Democritus and Epicurus attempt to formulate their own method of medical knowledge. Like the Empiricists, they claim that it is through the study and observation of the manifest symptoms of the disease that they can acquire medical knowledge; but, unlike them, they think that the study not of any manifest symptoms of disease, but of the excesses of constriction and dilation in the pores of the body, by virtue of which they understood the disease, could provide them with the practical medical knowledge they were looking for. Consequently, even though they take recourse to reason, as the Dogmatists do, nevertheless they do not conceive reason in terms of pre-existent, *a priori*, hidden causes (Carrick 2001, 41). Finally, the Pneumatists, the fourth major medical school of antiquity, were mainly eclectic and were influenced equally by the stoic school and the theory of four humours (*ibid.*). They are in total agreement with the Methodists when they argue that it is through the observation of the particular manifest symptoms of the body that they can understand the disease. But they disagree with them as to what these particular symptoms are. For while the Methodists understand the disease in terms of the excesses of constriction and dilation in the pores of the body, the Pneumatists put forward the view that the disease is determined by the particular condition of pneuma or 'vital air' which each man breathes; something which, in its turn, is dependent upon the particular balance or imbalance of the four humours (*ibid.*).

As becomes obvious, all the medical sects of antiquity were closely interrelated with various philosophical theories. It is not so much, therefore, that the author of the treatise *On Ancient Medicine* is attacking philosophy because it intrudes into the medical science of the time, as that he attacks the particular philosophical theory which seeks to deduce the observables from the unobservables. But if this is what he has been doing, then he was not trying to distinguish medicine from philosophy and thus render it autonomous. Medicine was autonomous in any case. On the contrary, what he was trying to do was to provide medicine with a more appropriate theory of knowledge with which to operate. But this is not to intrude into medical science nor to violate its autonomy.

Looking at the issue in modern terms, we could say that it is unavoidable, I think, that philosophy and medicine are interrelated. Philosophy deals with the issue of knowledge, it is concerned with methodological problems. In other words, philosophy poses the conceptual framework within which we can operate and do our research. This logical framework is unavoidably shared by all disciplines, if our research is to make sense. In the last analysis, the same logical framework employs the positive scientist, the social scientist and the art critic. And this logical framework is the philosopher's job to provide. So there is a sense in which no science, no discipline whatever can operate independently of it, i.e. independently of a philosophical scheme. For each particular science, whether it is medicine or physics, astronomy or literary criticism, has its own *constitutive notion* which determines the rules of reasoning and argument we employ in each particular field. Thus, even though we follow, strictly speaking, the same rules of reasoning, in medicine we are arguing about health and disease, in geometry about space, in history about the knowledge of the past. So for a philosopher it is quite understandable how each of these disciplines retains its autonomy, while at the same time it presupposes a logical framework provided by philosophy. And I think the situation is similar with regard to medicine in antiquity. If Hippocrates was such an important man for both his philological ability and his medical talent, as Celsus describes him, then he should have understood that in medicine one cannot get away from philosophy. Philosophy necessarily provides us with the logical foundation which enables us to reason in medicine. And if he had realised this, then he could not have attacked philosophy in the two treatises mentioned above. What he had most probably attacked was the rationalist logical framework, since he found it unhelpful in medical research, and because he and his contemporary physicians and philosophers were gradually looking for a different, more applicable conceptual scheme.

Acknowledgement

I wish to express my sincerest thanks to Professor Philip J. Van der Eijk for his constructive remarks and comments during the conference which helped me to reconsider some of the issues I discuss in this paper.

Bibliography

Aristotle 1986: *On the Soul, Parva naturalia, On breath,* transl. W. S. Hett, London.

Aristotle 1989: *Metaphysics,* 2 vols, trans. Hugh Tredennick, Cambridge, MA., London.

Carrick, P. 2001: *Medical Ethics in the Ancient World,* Washington.

Celsus 1971: *De medicina,* 3 vols, transl. W. G. Spencer, London, Cambridge, MA.

Diels, H. and Kranz, W. 1989: *Die Fragmente der Vorsokratiker,* vol. I, Zurich.

Diogenes Laertius 1991: *Lives of Eminent Philosophers,* 2 vols, transl. R. D. Hicks, Cambridge, MA., London.

Edelstein, L. 1987: *Ancient Medicine,* Baltimore and London.

Frede, M. 1987: *Essays in Ancient Philosophy,* Minneapolis.

Hippocrates 1984: 7 vols, transl. W. H. S. Jones, Cambridge, MA. and London.

Kuczewski, M. G. and Polansky, R. (eds), 2000: *Bioethics* (Ancient Themes in Contemporary Issues), Cambridge, MA., London.

Lloyd, G. E. R. 1963: 'Who is attacked in *On Ancient Medicine?*', *Phronesis* 8, 108–26.

Longrigg, J. 1993: *Greek Rational Medicine,* London, New York.

Plato, *Timaeus, Critias, Cleitophon, Menexenous, Epistles*, 12 vols, transl. R. G. Bury, London, 1981.

12. The Threshold of Pain: the Literary Embodiment of Pain and its Cognates in the Hippocratic Corpus

Nicholas A. E. Kalospyros

This paper aims to develop discussion of the complexity of pain-grief as a psychosomatic phenomenon awaiting its medical and humanistic treatment and relief in the so-called Hippocratic corpus. The issue towards the philological attestation as well as the semantic documentation of pain symptoms and signs, especially in the context of Hippocratic research, cannot be further detached from ancient medicine studies. Therefore, its presentation in the forms of pain and its cognates in varying cases cannot but apply for both the history of medicine in ancient Greece and the appreciation of Hippocratic data. The emergence of pain symptoms, factors or mind attitudes towards the necessity of dealing with them, along with the understanding of the first registration of diseases in the classical world, are of great importance to the modern status of knowledge in Hippocratic studies. The literary aspects and the versatility of medical information are for the first time examined within Hippocratic bibliography and special publications, this being an ambition, no less a desideratum, of my proposed discussion.

The *Corpus Hippocraticum* (*CH*), which most probably originated in Hellenistic Alexandria as the result of Ptolemaic diligence in collecting, written in the Ionic dialect of Greek, forms a collection recorded in AD 1526, when the first edition of the complete works of Hippocrates in Greek was printed by the Aldine press in Venice (Aldus Manutius). As we can conclude from the surviving manuscripts themselves and from the work of ancient commentators and compilers of Hippocratic dictionaries, the great majority of the texts printed in 1526 were already circulating together under the name of Hippocrates by the 1st century AD, if not three centuries earlier. However, the total number of treatises in the *CH* – some of which were already combined or separated in antiquity – remains uncertain (Nutton 2004, 60). All the same, scholars interested in the validity of medicine and the actual Hippocratic ideals, unfettered by doctrines, instead of concentrating on a small group of the so-called 'genuine' writings, are now free to consider the *CH* in all its diversity of attitudes and indeed purposes (see Haeser 1875, 109–210 for the appraisal of Hippocrates' contribution to the conditions of medical science), whereby the relation between physician and patient rests on the mutual interest and benefit of the first according to the famous maxim of *Epidemics* 1 2.5.9–10: ἀσκέειν, περὶ τὰ νουσήματα, δύο, ὠφελέειν, ἢ μὴ βλάπτειν – to help or at least make no harm is a clear assertion that the uttermost medical target is the protection of the patient's interests, although the injunction to 'do good' cannot always be attained by the physician.

This antithetical definition of the certain medical target reflects upon a dynamic intervention in medicine through lived experience. In the same sincerity of tone and profound exactness of argument in the preamble to *Breaths* (1.1–8) we read the following passage:

> 'Εἰσί τινες τῶν τεχνέων, αἳ τοῖσι μὲν κεκτημένοισίν εἰσιν ἐπίπονοι, τοῖσι δὲ χρεομένοισιν ὀνηισταί, καὶ τοῖσι μὲν ἰδιώτῃσι ξυνὸν ἀγαθόν, τοῖσι δὲ μεταχειριζομένοισι σφᾶς λυπηραί. Τῶν δὴ τοιουτέων ἐστὶ τεχνέων, καὶ ἣν οἱ Ἕλληνες καλέουσιν ἰητρικήν· ὁ μὲν γὰρ ἰητρὸς ὁρῇ τε δεινά, θιγγάνει ἀηδέων, ἐπ' ἀλλοτρίῃσί τε ξυμφορῇσιν ἰδίας καρποῦται λύπας· οἱ δὲ νοσέοντες ἀπαλλάσσονατι τῶν μεγίστων κακῶν διὰ τὴν τέχνην, νούσων, πόνων, λύπης, θανάτου· πᾶσι γὰρ τουτέοισιν ἄντικρυς ἰητρικὴ εὑρίσκεται ἀκεστορίς'

a passage enunciating a conception of medical art to the benefit of the one who is treated under such vigilance and concern.

My paper aims to develop discussion of the complexity of pain-grief-suffering pain as a psychosomatic phenomenon awaiting its medical and humanistic treatment – and relief

– in the *CH*; the entire issue towards the philological attestation as well as the semantic documentation of pain symptoms and signs, especially in the context of Hippocratic research, cannot be further detached from ancient medicine studies and narrative. For instance, we could begin with a passage from the *Epidemics*, which is actually a case report about an incident in Larissa, regarding the young servant of Dyseris, who suffered much pain whenever she had sexual intercourse:

> 'Ἐν Λαρίσσῃ, ἀμφίπολος Δυσήριδος, νέη ἐοῦσα, ὁκότε λαγνεύοιτο, περιωδύνεεν ἰσχυρῶς, ἄλλως δὲ ἀνώδυνος ἦν. Ἐκύησε δὲ οὐδέποτε. ἑξηκονταέτης δὲ γενομένη, ὠδυνᾶτο ἀπὸ μέσου ἡμέρης, ὡς ὠδίνουσα ἰσχυρῶς· πρὸ δὲ μέσου ἡμέρης αὕτη πράσα τρώγουσα πουλλά, ἐπειδὴ ὀδύνη αὐτὴν ἔλαβεν ἰσχυροτάτη τῶν πρόσθεν, ἀναστᾶσα ἐπέψαυσέ τινος τρηχέος ἐν τῷ στόματι τῆς μήτρης' (*Epidemics* 5, 1.25.1–6).

In fact, we read the author's main focus on Hippocratic prognosis, that is not a potentially embarrassing case report from the distant past but the physician's ability to state present observations and consequently offer a suitable medical treatment by providing explanations for different symptoms. The possible differentiation will lead to their alleviation in a congruent explanatory model which may amount to a cultural identity of medical reasoning that has undergone philological documentation. Helen King focused on plausible stories told in narrative forms and therefore useful as linking visions of health and recovery in cultural environments suggested by medical anthropologists like Arthur Kleinmann, 'that the search for meaning in suffering – whether carried out through what we should categorise as 'medicine' or as 'religion'– should be seen in terms of narrative' (King 1998, 111). This narrative kind with possible placebo-healing expectations of pain incidents and the recovery from these painful experiences may provide expectations for the medical future. Whether treated by fomentation or orally administered substances, a study of Hippocratic pharmacopoeia introduces the issues of change and corruption of the natural constitution (φύσις), upon which a physiology system could be based. In another passage from the *CH* treatise *Nature of Man* (4.1–10) we read that:

> 'τὸ δὲ σῶμα τοῦ ἀνθρώπου ἔχει ἐν ἑωυτῷ αἷμα καὶ φλέγμα καὶ χολὴν ξανθήν τε καὶ μέλαιναν, καὶ ταῦτ' ἐστὶν αὐτέῳ ἡ φύσις τοῦ σώματος, καὶ διὰ ταῦτα ἀλγέει καὶ ὑγιαίνει. Ὑγιαίνει μὲν οὖν μάλιστα, ὁκόταν μετρίως ἔχῃ ταῦτα τῆς πρὸς ἄλληλα κρήσιος καὶ δυνάμιος καὶ τοῦ πλήθεος, καὶ μάλιστα μεμιγμένα ᾖ· ἀλγέει δὲ ὁκόταν τι τουτέων ἔλασσον ἢ πλέον ᾖ ἢ χωρισθῇ ἐν τῷ σώματι καὶ μὴ κεκρημένον ᾖ τοῖσι ξύμπασιν. Ἀνάγκη γάρ, ὁκόταν τι τουτέων χωρισθῇ καὶ ἀφ' ἑωυτοῦ στῇ, οὐ μόνον τοῦτο τὸ χωρίον, ἔνθεν ἐξέστη, ἐπίνοσον γίνεσθαι, ἀλλὰ καὶ ἔνθα ἂν ἐπιχυθῇ, ὑπερπιμπλάμενον ὀδύνην τε καὶ νόσον παρέχειν'.

Here it is clearly stated that health and illness are radically opposed: the first defined by mixing (κρῆσις) of the constituent elements of the human body, and illness by the contrary concepts of separation and isolation of one element from the others. Whenever this sort of balance is disturbed, the elements of pain and its cognates constitute a pathological state. Without the characteristic sign of pain a diagnosis could easily be disputed, for only a few diseases do not present pain-sore stages. The prognostic value of some symptoms indicating a nosological state is of high importance to the ancient physicians. Such a description cannot but contain the perceptible signs or symptoms of the disease, which almost exclusively can be observed directly by the senses (Langholf 1990, 55–6), beyond the fact that some symptoms occur under specific circumstances and the simultaneous occurrence of symptoms when a patient performs certain movements of his body. Thus, the notion of the ancient medical diagnosis points towards the understanding of certain nosological syndromes,[1] as we would call them in modern medical terminology. Although medical progress cannot always derive from observation forwarded from the viewpoint of Western biomedicine, since there is no recognisable 'pain thermometer' and variably proposed pain scales lack objectivity (Good *et al.* 1992, 5–6), the sort of cultural or even scientific criteria, available to the writer(s) of the *CH*, against which to judge pain, may prove misleading or complicated if based simply on drug materials, since pain accompanies not only injury, disease and harmful situations, but also, for example, normal physiological childbirth. Sometimes pain can be encouraged in order to activate diagnostic processes or healing effects. Without taking into account the origin of the theories of its treatment, pain was regarded by the authors of the *CH* as a central element in diagnosis, usually first in the list of symptoms and viewed as an important indicator of the precise location of various diseases acknowledged by the ancient physicians.

> 'Health is defined both negatively, by the absence of suffering, and positively, by the balanced mixture of the constitutive elements of man. But insofar as this mixture holds together, the elements do not manifest themselves. In its negative aspect this definition was to inspire a certain number of modern definitions of health. "When we are well," Diderot was later to observe, "no part of the body tells us of its existence; if no one informs us of it through pain, this is a sure sign that we are ill"' (Jouanna 1999, 326[2]).

Then, how could we possibly avail ourselves of an ancient notion of pain's functionality like that attested in *CH*? As we know, the standard definition of pain is currently that approved by the International Association for the Study of Pain (IASP) in 1979:

> 'an unpleasant sensory and emotional experience associated with actual or potential tissue damage, or described in terms of such damage. Pain is always subjective. Each individual learns the application of the word through experiences related

to injury in early life. It is unquestionably a sensation in a part of the body, but it is also unpleasant, and therefore also an emotional experience. Many people report pain in the absence of tissue damage or any likely pathophysiological cause; usually this happens for psychological reasons. There is no way to distinguish their experience from that due to tissue damage, if we take this subjective report' (Brenner 2006, 3).

The neuroanatomy and neurochemistry of the pain – either nociceptive or neuropathic – processing system are extremely complex (Anand and Carr 1989) and, therefore, we access only a basic understanding of the physiology of pain along with its fundamental pathological mechanisms which result through nociception in persistent hyperexcitable states in the presence of acute and chronic pain. Even today, we access such definitions of pain with the goal of improving the success of our therapeutic interventions. Furthermore, we should deliberately explore the complex structures that mediate our appreciation of and response to pain, in order to find that we can conveniently categorise them into two groups: those dealing with the response to pain as an unpleasant sensation, and those more concerned with sensory/discriminative aspects of pain – to inspect a plethora of neurotransmitters mediating transmission of the sensations of pain in both brain and spinal cord. Anyway, we should not forget that cases with chronic pain lasting over six months, for which there is no detectable organic cause (Morris 1991, 70), challenge every possible ideal of medical progress by their resistance to current treatments and by the bewildering complexity of pain pathways.

In confronting this complexity, we tend to forget that fundamentally, above all else, pain is *sore*, and that Hippocrates was right to ascribe it to a nosological state. The Hippocratic localisation of a painful stimulus, long before our ancestors acquired the high-tech pathways necessary to perceive the sensory-discriminative aspects of pain, did not lead to a definition of pain, because definitions tend to force scientists into particular ways of thinking. By concentrating on the subjective nature of pain, the IASP definition allows us to conveniently ignore individuals whose physical findings are all consistent with a diagnosis of pain, but who cannot relate a subjective feeling of pain. Above all, it is still clinically, and will always be, vitally important to listen to the patient who reports pain. We naturally conclude that pain is primarily a symptom warning of injury and at the same time protecting against further injury by causing a reflexive withdrawal from the source of injury; finally, by leading to a period of reduced activity, pain enables injuries to heal more efficiently, apart from its emotional or psychological components. In the *CH* we testify the variation of a case study, in which each person perceives pain a little differently and so responds to painful stimulation differently. In *Diseases* 1 22.17–20, 'καὶ ὅσοι μὲν νεώτεροι πάσχουσί τι τούτων, ὅσα εἴρηται ἀπὸ πόνων παθήματα γίνεσθαι, πάσχουσι πλέω τε καὶ ἰσχυρότερα καὶ ἀλγέουσι μᾶλλον τῶν ἄλλων', we read that young men subject to one of the affections that were said to arise from exertions, suffer in more ways and more severely than others do. Due to the Hippocratic conception of medicine as a '*ganzheitlich orientierte Allgemeinmedizin*' towards the diagnosis of every possible disease (Golder 2007; Preiser 1976), the search for true healing beyond the mere application of remedies to the possession of an appropriate epistemology of health and disease aims at ensuring recovery and preventing any further deterioration, while asserting its superiority over mere chance or to empiricism. For instance, the question of whether the investigation of hidden causes and underlying reality is relevant to the study of pain, and, if so, whether a responsible physician should try to deduce treatments for such cases or just apply what has proved efficacious in what appeared to be similar cases in the experience of the 'scientific' past, being a type of epistemological question we should have been concerned with (Lloyd 1995, 37), suggests a further inquiry over clinical practice of Hippocrates' era. Otherwise, the senses were also to be questioned as reliable guides to enable the credibility of the known, i.e. body's systematical reading, beyond the existing possibilities of deceiving its more or less inexperienced readers. In his philosophical attitude, to refute the monists' theories the author of the treatise *Nature of Man* holds that if man were a unity he would never feel pain, for there would be nothing from which a unity could suffer pain. Pain seems inexplicable upon a scientific hypothesis for it entails an interaction of different substances, which is impossible on the hypothesis that the human body is formed of a single substance (Longrigg 1993, 86–87):

> 'ἐγὼ δέ φημι, εἰ ἓν ἦν ὥνθρωπος, οὐδέποτ' ἂν ἤλγεεν· οὐδὲ γὰρ ἂν ἦν ὑφ' ὅτου ἀλγήσειεν ἓν ἐών· εἰ δ' οὖν καὶ ἀλγήσειεν, ἀνάγκη καὶ τὸ ἰώμενον ἓν εἶναι· νῦν δὲ πολλά' (*Nature of Man* 2.13–16).

The Hippocratics regard the most significant aspect of their knowledge is to know the normal behaviour of the human body (Haeser 1875, 130), along with its physiological state. The assessment of pain should be systematic and thus requires re-evaluation throughout the course of the illness in the cognitive development of medical art; it is, therefore, necessary (i) to study and describe with scientific exactitude, detailed history and careful physical examination the course of disease, including inspection, palpation and auscultation, (ii) to record the epidemiological history including weather information and local conditions prevailing at the time of the epidemic, (iii) to elucidate the pathophysiology of the disease, and (iv) to view the physician as an instructor of the public for a hygienic life, by emphasising the significance of diet and the impulsive compassion for the suffering patient. Toward these aims and to medical etiquette we attribute the stylistic devices of most of the treatises of the *CH*, evidently composed for novices by an experienced practitioner: detailed instructions magisterially given by the verbs χρὴ or δεῖ and by imperatives, imperatival infinitives and gerunds in a more or less dogmatic stance. Technical terms are also used in the didactic tenor of the *CH* treatises.

> 'Another Hippocratic text, *Epidemics* 6.6.3, gives a series of general principles of relieving pain anywhere in the body; you should purge the nearest cavity of blood, using cautery or incision, or apply hot or cold substances, or induce sneezing, or use vegetable juices where these have power, or use the ancient multipurpose remedy called *kykeôn*, a mixture of wine and barley-flour (Loeb VII, 262). For ever worse pains, milk, garlic, boiled wine, vinegar and salt are recommended. I would emphasise that the vegetable juices (*phytôn chymoi*) are to be used "where these have power" – again implying that certain types of ancient medicine would regard as alien the idea of a single drug having the same properties in all cases and situations. Another passage, *Aphorisms* 2.46, says that if someone has two pains (*ponoi*), in different places, the strongest will cancel out the weaker; the implications of this position for pain relief would suggest that you create a worse pain somewhere else to remove the one you started with, rather than considering a drug (Loeb IV, 118; Rey 1993, 31). There is thus no single medical attitude to pain or to the use of pain-relieving substances in Hippocratic medicine' (King 1998, 121–2).

We could also wonder about other applications of pain management treatments, either *ex silentio* or *in expressis verbis*:

> 'The almost total silence regarding the pain of the one being operated on, whether in the case of common procedures such as venesection and cauterisation, or in the case of more dangerous ones such as trephination, is surprising. After all, these patients were not operated on under anaesthesia. It is all the more surprising since the Hippocratic Collection is filled with their pain, and sometimes, too, with their anguished cries. One of the words used to refer to pain (*odunè*) occurs more than seven hundred times in the treatises. But it almost always signifies the pain felt by the patient on account of his illness. This pain interested the physician insofar as it was a meaningful symptom for establishing the diagnosis or prognosis of the illness. The pain of the patient when he was being operated on was of another kind: it was a necessary evil that did not enter into the language of signs and symptoms'.

as Jouanna (1999, 127–28) mentions it. Actually, there is a certain passage in *Physician* 5.1–9:

> 'Ἐπὶ δὲ τῶν χειρουργιῶν, ὅσαι διὰ τομῆς εἰσιν ἢ καύσιος, τὸ ταχέως ἢ βραδέως ὁμοίως ἐπαινεῖται· χρῆσις γάρ ἐστιν ἀμφοτέρων αὐτῶν. Ἐν οἷς μὲν γάρ ἐστι διὰ μιῆς τομῆς ἡ χειρουργία, χρὴ ποιέεσθαι ταχεῖαν τὴν διαίρεσιν· ἐπεὶ γὰρ συμβαίνει τοὺς τεμνομένους πονέειν, τὸ λυπέον μὲν ὡς ἐλάχιστον χρόνον δεῖ παρεῖναι· τοῦτο δὲ ἔσται ταχείης τῆς τομῆς γενομένης. Ὅπου δὲ πολλὰς ἀναγκαῖον γενέσθαι τὰς τομάς, βραδείῃ χρηστέον τῇ χειρουργίᾳ· τὸ μὲν γὰρ ταχὺ ξυνεχῆ ποιέει τὸν πόνον καὶ πουλύν· τὸ δὲ διαλιπὸν ἀνάπαυσιν ἔχει τινὰ τοῦ πόνου τοῖς θεραπευομένοις'

whereby it is stated that the rhythm of the operation should be guided by the desire to ease the patient's suffering in an unavoidable painful condition. Moreover, we should notice that the order of the senses relevant to observation given in the surgeon's memorandum indicates touch next after sight (Jouanna 1999, 298–9); by palpating, e.g. the hypochondria. The physician can judge the possible warnings of an illness latent in signs of pain (see *Prognostics* 7). This could be done in order to determine the sensitivity of a body's part to pain or to solicit other useful observations. Such a clinical account seems to be a physical talent augmented by experience and the acute perceptibility of the exercised senses, but without the knowledge of the invisible world of the internal body. It is explicable to view the identification of medicine as a τέχνη (art) and to maintain its boundaries against ignorance, as it is stated in some Hippocratic texts.

Actually, the types of text and variations included in the *CH* have made it a valuable source for those seeking the authority of medical terminology of the past, so as to delineate the vast knowledge of any new medical development. By anchoring the meaning of suffering to the patient's own experience and sensory perception, Hippocratic medicine allows us to decipher the creation and application of meaning in a philological methodology: the pain of being human and of possessing human feelings and sentiments readable for interested experts of medical terminology. So, in the *CH* we enumerate the following terms[3] denoting pain, grief, distress and suffering from pain: ἀλγεινός, ἀλγέω, ἀλγηδών, ἄλγημα, ἄλγος, λύπη, λυπηρός, ὀδυνάω, ὀδύνη, ὀδύνημα, ὀδυνηρός, ὀδυνηρῶς, ὀδυνώδης, ἐπώδυνος, ἐπωδύνως, περιωδυνέω, περιωδυνία, περιώδυνος, πονέω, πόνημα, πόνος.

In their work Fabrega and Tyma (1976) suggest, beyond the case of authorship and date of single treatises, another class of factors governing the selection of words. Namely cultural considerations which allow us to deduce something of a certain culture's attitude to pain from the choice of the words describing it, since the vocabulary of pain shapes the phenomenon of pain itself. Upon the etymology of the English word 'pain', deriving from the Latin *poena*, 'punishment', they argue that the idea of disease caused by divine vengeance still hovers behind the modern word's use, whereas Scarry (1985, 16) argues that the pain/*poena* connection suggests a search for a cause of pain external to the interior sensation. It is almost impossible to find a perfect match between words and feelings like pain, i.e. feelings variably complicated and subject to subtle physiological or psychological distinctions. Helen King was right to attest the variability of pain viewed as a normal part of human life in the social context of ancient Greece:

> 'In the medical texts, *ponos* seems to be used for long-lasting pain, or dull pain: *odynê* for sharp pain, pain which pierces the body. Rey (1993, 21) argues that *odynê* is "a sharp, shooting

> pain" associated with cutting. In this, it corresponds to the Thai term Diller classifies as $PAIN_3$, a "sudden piercing or stabbing pain, highly focused" (see Diller 1980 on the study of Thai terms for pain). To understand the full field of meanings for *ponos* in classical Greece we must however look outside the medical texts. Hippocratic medicine may be seen as the medicine appropriate to the Greek *polis*, a city-state within which there is an emphasis on particular parts of the body; the arms and hands which bear weapons and practise crafts, and the voice which is central to the oral culture of the *polis*, based as it is on the ideal of participation by all citizens. Activities such as athletics and body-building, which in our society are performed for the sake of the individual, were performed for the state' (King 1998, 123).

In classical Athens, an exemplary *polis* indeed, the male body should be maintained in a healthy condition primarily for military service and the defence of the city; Aristotle's *Constitution of Athens* (*Ath. Pol.* 49.4) provides us with a certain notion of *δοκιμάζω* meant for the proper maturation of male bodies and a relevant state allowance to the conditions fulfilled. Moreover, Spartan women, being unique among Greek women in training their bodies in a respective way, Plutarch (*Life of Lycurgus* 14) suggested physical fitness was seen as necessary both in order to facilitate their own particular service to the state, that is bearing healthy children, and to prepare Spartan *parthenoi* exercising themselves for the *ôdines* of giving birth.

> '*ôdines* has as its primary meaning "labour pains", and is then used figuratively for other mental and physical suffering. In ancient Greek culture further parallels were drawn between fighting and, if necessary, dying for his city, as the most highly valued male social activity, and childbirth, as the corresponding activity by which women prove themselves to be proper women [...]. According to Plutarch (*Life of Lycurgus* 27.2–3), the Spartans were allowed to commemorate only two classes of death by inscriptions on the tomb: men dying in battle, and women dying in childbirth. In a famous passage from Greek tragedy, Medea draws an explicit comparison between the two spheres of activity when she says that she would rather stand in the line of battle three times than give birth once (Eur. *Medea* 248–51). This should probably not be taken as evidence that the Greeks expected normal childbirth to be even more painful than battle injuries; Medea is not a typical Greek woman, but a foreign sorceress who murders her own children, and these lines occur in a long speech on the miserable condition of women, written by a man. However, a fragment of Aeschylus' play *Europê* (fr. 99. 7–8 Nauck[2]) includes the lines "Three times in childbirth, I have endured *gynaikeioi ponoi*", making it clear that the pains of labour are most definitely classified as *ponoi*. Both war and childbirth were viewed as forms of combat involving pain, but in childbirth the enemy was labour itself [...]. Loraux (1982) argues that, for the classical Greek city, *ponos* became a positive, glorious sensation linked to war and childbirth; outside the civic context, however, *ponos* kept its earlier associations of pain and fatigue' (King 1998, 124).

In order to understand Hippocratic perceptions of pain-terms we need to translate semantic uses in former classical literature. Even in Homeric epic (*Iliad*) and though absent from scenes of death, ὀδύναι as pains usually caused by weapons appear in descriptions of wounding and offer the warrior a chance to display his bravery in the context of ἀρετή. The wound of Agamemnon (11.267–72) challenges conventional representations of ὀδύναι and blood by invoking the simile of a woman in labour. The simile implicitly challenges an economy in which τιμή is traded in blood and pains, e.g. in Hecuba's words at 24.212–14. The epic's use of mothers to represent pain anticipates tragic appropriations of the feminine (Holmes 2007). We owe much to the processing and the denoting of pain in the *CH* to King (1998, 114–31; also 1988), who stresses three more aspects in this semantic area of the term *ponos*: i) when used in the plural, in medical texts, for the strengthening exercises, that is for the training necessary for those who want to face the situations in which pain will occur, although 'exertions' of any kind could also cause disease, if undertaken with insufficient care; ii) when, in a wider use, pain has a goal, a means to an end (Loraux 1982, 172); e.g. in *Epidemics* 5.2, whence Timocrates of Elis suffering from madness took the necessary purgative drug to cure his excess of black bile, having undergone 'excessive pain in the purging', but was cured in the end. This case may be contrasted with the fatal condition of Eupolemos of Oineiadae whose critical situation began with severe *odynai* in the hip and groin. Although he drank a purgative, and was given at first the impression of an improvement, 'the pains (*odynai*) did not leave him' (*Epidemics* 5.7) and they remained untouched by the treatment; and iii) in the early gynaecological and other medical texts, when pains during childbirth can be described either as *ponoi* or as *odynai* and could signify either something to be endured or something excessive and thus demanding special attention. For instance, if a woman in labour has pain (*odynê*) in her womb and she worsens or even dies, although her physician 'gives her something' (*Diseases* 1.8):

> 'the particular problem here could be that the doctor defines the woman's pain as being in excess of what is needed, but those members of the family and neighbourhood involved in the birth believe that the pain falls within the limits of "normal and necessary". The particular problem here could be that the doctor defines the woman's pain as being in excess of what is needed, but those members of the family and neighbourhood involved in the birth believe that the pain falls within the limits of "normal and necessary" ' (King 1998, 126).

The Hippocratic treatise *Coan Prognoses* (19.364) states that 'pains which are accompanied by no certain cause are fatal'. Therefore, we could not locate any single medical attitude to pain in Hippocratic writings. Apart from its epistemological state, the perception of pain in the biological root of αἴσθησις and the link between perception and knowledge allow us to argue against an empiricist representation of Hippocratic views on sense perception (so Lo Presti 2007). Though a central element in diagnosis, pain should be viewed as a bodily process and a prominent symptom concerning either the possible location of the disease or its hypothesised mechanism towards a clear conception of the fundamental anatomical and/or physiological disturbance causing the disorder under question. Pain should function as an important indicator of the precise location of a disease (Siegel 1970, 184–93), whilst it does not only accompany injury and pathophysiological disorders. Otherwise, a structural analysis of the Hippocratic data will not point to infinite configurations, as they lack inference to a quaternary system of humoral pathology. Which are the exact cultural criteria of pain or pain-relief in a systemical approach? For instance, in the exhausting discussion of pain (*odynê*) in *Places in Man* 42, it is stated that pain is produced by antithetical conditions: cold and hot, excess and deficiency, whenever a change of the natural constitution (*physis*) takes place within bodily metres; and that pains are cured by contraries in the major Hippocratic dogma.

> 'Where too much exercise is taken in relation to the food intake, the regimen proposed is "soft" and feminine (Loraux 1982: 175); warm baths, soft beds, sex and alcohol, and easing of the *ponoi* (*Regimen* 3.85). I would therefore argue that Hesiod's foregrounding of *ponos* as an essential part of the world of the present, the Age of Iron, continues to influence the choice of pain terminology in the early medical writers. This would in turn suggest that, if a pain is defined as *ponos* at the onset, it may be considered culturally inappropriate to offer pain relief for it. [...] What of chronic illness and chronic pain in the Hippocratic medical texts? Chronic illness is recognised in Hippocratic medicine; there is the belief that it arises from minor conditions which are wrongly treated (e.g. *Aff.* 18). Acute diseases are, however, said to cause the most deaths and to be the most painful or most wearisome (*epiponotatai*, *Aff.* 13). Sciatica is considered long and painful (*epiponos*), but not fatal; arthritis –in sharp much higher than in classical Greece– is described as short, acute, not fatal and affecting the young; gout is the "most chronic" (*polychronios*) and the most intractable condition (*Aff.* 29–30). *Diseases* 1 gives a full classification of conditions according to whether they are invariably fatal, only fatal if there are complications, long-lasting, quick, and so on (1.3). Taken with the example of labour pain, these observations and the difficulty of knowing whether the disease labels or even the experience are translatable suggest some of the limitations of any study of pain in the ancient world. Where much pain was seen as a normal part of human life, and was regarded as "warming" in a system in which heat was considered essential to many bodily processes, patients may have been as reluctant to complain as healers were reluctant to administer painkilling treatments' (King 1998, 126).

In different treatises of the *CH* we can trace the stylistic use of pain terms. In *Places in Man*

> 'there is a tendency for ὀδύνη to be used of localized pain (joints, here; belly, 20; side, 26.1, 2; head, 40.2; pelvic region, 47.3, 4); but it may also be used generally (33.3; 42.1). Πόνος may be used of an accident (as probably implied in the verb πονησάσης τι here; this is a rare reference in *Loc.* to an external cause of illness, rather than the internal cause of belly flux); also for exercise or physical labour. Preference for one term or another for 'pain' is stylistically rather than semantically significant [...]. Pain was a significant guide to prognosis (e.g., as an indicator of the accumulation of 'pus', *Aph.* 2.47) and to treatment (e.g., pains above diaphragm indicate that emetics should be prescribed; below that laxatives are appropriate, *Aph.* 4.18)' (Craik 1998, 129).

In another chapter from the same work, a chapter whose style is rhetorical with highly wrought use of chiasmus and antithesis and a content which could easily be regarded as Gorgianic, the causes and treatment of pain and illness are defined:

> 'ὀδύνη τε γίνεται καὶ διὰ τὸ ψυχρὸν καὶ διὰ τὸ θερμόν, καὶ διὰ τὸ πλέον λίην καὶ διὰ τὸ ἔλασσον· καὶ ἐν μὲν τοῖσιν ἐψυγμένοισι τοῦ σώματος διὰ τὸ θερμαῖνον, ἐν δὲ τοῖσι τεθερμασμένοισι διὰ τὸ ψυχραῖνον ὀδύνη γίνεται· καὶ ἐν μὲν τοῖσι ψυχροῖσι φύσει διὰ τὸ θερμόν, ἐν δὲ τοῖσι θερμοῖσι φύσει διὰ τὸ ψυχρόν· καὶ ἐν μὲν τοῖσι ξηροῖσι φύσει ὑγραινομένοισιν, ἐν δὲ τοῖσιν ὑγροῖσι φύσει ξηραινομένοισι· τὴν γὰρ φύσιν διαλλασσομένοις ἑκάστοισι καὶ διαφθειρομένοις αἱ ὀδύναι γίνονται· ὑγιαίνονταί τε αἱ ὀδύναι τοῖσιν ὑπεναντίοισιν· ἴδιον ἑκάστῳ νοσήματί ἐστι· τοῖσι θερμοῖσι φύσει, διὰ δὲ τὸ ψυχρὸν νοσέουσι, θερμαῖνόν τε καὶ τἆλλα τούτων κατὰ λόγον' (*Places in Man* 42.1–10).

It is obvious that the conception of nature implicit in certain texts of the *CH* has prepared the separation of medicine and natural philosophy (according to Steiger 1982).

What about pain relief or prognosis in an unsuccessful confrontation? In *Ancient Medicine* it is stated that the strongest foods hurt a man most and affect the situation of his health, whether he be well or not, and that all the causes of pain can be reduced to this particular:

> 'πάντα δὴ τὰ αἴτια τοῦ πόνου ἐς τὸ αὐτὸ ἀνάγεται, τὰ ἰσχυρότατα μάλιστά τε καὶ ἐπιφανέστατα λυμαίνεσθαι τὸν ἄνθρωπον καὶ τὸν ὑγιᾶ ἐόντα καὶ τὸν κάμνοντα' (*Ancient Medicine* 6.15–18).

In the same treatise we read that the use of a concrete diet will lead to the experience of harsh and severe suffering and physical weakness, and that the patient's digestion will be ruined to the threshold of death:

> 'ταύτῃ χρεώμενος τῇ διαίτῃ εὖ οἶδ' ὅτι πείσεται πολλὰ καὶ δεινά· καὶ γὰρ πόνους πονήσει καὶ τὸ σῶμα ἀσθενὲς ἔσται καὶ ἡ κοιλίη φθαρήσεται καὶ ζῆν πολὺν χρόνον οὐ δυνήσεται' (*Ancient Medicine* 13.11–15).

Besides, in the treatise *Nature of Man* (10.1–5)

> 'ὅσα δὲ τῶν νοσημάτων γίνεται ἀπὸ τοῦ σώματος τῶν μελέων τοῦ ἰσχυροτάτου, ταῦτα δὲ δεινότατά ἐστιν· καὶ γὰρ ἢν αὐτοῦ μένῃ ἔνθα ἂν ἄρξηται, ἀνάγκη, τοῦ ἰσχυροτάτου τῶν μελέων πονεομένου, ἅπαν τὸ σῶμα πονεῖσθαι'

he states that the most dangerous diseases arise from the strongest part of the body and that the sensitivity of the whole body is affected if the disease remains where it began. In the *Regimen* 1 15.7–9, 'καὶ τόδε ἰητρικῆς· τὸ λυπέον ἀπαλλάσσειν, καὶ ὑφ' οὗ πονεῖ ἀφαιρέοντα ὑγιέα ποιεῖν', we read that part also of the physician's art is to do away with that which causes pain and by taking away the cause of the patient's suffering to make him sound. Medical treatment produces moral conclusions for the first registration of diseases in the classical world, when something biologically harmful is happening to our bodies (Melzack 1977, 15–6).

Pain has its cultural as well as its medical history. Rey in her *History of Pain* has described the development of thought around pain from Plato until modern times;[4] it is undisputable that the notion of pain being of a distinct use, and especially that it is protective and a warning, developed in the last century (Melzack and Wall 1982, 15–9; Sternbach 1968, 95–115). Beyond the Stoic doctrine of the four generic πάθη, pain, pleasure, desire and fear (Rabel 1977), and pain's use in Aristotle's *Nicomachean Ethics* (Lindenmuth 1981), the narrative representation of pain in the Christian era (Perkins 1995) or the philosophical conception of ideal death with the absence of pain and fear in Roman times (Beagon 2005), we have to accept that through Galen's systematisation of physiology in his commentaries – where the physician from Pergamon also claimed that Hippocrates' style was ideal for the specific didactic genre he was involved in, sharing a pronounced philological-literary character (Sluiter 1995) – Hippocrates formed the primary scientific source for European medicine (Siegel 1970). In the Heroic Age of Greece, depicted in Greek mythological references, diseases were attributed to divine wrath: they emerged out of Pandora's jar, a mythical symbol the ancient world was acquainted with (Panofsky and Panofsky 1956). We should not forget that one of the earliest uses of *ponos* is with the meaning of agricultural labour and that in Hesiod it is associated with Pandora opening her jar to release the evils which entered the world. Thus, *ponos* is ordained by the gods and forms an inescapable (*Erga* 92, 113) as well as integral part of human existence. 'It hurts but, whether experienced as war for men or as childbirth for women, it remains part of a process necessary for the continuation of human life' (King 1998, 124). Nevertheless, a genuine physician's treatment must enable the solacious present left inside: hope; she is not to disperse in E. Scarry's aphorism that 'severe pain is world destroying' (Scarry 1985) and thus apply for the patient's increased self-reliance and eliminating catastrophising. Since in the advent of Ionian rationalism man was regarded subject to the same natural laws and not to arbitrary supernatural interference, and since pain does not have age, sex, race, country, religion or social identity, we must perhaps consider it a modality to test our humanity or scientific skill. At least, it should be our last obligation towards the suffering people – i.e. in ἀλγεινὴ διάθεσις, to imitate Hippocrates' vocabulary – among other divine remedies – to contextualise his proverbial compassion.

Notes

1 See Graumann 2000, 63-6; esp. 65: '*Unter dem Ergebnis einer antiken Diagnose, also dem Zuordnen eines Namens als Ausdruck des Krankheitserkennens, darf man sich heute nicht eine klar definierte Krankheitsentität vorstellen, sondern vielmehr eine Beschreibung eines mehr oder weniger regelmäßigen, gleichzeitigen Auftretens von bestimmten Krankheitszeichen, somit am ehesten ein Syndrom im heutigen Sinne*'.

2 D. Diderot's words cited from his treatise *Lettre sur les sourds et muets à l'usage de ceux qui entendent et qui parlent*, Paris 1751.

3 See the *Index Hippocraticus* (Kühn and Fleischer 1986) s.v. and the *Concordance* in *CH* (Maloney and Frohn 1986) s.v.

4 Rey 1993 offers interesting reading in the philosophy of science and social psychology by providing a brief overview of concepts of pain throughout history. The author addresses the major scientific contributions and therapies for treating pain, as well as the scientific and institutional conditions under which these approaches were promulgated in France.

Bibliography

Aldus Manutius 1526: *Hippocrates, Opera Omnia* (in Greek), Venice.

Anand, K. J. and Carr, D. B. 1989: 'The neuroanatomy, neurophysiology, and neurochemistry of pain, stress, and analgesia in newborns and children', *Pediatric Clinics of North America* 36(4), Aug. 1989, 795–822.

Beagon, M. 2005: 'Mors repentina and the Roman art of dying', *Syllecta Classica* 16, 85–137.

Brenner, G. J. 2006: 'Neurophysiologic basis of pain', 3–18 in J. C. Ballantyne (ed.), *The Massachusetts General Hospital of Pain Management* (Lippincott Williams and Wilkins Handbooks), 3rd ed., Philadelphia.

Craik, E. M. 1998: *Hippocrates*, Places in Man, *Edited and Translated with Introduction and Commentary*, Oxford.

Cross, S. A. 1994: 'Pathophysiology of pain', *Mayo Clinic Proceedings* 69, 375–83.

DelVecchio Good, M.-J., Brodwin, P. E., Good, B. J. and Kleinman, A. (eds) 1992: *Pain as Human Experience: An Anthropological Perspective*, Berkeley, Los Angeles and London.

Diller, A. 1980: 'Cross-cultural pain semantics', *Pain* 9, 9–26.

Fabrega, H. F. and Tyma, S. 1976: 'Culture, language and the shaping of illness: an illustration based on pain', *Journal of Psychosomatic Research* 20, 323–7.

Golder, W. 2007: *Hippokrates und das Corpus Hippocraticum. Eine Einführung für Philologen und Mediziner*, Würzburg.

Graumann, L. A. 2000: *Die Krankengeschichten der Epidemiebücher des Corpus Hippocraticum. Medizinhistorische Bedeutung und Möglichkeiten der retrospektiven Diagnose* (Berichte aus der Medizin) (Dissertation Medizinischen Fakultät der Universität Leipzig), Aachen.

Haeser, H. 1875: *Lehrbuch der Geschichte der Medizin und der epidemischen Krankheiten*, Vol. I: *Geschichte der Medizin im Alterthum und Mittelalter*, 3rd ed., Jena (repr. 1996, Hildesheim, Zürich, New York).

Jouanna, J. 1999: *Hippocrates (Medicine & Culture)*, transl. by M. B. DeBevoise, Baltimore and London.

King, H. 1998: *Hippocrates' Woman. Reading the Female Body in Ancient Greece*, London and New York.

Kühn, J.-H. and Fleischer, U. 1986–1989: *Index Hippocraticus.* Curas postremas adhibuerunt K. Alpers, A. Anastassiou, D. Irmer, V. Schmidt, Göttingen.

Langholf, V. 1990: *Medical Theories in Hippocrates. Early Texts and the 'Epidemics'* (Untersuchungen zur antiken Literatur und Geschichte 34), Berlin and New York.

Lindenmuth, D. C. 1981: *The Treatment of Pleasure and Pain in Aristotle's* Nicomachean Ethics, New York.

Lloyd, G. E. R. 1995: 'Epistemological arguments in early Greek medicine in comparativist perspective', 25–40 in D. Bates (ed.), *Knowledge and the Scholarly Medical Traditions*, Cambridge.

Longrigg, J. 1993: *Greek Rational Medicine: Philosophy and Medicine from Alcmaeon to the Alexandrians*, London and New York.

Loraux, N. 1982: 'Ponos. Sur quelques difficultés de la peine comme nom du travail', *Annali dell'Istituto Orientale di Napoli* 4, 171–92.

Maloney, G. and Frohn, W. (eds) 1986: *Concordantia in Corpus Hippocraticum/ Concordance des oeuvres Hippocratiques* (Alpha-Omega. Reihe A: Lexika-Indizes. Konkordanzen zur Klassischen Philologie 75), vols I–IV, Hildesheim, Zürich, New York.

Melzack, R. 1977: *The Puzzle of Pain*, Harmondsworth.

Melzack, R. and Wall, P. 1982: *The Challenge of Pain*, Harmondsworth.

Morris, D. B. 1991: *The Culture of Pain*, Berkeley.

Nutton, V. 2004: *Ancient Medicine*, London and New York.

Panofsky, D. and Panofsky, E. 1956: *Pandora's Box: The Changing Aspect of a Mythical Symbol*, London.

Perkins, J. 1995: *The Suffering Self: Pain and Narrative Representation in the Early Christian Era*, New York.

Preiser, G. 1976: *Allgemeine Krankheitsbezeichnungen im Corpus Hippocraticum. Gebrauch und Bedeutung von Nousos und Nosema* (Ars Medica. Texte und Untersuchungen zur Quellenkunde der Alten Medizin 5), Berlin and New York.

Rabel, R. J. 1977: 'The Stoic doctrine of generic and specific pathē', *Apeiron* 11, 40–2.

Rey, R. 1993: *The History of Pain*, transl. by L. E. Wallace, J. A. Cadden and S. W. Cadden, Cambridge, MA. (French orig. *Histoire de la douleur*, 1993, Paris).

Scarry, E. 1985: *The Body in Pain: The Making and Unmaking of the World*, Oxford.

Siegel, R. E. 1970: *Galen's System of Physiology and Medicine, II: Galen on sense perception. His doctrines, observations and experiments on vision, hearing, smell, taste, touch and pain, and their historical sources*, Basel.

Sluiter, I. 1995: 'The embarrassment of imperfection: Galen's assessment of Hippocrates' linguistic merits', *Clio Medica* 28, 519–35.

Steiger, K. 1982: 'Hippocrates, philosophy and medicine', *Annales Universitatis Scientiarum Budapestinensis* (Phil.) 16, 177–84.

Sternbach, R. A. 1968: *Pain: A Psychophysiological Analysis*, New York.

Willis, W. D. and Westlund, K. N. 1997: 'Neuroanatomy of the pain system and of the pathways that modulate pain', *Journal of Clinical Neurophysiology* 14, 2–31.

13. Le Traité de Galien *De pulsibus ad tirones* : Pratique Médicale et Représentation du Corps Humain

Dina Bacalexi

The treatise De pulsibus ad tirones, *composed during Galen's first stay in Rome (162–166 AD), is intended to teach novice physicians how to 'read' the pulse and establish a diagnosis and a prognosis. We first examine how the pulse doctrine provides the physician with a global perception of the human body, combining the empiric data with a theoretical knowledge fully independent from the medico-philosophical schools. Secondly, we present a description of the different kinds of pulse (single pulse/ succession of pulses). Then we study the causes of the pulse change, in order to find out how their threefold classification (natural/non natural/contra natural) can also be regarded as a twofold one, based on* μέτρον *and excess.*

Comparison with the four treatises De morbo et accidenti, *not intended for beginners, focuses on the different ways and methods Galen uses to reach the same (pedagogical) goal, despite the different target public.*

The wide reception of this treatise from Late Antiquity until the Renaissance shows that it has been instrumental in the diffusion of Galen's theory and praxis.

Destiné aux médecins débutants (*tirones*), adressé à Teuthras, son ami et condisciple, ce court traité, composé lors du premier séjour à Rome du médecin de Pergame (162–166 apr. J.-C.), relu, corrigé et diffusé sous sa forme achevée lors de son second séjour (qui commence en 169 et se poursuit au moins jusqu'en 193) vise, comme il est indiqué dans le c. 1 (K. VIII, 453), à 'exposer toutes les connaissances sur le pouls utiles aux débutants', tout en les incitant, grâce à de nombreuses allusions qui y sont disséminées, à ne pas s'arrêter à ce condensé de science du pouls, mais à consulter ses autres ouvrages y afférents, où ils trouveront 'l'ensemble de l'art le concernant'.[1] Le médecin débutant passera ainsi, grâce à l'acquisition du savoir, de l'état de ἰδιώτης à celui de τεχνίτης, maîtrisant sa τέχνη, en artisan ou artiste accompli, pétri de longue expérience et de réflexion créatrice.

Que ce soit en réponse à une question posée par Teuthras, comme le prétend Agnellus de Ravenne, ce qui n'apparaît pourtant pas clairement dans le texte, ou bien, plus probablement, à la suite d'une conversation que Galien semble poursuivre ici, en commençant son traité *in medias res*, sans exposé théorique préalable sur la santé et la maladie (ce qui est le cas dans les traités *Sur les différences et les causes des maladies et des symptômes*), nous reconnaissons facilement la démarche pédagogique du médecin de Pergame, 'maître sans école et sans disciples', particulièrement attentif à ce que les débutants soient formés de la meilleure façon possible à la science du pouls.[2] Les *tirones*, qui ne sont pourtant pas de profanes, auront à effectuer une lecture du pouls comme signe de l'état de leur patient (diagnostic) et de son évolution (pronostic), dans le contexte réel de la vie dans l'empire romain du 2e s. apr. J.-C. C'est pourquoi la première préoccupation de Galien sera de préciser où et selon quel critère le médecin effectuera une lecture du pouls qui permettra de lire le grand livre du corps humain. La description des variations et la présentation des causes viennent ensuite, sans être jamais exemptes de cet esprit rigoureux et polémique qui caractérise le médecin de Pergame.

Notre présentation aura donc pour but, dans un premier temps, d'examiner la pratique médicale, c'est-à-dire la méthode, les modalités du toucher, les différences du pouls décelées. L'examen des causes et leur classement permettra ensuite d'esquisser une conception du corps humain qui, tout en étant basée sur la célèbre distinction tripartite de Galien, κατὰ φύσιν/οὐ κατὰ φύσιν/παρὰ φύσιν, mettra en évidence un schéma binaire, celui de la mesure et de l'excès, συμμετρία/ἀμετρία, μέτρον/ὑπερβολή. Dans un troisième temps, nous présenterons un aperçu de la diffusion de ce traité, inversement proportionnelle à sa taille, depuis l'Antiquité tardive jusqu'à la fin du 16ᵉ s.

1. Pratique médicale : la méthode, le toucher et les variations du pouls

Dans son traité *De ordine librorum suorum* (K. XIX, 54 = Boudon II, 1, p. 91), Galien conseille tout naturellement aux hommes 'sages et amis de la vérité' (συνετοὶ καὶ ἀληθείας ἑταῖροι) de commencer la lecture de ses traités (logiquement) par ceux destinés aux débutants. Parmi ceux-ci, le *De pulsibus* occupe la deuxième place, juste après le *De sectis*. Les quatre traités *Sur les différences et les causes des maladies et des symptômes* suivent loin derrière. Cela montre l'importance capitale de ce traité, mais aussi sa place méthodologique, car la connaissance des préceptes des 'sectes/écoles' médicales de son époque permettra au futur médecin d'appréhender tant les consignes méthodologiques données dans le *De pulsibus*, que les allusions polémiques aux médecins dont la méthode induit en erreur. Mais quelle est, pour Galien, la méthode la plus sûre de la prise du pouls ?

Au c. 1 du traité, le vocabulaire employé est celui de la sensation, αἰσθάνομαι, αἴσθησις, qui donnera le mouvement de l'artère σφύζουσα, l'αἰσθητὴ κίνησις. C'est le toucher, ἡ ἁφή, du médecin qui sera mis à contribution, et l'endroit du corps le plus propice à ce geste médical est le carpe. La raison est évidente :

> 'parce que l'endroit n'est pas charnu – il n'est donc nécessaire de dénuder aucun membre du corps, comme c'est le cas pour plusieurs autres – et parce qu'elles [les artères des carpes] sont disposées en ligne droite. Et ce dernier point n'est pas négligeable pour l'exactitude du diagnostic' (K. VIII, 454, 14–18).[3]

Une méthode empirique, pourrait-on dire, peut-être plus facile pour un débutant que l'acquisition de connaissances théoriques, travail plus ardu et de longue haleine. Or, si le toucher du médecin reçoit ces données fournies par le corps de son patient 'gratuitement', sans élaboration préalable, en quelque sorte à l'état brut, le diagnostic et le pronostic sont des opérations intellectuelles, qui présupposent une exploitation 'utilitaire' des 'entités gracieuses' (selon l'expression de Michel Serres), la réconciliation du 'gratuit' et du 'rentable', du sensoriel et du rationnel : le médecin, même débutant, aura comme mission l'analyse rationnelle et systématique de ce capital de connaissances 'à l'état pur'.[4] C'est d'ailleurs la réalité de la vie des patients qui conduira le médecin à adopter la bonne méthode, comme le dit Galien au c. 9 (K. VIII, 462–463) :

* premièrement, la bonne connaissance du pouls 'conforme à la nature' (κατὰ φύσιν) sera le point de référence. Mais cette situation 'de santé et de repos parfaits' (ὑγιαίνοντος ἀμέμπτως καὶ ἐν ἡσυχίᾳ πάσης σφοδρᾶς κινήσεως) est un idéal qu'on ne risque pas de rencontrer souvent lors de la pratique quotidienne avec les patients. Même si le conseil de 'tâter souvent l'artère' (δεῖ πολλάκις ἧφθαι τῆς ἀρτηρίας) lors d'un tel état est valable dans l'absolu, une longue expérience a enseigné à Galien qu'on ne peut pas se limiter à cela.
* deuxièmement, l'exercice, la pratique, la fréquence des cas fourniront la palette des pouls correspondant à celle des états précis des patients (τὸ μὲν ἴδιον ἑκάστου ἀκριβῶς ἄν τις πειραθεὶς μάθοι). Galien insiste sur ce point, et sur la fréquence du geste. Mais le nœud du problème consiste en une combinaison de l'expérience et de la raison, et non, comme le prétendent les médecins empiriques, en une simple constatation ou analogie. C'est pourquoi, dans le *De sectis* (K. I, 67), Galien critique de l'empirisme pur, qui distingue les affections en φυσικὰ, τυχικὰ et μιμητικά, ces derniers étant une transposition du semblable au semblable ; et dans le *Ad Thasybulum* (K. I, 133), la critique se poursuit contre la distinction des symptômes en 'utiles' et 'inutiles'.[5]
* troisièmement, le médecin prendra conscience du fait que, dans le monde complexe où il vit, ni l'expérience seule, ni l'exercice fréquent dans les mêmes conditions ne pourront l'aider efficacement pour son diagnostic :

  'puisqu'il n'est pas possible que tout soit accessible par l'expérience et que plusieurs personnes ont eu souvent besoin de médecins à qui elles n'avaient pas eu affaire quand elles étaient en bonne santé, le mieux dans ces cas-là aussi est que l'expert (τεχνίτης) surpasse le profane (ἰδιώτης). Et il peut le surpasser s'il puise sa science (ἐπιστήμη) dans les ressemblances qui existent entre plusieurs individus' (K. VIII, 463).

La connaissance du fonctionnement du pouls correspond donc à une nécessité qu'on pourrait qualifier de 'professionnelle', liée aux conditions d'exercice de l'art médical. C'est précisément pour cette raison qu'un débutant doit être bien orienté, dans le dédale des obédiences qui constituent l'offre d'enseignement des sectes médicales : Galien critique l'expérience pure, mais ne prône jamais son contraire, le rationalisme pur, se démarquant ainsi des dogmatiques ou rationalistes. Il incite ses futurs collègues :

> 'à exercer en même temps le raisonnement (τὸν λογισμόν) et le toucher (τὴν ἁφήν), parce que c'est précisément par la pratique (ἀπ᾽ αὐτῶν τῶν ἔργων) qu'on pourra reconnaître le pouls et non seulement le distinguer en théorie (λόγῳ). Le fondement de l'exercice pratique est l'enseignement théorique. Mais il est bien sûr impossible d'expliquer par la théorie combien dense est le pouls, même s'il existe une grande

différence entre le fait que la pleurésie dépasse son seuil habituel ou ne l'a pas encore atteint. [...]. Il en est de même pour les différentes espèces d'inégalité' (K. VIII, 478).

Voilà donc comment le médecin pourra être vraiment utile, connaisseur, ἐπιστήμων. Il étudiera plusieurs groupes de personnes semblables, hommes ou femmes, enfants, adultes ou vieillards, en plusieurs moments de l'année, été, automne, hiver, printemps, et, ce qui est tout à fait probable dans un empire romain favorisant les contacts et les voyages, dans des contrées à climat tempéré, ou chaud ou froid. Même s'il n'arrive pas à avoir toutes ces expériences de première main, la méthode et l'acquisition du savoir sauront compenser ce manque. Il est important à noter ici que cette acquisition du savoir médical se fera de première main, le médecin puisant dans le réservoir des 'signes' donnés par le corps de son patient et essayant de les interpréter grâce au savoir théorique qu'il aura acquis.[6] Il s'agit là d'une très haute conception de l'art médical que le médecin de Pergame transmet aux débutants, en les préservant ainsi du scepticisme, comme il l'avait été lui-même préservé, grâce à ses études mathématiques.[7]

Si la méthode est tellement importante, il en va de même pour l'expertise manuelle, car en lisant ce traité le médecin débutant comprendra qu'il n'a pour lire le pouls de son patient qu'une seule arme concrète, fournie non par un instrument extérieur, mais par son propre corps : c'est son toucher qui recevra le coup (la diastole) ou percevra le repos (la systole). C'est donc grâce à un contact direct que circuleront les informations entre les deux corps dont chacun pourra être conçu comme la continuité de l'autre. La description détaillée des changements du pouls, et l'insistance sur leur multiplicité (πολυειδῶς οἱ σφυγμοὶ τρέπεσθαι πεφύκασιν, οὐδὲν γὰρ εὔροις... αἴτιον ὃ μὴ καὶ τούτους τρέπει , K. VIII, 462), ainsi que l'absence, chez Galien, d'un instrument de mesure du pouls (Hérophile avait inventé une sorte de clepsydre pour mesurer le rythme du pouls) suggèrent le haut niveau d'exigence requis pour les débutants, dont le toucher doit être le plus exercé possible, l'attention au patient et la compétence technique portées au plus haut degré.[8]

Cependant, la question a été souvent posée : malgré la précision dans la description, malgré le soin que met Galien à former ses collègues débutants à la meilleure lecture du pouls, comment serait-il humainement possible que toutes les nuances du pouls qu'il nous présente soient clairement établies ? N'est-ce pas là une pure spéculation, une construction intellectuelle, sans fondement réel ?

Sans tomber dans des considérations anachroniques, à savoir celles qui comparent Galien et les médecins de notre temps, en oubliant qu'on ne peut comparer que des choses comparables et que, même avec des similitudes dans le mode de vie et de déplacement l'époque des Antonins n'est pas la nôtre, et sans verser dans l'excès contraire et considérer toute médecine non occidentale comme une médecine parfaite, qui nous aiderait à retourner dans un hypothétique 'état de nature' à jamais disparu, il est légitime d'une part de s'interroger sur la capacité à déceler les variations que nous allons présenter, et d'autre part de chercher des parallèles réels dans les pratiques des médecines traditionnelles extrême-orientales.[9] Loin d'être 'plus mystiques' ou 'moins rationnelles', ces médecines, tout en présentant d'incontestables différences avec la médecine grecque, conçoivent l'organisme humain comme un ensemble, et trouvent dans le pouls l'un des signes les plus accomplis de sa lecture, peut-être parce qu'elles prennent en considération des facteurs plus complexes que le simple toucher ou que la distinction mécanique entre la diastole et la systole. La méthode de poser les doigts, la distinction de différents 'lieux' du carpe, chacun correspondant à une information précise venant d'un 'lieu' du corps, une conception du rythme, une technique de palpation, tout cela suggère que des descriptions du pouls comme celle que fournit Galien aux débutants ne sont pas le produit d'une imagination débordante, mais le fruit d'un effort du médecin de Pergame pour donner la vision la plus complète du corps à soigner. Par ailleurs, la science moderne peut aujourd'hui expliquer la spécificité du toucher, grâce à des données physiologiques observées chez l'homme et chez certains animaux : une sensibilité particulière existerait chez les humains, dans certaines conditions (Barras 2005, 55–6). Mais ce qui nous intéresse ici n'est pas tant l'aspect biomédical de la question que son aspect philosophique : la lecture du pouls est un acte conscient effectué par le médecin galénique, c'est-à-dire une association de la nature et de la culture, des données sensorielles et de leur exploration intellectuelle en vue d'un diagnostic qui ne dépend plus des sens, mais de l'esprit, et, si possible, d'un pronostic, qui dépend encore plus de la capacité d'appropriation intellectuelle de ces données. Nous constatons d'ailleurs que, dans la postérité de Galien, comme, par exemple, dans le traité sur le pouls du Pseudo-Soranos (5e–6e s.), il existe, certes, une explication détaillée de la façon de poser les doigts du médecin sur la main du patient etc. Mais le fait que de telles explications ne sont pas reprises par d'autres auteurs qui ont lu et commenté les traités de Galien sur le pouls, et notamment le *De pulsibus ad tirones* (Agnellus, Théophile protospathaire, Ioannes Grammaticus), suggère que l'accent est mis ailleurs que sur la technique (Palmieri 2003, 78–9).

Le médecin débutant ne trouvera pas dans ce traité une explication détaillée de la position des doigts du médecin qui tâte le pouls, comme c'est le cas dans le *De dignoscendis pulsibus* par exemple (K. VIII, 803–804), où l'on apprend de quelle façon il convient de placer sa main (τὴν ἐπιβολὴν τῆς χειρὸς προσήκει ποιεῖσθαι), et de quelle façon ce contact sera le plus efficace en matière de diagnostic. Il ne trouvera pas non plus la distinction entre le simple contact, ἅπτομαι, et l'exploration, ψαύω, qui s'effectuent tous les deux grâce au toucher (le verbe ψαύω désigne souvent le toucher de la sage-femme, comme par exemple dans la collection hippocratique, *De natura muliebri, De morbis mulierum*).[10] Mais il trouvera une description très précise des variations du pouls tant isolé (un fait précis survenu à un moment précis) qu'en situation (une succession de pouls pendant une période temporelle). Mémoriser ces variations sera déjà le premier pas pour devenir expert.

Paramètres de changement du pouls isolé (c. 2, 3 et 4) (Tableau 13.1)

La description des changements du pouls se poursuit avec l'examen du pouls 'en situation', c'est-à-dire de la succession des pouls : les paramètres examinés pour le pouls isolé serviront de base pour mieux appréhender cette succession, ce qui aidera le médecin à établir son diagnostic quand il se trouvera, lui aussi, 'en situation', face à son patient. Selon chacun des paramètres précités (taille, mouvement, durée de la systole et de la diastole), Galien examinera l'égalité et l'inégalité du pouls. Et selon la périodicité ou non de l'apparition de ces différences, il établira l'ordre ou le désordre, la régularité ou l'irrégularité.

Paramètres de changement du pouls en succession (c. 5, 6, 7 et 8) (Tableau 13.2)

La partie descriptive s'achève sur une conclusion partielle à la fin du c. 9 (K. VIII, 461), qui sert d'une part à introduire la partie étiologique du traité, et d'autre part à rappeler que, malgré cet exposé détaillé, ce traité ne donne qu'un condensé de sphygmologie, un *Grundriss* (Ilberg 1889), et qu'il serait utile d'approfondir ses connaissances grâce au 'livre entier' écrit par Galien sur les différences du pouls (*De differentia pulsuum).*

Après avoir examiné cette description du pouls si détaillée et précise, destinée pourtant 'aux débutants', il est légitime de se poser la question du public réel de ce traité et du niveau d'instruction de ces 'débutants', capables de tant de finesse afin de se retrouver dans un phasme si étendu de variantes. Galien ne donne pas de précision, mais il est facile de comprendre, compte tenu des références à ses traités sur le même sujet qui ne sont pas destinés aux débutants qu'il a souhaité d'une part fournir aux médecins des connaissances indispensables, d'autre part contribuer à la diffusion du savoir médical. On pourrait même avancer l'hypothèse qu'un tel traité serait fort utile à des médecins qui voyagent beaucoup (comme Galien lui-même) et qui ne peuvent donc pas emporter avec eux de livres volumineux. Dans ce cas, ce ne serait pas uniquement un public d'étudiants ou d'apprentis médecins (sorte d'internes de nos jours), mais un public de médecins confirmés qui aurait besoin à tout instant d'un manuel de référence.[11]

Tableau 13.1. Paramètres de changement du pouls isolé (c. 2, 3 et 4)

	pouls conforme à la nature quant à la diastole (κατὰ φύσιν = σύμμετρος διαστολή)	***pouls conforme à la nature quant à la systole*** (μέσος, entre le rare et le dense)
pouls non conforme à la nature (παρὰ φύσιν)		
1. quant à sa quantité (ποσόν)		
A. chacune des trois dimensions de l'artère toute seule		
large (πλατής)	*étroit (στενός)*	
long (μακρός)	*court (βραχύς)*	
profond (ὑψηλός)	*bas (ταπεινός)*	
B. les trois dimensions de l'artère ensemble		
petit (μικρός)	grand (μέγας)	
2. quant au mouvement *(κίνησις)*		
rapide (ταχύς)	*lent* (βραδύς)	
3. qualité du coup ressenti au toucher (ποιὸν τῆς προσβολῆς)		
vigoureux (σφοδρός)	*faible* (ἀμυδρός)	
4. qualité de la paroi de l'artère (ποιότης τοῦ χιτῶνος τῆς ἀρτηρίας)		
doux au toucher (μαλακός)	*dur au toucher* (σκληρός)	
5. intervalle des battements (ἡσυχία ἢ διάλειμμα ἢ πληγῶν διαστολή)		
dense (πυκνός)	*rare* (ἀραιός)	

Tableau 13.2. Paramètres de changement du pouls en succession (c. 5, 6, 7 et 8)

battements successifs					
égal (ὁμαλός)	*inégal* (ἀνώμαλος)				
périodicité (battements inégaux après une série d'égaux)					
ordonné (τεταγμένος)	*désordonné* (ἄτακτος)				
inégalités simples					
1. quant à la position (θέσει) **des parties de l'artère**					
haut/bas (ἄνω/κάτω)	*devant/derrière* (πρόσω/ὀπίσω)	droite/gauche (δεξιά/ἀριστερά)			
2. quant au mouvement (κινήσει) **des parties de l'artère**					
plus rapide/ plus lent (θᾶττον/βραδύτερον)	plus précoce/ plus tardif (πρωιαίτερον/ ὀψιαίτερον)	plus durable/ plus bref (ἐπὶ πλείονα/ ἐλάσσονα χρόνον)	perpétuel/absent complètement (ἀεί/οὐδ'ὅλως)	nette interruption (διακεκόφθαι σαφῶς)	palindromique (παλινδρομεῖν)
				« capricant » (δορκαδίζων)	*« dicrote » (δίκροτος)*
inégalités complexes (qui n'ont pas toutes un nom)					
vermiculaire (σκωληκίζων), petite diastole	*ondoyant* (κυματώδης), *grande diastole*				
formicant (μυρμηκίζων)					
hectique (ἑκτικός)[1]					

[1] Il est à noter que l'adjectif 'hectique' (le pouls, comme la fièvre) n'a pas le même sens chez Galien et en français, où il est également utilisé dans le vocabulaire médical. Ἑκτικός, dérivé de ἕξις, le caractère de ce qui est habituel, sans variations importantes, désigne un pouls qui ne change pas beaucoup. Or selon le *Petit Robert*, une 'fièvre hectique' est au contraire une fièvre qui présente des oscillations importantes, de très importants frissons suivis de bouffées de chaleur et de sudation conséquentes.

2. Causes, juste mesure et excès : quelle conception du corps humain ?

L'examen des causes nous conforte dans l'idée que le médecin débutant est quelqu'un qui agit mais qui réfléchit en même temps, puisque pour Galien *le meilleur médecin est aussi philosophe,* pourvu d'une 'culture générale' acquise grâce à une éducation complète. Signe clinique par excellence, mais aussi clé de lecture du corps humain, le pouls subit des changements liés à toute une série de pathologies ou d'états non pathologiques, classés dans les trois catégories bien connues : *conformes à la nature/non conformes à la nature/contre nature.* On pourrait établir ici un parallèle (comme le fait Agnellus de Ravenne dans son commentaire) avec la distinction tripartite aristotélicienne entre φυσιολογικόν/αἰτιολογικόν/σημειωτικόν, ou supposer l'existence d'un 'état intermédiaire' entre la santé et la maladie, cet οὐδέτερον auquel Galien fait référence dans d'autres traités (*Ars medica*) et qui correspondrait aux causes 'non conformes à la nature' du *De pulsibus.*[12] Or, ce qui frappe dans notre traité ce sont les références constantes aux notions de symétrie et d'amétrie, et, par conséquent, l'évaluation du pouls selon une 'juste mesure', qui, elle, ne serait pas 'non conforme', mais bien 'conforme' à la nature. La tripartition des causes subit une première entorse au c. 8 du *De pulsibus*, car Galien avoue lui-même que :

> « ce n'est pas un secret que, pour les autres oppositions de pouls, il existe à chaque fois une voie médiane ; mais il n'en existe aucune entre l'égal et l'inégal, ni entre l'ordonné et le désordonné. Aussi pour tous les autres cas la voie médiane est conforme à la nature, mais pour ces deux-là c'est uniquement l'égal qui est conforme à la nature, les autres, à savoir l'inégal et le désordonné, ne sont pas conformes à la nature » (K. VIII, 461–62).

Selon leur rapport à la juste mesure, les causes 'non naturelles', qui ne sont pas une catégorie fermée, appartiendraient tantôt à la partie 'naturelle', tantôt à la

Tableau 13.3. Causes non naturelles de changement du pouls et notion d'excès

exercices corporels	μέχρι τοῦ **μετρίου**	ὑπερβαλλόντως δ'**ἄμετρα**
bains chauds	**σύμμετρα**	**ἄμετρα**
bains froids	παραχρῆμα	εἰς ὕστερον
nourriture	**σύμμετρα**	**πολλά**, ὥστε βαρύνειν τὴν δύναμιν/**ἐλάττονα**, ὥστε μὴ τρέφειν
vin (παραπλησίως σιτίοις)		
eau (ἀνάλογον σιτίοις)		

partie 'contre nature', car elles produisent des changements du pouls tantôt semblables aux causes naturelles, tantôt à ceux provoqués par les causes contre nature, les causes pathologiques.[13]

En énumérant les causes 'non naturelles', Galien introduit déjà la notion d'excès (Tableau 13.3).

Le dépassement de la juste mesure (surplus ou manque) transforme donc ces causes en 'contre nature' et appuie l'idée que le diagnostic par le pouls doit être fondé sur le rapport qu'entretient le médecin avec le μέτρον.

3. Le diagnostic et le pronostic

À chaque cause présentée dans cette seconde partie correspondent une ou plusieurs variantes du pouls citées dans la première partie du traité ; le médecin, qui les reconnaît au toucher, est donc capable de statuer sur le type de pathologie et sur ses nuances, mais aussi d'aller plus loin, car le pouls prédit (pronostique) l'évolution et la fin de chaque maladie, sa curabilité ou son caractère fatal. Cependant, ce qui manque dans le *De pulsibus*, ce sont les conseils de thérapie : il n'y a aucune mention de remèdes, justement parce que l'objectif du 'maître' est de procéder par étapes et de développer d'abord chez ses 'élèves' le sens de l'observation et de l'analyse. C'est aussi une preuve que, comme pour la médecine tibétaine, le diagnostic et le pronostic constituent une branche de la médecine séparée de la thérapeutique. Ce n'est d'ailleurs pas un hasard si, dans la médecine arabe, par exemple (Haly Abbas †944, Avicenne), ainsi que dans les temps modernes (William Harvey, qui applique les principes de changement du pouls à ceux de la régulation de la circulation sanguine), la réflexion sur les causes 'naturelles' et 'non naturelles' du *De pulsibus* est reprise dans des traités concernant l'hygiène (facteur de régulation des différentes causes), et non la pathologie pure.[14]

Plus spécifiquement pour le pronostic, notons ici que, dans les c. 11 et 12 qui concernent les changements dus aux causes contre nature, Galien explique qu'il existe des étapes que le médecin pourra reconnaître grâce au pouls qui leur est propre. Chaque étape aura une incidence sur la faculté vitale (ζωτικὴ δύναμις) que les causes contre nature compriment ou surchargent (θλίβειν/βαρύνειν) ou bien qu'elles anéantissent ou dispersent (λύειν/σκεδαννύειν) (K. VIII, 471). La distinction des étapes concerne tant l'évolution de la maladie dans le temps, c'est-à-dire le début, le milieu et la fin (K. VIII, 471–472, où l'on parle de la βλάβη en général ; VIII, 474, de la douleur ; VIII, 475, de l'inflammation ; VIII, 479, des abcès etc.), que son caractère aigu ou chronique (K. VIII, 473, sur les affections entraînant des évacuations aiguës, ὀξέως κενωτικὰ πάθη ; VIII, 473–474 sur la peur, qui vient en dernier lieu d'une courte énumération comprenant aussi la colère, le plaisir, la tristesse) ou bien l'évolution d'une maladie vers un état qu'on pourrait appeler 'terminal' ou 'fatal' (le cas de l'angine, K. VIII, 488 ; le cas de l'orthopnée aiguë, moyennement violente, extrêmement violente ou 'sur le point d'emporter' le malade, VIII, 489 ; le cas de la suffocation hystérique qui pourrait devenir ὀλεθρία, VIII, 489) etc.

Armé pour le diagnostic et pour le pronostic, le médecin débutant ne connaît pourtant que des rudiments concernant les causes des maladies citées dans ce traité, et pratiquement rien de leurs symptômes. Il les connaîtra grâce aux quatre traités détaillés que Galien a composés sur ce sujet : *De morborum differentiis, De morborum causis, De symptomatum differentiis, De symptomatum causis*. Leur diffusion a été comparable à celle du *De pulsibus*, car ils ont également été perçus par les galénistes (dès l'époque alexandrine, ils font partie du *Canon* comme le *De pulsibus*) comme des instruments pédagogiques utiles à la formation des médecins.[15] L'objectif pédagogique commun est le premier point de comparaison entre le *De pulsibus* et les quatre traités souvent regroupés sous le titre collectif *De morbo et accidenti*.[16] Mais cet objectif n'est explicite que dans le *De pulsibus*, non dans les traités sur les maladies et les symptômes. Il est par ailleurs atteint par des voies différentes :

1. Au début du *De morborum differentiis* (K. VI, 836–837 et 838) et du *De symptomatum differentiis* (K. VII, 49–50), la définition de la santé et de la maladie constitue un préalable à un développement technique détaillé. C'est là où l'on retrouve, d'ailleurs, les notions de symétrie et d'amétrie, correspondant la première à la santé et la seconde à la maladie :

εἴη ἂν οὖν ἡ μὲν ὑγεία συμμετρία τις, ἡ δὲ νόσος ἀμετρία [...].

Tableau 13.4. Diffusion du De pulsibus : Antiquité tardive et haut Moyen Âge

Chronologie	Nature	Personne(s)	Langue	Objectif	Témoignages ou sources
6e s. (avant 536)	*Canon* d'Alexandrie	Anquilâûs (publie) ; Stéphanos, Ges(s)ios, Marinos (ordonnent et commentent)	grec (textes originaux)	Pédagogique (16 traités à l'usage des médecins débutants)	*Synopsis* de Ioannes 'Grammaticus' (6e ou 7e s.) ; Hunain ibn Ishaq (ob. 873) ; Ali ibn Ridwan (9e s.)
6e-7e s.	*Εἰσαγωγαί* : subdivision du *Canon* d'Alexandrie comprenant 4 traités		grec (textes originaux)	Introduction à l'apprentissage de la médecine	ms Milan, Bibl. Ambrosiana, G 108 inf. (9e s.)
6e s.	Commentaire du *De pulsibus*	Ioannes 'Grammaticus'[1]	grec (perdu), arabe (conservé)	Exégèse	Traduction arabe par Al-Dimashqî (10e s.), ms Berlin, Staatsbibl., ar. 6230 (12e s.)
6e s.	Commentaire lemmatique du *De pulsibus* 'ex uoce Agnello'[2]	Agnellus de Ravenne 'iatrosophiste' (le maître) ; Simplicius (médecin ; l'élève/transcripteur)	latin	Exégèse à partir de 'notes de cours'	ms Milan, Bibl. Ambrosiana, G 108 inf. (9e s.)
6e s.	*Summaria Alexandrinorum*		grec (perdu), syriaque et arabe (conservé)	Extraction de 'quintessence'	Hunain (9e s.) (traduit) ; Razès (9e-10e s.) (en cite le texte)
6e-7e s.	Résumés (plus courts que les *Summaria*) des traités du *Canon*	Ioannes 'Grammaticus'	grec (perdu), arabe (conservé)	Exégèse synthétique	Ms Londres, British Libr., Arundel Or. 17 = 444
	Διαιρέσεις ou *Tabulae* (divisions stemmatiques basées sur les *Sommaires*)[3]		grec : *Σφυγμικάριον τὸ πρὸς Τεῦφραν* (sic)	Présentation schématique des traités du *Canon*	Ms Vienne, ÖNB, Med. gr. 16, (ff. 329r-359v) (13e-15e s.)
11e s.	Commentaire	Al-Taiyib ob. 1043	arabe	Éxegèse	Ms Princeton-Garrett 1095

[1] Pormann 2003, 248-50, passe en revue les différents 'Jean' de l'Antiquité tardive, dont la liste est dressée par Garofalo 1999, afin de déterminer qui est ce 'Jean le Grammairien' qui a rédigé le commentaire du *De pulsibus.* En fait, nous ne savons pratiquement rien sur lui, sauf qu'il a vécu au 6e ou au 7e s.

[2] Palmieri 2005.

[3] Pour les *Tabulae Vindobonenses* et leur apport dans la réception de Galien : Gundert 1998.

> εἰ μὲν οὖν ἐν πόρων συμμετρίᾳ τὸ ὑγιαίνειν ἐστίν, ἐν πόρων ἀμετρίᾳ γενήσεται καὶ τὸ νοσεῖν (K. VII, 838, 8–12).[17]

Rien de tel, comme nous l'avons vu, dans le *De pulsibus,* où l'accent est mis sur l'énumération et la description.

2. Ainsi que nous l'avons déjà noté, et même sans s'attarder sur la méthode de la prise du pouls, le fait de tâter le carpe du patient, peut-être aussi d'autres endroits du corps, le carpe constituant le 'meilleur endroit à toucher' pour des raisons pratiques, c'est-à-dire parce qu'il n'est pas couvert, et scientifiques, parce que c'est là où le pouls est le plus 'lisible', comme la chair qui le recouvre n'est pas épaisse (K. VIII, 454) est l'élément clé de la pratique médicale enseignée dans ce traité. Toucher son patient signifie pour le médecin établir une communication directe entre les deux corps, comme si l'un se prolongeait par l'autre.[18] La perspective est différente dans les traités *Sur les maladies et les symptômes,* où nous n'avons pas de 'lecture' directe, mais où nous pouvons comprendre le fonctionnement du corps si l'on suit le liquide et le souffle dont la circulation structure le 'réseau' interne du corps humain et dont la modification de la consistance ou l'accumulation dans des endroits stratégiques, les 'conduits' (πόροι), ont des conséquences pathologiques, l'obstruction (ἔμφραξις) interrompant la fluidité de la communication des informations à l'intérieur, ou de l'intérieur vers l'extérieur. Le retour à la normale, la désobstruction (ἔκφραξις), se fait lorsque ces

Tableau 13.5. Traductions en langue orientale

Chronologie	Personne	Langue	Public
9e s.	Hunain ibn Ishaq	Syriaque	Traduction à l'usage des non-hellénophones
9e s.	Hunain ibn Ishaq	Arabe	Traduction à l'usage des non-hellénophones

Tableau 13.6. Éditions des 12e–16e siècles : texte grec

Édition princeps 1525	Édition 1529	Édition 1538	Édition 1543
Alde Manuce éditeur et imprimeur, Venise	Simon de Colines, imprimeur, Paris	Leonhart Fuchs, Hieronymus Gemusaeus, Joachim Camerarius, éd. ; Andreas Cratander, imprimeur, Bâle	Chrétien Wechel, imprimeur, Paris
Galeni librorum pars quinta, doubles pages 1-5		*Galeni librorum pars tertia*, p. 1-7, premier traité du volume avant le *De differentiis pulsuum* I	
BIUM numérisé	BNF 8-TD3-2(2)	BIUM numérisé	Paris, Faculté de la médecine

mêmes substances retrouvent leur état premier et que la fluidité de la circulation des informations est rétablie : le réseau fonctionne donc à nouveau, le corps humain recouvre la santé.

5. La diffusion du *De pulsibus* depuis l'antiquité tardive jusqu'à la fin du 16e s.

On est frappé de constater combien un traité si court et parfois assez elliptique, sans développements théoriques ou approfondissements, a fait l'objet de lectures, de relectures (commentaires ou rédaction de traités semblables qu'il a influencés), d'éditions et de traductions pendant une période si longue, sans interruption. Son caractère pédagogique aidant, et malgré le fait qu'à la fin le lecteur ne retrouve pas de conclusion ou de synthèse, le *De pulsibus* a été remarqué d'abord par les médecins alexandrins, qui l'ont intégré dans le *Canon* des 16 traités de Galien indispensables pour l'enseignement, ensuite par les Arabes, qui en ont fait des *Sommaires*, des résumés et des commentaires, enfin par les traducteurs qui, dès le Moyen Âge (11e–12e s.) l'ont traduit en latin, ce qui suggère une diffusion large dans les milieux érudits et universitaires.[19] Les Tableaux 4, 5, 6 et 7 donnent un aperçu de cette diffusion.

Une si large diffusion, tant de traductions et de commentaires (sans compter tous les traités 'Sur le pouls' inspirés ou influencés par le *De pulsibus* qui ne sont pas répertoriés ici), est étonnante de première vue. En comparaison, si l'on tient compte seulement des traductions latines de la Renaissance, les quatre traités *Sur les différences et les causes des maladies et des symptômes* ont eu une diffusion semblable, tout en étant plus étendus, plus détaillés, plus approfondis au niveau de la doctrine de Galien (nous avons 23 traductions latines de ces traités, dont certaines ne concernent qu'un seul ou deux d'entre eux, tandis que nous recensons ci-dessous 18 traductions du *De pulsibus*, plus deux réimpressions). Cela peut paraître étonnant, de première vue, mais nous pensons que les raisons qui ont favorisé une telle réception de ce traité tiennent à son caractère et à sa spécificité, déjà évoquées précédemment, lorsque nous parlions des *tirones* à qui Galien le destine. Commodité de consultation due à sa brièveté, détail de la description du pouls 'dans tous ses états', mais en même temps souci pédagogique et présence des grands traits de la doctrine galénique, c'est-à-dire simplicité sans aucune simplification : voilà la recette du succès, la même qui aiguise l'intérêt du lecteur moderne pour ce 'petit' traité. Ajoutons à cela l'importance de la prise du pouls dans la pratique médicale de la Renaissance. Comme le souligne Guinterius dans l'épître dédicatoire de l'édition de 1532,

> 'Malgré tout le savoir médical que les contemporains ont bien acquis, le pouls demeure un point très difficile et encore obscur, même s'il est très utile et nécessaire pour acquérir d'autres connaissances afin de différencier la nature [des hommes] et les maladies. C'est d'une extrême absurdité que de prétendre connaître les maladies en se fiant uniquement aux urines (même si le *uulgus medicorum* aujourd'hui ne fait pas autre chose). Mais le pouls est considéré comme la dernière chose, tandis qu'il devrait être appris en premier, et le médecin le tâte plutôt par habitude que pour se rendre vraiment compte de l'état de la maladie'.

En tant que traité-outil, utile au praticien dans l'exercice quotidien de son art, en tant que vulgarisation qui n'est pourtant pas simpliste et garde en arrière-plan toute l'exigence théorique et la compétence que Galien demande à ses 'disciples' et futurs collègues, le *De pulsibus* démontre encore une fois l'attachement de Galien à une médecine 'scientifique' basée sur les données physiologiques et sur la recherche des causes, ainsi que sur les données 'environnementales' ou ayant trait à la réalité de la vie quotidienne de son époque, dans la lignée de l'héritage hippocratique.[20] Libéré des impératifs ou préjugés des écoles médicales, le médecin débutant qui suivra la méthode enseignée dans ce traité

Tableau 13.7. Éditions des 12e–16e siècles : texte latin

Année	Traducteur	Éditeur (si différent du traducteur)	Imprimeur, lieu d'impression	Titre livre	Localisation	cote
12e s.	Marcus Toletanus (vers 1191–1216)			*Liber Galieni de tactu pulsus quem transtulit Johannicius de greco in arabicum et Marcus Toletanus de arabico in latinum*	Bibliothèque interuniversitaire Montpellier, section médecine, recueil de 17 traités de Galien en latin[1]	Ms H 18
12e s.	Burgundius Pisanus (vers 1110–1193)			*Liber Galieni de introducendis in pulso a Burgundione judice Pisano de greco in latinum translatum*	Paris, Académie nationale de médecine, 51(1005), f. 262–273, 15e s.	
1490	Burgundius Pisanus	Diomedes Bonardus (*Opera omnia* en 2 vol.)	Philippus Pincius (Filippo Pinzi), Venise	*Liber de pusibus qui dicit introductorius ad theucrum.* Dans le même volume, après les *Liber de differentiis pulsuum* et *Liber de juvamento pulsuus*, un *Commentarius Galeni super librum ejus introductorium de pulsibus* (anonyme)	BIUM numérisé (original : Paris, Académie nationale de médecine, coll. Daremberg)	Acad. Méd. A 11
1515	Burgundius Pisanus	Rusticus Placentinus (préf.)	Giovanni Battista de Burgofranco, Pavie	*Quarta impressio ornatissima : continens omnes Galeni libros alias impressos...* (contient aussi le *Commentarius Galeni super librum ejus introductorium de pulsibus*)	The Wellcome Library	
1528		Scipio Ferrarius († entre 1500 et 1525)	Giunta, Venise	*Operum impressio novissima*	The Wellcome Library (4 vol. fol.)	
1531	Winter, Johann (Johannes Guinterius Andernacus, 1505–1574)		Simon de Colines, Paris	*Claudii Galeni Commentariolus de pulsibus ad medicinae candidatos*	BNF	8-TD16-3
1531	Winter, Johann (Johannes Guinterius Andernacus)		Andreas Cratander, Bâle	*De pulsibus ad medicinae candidatos* (précédé de : *De anatomicis administrationibus ; De constitutione artis medicae ; De theriaca ad Pisonem*)	Faculté de médecine, Paris	

[1] *Liber Galieni de elementis secundum sententiam Ypocratis ; Liber Galieni de complexionibus ; Liber Galieni de mala complexione diversa ; Liber Galieni de virtutibus naturalibus ; Liber Galieni de voce ; Liber Galieni de tactu pulsus quem transtulit Johannicius de greco in arabicum et Marcus Toletanus de arabico in latinum ; Liber Galieni de morbo et accidente ; Liber Galieni de crisi ; Liber de diebus criticis ; Galieni de heresibus his quæ introducuntur liber incipit de greco in latinum domino Henrico regi a Burgundico judice Pisano anno incarnationis MCLXXXV fideliter translatus.*

Année	Traducteur	Éditeur (si différent du traducteur)	Imprimeur, lieu d'impression	Titre livre	Localisation	cote
1532	Cruser, Hermann (Hermannus Cruserius, vers 1510–1575)		Simon de Colines, Paris	*De Pulsibus libellus ad tirones*, (suivi de : *De Pulsuum differentiis* ; *De Dignoscendis pulsibus* ; *De Causis pulsuum* ; *De Praesagitione ex pulsibus* ; *De Pulsuum usu* le dernier trad. par Thomas Linacer)	BNF	VELINS-511 et NUMM-53722
1534	Winter, Johann (Johannes Guinterius Andernacus)		Simon de Colines, Paris	*Varia Claudii Galeni opera*	BNF	FOL-T23-72 ou NUMM-53811
1537	Grégoire, Martin (Martinus Gregorius, † 1552)		Chrétien Wechel, Paris	*Introduction in pulsus* (suivi de : *De pulsuum usu*, trad. par Th. Linacer)		
1541	Grégoire, Martin (Martinus Gregorius)		Chrétien Wechel, Paris	*Introduction in pulsus ad Teuthram* (suivi de : *De pulsuum usu*, trad. par Th. Linacer)	BNF	4-TD16-4(1)
1541	Winter, Johann (Johannes Guinterius Andernacus)	J. B. Montanus	Giunta, Venise	In *Opera omnia*		
1544	Grégoire, Martin (Martinus Gregorius)	A. Ricco et V. Trincavelli	'ex officina Farrea ', Venise	In *Opera omnia*	BNF	8-T23-57 ou NUMM-60526
1549	Janus Cornarius (1500 1558)			*Opera omnia,* vol. 4, p. 164–80	BIUM numérisé	
1549, réimpr. 1550	Grégoire, Martin (Martinus Gregorius)		G. Rouillé, Lyon	*Introductio in pulsus ad Teuthram* (suivi de : *De pulsuum usu*, trad. par Th. Linacer)	BNF (format in-16°)	8-TD16-5
1553	Mena, Ferdinando († vers 1580)		J. Brocar, Alcalá de Henares	*Claudii Galeni de pulsibus ad tirones liber*	Madrid, Biblioteca Complutense	
1556	Cruser, Hermann (Hermannus Cruserius)	Leo Roganus († 1558)	R. de Amato, Naples	*In Galeni libellum de pulsibus ad tirones commentarium*	The Wellcome Library	
1565	Cruser, Hermann (Hermannus Cruserius)	A. Gadaldini (corrections et améliorations 'd'après des mss grecs')	Giunta 4	*De pulsibus libellus ad tirones* (fait partie de la *Quarta classis*, f. 43r–46v)	BIUM numérisé	
1575	Cruser, Hermann (Hermannus Cruserius)	Leo Roganus, commentateur	'ad instantiam J. Anelli de Maria', Naples	*In Galeni libellum de pulsibus ad tirones commentarium*	BNF	8-TD16-6
1597 (réimpr. de 1575)	Cruser, Hermann (Hermannus Cruserius)	Leo Roganus	Héritiers de M. Sessa, Venise	*In Galeni libellum de pulsibus ad tirones commentarium*		

adoptera du même coup l'éclectisme du maître, qui le conduira à combiner de la façon la plus efficace possible empirisme et rationalisme et de tenir compte aussi de l'évolution des maladies dans la durée. Son objectif sera d'avoir la capacité et le savoir de 'sentir' jusqu'au fond de son être cet 'autrui', son patient, qui n'est autre que son propre reflet, son miroir. La continuité entre les deux organismes s'établira à l'aide de la peau/frontière (comme le dit Vincent Barras) : à notre époque où la notion de 'frontière' est si souvent utilisée pour exclure et marginaliser, l'étude de Galien pourrait ainsi servir à rétablir ce contact si nécessaire à la santé des êtres humains, au propre, comme au figuré. Sans cultiver la nostalgie d'un 'toucher exceptionnel', d'une finesse perdue à jamais à l'époque de la technique, la lecture du traité destiné aux débutants inciterait le lecteur moderne à réfléchir sur le sens du toucher et sur les moyens d'atteindre les profondeurs du corps humain à l'aide de l'expérience et de la raison, pour arriver à devenir enfin un médecin, c'est-à-dire un 'artiste' complet.

Remerciements

Remerciements chaleureux d'abord au professeur Demetrios Michaelides et à tous les organisateurs du colloque *Medicine in the Ancient Mediterranean World* qui ont accepté ma participation. Leur accueil, leur disponibilité et leur compétence scientifique ont contribué à ce que les jours passés à Chypre soient riches en échanges et expériences entre collègues de différentes disciplines et de plusieurs pays. Mes remerciements également aux participants du colloque, qui ont formulé des questions et des remarques visant à approfondir et à améliorer ce texte. Merci aussi à Pierre-Paul Corsetti, directeur à l'époque de *L'Année Philologique*, qui a eu l'amabilité de relire la première version de cette communication. Il est bien évident que toute erreur ou omission sont de notre propre responsabilité.

Notes

1 Comme nous n'avons pas d'éléments de datation précis, nous pouvons dater ce traité par rapport aux autres traités de Galien sur le pouls et en tenant compte de ce que Galien lui-même dit dans le *De propriis libris*. Agnellus de Ravenne suppose que le traité abrégé a été rédigé *a posteriori*, et qu'ensuite Galien est revenu sur la *Maior Sfigmici*, c'est-à-dire l'ensemble des 16 livres, pour la compléter et la corriger (Garofalo 1998, 386–7). L'emploi de ὅλον (τὴν δ' ὅλην ὑπὲρ αὐτῶν τέχνην, K. VIII, 453 ; βιβλίον ὅλον ἔχει περὶ τῆς τῶν σφυγμῶν διαφορᾶς ὑφ'ἡμῶν γεγραμμένον, K. VIII, 461) confirme le caractère sommaire du traité destiné aux débutants, ainsi que l'interdépendance entre l'ensemble des écrits galéniques sur le pouls. Voir à ce sujet Ilberg 1889, 220–1 et Mavroudis 2000, 98 n. 241. Mavroudis étudie le rapport entre la théorie d'Archigène et celle de Galien sur le pouls.

2 Voir à ce sujet Boudon-Millot 2008, 259–81.

3 Tous les passages du *De pulsibus* sont traduits par nous-mêmes et font partie d'une traduction française inédite de l'ensemble du traité. Il existe par ailleurs une traduction anglaise du *De pulsibus* (Singer 1997).

4 Serres 1985, 362–3, pour un développement plus détaillé de ces notions.

5 La critique des principes méthodologiques des médecins empiriques, mais aussi des rationalistes et des méthodiques est développée notamment par Boulogne 2004.

6 Sur le fondement épistémologique de la science de Galien et sur ses préceptes méthodologiques, voir Barras 2005. Sur l'importance des *signes*, γνωρίσματα ou σημεῖα, et le parallèle avec les signes de reconnaissance par exemple dans l'*Odyssée* : Deichgräber 1984, 312–3.

7 Examen du milieu familial, de la société de Pergame et des études de Galien : Moraux 1985.

8 Von Staden 1989, 280–2, sur le parallèle entre le rythme du pouls et le rythme musical chez Hérophile et sur son idée d'inventer un instrument pour le mesurer. Des médecins des 16e–18e s. avaient également tenté de figurer le pouls à l'aide de notes musicales (Kuriyama 1999, 81–4 et ill. 9–12). Voir aussi Bacalexi 2001, 139 et n. 10. Mais chez Galien il n'existe pas de μιμήματα de pouls, comme il l'explique dans le *De dignoscendis pulsibus* (K. 9, 768). Voir à ce sujet Deichgräber 1984, 291–3.

9 Unschuld 2001, 110–1 sur le 'marketing actif' visant à promouvoir une image idéalisée de la médecine chinoise et sur la conception du corps dans cette médecine. Voir aussi Kuriyama 1999 et Bacalexi 2001, 134, n. 6 avec des références bibliographiques sur la prise du pouls dans la médecine tibétaine.

10 Sur le toucher dans la médecine grecque et sur les termes qui le désignent, voir Jouanna 2003 et Boehm 2003. Sur le toucher de la sage-femme plus particulièrement : Bacalexi 2005, 10–1, avec les références des textes antiques et un aperçu bibliographique.

11 Sur la fonction pédagogique et initiatique des traités de Galien pour les débutants, ainsi que sur l'enseignement de la médecine à Rome et par la suite (Alexandrie), voir Boudon 1994.

12 Palmieri 1998, 396–7 et 400. Le commentaire d'Agnellus de Ravenne a été publié par Palmieri 2005.

13 Pour plus de détails, voir Bacalexi 2001, 140–3.

14 Sur le rapport entre la doctrine galénique et la science moderne, notamment la cardiologie, ainsi que sur les 'erreurs' de Galien concernant la circulation du sang : Pino Campos 2006.

15 Sur la tradition alexandrine du *De pulsibus* : Palmieri 2003, 76. Sur le *Canon*, voir entre autres Iskandar 1976 et Garofalo 2003.

16 L'importance de ces quatre traités pour l'enseignement universitaire de la médecine au Moyen Âge et à la Renaissance montre qu'ils ont été considérés pendant longtemps comme des instruments pédagogiques. Voir à ce sujet Jacquart 1998 et Bacalexi 2009.

17 'Par conséquent, la santé serait un état de symétrie et la maladie d'amétrie [...]. Si le fait d'être en bonne santé correspond donc à la symétrie des conduits, le fait d'être

malade correspondra, quant à lui, à l'amétrie des conduits' (traduction personnelle).

18 Barras 2005, 70–1 : analyse du rôle primordial de la peau et du 'rapport spéculaire' entre le corps du médecin et celui du patient, établi grâce au toucher.

19 La diffusion et la réception de l'œuvre de Galien est étudiée en détail dans Boudon-Millot 2007. Voir aussi Palmieri 2003, Garofalo 2003 et Pormann 2003. Pour les traductions de la Renaissance voir le *Census* de Durling (1961) et les compléments dans Fortuna et Raia 2006. En ce qui concerne la tradition arabe : Ullmann 1970 et Sezgin 1970.

20 Examen du facteur environnement et parallèle entre le *De pulsibus* et le traité hippocratique des *Airs, Eaux, Lieux* : Bacalexi 2001, 144 et n. 19.

Bibliographie et Abréviations

Bacalexi, D. 2001 : '*De pulsibus ad tirones* : Galien et les médecins débutants : le pouls comme moyen de diagnostic et de pronostic', *Bulletin de l'Association Guillaume Budé* 2001 (1), 131–52.

Bacalexi, D. 2005 : 'Sages-femmes, nourrices et mères chez quelques médecins de l'Antiquité et de la Renaissance', *Gesnerus* 62 (1–2), 5–32.

Bacalexi, D. 2009 : 'Trois traducteurs de Galien au XVIe siècle et leur regard sur la tradition arabe', 202–22 dans J. Vons (éd.), *Pratique et pensée médicales à la Renaissance, Actes du 50e colloque international d'études humanistes, Tours, 2–7 juillet 2007* (collection Medic@), Paris.

Barras, V. 2005 : 'Le "Galen's touch" : peau, objet et sujet dans le système médical galénien', 55–73 dans *La pelle umana = The human skin* (Numéro monographique de *Micrologus: natura, scienza e società medievali* 13), Tavarnuzze.

Boehm, I. 2003 : 'Toucher du doigt : le vocabulaire du toucher dans les textes médicaux grecs et latins', 229–40 dans F. Gaide et F. Biville (éds), *'Manus medica'. Actions et gestes de l'officiant dans les textes médicaux latins. Questions de thérapeutique et de lexique. Actes du colloque tenu à l'Université Lumière-Lyon II, les 18 et 19 septembre 2001*, Aix-en-Provence.

Boudon, V. 1994 : 'Les œuvres de Galien pour les débutants (*De sectis, De pulsibus ad tirones, De ossibus ad tirones, Ad Glauconem de methodo medendi* et *Ars medica*) : médecine et pédagogie au II s. ap. J.-C.', 1421–67 dans W. Haase (éd.), *Aufstieg und Niedergang der römischen Welt: Geschichte und Kultur Roms im Spiegel der neueren Forschung. 2, Principat. 37, Philosophie, Wissenschaften, Technik. 2, Wissenschaften (Medizin und Biologie)*, Berlin, New York.

Boudon-Millot, V. 2007 : *Introduction générale ; Sur l'ordre de ses propres livres ; Sur ses propres livres ; Que l'excellent médecin est aussi philosophe*/Galien ; texte établi, trad. et annoté (Collection des universités de France. Série grecque 450), Paris.

Boudon-Millot, V. 2008 : 'Un étudiant sans école, un maître sans disciples : l'exemple paradoxal de Galien de Pergame', 259–81 dans H. Hugonnard-Roche (éd.), *L'enseignement supérieur dans les mondes antiques et médiévaux. Aspects institutionnels, juridiques et pédagogiques (Actes du Colloque international de Paris, 6–8 Octobre 2005)*, Paris.

Boulogne, J. 2004 : 'Du bon usage de la raison chez Galien', 83–92 dans V. Naas (éd.), *En deçà et au delà de la 'ratio' ; Actes de la journée d'études, Université de Lille III, 28 et 29 septembre 2001* (Collection UL3 : travaux et recherches), Villeneuve-d'Asq.

Deichgräber, K. 1984 : 'Galen als Erforscher des menschlichen Pulses : ein Beitrag zur Selbstdarstellung des Wissentschaftlers (*De dignotione pulsuum* I 1)', 288–326 dans H. Gärtner, E. Heitsch et U. Schindel (éds), *Ausgewählte kleine Schriften*, Hildesheim, München, Zürich.

Durling R. 1961 : 'A chronological census of Renaissance editions and translations of Galen', *Journal of the Warburg and Courtauld Institutes* 24, 230–305.

Fortuna, S. et Raia, A. 2006 : 'Corrigenda and addenda to Diels' "Galenica" by Richard J. Durling. 3, Manuscripts and editions', *Traditio* 61, 1–30.

Garofalo, I. 1998 : 'Le commentaire ravennate du *De pulsibus ad tirones* de Galien : le commentaire et ses sources', 383–92 dans C. Deroux (éd.), *Maladie et maladies dans les textes latins antiques et médiévaux. Actes du Ve colloque international 'Textes médicaux latins', Bruxelles, 4–6 septembre 1995* (Collection Latomus 242), Bruxelles.

Garofalo, I. 1999 : 'La traduzione araba del comento di Ioannes Grammatikos al *De pulsibus* di Galeno', 185–218 dans A. Garzya et J. Jouanna (éds), *I testi medici greci, traduzione e ecdotica*, Napoli.

Garofalo, I. 2003 : 'I sommari degli Alessandrini', 203–31 dans I. Garofalo et A. Roselli (éds), *Galenismo e medicina tardoantica : fonti greche, latine e arabe. Atti del seminario internazionale di Siena, Certosa di Pontignano, 9 e 10 settembre 2002* (Annali dell'Istituto Universitario Orientale di Napoli, Dipartimento di Studi del Mondo Classico e del Mediterraneo Antico, Sezione Filologico-Letteraria, Quaderni 7), Napoli.

Gundert, B. 1998 : 'Die *"tabulae Vindobonenses"* als Zeugnis alexandrinischer Lehrtätigkeit um 600 n. Chr.', 91–144 dans K.-D. Fischer, D. Nickel and P. Potter (éds), *Text and tradition : studies in ancient medicine and its transmission presented to Jutta Kollesch* (Studies in Ancient Medicine 18), Leiden and Boston.

Ilberg, J. 1889 : 'Über die Schriftstellerei des Klaudios Galenos', *Reinisches Museum* 44, 207–39.

Iskandar, A. Z. 1976 : 'An attempted reconstruction of the late Alexandrian medical curriculum', *Medical History* 20, 235–58.

Jacquart, D. 1998 : *La médecine médiévale dans le cadre parisien : XIV–XVe siècle,* Paris.

Jouanna, J. 2003 : 'Sur la dénomination et le nombre des sens d'Hippocrate à la médecine impériale : réflexions à partir de l'énumération des sens dans le traité hippocratique du "Régime", c. 23', 9–20 dans I. Boehm et P. Luccioni (éds), *Les cinq sens dans la médecine de l'époque impériale : sources et développements : actes de la table ronde du 14 juin 2001* (Collection du Centre d'études et de recherches sur l'Occident romain, Nouvelle série 25), Paris.

K. : Kuhn, C. G. 1821–33 : *Claudii Galeni Opera Omnia*, Leipzig (réimpr. Hildesheim 1964–65).

Kuriyama, S. 1999 : *The expressiveness of the body and the divergence of Greek and Chinese medicine*, New York.

Mavroudis, 2000 : Μαυρουδῆς, Αἰμ. Δ. 2000 : *Ἀρχιγένης Φιλίππου Ἀπαμεύς : ὁ βίος καὶ τὰ ἔργα ἑνὸς Ἕλληνα γιατροῦ στὴν αὐτοκρατορικὴ Ρώμη* (Πονήματα 3), Ἀθῆναι.

Moraux, P. 1985 : *Galien de Pergame. Souvenirs d'un médecin*, Paris.

Palmieri, N. 1998 : 'La structure du commentaire ravennate au *De pulsibus ad tirones* de Galien', 393–405 dans C. Deroux (éd.), *Maladie et maladies dans les textes latin antiques et médiévaux. Actes du Ve colloque international 'Textes médicaux latins', Bruxelles, 4–6 septembre 1995* (Collection Latomus 242), Bruxelles.

Palmieri, N. 2003 : 'L'*inspectio pulsus* dans le premier galénisme gréco-latin ou Les artifices du toucher', 75–92 dans F. Gaide et F. Biville (éds), *'Manus medica'. Actions et gestes de l'officiant dans les textes médicaux latins. Questions de thérapeutique et de lexique. Actes du colloque tenu à l'Université Lumière-Lyon II, les 18 et 19 septembre 2001*, Aix-en-Provence.

Palmieri, N. 2005 : *Agnellus de Ravenne : lectures galéniques, le 'De pulsibus ad tirones'*, traduction et notes explicatives ; introduction, texte latin adiuuante I. Garofalo (Mémoires du Centre Jean-Palerne 28), Publications de l'Université de Saint-Étienne.

Pino Campos, L. M. 2006 : 'Observaciones al tratado de Galeno *Acerca de la diferencia de los pulsos*', *Fortunatae* 17, 99–115.

Pormann, P. E. 2003 : 'Jean le Grammairien et le *De sectis* dans la littérature médicale d'Alexandrie', 233–63 dans I. Garofalo et A. Roselli (éds), *Galenismo e medicina tardoantica : fonti greche, latine e arabe. Atti del seminario internazionale di Siena, Certosa di Pontignano, 9 e 10 settembre 2002* (Annali dell'Istituto Universitario Orientale di Napoli, Dipartimento di Studi del Mondo Classico e del Mediterraneo Antico, Sezione Filologico-Letteraria, Quaderni 7), Napoli.

Serres, M. 1985 : *Les cinq sens*, Paris.

Sezgin, F. 1970 : *Geschichte des arabischen Schrifttums. 3, Medizin-Pharmazie, Zoologie-Tierheilkunde*, Leiden.

Singer, P. N. 1997 : *Selected works : Galen; translated with an introduction and notes* (World's classics), Oxford, New York.

Ullmann, M. 1970 : *Die Medizin im Islam*, Leiden.

Unschuld, P. U. 2001 : *Médecines chinoises : une exposition produite par l'établissement public du Parc et de la Grande halle de la Villette, au Pavillon Delouvrier du 18 avril au 8 juillet 2001*, Paris.

Von Staden, H. 1989 : *Herophilus: the art of medicine in early Alexandria*, Cambridge.

14. Γαληνού της Περγάμου «*Τέχνη Ἰατρική*»: Επιτομή της Ιατρικής και των Τομέων της

Δημήτριος Χρ. Κουτρούμπας και Γιώργιος Παπαδόπουλος
(Dimitrios C. Koutroumpas and Giorgos Papadopoulos)

Galen's Art of Medicine *was one of the most well-known medical handbooks in medieval and Renaissance times. As it was the main textbook used for the teaching of medical practice, it had a tremendous impact on the science of medicine. The* Art of Medicine *or* Microtegni, *as it was called by the medical world of the medieval west, contains in summary form the entire fundamental, theoretical and practical teachings of Galen. According to Galen the* Art of Medicine *was intended to play a special role. Its aim is to introduce the reader through categorisation to the different fields of medicine: physiology, stoicheiology, anatomy, diagnostics, hygiene, analepsy and finally preventive medicine.*

Ο Γαληνός της Περγάμου (129–210/216 μΧ) αποτελεί τη σημαντικότερη ιατρική φυσιογνωμία της ελληνορωμαϊκής περιόδου και είναι ο μεγαλύτερος ιατρός της αρχαιότητας, μετά τον Ιπποκράτη. Υπήρξε ο κορυφαίος ανατόμος, φυσιολόγος, παθολογοανατόμος και φαρμακολόγος της εποχής του, αφήνοντας ανεξίτηλη τη σφραγίδα του σε όλες τις προαναφερόμενες ιατρικές ειδικότητες. Αναμφίβολα ήταν πολυγραφότατος καθώς ασχολήθηκε όχι μόνο με την ιατρική αλλά και με τη φιλοσοφία, τη ρητορική και τη φιλολογία, με αποτέλεσμα να εγγραφεί στη συνείδηση των μεταγενέστερων όχι μόνο ως ιατρός αλλά και ως φιλόσοφος. Σύμφωνα με τον καθηγητή Jean Irigoin (1997, 211) το τεράστιο έργο του εκπροσωπεί το 1/8 της αρχαίας ελληνικής λογοτεχνικής παραγωγής που μας έχει διασωθεί από τον Όμηρο έως και τα τέλη του 2^ου^ μΧ αιώνα.

Αναντίρρητα, η φήμη του επηρέασε καθοριστικά την ιατρική, και τα έργα του, παρά τις όποιες αδυναμίες τους, περιεβλήθησαν με το κύρος της αυθεντίας. Είναι ο επιστήμονας-ιατρός που, για πρώτη φορά μέχρι τότε, θεμελίωσε με την συγγραφή των έργων του ένα μεγαλόπνοο σύστημα θεραπευτικής, το οποίο για περισσότερα από 1500 χρόνια επηρέαζε την ιατρική σχεδόν αποκλειστικά, ενώ τελικά η επιρροή του δεν εξασθένισε παρά μόνο τον 17^ο^ αιώνα.

Ένα από τα έργα του, που άσκησε τεράστια επίδραση στη δυτική ιατρική παράδοση είναι το «*Τέχνη Ἰατρική*». Πρόκειται για την πραγματεία που χρησιμοποιήθηκε ως κορυφαίο ιατρικό σύγγραμμα τον ύστερο Μεσαίωνα και την Αναγεννησιακή περίοδο (Hankinson 2008, 22). Το έργο αυτό αποτελεί είδος επιτομής της ιατρικής και των τομέων της με ταυτόχρονη συνοπτική παρουσίαση των διαγνωστικών και θεραπευτικών μεθόδων που χρησιμοποιούσε ο Γαληνός. Έχαιρε εξαιρετικής δημοτικότητας από την ύστερη αρχαιότητα, καθώς είχε επιλεγεί ως εισαγωγικό εγχειρίδιο, κατάλληλο για αρχάριους, στα πλαίσια της ύστερης Αλεξανδρινής Ιατρικής Σχολής.

Αν και ο χρόνος συγγραφής της πραγματείας «*Τέχνη Ἰατρική*» δεν μπορεί να καθοριστεί με ακρίβεια, θα πρέπει να τοποθετηθεί μετά το 207 μΧ και πιθανότατα η συγγραφή του να πραγματοποιήθηκε τα τελευταία χρόνια της ζωής του Γαληνού. Σίγουρα όμως η συγγραφή του είχε ολοκληρωθεί πριν από το έργο «*Περὶ τῶν ἰδίων βιβλίων γραφή*», για το οποίο με σαφέστατα ρομαντική διάθεση ο Vivian Nutton αναφέρει ότι γράφτηκε πάνω στην νεκρική κλίνη (Nutton 1999, 217–8). Ο ίδιος ο Γαληνός άλλωστε, στο τέλος τής εν λόγω πραγματείας αναφέρει ότι πρόκειται να συγγράψει ένα ή δύο βιβλία που θα έχουν τον τίτλο «Γαληνοῦ, *Περὶ τῶν ἰδίων βιβλίων γραφή*» (I, 411, 16–412, 3, έκδοση Kühn 1819–33, εφεξής K).

Ευθύς αμέσως μετά το θάνατο του Γαληνού η συστηματική μελέτη και σχολιασμός της πραγματείας «*Τέχνη Ἰατρική*», από μέλη της αλεξανδρινής ιατρικής κοινότητας, γίνεται αισθητή. Οι τελευταίοι, ερχόμενοι αντιμέτωποι με την ογκωδέστατη ιατρική παραγωγή του Γαληνού αισθάνθηκαν την ανάγκη να επιλέξουν κάποια από τα σημαντικότερα έργα του για μελέτη και σχολιασμό. Η διαδικασία της συλλογής των σπουδαιοτέρων γαληνικών πραγματειών μοιραία διαδραμάτισε τον πλέον καθοριστικό και κρίσιμο ρόλο στην ανάπτυξη της ιατρικής από τον 6ο μΧ αιώνα έως και την οριστική κατάρρευση του Γαληνισμού.

Πρόκειται για ένα εγχείρημα που δεν μπορεί να θεωρηθεί πρωτόγνωρο στο χώρο της αλεξανδρινής ιατρικής, καθώς παρόμοια διαδικασία συλλογής ιατρικών κειμένων υιοθετήθηκε και για τις ανάγκες διδασκαλίας της Ιπποκρατικής Ιατρικής, οδηγώντας στη δημιουργία της *Ιπποκρατικής Συλλογής*. Βέβαια δεν πρέπει να παραλείψουμε ότι προς την κατεύθυνση αυτή νοερά αλλά επιτακτικά «συνηγορούσε» και ο ίδιος ο Γαληνός, καθώς σε αρκετά έργα του υποδείκνυε όχι μόνο τις πραγματείες που ήταν οι σημαντικότερες, αλλά και την ακριβή σειρά που πρέπει να μελετούνται τα έργα του, με αντίστοιχες αναφορές στα έργα «*Τέχνη Ἰατρική*», «*Περὶ τῆς τάξεως τῶν ἰδίων βιβλίων πρὸς Εὐγενιανόν*» και κυρίως στο «*Περὶ τῶν ἰδίων βιβλίων γραφή*». Στο τελευταίο μάλιστα προσπαθεί κατά τρόπο συστηματικό να καταγράψει το σύνολο των έργων του.

Η ενότητα αυτών των επιλεγμένων πραγματειών του Γαληνού αρχικά αποκαλούνταν *Summaria Alexandrina*, και το «*Τέχνη Ἰατρική*» κατείχε μεταξύ των άλλων κεντρική θέση ως εισαγωγικό στην ιατρική σπουδή. Δεν πρέπει να διαφεύγει της προσοχής μας ότι η διαμόρφωση του γαληνικού προγράμματος σπουδών, εντός του οποίου εμπεριέχονταν και το έργο «*Τέχνη Ἰατρική*», ήταν μια αρκετά αργόσυρτη και εργώδης διαδικασία που διήρκησε περί τους τρεις αιώνες, και τα πρώτα δείγματα της μορφοποίησης του δεν εντοπίζονται παρά τον 6ο μΧ αιώνα στην Αλεξάνδρεια. Αυτή η συλλογή κειμένων είχε μεγάλη παιδαγωγική επίδραση και αποτέλεσε το γαληνικό ιατρικό πρόγραμμα σπουδών, που επιβίωσε με μικρές τροποποιήσεις τους επόμενους αιώνες, περίοδο κατά την οποία γιγαντώθηκε ο γαληνισμός ως το κυρίαρχο ιατροφιλοσοφικό ρεύμα.

Σε όλους τους μετέπειτα αιώνες, πάντα συμπεριλαμβανόταν η πραγματεία «*Τέχνη Ἰατρική*» ως τμήμα της συλλογής των 16 κορυφαίων γαληνικών έργων, που παρά τις όποιες επιμέρους τροποποιήσεις της είχε μορφή «κανόνα» και στην ουσία αποτελούνταν από 24 πραγματείες.[1] Οι περισσότερες πραγματείες που περιέχονταν στον 'Αλεξανδρινό Κανόνα' του Γαληνού ήταν συνήθως ακέραιες, όμως ορισμένες που ήταν ογκώδεις εμφανιζόταν υπό τη μορφή περιλήψεων ή συνόψεων και κατά συνέπεια συχνά απλοποιούνταν ή αλλοιώνονταν.

Στην ανωτέρω συλλογή έργων του Γαληνού την πρώτη θέση κατείχαν οι βασικές αρχές της ιατρικής, όπως περιγράφονται στα έργα «*Περὶ αἱρέσεων τοῖς εἰσαγομένοις*» και «*Τέχνη Ἰατρική*» (Nutton 2008, 362–3). Ακολουθούσαν συνοπτικές οδηγίες για τις θεραπευτικές μεθόδους και για τη λήψη των σφυγμών, πριν οι σπουδαστές εντρυφήσουν σε πιο εξειδικευμένες και σημαντικότερες πραγματείες. Με σύγχρονους όρους, ο σπουδαστής διδασκόταν ανατομία, φυσιολογία, παθολογία, θεραπευτική, και η σπουδή του ολοκληρωνόταν πιθανότατα με διαιτητική και υγιεινή. Αν και οι σπουδαστές ενθαρρύνονταν να μελετήσουν και άλλες πραγματείες του Γαληνού, αυτή η διδακτέα ύλη από μόνη της εξασφάλιζε μια γενική επισκόπηση της γαληνικής ιατρικής και ήταν ικανοποιητική για τους σκοπούς της, καθώς περιελάμβανε σε αδρές γραμμές ότι ήταν αναγκαίο να γνωρίζει ένας σπουδαστής. Είχε το σπάνιο πλεονέκτημα να είναι ταυτόχρονα περιεκτική και περιληπτική.

Η επίδραση της συλλογής μπορεί να αξιολογηθεί από την αξιοσημείωτη διαχρονικότητα και τη γεωγραφική της εξάπλωση. Μέχρι το 550 μΧ είχε μεταφραστεί στα συριακά και περίπου την ίδια εποχή ή μερικές δεκαετίες αργότερα μεταλαμπαδεύτηκε στην δυτική ιατρική παράδοση, καθώς μεταφέρθηκε και μεταφράστηκε στα λατινικά, πιθανότατα στην ευρύτερη περιοχή της Ραβέννας, ίσως και στην ίδια την πόλη, που αποτελούσε το κέντρο της βυζαντινής διοίκησης στην Ιταλία (Irigoin 1997, 223–4).

Πράγματι το έργο «*Τέχνη Ἰατρική*» είναι από τα πρώτα έργα που μεταφράζεται στα λατινικά απευθείας από τα αρχαία ελληνικά αρκετά πριν από το τέλος του 9ου μΧ αιώνα, αν και ο ακριβής χρόνος δεν μπορεί να προσδιοριστεί με ασφάλεια (Temkin 1935, 179–82). Όμως, απτές ενδείξεις αυτής της πρώιμης μεταβίβασης πιστοποιούνται στον Αμβροσιανό κώδικα G 108 inf. (*codex Ambrosianus* G 108 inf., fol. 22r–130r) όπου εμπεριέχονται τμήματα των έργων α) «*Περὶ αἱρέσεων τοῖς εἰσαγομένοις*», β) «*Τέχνη Ἰατρική*», γ) «*Περὶ τῶν σφυγμῶν τοῖς εἰσαγομένοις*» και δ) «*Τῶν πρὸς Γλαύκωνα θεραπευτικῶν*».

Τόσο ο Sigerist, στις αρχές του προηγούμενου αιώνα, που ανακάλυψε τα κείμενα, όσο πολύ περισσότερο ο Temkin, που τα μελέτησε συστηματικά και ασχολήθηκε με την κριτική τους, πιστοποιούν ότι αν και το χειρόγραφο είναι προϊόν του 9ου μΧ αιώνα, αποτελεί αντίγραφο παλαιότερου χειρογράφου που πρέπει να γράφηκε στην περιοχή της Ραβέννας και ανάγεται τουλάχιστον στον 6ο μΧ. αιώνα. Παρόμοια μεταφορά της πραγματείας «*Τέχνη Ἰατρική*» στη λατινική δυτική παράδοση από την Αλεξανδρινή Ιατρική Σχολή της ύστερης αρχαιότητας ενισχύεται και από τα κείμενα του κώδικα *Vindobonensis medicus Graecus* 16 (Hunger and Kersten 1969 = 35 Lambeck/Kollar 1780) που αν και δεν μπορεί να χρονολογηθεί με ακρίβεια εντούτοις έχει αποδειχτεί ότι το κείμενο σχετίζεται σε ευθεία γραμμή με την αλεξανδρινή παράδοση (Temkin 1935, 180–1).

Αυτή η πρώιμη επαφή της δυτικής ιατρικής με την πραγματεία «*Τέχνη Ἰατρική*» αποτελεί εξαίρεση στη συνηθισμένη διαδρομή μεταβίβασης της γαληνικής γνώσης μέσω της αραβικής ιατρικής. Βέβαια, αυτή η πρώιμη μεταφορά δημιουργεί τις προϋποθέσεις για τη μεταγενέστερη διάδοση και κυρίαρχη επίδραση του έργου. Με αποτέλεσμα να θεωρείται γύρω στο 1450 μΧ απαραίτητη προϋπόθεση η γνώση του έργου για κάθε τελειόφοιτο σπουδαστή της ιατρικής, ιδιαίτερα στα τρία σπουδαία ευρωπαϊκά πανεπιστημιακά κέντρα της ιατρικής, του Μονπελιέ, της Μπολόνια και του Παρισιού. Ακόμα και στην περίπτωση που κάποιος γιατρός δεν είχε σπουδάσει σε πανεπιστημιακή ιατρική σχολή έπρεπε να έχει οπωσδήποτε μελετήσει συστηματικά την πραγματεία «*Τέχνη Ἰατρική*» ως τμήμα της διάσημης μεσαιωνικής ανθολογίας *Articella* (Temkin 1973, 100–1), η οποία περιελάμβανε ως εκπαιδευτικό υλικό μια συλλογή εκλατινισμένων κλασσικών, βυζαντινών και αραβικών ιατρικών κειμένων.

Ήταν τόσο μεγάλη η δημοτικότητα της πραγματείας «*Τέχνη Ἰατρική*», ώστε όταν ο Δάντης έγραφε για αταίριαστα δώρα χρησιμοποίησε το ακόλουθο παράδειγμα ως ενδεικτικό της επιρροής του έργου «*Τέχνη Ἰατρική*» : «*Αν ένας ιππότης δώριζε μια ασπίδα σε ένα ιατρό, ή ο ιατρός δώριζε στον ιππότη ένα αντίγραφο των Αφορισμών του Ιπποκράτη ή της Τέχνης του Γαληνού*» (Dante, *Il Convivio* I. VIII. 5).

Αναντίρρητα το έργο «*Τέχνη Ἰατρική*» πρόκειται για πραγματεία που επηρέασε βαθύτατα τη λόγια μεσαιωνική και αναγεννησιακή ιατρική. Εδώ θα πρέπει να αναζητήσουμε το θεωρητικό υπόβαθρο της διδασκαλίας των τεσσάρων «κράσεων», που εμφανίστηκε στη μεσαιωνική ιατρική γραμματεία. Η επίδραση του έργου παρέμενε σημαντική ακόμα και όταν ο Γαληνισμός έφθινε ως κυρίαρχη ιατρική και φιλοσοφική θεώρηση. Η μελέτη της αλλά και η αξία της ως ιατρικό εγχειρίδιο εξακολουθούσε να θεωρείται σημαντική ακόμα και από τους αντιπάλους του γαληνικού δόγματος. Είναι χαρακτηριστικό ότι ο Ioannes Argenterius (Pedemontanus) (1513–1572), ο οποίος ως ακαδημαϊκός ιατρός αποτελούσε έναν από τους σφοδρότερους πολέμιους του Γαληνού, αντιμετώπιζε το έργο «*Τέχνη Ἰατρική*» με σεβασμό. Στο έργο του *In artem medicinalem Galeni*, που συνέγραψε το 1566 στη Φλωρεντία, αναφέρει στον πρώτο τόμο των σχολίων του σχετικά με την «*Τέχνη Ἰατρική*» του Γαληνού ότι το έργο αυτό είναι χρήσιμο και απαραίτητο τόσο σε εκείνους που ασκούν την ιατρική, όσο και στους φιλοσόφους και όλους όσους αρέσκονται στη γνώση των πραγμάτων (Argenterius, *In artem medicinalem Galeni*, I. I).

Τέλος, η χρησιμότητα του έργου «*Τέχνη Ἰατρική*» εξακολουθεί να θεωρείται σπουδαία ακόμα και όταν η ιατρική κινούνταν εμφανώς προς μια νέα επιστημονική πορεία και πλέον ο Γαληνισμός ως ιατρική φιλοσοφία είχε καταστεί παρωχημένος. Το 1652 ο Nicholas Culpeper (1616–1654) μετέφρασε στην αγγλική γλώσσα το έργο «*Τέχνη Ἰατρική*», στο βιβλίο '*Galens Art of Physick*' που εκτός των άλλων περιείχε και σχόλια σε αυτή την πραγματεία. Ο Culpeper αναφέρει ότι προσφέρει το βιβλίο ως «*ένα αλφαβητάρι για την εκμάθηση της Ιατρικής*» καθώς θεωρούσε ότι το έργο περιλαμβάνει τις βασικές αρχές της Ιατρικής Τέχνης. Πίστευε δε ότι ήταν το τελευταίο έργο το οποίο έγραψε ο Γαληνός το οποίο αποτελεί μια επιτομή όλων των έργων (Culpeper 1652, 25).

Σε αυτά ακριβώς τα λόγια του Culpeper αποκαλύπτεται η δημοφιλία και η διαχρονική εκπαιδευτική αξία του έργου από τον 3ο μ.Χ. αιώνα ως και τον 17ο αιώνα. Επί δεκατέσσερις αιώνες ιατροί και λόγιοι της ύστερης Αλεξανδρινής Ιατρικής Σχολής, Βυζαντινοί, Σύριοι, Πέρσες, Άραβες και Δυτικοευρωπαίοι μελετούσαν τις βασικές αρχές, καθόριζαν τους κλάδους και τα όρια του γνωστικού πεδίο της ιατρικής έχοντας ως οδηγό το έργο «*Τέχνη Ἰατρική*».

Πράγματι το υπό εξέταση έργο αποτελεί μια επιτομή της ιατρικής και ως έργο έχει κατά τον Γαληνό έναν ξεχωριστό ρόλο. Στόχος του είναι να εισαγάγει τον μελετητή του χρησιμοποιώντας την μέθοδο των διαιρέσεων σε είδη, στους επιμέρους τομείς της ιατρικής τέχνης: σημειωτικής, φυσιολογίας, αιτιολογίας, θεραπευτικής και υγιεινής, με τους επιμέρους κλάδους κάθε τομέα.

Στον πρόλογο του έργου, ο Γαληνός, εισάγει τον αναγνώστη στην τέχνη της ιατρικής μέσω της ανάλυσης του ορισμού της (I, 306, 7–14, K). Η παρουσίαση της ιατρικής με τη μέθοδο αυτή θεωρούσε ότι συμβάλλει στην ευκολότερη απομνημόνευση όλων όσων είναι ουσιώδη επειδή ο τέλειος ορισμός περιλαμβάνει όλα τα βασικά σημεία της τέχνης. Για τον ίδιο η ιατρική ως επιστημονικός κλάδος είναι «*η επιστήμη των υγιεινών, των νοσωδών*[2] *και των ουδετέρων*» (I, 307, K). Κάθε ένα από τα τρία αυτά συστατικά της ιατρικής αναφέρονται τόσο στο ανθρώπινο σώμα όσο στα αίτια και τα γνωρίσματα αυτών.

Όμως, ως ορισμός είναι αρκετά λακωνικός για τα μέτρα και τα σταθμά του Γαληνού και απαιτεί πληθώρα διευκρινήσεων για να καταστεί κατανοητός. Για τον Περγαμηνό «πολυλογά», ένα προσωνύμιο που πρέπει να το απέκτησε όσο ήταν ακόμα στη ζωή, ο ορισμός της ιατρικής σε μόλις οκτώ λέξεις συμπεριλαμβανομένων των άρθρων χρειάζεται ενδελεχή αλλά επίπονη για τον αναγνώστη ανάλυση.

Η αναλυτική προσέγγιση των όρων «υγιεινών», «νοσωδών» και «ουδετέρων» οδηγεί σε θεωρήσεις πολλαπλών συνδυασμών που εν τέλει σκιαγραφούν τους επιμέρους κλάδους της ιατρικής. Ένα σώμα είναι υγιές όταν υπάρχουν τα αίτια, δηλαδή οι υγιεινοί παράγοντες, και γίνεται εμφανές ότι είναι υγιές από τα εξωτερικά του γνωρίσματα. Κατά παρόμοιο τρόπο ο ανθρώπινος οργανισμός νοσεί όταν ο ίδιος φέρει τις νόσους και τα αίτια που όχι μόνο τις προκαλούν αλλά και τις διατηρούν ενώ ταυτόχρονα το σώμα εμφανίζει τα γνωρίσματα της νόσου (I 307, 7–12, K).

Το ανθρώπινο σώμα μπορεί να χαίρει άκρας υγείας όταν οι τέσσερεις ποιότητες (θερμό, ψυχρό, υγρό, ξηρό) βρίσκονται σε πλήρη αρμονία ως αποτέλεσμα της ισορροπίας – ευκρασίας των τεσσάρων χυμών. Σε αντιδιαστολή όταν το σώμα νοσεί τότε οι τέσσερεις χυμοί βρίσκονται σε ανισορροπία – δυσκρασία. Ενώ, ο πόνος ως παράγωγο της νόσου αποτελεί λύση της συνοχής ή μαζικής μεταβολής των ποιοτήτων της περιοχής στην οποία εντοπίζεται (I 357, K). Στην ενδιάμεση κατάσταση, κατά την οποία το σώμα δεν νοσεί αλλά και δεν είναι υγιές χαρακτηρίζεται ως ουδέτερο.

Ο Γαληνός, λοιπόν, παραμένει πιστός στην Ιπποκρατική θεωρία των τεσσάρων χυμών, όπως περιγράφεται στο έργο «*Περί Φύσιος Ἀνθρώπου*» της *Ιπποκρατικής Συλλογής*. Την προεκτείνει και συνδυάζοντας μοναδικά τους ιπποκρατικούς χυμούς με τις αριστοτελικές ποιότητες διατυπώνει τις δικές του θεωρήσεις (Nutton 2005, 111–21).

Ο Γαληνός δεν είναι ικανοποιημένος απλώς με την παρουσίαση της ιατρικής ως επιστημονική γνώση των υγιεινών, των νοσηρών και των ουδετέρων. Αισθάνεται την ανάγκη να εμβαθύνει τη σκέψη του ώστε να μπορέσει ο αναγνώστης να συλλάβει την ιατρική τέχνη ως μια ολότητα, όπως ακριβώς την αντιλαμβάνεται και τη βιώνει ο ίδιος μέσω της εμπειρικής παρατήρησης και της λογικής.

Εισάγει στον ορισμό της ιατρικής επιπλέον τη γνώση των επιμέρους χαρακτηριστικών γνωρισμάτων και τύπων των τριών καταστάσεων του σώματος. Κάθε ένας από τους τρεις επιμέρους τύπους διακρίνεται αρχικά σε «*ἁπλῶς*» και «*νῦν*» (I, 308, 7–12, K). Το ανθρώπινο σώμα διακρίνεται σε «*Ὑγιεινόν ἁπλῶς*» και «*Ὑγιεινόν νῦν*», δηλαδή σε «γενικά» υγιές σώμα και υγιεινό «προς το παρόν» (I, 309, 16–310, 3, K). Κατά παρόμοιο τρόπο ένα σώμα μπορεί να είναι «γενικά» νοσηρό ή «γενικά» ουδέτερο και «προς το παρόν» νοσηρό ή «προς το παρόν» ουδέτερο.

Απαρχή αυτής της πρώτης διάκρισης του ανθρωπίνου σώματος ως προς την κατάσταση της υγείας του είναι για μεν την «γενικά» η εκ γενετής ιδιοσυστασία του σώματος ως προς την κράση του, για δε την «προς το παρόν» η κατάσταση του στη δεδομένη χρονική στιγμή. Για παράδειγμα, στην περίπτωση του νοσηρού σώματος, αυτό διακρίνεται σε «γενικά» νοσηρό, όταν από την γέννησή του παρουσιάζει δυσκρασία, δηλαδή δεν εμφανίζει καλή κράση. Ενώ η «προς το παρόν» νοσηρή κατάσταση του σώματος υποδηλώνει ότι στη συγκεκριμένη χρονική περίοδο το σώμα νοσεί και θα συνεχίσει να ονομάζεται κατά αυτό τον τρόπο για όσο νοσεί.

Η κατηγορία της περίπτωσης «*ἁπλῶς*», δηλαδή, όταν αναφερόμαστε ότι το σώμα είναι «*Ὑγιεινόν ἁπλῶς*», διαχωρίζεται σε δύο επιμέρους υποκατηγορίες, στην «*διὰ παντός*», δηλαδή «πάντοτε», και στην υποκατηγορία «*ὡς ἐπὶ τὸ πολύ*», δηλαδή «ως επί το πλείστον» (I, 310, 10–311, 4, K). Αναφερόμενοι, επί παραδείγματι, στην περίπτωση του νοσηρού σώματος, αυτό θα είναι δια παντός νοσηρό όταν δεν έχει, από τη γέννηση του, καλή κράση σε υπερθετικό βαθμό, είναι δηλαδή «*δυσκρατότατον*», σε αντίθεση με την περίπτωση του «γενικά» νοσηρού που είναι απλά «*δύσκρατον*» εκ γενετής. Η διάκριση της γενικής κατηγορίας «*ἁπλῶς*» και της υποκατηγορίας «*διὰ παντός*» είναι ως προς τον βαθμό «*δύσκρατον*» και «*δυσκρατότατον*», χωρίς ο Γαληνός να προχωρά σε καμία περεταίρω διευκρίνιση. Στην περίπτωση της υποκατηγορίας «*ὡς ἐπὶ τὸ πολύ*» είναι το νοσηρό σώμα που υπολείπεται σε κακή κατασκευή από το «*διὰ παντός*», χωρίς όμως να έχει κατορθώσει να φτάσει σε ισορροπημένη κατάσταση.

Η συγκεκριμένη διαβάθμιση των τριών καταστάσεων της υγείας αν και κατά τη θεώρηση του Γαληνού είναι αναγκαία εντούτοις προκαλεί σύγχυση στον αναγνώστη. Είναι ένα γεγονός που σιωπηρά αποδέχεται ο Γαληνός καθώς στη συνέχεια επανέρχεται και συγκεφαλαιώνει τις επιμέρους κατηγορίες και υποκατηγορίες. Αφετηρία σε αυτή την επαναληπτική αλλά περιληπτική αναφορά είναι η περίπτωση της ουδέτερης κατάστασης του ανθρωπίνου σώματος. Γενικά, ουδέτερο είναι το σώμα που από τη γέννησή του και ως προς την κράση του είναι ουδέτερο. «Προς το παρόν» ουδέτερο είναι το σώμα που εμφανίζεται ουδέτερο στην παρούσα κατάσταση. Πρέπει να ξεκαθαρίσουμε ότι το ουδέτερο δεν σημαίνει σε καμιά περίπτωση ευκρασία, δηλαδή δεν σημαίνει ότι οι ποιότητες των χυμών είναι σε απόλυτη ισορροπία. Απλά πρόκειται για μια ενδιάμεση κατάσταση μεταξύ του υγιούς σώματος και του νοσώδους. Η διάκριση ανάμεσα στην περίπτωση του «γενικά» ουδέτερου σώματος ως προς την υγεία και του «δια παντός» ουδέτερου σώματος σχετίζεται με τη διάρκεια στο χρόνο και πάντα σε σχέση με την ηλικία του ανθρωπίνου σώματος (I, 312, 7– 14, K). «Δια παντός» ουδέτερο είναι το σώμα που πάντοτε διατηρείται ουδέτερο σε όλες τις ηλικίες. Αυτό αποτελεί την ακριβή διάκριση από το «γενικά» ουδέτερο σώμα που μπορεί σε κάποια ηλικία και κάτω από συγκεκριμένους παράγοντες να μεταβληθεί.

Οφείλουμε να αναφέρουμε ότι η ουδέτερη κατάσταση του ανθρωπίνου σώματος εμφανίζει μια επαμφοτερίζουσα «συμπεριφορά», καθώς το ουδέτερο σώμα αποτελεί μια ενδιάμεση κατάσταση μεταξύ του υγιεινού σώματος και του νοσηρού. Άλλοτε το ουδέτερο σώμα είναι υγιές και άλλοτε μεταπίπτει στην κατάσταση του νοσηρού.

Με την ακριβή κατάταξη σωμάτων σε μια από τις τρείς κύριες κατηγορίες, υγιές, ουδέτερο ή νοσώδες σώμα, ασχολείται ο πρώτος τομέας της «*Ιατρικής Τέχνης*», που είναι η σημειωτική. Ως σημεία κατά τον Γαληνό είναι σε αδρές γραμμές τα κλινικά χαρακτηριστικά της εικόνας του ανθρώπου. Διακρίνονται σε διαγνωστικά, προγνωστικά και αναμνηστικά, και σχετίζονται τόσο με τις τρείς καταστάσεις του ανθρωπίνου σώματος όσο και με τις τρεις χρονικές βαθμίδες παρόν, μέλλον και παρελθόν (I, 313, 5–3 14,1, K). Άξιο αναφοράς είναι και το γεγονός ότι κατά τον Γαληνό τα «σημάδια» των υγιεινών, των νοσωδών και των ουδετέρων διαιρούν το εύρος της υγείας σε τρία αντίστοιχα μέρη, δηλαδή υπάρχει το νοσηρό, το υγιεινό και το ουδέτερο μέρος της υγείας (I, 316, 17–317, 4, K).

Τα διαγνωστικά σημεία είναι τα κλινικά χαρακτηριστικά που βοηθούν στη διάγνωση της υγείας ή της νόσου που υπάρχει. Τα προγνωστικά σημεία είναι τα κλινικά ευρήματα που συμβάλλουν στην πρόγνωση της υγείας ή της νόσου που πρόκειται να αποκτήσει το ανθρώπινο σώμα. Τα αναμνηστικά σημεία είναι τα κλινικά ευρήματα που υπενθυμίζουν την υγεία ή τη νόσο που έχει υπάρξει. Σημαντικότερα όμως είναι τα διαγνωστικά και τα προγνωστικά καθώς χάρη σε αυτά οδηγούμαστε στη σωστή αξιολόγηση, την έγκαιρη διάγνωση της νόσου, την αντιμετώπισή της και την πρόγνωση της πορείας της (I, 314, 3–5, K).

Κατά παρόμοιο τρόπο ο Γαληνός διακρίνει και τα σημεία των ουδετέρων. Επειδή όμως η συγκεκριμένη κατηγορία κλινικών χαρακτηριστικών ίσως παρουσιάζει δυσκολίες στην ακριβή σύλληψη καταφεύγει σε ένα αρκετά χρηστικό παράδειγμα. Ο Γαληνός θέτει σε έναν άξονα δύο ακρότατα όρια που είναι αντίθετα μεταξύ τους. Στο ένα άκρο τοποθετεί τα σημάδια των υγιεινών που αντιστοιχούν στην τέλεια κατασκευή του ανθρώπινου σώματος, και στο άλλο άκρο, που αποτελεί το αντίθετό του, τοποθετεί τα σημάδια των νοσηρών σωμάτων. Στο μέσο και των δυο, που απέχει ίσες αποστάσεις και από τα δυο άκρα, τοποθετεί τα σημάδια των ουδετέρων σωμάτων.

Δεύτερος τομέας που εμφανίζεται ονομάζεται φυσιολογικός και καταλαμβάνει περίπου το ένα τρίτο του συνολικού έργου. Το τμήμα αυτό της πραγματείας μπορούσαμε να θεωρήσουμε ότι αποτελεί προέκταση ή συμπλήρωμα του έργου «*Περὶ Κράσεων*» καθώς αναφέρονται οι «τέσσαρες ἀρχαί» και οι κράσεις τους (I, 318, 15–319, 4, K). Οι αρχές αυτές αποτελούν τα κύρια μέρη του ανθρωπίνου σώματος, διέπουν τη λειτουργία στην ολότητά του και καθορίζουν τη συνολική κράση του υπό προϋποθέσεις.

Ο Γαληνός θεωρεί δεδομένη τη γνώση που εμπεριέχεται στο «*Περί Κράσεων*» και αφού ορίσει τις τέσσερεις αρχές, τμήματα του ανθρωπίνου οργανισμού, που είναι: α) ο εγκέφαλος, β) η καρδιά, γ) το ήπαρ και δ) οι όρχεις, προχωρά στην παρουσίαση των επιμέρους εννέα τύπων κράσεων κάθε αρχής και των εκδηλώσεών τους.

Απαρχή της μελέτης του Γαληνού αποτελεί ο εγκέφαλος και κυρίως η μελέτη των φυσικών γνωρισμάτων ως απόρροια της κράσεώς του. Κατά τον Γαληνό τα είδη των φυσικών γνωρισμάτων του είναι πέντε: η κατάσταση όλου του εγκεφάλου, η τέλεια ή κακή εκτέλεση των ενεργειών των αισθήσεων, οι ενέργειες που πράττουν, οι ενέργειες που διοικούν, οι αισθήσεις και, τέλος, οι φυσικές ενέργειες (I, 319, 14, 320–3, K). Ας αναφερθούμε στο παράδειγμα του εγκεφάλου που έχει ψυχρή και ξηρή κράση. Ανήκει, δηλαδή, στην κατηγορία των σύνθετων κράσεων, όπου τα αντιθετικά ζεύγη των ποιοτήτων ψυχρό–θερμό και ξηρό υγρό βρίσκονται σε ανισορροπία και υπερτερούν οι ποιότητες της ψυχρότητας και της ξηρότητας. Όσα άτομα έχουν εγκέφαλο με τη σύνθετη κράση ψυχρού–ξηρού παρουσιάζουν ασταθή υγεία στους οφθαλμούς. Εμφανίζουν στην ηλικία της νεότητας οξείες αισθήσεις ενώ με την πάροδο των χρόνων η οξύτητα μειώνεται. Παράλληλα όταν επικρατούν υγρές και ξηρές κράσεις του εγκεφάλου προκαλείται βαθύς ύπνος, υπνηλία, ευαισθησία στις καταρροές και συνάχια, ενώ γενικά είναι υπεύθυνες για πληθώρα χαρακτηριστικών τόσο στην ψυχοσύνθεση του ανθρώπου όσο και στη φυσιολογία του εγκεφάλου του συγκεκριμένου τύπου κράσεως. Ανάλογα χαρακτηριστικά εμφανίζουν και οι υπόλοιποι οκτώ τύποι κράσεως και πάντα τα γνωρίσματα της μορφολογίας και της φυσιολογίας του εγκεφάλου είναι αποτέλεσμα της ποιότητας που επικρατεί και καθορίζει την κράση του (I 328–329, K).

Στο ίδιο πλαίσιο παρουσιάζεται και η φυσιολογία της καρδιάς πάντα κατά τα μέτρα και τα σταθμά του Γαληνού και της εποχής στην οποία ζει. Οι κράσεις της καρδιάς είναι αυτές που καθορίζουν σε σημαντικό βαθμό τη λειτουργία της, και πάντα η κράση της καρδιάς είναι πιο θερμή και από την πιο θερμή κράση του εγκεφάλου (I, 332, 1–2, K). Στην περίπτωση που ένας άνθρωπος έχει ψυχρή την κράση της καρδιάς τότε οι σφυγμοί είναι πιο μικροί από τους κανονικούς, χωρίς αναγκαστικά να είναι πιο αραιοί (I, 333, 14–334, 2, K). Συνέπεια της ψυχρής κράσης της καρδιάς κατά τον Γαληνό είναι το άτομο να παρουσιάζει από τη φύση του άτριχο στέρνο, ενώ ως προς τις εξωτερικές του εκδηλώσεις να εμφανίζεται δειλό, άτολμο και αναβλητικό. Ιδιαίτερα σε αυτό το τμήμα του έργου που αναφέρεται στις κράσεις της καρδιάς και την επακόλουθη φυσιολογία της εντοπίζεται έντονα τόσο η χρήση της λογικής του Γαληνού όσο και η προφανής θεωρητική επινόηση ορισμένων εμπειρικών δεδομένων, όπως το παράδειγμα της καρδιάς που εμφανίζει θερμή–ξηρή κράση (I, 334, 14–335, 5, K).

Η κράση της καρδιάς καθορίζει τη συνολική κράση του ανθρώπινου οργανισμού εκτός και αν η κράση του ήπατος «αντιστέκεται» σε αυτή (I, 332, 9–11, K). Για παράδειγμα η κράση του ανθρωπίνου σώματος θα είναι θερμή αν η θερμότητα που ξεκινά από την καρδιά κυριαρχήσει επί της ψυχρότητας του ήπατος (I, 338, 2–4, K). Ενώ αν τόσο η καρδιά όσο και το ήπαρ συμπέσουν στην κράση τους η συνολική κράση του οργανισμού δεν θα είναι το αποτέλεσμα του αθροίσματος ή της διαφοράς αλλά θα διαμορφωθεί απολύτως σύμφωνα με αυτές (I, 338, 10–12, K). Αν δηλαδή τόσο η κράση της καρδιάς όσο και η κράση του ήπατος είναι ψυχρή, τότε και η συνολική κράση του οργανισμού θα είναι ψυχρή, με την ίδια αρχή να ισχύει και στην περίπτωση της θερμής κράσης καρδιάς και ήπατος.

Ο τομέας της ιατρικής που έπεται είναι ο αιτιολογικός. Σύμφωνα με τη θεώρηση του Γαληνού η υγεία είναι αποτέλεσμα της δράσης κάποιου αιτίου. Τα υγιή αίτια διακρίνονται κυρίως σε τρείς κατηγορίες, α) σε αυτά που συμβάλλουν στη διατήρηση της καλής υγείας, β) στα αίτια που προλαμβάνουν την εκδήλωση των νόσων, και γ) εκείνα που έχουν τη δυνατότητα να επαναφέρουν έναν άρρωστο στην προγενέστερη κατάσταση καλής υγείας (I, 366, 9–14, K).

Βέβαια υπάρχουν και τα αίτια που μεταβάλλουν τον οργανισμό. Γιατί αν δεν υπήρχαν τα αίτια θα ήταν αμετάβλητος, θα παρέμενε η τέλεια κατασκευή και δε θα υπήρχε η ανάγκη της ιατρικής τέχνης για να τον προστατεύει. Η επίδραση των αιτιών είναι αναπόφευκτη (I, 367, 13–368, 1, K) για τον ανθρώπινο οργανισμό και κατηγοριοποιούνται σε πέντε τύπους:

1 Η επαφή με τον περιβάλλοντα αέρα.
2 Η κίνηση και η ηρεμία του σώματος ή κάποιων μερών του.

3 Ο ύπνος και η αγρυπνία.
4 Η τροφή.
5 Τα εκκρινόμενα και αυτά που κατακρατούνται από τον οργανισμό.
6 Τα πάθη της ψυχής.

Τα ανωτέρω αίτια μεταβάλλουν το ανθρώπινο σώμα ανάλογα με την χρήση τους. Αποτελούν τμήμα των υγιεινών αιτιών αν χρησιμοποιούνται κατάλληλα και συμβάλλουν στην υγεία. Αν όμως ξεπεράσουν το μέτρο τότε γίνονται νοσηρά καθώς μεταβάλλουν και φθείρουν το σώμα.

Ο θεραπευτικός ως τομέας της ιατρικής διαιρείται κατά τον Γαληνό στον περί των φαρμάκων τομέα, τη χειρουργική, την ανατομική και μια γενικότερη υποκατηγορία όπου εντάσσονται όλες οι υπόλοιπες μορφές αντιμετώπισης των νόσων που σχετίζονται με τη δυσκρασία των χυμών (I, 381, 1–6, K). Σκοπός του θεραπευτικού τομέα είναι η αποκατάσταση της υγείας του ατόμου που νοσεί. Στη θεώρηση του Γαληνού η νόσος, η οποία έχει ήδη προκληθεί, θα θεραπευτεί αν αναιρεθεί η κατάσταση από την οποία πρωταρχικά βλάπτεται ο οργανισμός. Προκειμένου να γίνει πλήρως αντιληπτός ο στόχος της θεραπευτικής ο Γαληνός περιγράφει με μεγάλη λεπτομέρεια τις βασικές αρχές της εναντιοπαθολογίας. Βασικός σκοπός της θεραπείας είναι η αναίρεση του αιτίου που προκαλεί τη νόσο με τη χρήση του αντιθέτου του.

Για τη θεραπεία των ασθενειών που σχετίζονται με ανισορροπία των τεσσάρων χυμών και κατ' επέκταση με προβλήματα της κράσης του ανθρώπινου οργανισμού ο Γαληνός ακολουθεί πιστά το δόγμα της εναντιοπαθολογίας «*Τά ἐνάντια τοῖς ἐναντίοις εἰσὶν ἰήματα*». Η άρση της ανισορροπίας των χυμών επιτυγχάνεται με δύο τρόπους. Είτε με τη χορήγηση τροφών και φαρμάκων στα οποία υπερτερεί ο αντίθετος χυμός από αυτόν που είναι σε πλεόνασμα, είτε με την αποβολή του πλεονάζοντος χυμού. Η αποβολή πραγματοποιείται με φλεβοτομία, κλύσματα και καθαρτικά φάρμακα.

Εκτός από τον τομέα σχετικά με τα φάρμακα και τις αγωγές για την αποκατάσταση της ισορροπίας των χυμών στον τομέα της θεραπευτικής εντάσσεται και η χειρουργική, η ανάταξη καταγμάτων και επούλωση πληγών. Η χειρουργική ως τεχνική έχει περιορισμένη χρήση στην ιατρική τέχνη του Γαληνού. Η χρήση του νυστεριού αναφέρεται σε ελάχιστες πλην όμως πολύ συγκεκριμένες περιπτώσεις, όπως όταν περιέχεται κάτι αφύσικα σε κάποιο μέλος. Ακόμα και σε αυτή την περίπτωση προτιμείται η μετατόπιση ή η χρήση φαρμάκων, και σε επόμενο στάδιο η χρήση της χειρουργικής.

Ως τελευταίο τομέα της πραγματείας «*Τέχνη Ιατρική*» θα πρέπει να αναφέρουμε τον τομέα της υγιεινής. Ο υγιεινός τομέας είναι ο πλέον πολυδιάστατος και διεισδύει σε όλους τους υπόλοιπους τομείς καθώς αυτός είναι ο σκοπός της ιατρικής, η διατήρηση της υγείας του ανθρώπινου οργανισμού. Ο τομέας αυτός διακρίνεται στον προφυλακτικό ή προληπτικό υγείας, τον αναρρωτικό και τον αναθρεπτικό.

Ο προληπτικός είναι ο τομέας της υγείας που σχετίζεται με τα αίτια που συμβάλλουν στη διατήρηση της υγείας κάθε προβληματικής κράσης. Ο αναρρωτικός τομέας και ο αναθρεπτικός τομέας σχετίζονται με τους ασθενείς, που αναρρώνουν από οποιαδήποτε πάθηση, και με τους γέρους (I, 405, 14–15, K).

Συμπερασματικά, η ιατρική τέχνη κατά τον Γαληνό διακρίνεται σε πέντε κυρίως τομείς, α) φυσιολογικό, β) σημειωτικό, γ) αιτιολογικό δ) θεραπευτικό, και τέλος ε) υγιεινό. Βέβαια, αρκετοί τομείς διακρίνονται και σε επιμέρους υποτομείς, όπως έχουμε ήδη διαπιστώσει από τα ανωτέρω.

Ακριβώς αυτή η διάκριση της ιατρικής κατά τον Γαληνό παρουσιάζει ενδιαφέρουσες ομοιότητες με την αντίστοιχη διαίρεση που εμφανίζεται στον κώδικα *Additicius* 23,407 του Βρετανικού Μουσείου και στον κώδικα *Vindobonensis Medicus Graecus* 16 (Hunger and Kersten 1969 = 35 Lambeck/Kollar 1780). Συγκεκριμένα στους δύο αυτούς κώδικες γίνεται αναφορά στη διαίρεση της ιατρικής, σύμφωνα μάλιστα με ορισμένους λογίους σε δύο τομείς, τον θεωρητικό και πρακτικό, και σύμφωνα με άλλους σε πέντε. Η διαίρεση της ιατρικής τέχνης σύμφωνα με τους δύο κώδικες φαίνεται και στο σχήμα (Εικ. 14.1).

Η περίπτωση της διαιρέσεως σε πέντε μέρη είναι ταυτόσημη με την αντίστοιχη που προτείνεται από τον Γαληνό. Η κύρια διαφορά εντοπίζεται στο ότι ο Γαληνός ξεκινά την παρουσίαση με τον σημειωτικό τομέα σε αντίθεση με την περίπτωση των δύο κωδίκων που ξεκινούν με τον φυσιολογικό.

Κατά τον Temkin η διαίρεση της ιατρικής σε πέντε κύριους τομείς ανάγεται πολύ πριν τον 6ο αιώνα μΧ και έχει ως υπόβαθρο ελληνικές πηγές χωρίς όμως να τις προσδιορίζει (Temkin 1935, 179–97).

Με βάση τις ενδείξεις που παρατηρούνται στην πραγματεία «*Τέχνη Ἰατρική*» θα πρέπει να αναθεωρήσουμε τη θέση Temkin, ως προς τον χρονικό προσδιορισμό της διαίρεσης, τουλάχιστον κατά τρεις αιώνες νωρίτερα. Δηλαδή η διαίρεση της ιατρικής σε πέντε τομείς, όπως σκιαγραφείται από τον Γαληνό σε αυτό το έργο, θα πρέπει να αναχθεί τουλάχιστον πριν από την πρώτη δεκαετία του 3ου μΧ αιώνα. Κατά συνέπεια η αναζήτηση των σχετικών πηγών θα πρέπει να στραφεί στην εποχή του Γαληνού και παλαιότερα.

Η πραγματεία «*Τέχνη Ἰατρική*» γράφηκε από το Γαληνό με στόχο την επιμέρους εξέταση και υπενθύμιση των βασικών σημείων προγενέστερων έργων του. Αποτελεί μια συγκεφαλαίωση της γαληνικής ιατρικής γνώσης και μια επιτομή της προσφοράς του στην ανάπτυξη της τέχνης. Επιγραμματικά το έργο «*Τέχνη Ἰατρική*» παρουσιάζει ένα περίγραμμα της ιατρικής υπό το πρίσμα των κατηγοριών της υγείας και της ασθένειας, των κατηγοριών που ενδιέφεραν

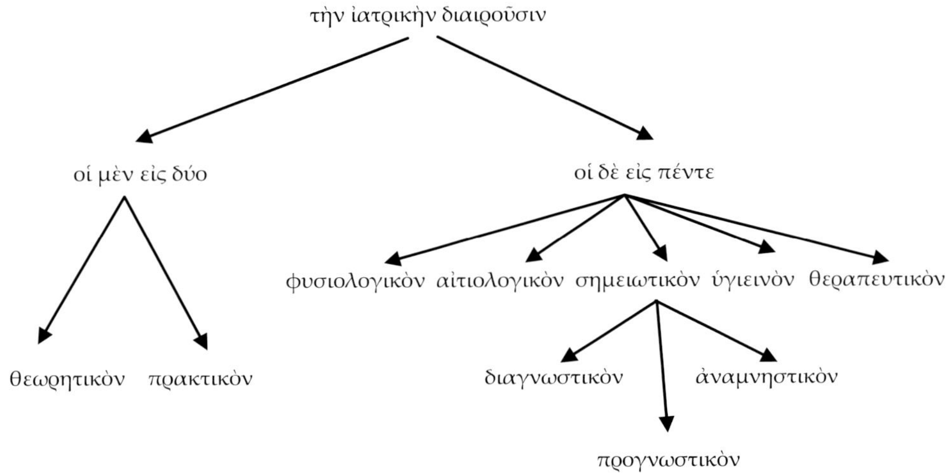

Figure 14.1.

κατά κύριο λόγο αυτόν που ασκούσε την ιατρική (I, 407, 6–9, K). Σε αυτόν ακριβώς τον λόγο θα πρέπει να αποδώσουμε τη μεγάλη διάδοση και αποδοχή του για περισσότερο από δεκαπέντε αιώνες.

Σημειώσεις

1 Το σύνολο των έργων που απαρτίζουν τον 'Αλεξανδρινό Κανόνα' του Γαληνού είναι τα ακόλουθα: «*Περὶ αἱρέσεων τοῖς εἰσαγομένοις*», «*Τέχνη Ἰατρική*», «*Σύνοψις περὶ σφυγμῶν ἰδίας πραγματείας*», «*Τῶν πρὸς Γλαύκωνα θεραπευτικῶν*», «Περὶ ἀνατομικῶν ἐγχειρήσεων», «Περὶ ὀστῶν τοῖς εἰσαγομένοις», «*Περὶ μυῶν κινήσεως*», «*Περὶ μυῶν ἀνατομῆς*», «*Περὶ νεύρων ἀνατομῆς*», «*Περὶ φλεβῶν καὶ ἀρτηριῶν ἀνατομῆς*», «*Περὶ τῶν καθ' Ἱπποκράτην στοιχείων*», «*Περὶ κράσεων*», «*Περί δυνάμεων φυσικῶν*», «*Περὶ αἰτίων συμπτωμάτων*», «*Περὶ τῶν πεπονθότων τόπων*», «*Περὶ διαφορᾶς σφυγμῶν*», «*Περὶ διαγνώσεως σφυγμῶν*», «*Περὶ τῶν ἐν τοῖς σφυγμοῖς αἰτίων*», «*Περὶ προγνώσεως σφυγμῶν*», «*Περὶ διαφορᾶς πυρετῶν*», «*Περὶ κρίσεων*», «*Περὶ κρισίμων ἡμερῶν*», «*Περὶ ὑγιεινῶν*», «*Περὶ θεραπευτικῆς μεθόδου*».

2 Για τον Γαληνό δεν υπάρχει διαφορά μεταξύ των νοσηρών και νοσωδών και προτιμά τη χρήση του τελευταίου όρου («οὐ διαφέρει δὲ οὐδ' εἰ νοσερῶν τις εἴποι», I 307, K)

Βιβλιογραφία

Alighieri D. 1989: *Dante: The Banquet*. Trans. Chr. Ryan., Saratoga, California: ANMA Libri.

Argenterius, J. 1566: *In artem medicinalem Galeni, commentarii tres*, Monteregali.

Culpeper, N. 1652: *Galen's Art of Physick*, London.

Hankinson, R.J. 2008: 'The man and his work', in R. J. Hankinson (ed.), *The Cambridge Companion to Galen*, Cambridge.

Hunger, H. and Kersten, O. 1969: *Katalog der griechischen Handschriften der Oesterreichschen Nationalbibliotek,* Vienna.

Irigoin, J. 1997: *Tradition et Critique des Textes Grecs*, Paris.

Kühn, C. G. (ed.) 1819–33: *Claudii Galeni Opera Omnia*, vols I–XX, Lipsiae.

Lambeck/Kollar 1766–1782: *Petri Lambecii Hamburgensis Commentariorum de Augustissima Bibliotheca Caesarea Vindobonensi,* ed. by A. F. Kollar, Vienna.

Nutton, V. 2005: 'The fatal Embrace: Galen and the History of Ancient Medicine', *Science in Context* 18, 111–21.

Nutton, V. 2008: 'The fortunes of Galen', 355–90 in R. J. Hankinson (ed.), *The Cambridge Companion to Galen*, Cambridge.

Temkin, O. 1935: 'Studies on Late Alexandrian Medicine', *Bulletin of the History of Medicine* 3, 405–30.

Temkin, O. 1973: *Galenism: Rise and Decline of a Medical Philosophy*, Ithaca & London.

15. An Episode in the Historiography of Malaria in the Ancient World

Philip van der Eijk

This paper provides a historiographical analysis of the theory of W. H. S. 'Malaria' Jones about the role of malaria in the history of the ancient Mediterranean world and its reception in subsequent scholarship on ancient medicine. This theory argued that malaria was introduced as a new disease into Greece in the mid-5th century BC, perhaps as a result of the Persian invasions, and that the disease, by its long-term debilitating effects on human society, was a main cause of the cultural decline that set in towards the end of the 5th century and culminated in the collapse of classical civilization in late antiquity. The paper analyses the historical background of Jones' theory and its connection with the research of people such as Angelo Celli and Major Ronald Ross and the Greek Anti-malaria League. It also analyses the presuppositions and the methodological peculiarities of Jones' theory and his use of the evidence, and concludes with some more general observations on the methodological problems involved in trying to determine the historical role of disease in ancient history.

> 'It was with diffidence and misgiving that I accepted the invitation to contribute this paper. A schoolmaster, without any medical training, whose life has been spent in the humble task of teaching little boys their Latin, what right can such an one have to address a conference of physicians and scholars? And, indeed, had it not been for Major Ross, who was the first to suggest that malaria influenced Greek history, and other physicians and scholars, whose help has been as generous as it was invaluable, I should never have been able to gather together the few facts about malaria in the ancient world which I am about to lay before you'.

Thus spoke William Henry Samuel Jones (Fig. 15.1[1]) at the beginning of his paper 'Disease and History', read before a joint meeting of the Liverpool Classical Association and the Liverpool School of Tropical Medicine on 25 January 1909 (Jones 1909b). Although more than a hundred years ago, the quotation is appropriate to this paper as well. For, like Jones, the present author is not a medical doctor, palaeopathologist or environmental historian, but a classicist and historian of thought, concerned with the Greeks' and Romans' reactions to, and understandings of, the nosological and ecological reality as these are reflected in ancient medical thought and practice, rather than with the reconstruction of this nosological reality itself.[2] Of course, history of disease and history of medicine are, or at least should be, two interrelated aspects of the integrated study of health and disease in classical antiquity. But it rarely happens that these two competences are united in one person, and interdisciplinary co-operation between the two specialisms is therefore necessary.

This paper, however, will be concerned with an even further meta-level of discourse in that it will study the historiography of malaria in the ancient world as found in Jones' work; and as such it will be devoted to an episode in the history of medico-historical scholarship — indeed, with a particular example of the kind of interdisciplinary collaboration just mentioned. The point here is not so much to assess the factual accuracy of Jones' work, but rather to shed light on some of its methodological and indeed ideological presuppositions.

In doing so, I should like to start by stressing that the study of ancient medicine owes a very great debt to Jones' work. A fellow of St Catherine's College, Cambridge, Jones is perhaps best known for his three volumes of Hippocratic writings (Greek text and English translation) for the Loeb Classical Library, first published in the 1920s and '30s (and reprinted many times), which have been widely used for many decades by scholars and students alike. True, these

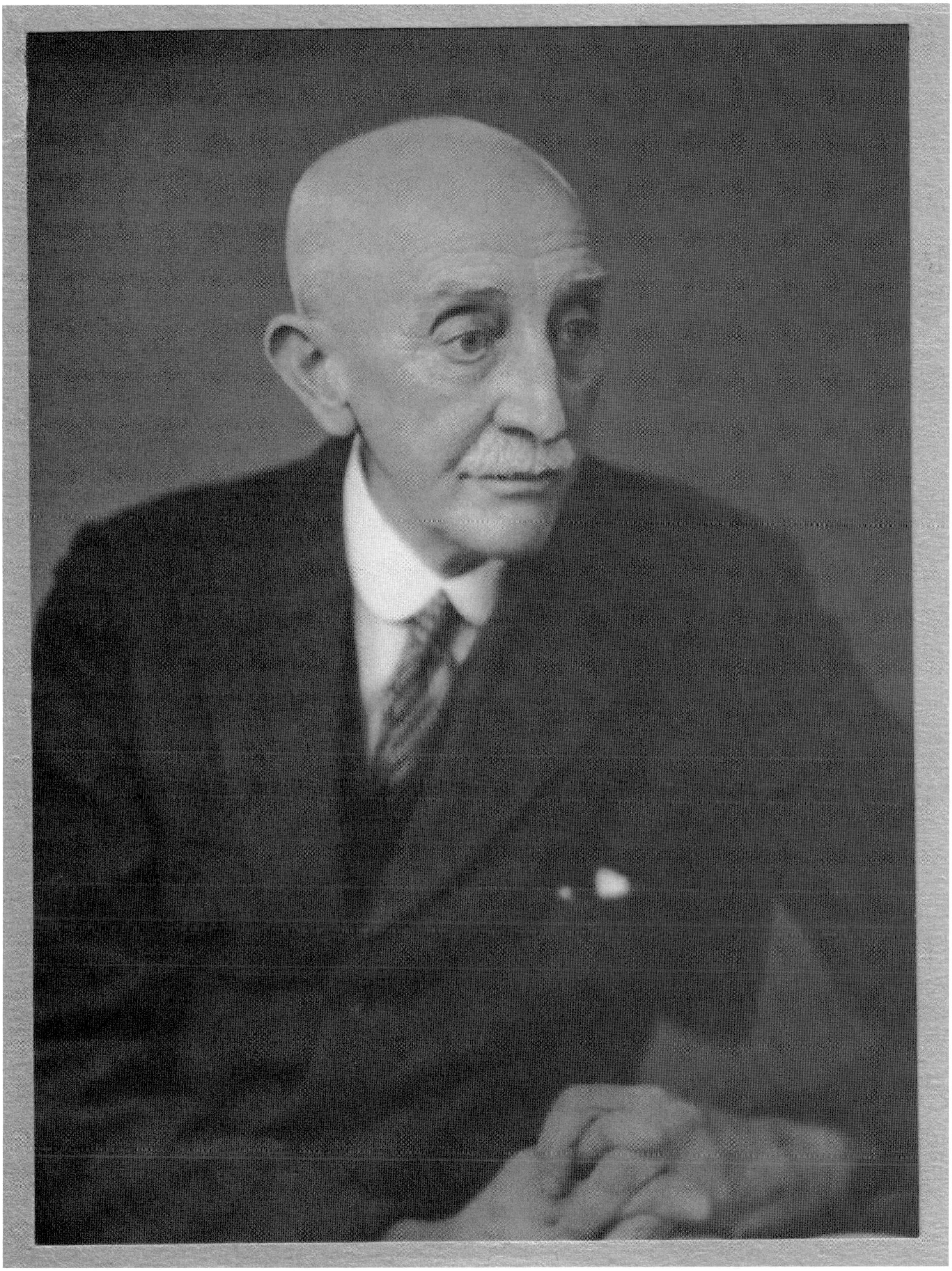

Fig. 15.1. W. H. S Jones in 1947, photographed by Walter Stoneman (St. Catharine's College, Cambridge, Reference: PHOT/7/Jones/1)

volumes do not always live up to the rigorous standards of classical philology, and they are somewhat idiosyncratic in their introductions to the individual Hippocratic writings. But it is nevertheless thanks to Jones that the Hippocratic writings emerged from the obscurity in which they had long been for lack of an accessible edition in English; and many a Classics teacher, as indeed many historians of medicine, will be grateful to him for providing just that (and to E. Withington, who translated the volume on Hippocratic surgery and with whom Jones had been co-operating from the malaria publications onwards). Jones is further known for his respectable translation and commentary of the Hippocratic work *On Ancient Medicine* (Jones 1946), for his edition and translation of the medical papyrus known as *Anonymus Londiniensis* (Jones 1947), and for a booklet discussing the various versions of the Hippocratic Oath (Jones 1924).

Yet Jones is probably best known for his theory on malaria in antiquity. His view that malaria was the catalyst of the decline of classical Greek civilization became so well-known, if not notorious, that it caused him to be called by the nickname 'Malaria Jones' – hardly meant as a compliment, it would seem. Yet when one looks at the reception of Jones' theory in subsequent scholarship, one will find that downright rejection has by no means been the only reaction – indeed, the theory found more resonance and acceptance than one may be inclined to think today. True, classicists and ancient historians have in the main thought poorly of it; but among historians of diseases, reactions have ranged from enthusiastic embracing, e.g. by F. Cartwright in *Disease and History* (1972) to cautious endorsement, e.g. by Mirko Grmek, who in his book on *Diseases in the Ancient Greek World* (1989) reviews Jones' theory in rather favourable terms and labels malaria as 'the disease par excellence' in antiquity.[3]

So what was this theory? To put it briefly, Jones argued that malaria was introduced as a new disease into Greece in the mid 5th century BC, perhaps as a result of the Persian invasions, and that the disease, by its long-term debilitating effects on human society, was a main cause for the cultural decline that set in towards the end of the 5th century and culminated in the collapse of classical civilization in late antiquity. Malaria was, in other words, a key factor in the decline and fall of the Roman Empire – although Jones later modified his views for the Roman period and attributed to malaria a more limited role.

Jones expounded his theory at the beginning of the 20th century in two books: *Malaria, a Neglected Factor in the History of Greece and Rome* (1907), followed by *Malaria and Greek History* (1909a), and in a number of related publications, such as the paper mentioned at the beginning of this contribution (Jones 1909b), and in '*Dea febris*' (a study of the cult of the goddess of fever), also from 1909 (Jones 1909c). Yet his theory also shines through in his commentaries on Hippocratic writings of the next decades; and it is still upheld in Jones' article on 'Ancient documents and contemporary life' (1953). So although Jones modified and corrected parts of his theory, on the whole he remained faithful to it until the 1950s.

Jones arrived at this theory, partly inspired by new discoveries of the aetiology and transmission of malaria and by the spread of the disease in modern Greece and central Italy at the end of the nineteenth century; and he was particularly motivated by the research of Angelo Celli and Major Ronald Ross, mentioned at the beginning of this paper. Thus Jones' book on *Malaria and Greek History* (1909a), dedicated to Ross, contains a long 'Appeal made to the Greek government by the Greek Anti-malaria league, Athens, 1907'. This is of some interest here, as one of Jones' presuppositions is that the ecological situation in contemporary Greece was roughly similar to that of classical Greece: 'Owing to the absence of statistics it is not possible accurately to measure the extent to which ancient Greece was infected; but, although changes favouring the disease have occurred since the classical period, these are counterbalanced by the improved treatment of modern times, and especially the use of quinine' (Jones 1909a, 21).

Whether this assumption was justified at the time is probably difficult to determine. Today, hardly any historian of disease will doubt that malaria was present in the ancient world and that it may have been of very considerable significance for the health and disease situation (the *pathocoenosis*, as Grmek would put it) of the ancient world. This is the view, for example, that one finds in the work of J. L. Angel (for full bibliography see Roberts *et al.* 2005) and also, more recently, in that of Robert Sallares (1991; 2002). Greek medical literature refers on numerous occasions to the typical tertian and quartan fever patterns; its doctrine of critical days seems to make good sense with reference to malaria; and its references to people suffering from, or prone to, the 'spleen-disease' may also be taken as a clear reference to malaria – although it should be stressed that in all these cases, alternative explanations cannot be ruled out and retrospective diagnosis remains problematic. The issues on which scholars are still divided are, as far as I can see, *when* malaria was introduced and what role it played in the course of history. Contemporary scholars seem to prefer to believe that malaria had its ups and downs, that it was present in the Iron Age (and perhaps even earlier than that), then disappeared and then reappeared. There seems broad agreement, however, concerning Jones' claim that the disease was not present in the Archaic period, and that it must have been introduced or re-introduced in the course of the 5th century.

Although informed by the medical and ecological knowledge of the time, Jones did not betray his background as a classicist and based his theory almost exclusively on the interpretation of Greek and Latin texts. This, alone, makes any contemporary application of his theory immediately problematic, for palaeopathology, environmental history and bio-archaeology have enormously enriched our knowledge of health and disease in the ancient world. Yet even as far as texts are concerned, we have increasingly become aware of the difficulties of disease identification and retrospective diagnosis on the basis of textual evidence alone; for texts, whether medical or non-medical, literary or non-literary, reflect perceptions and interpretations of nosological reality, and the ways in which they do so are manifold and very complicated — and here, it may be noted, even nowadays there is a sometimes alarming gap between the confidence of historians of diseases and the scepticism and relativism of social historians of medicine when it comes to the use of texts in the reconstruction of the nosological reality of the past.

Jones was of course not bothered by these typically postmodern methodological considerations about 'representation' and 'construction'. But a problem which he should have been aware of is that our picture may be distorted by the hazards of the transmission of the extant source material. Jones argues that Archaic Greek literature (Homer and Hesiod) nowhere refers to anything that might be identified with malaria; thus we may conclude that 'On the whole, the evidence is in favour of the view that malaria was unknown to Hesiod, for it is scarcely conceivable that, had it existed in his day where he lived, he would have omitted to mention it as one of the plagues of the farmer during the hot months' (Jones 1909a, 26). Mirko Grmek and even Paul Burke, in his 1998 survey article, seem to accept Jones' view on the absence of malaria in the early period; yet as P. Brunt points out, this use of the *argumentum e silentio* is highly dubious:

> 'Outside medical writings, clear references to malaria are uncommon in Greek and Latin even from the time when its presence is beyond doubt. There was no reason why epic or lyric poets should speak of periodic fevers or any of the other specific symptoms' (Brunt 1971, 613–4).

And as Brunt goes on to note, the fact that from the late 5th century onwards, references to fever, including the characteristically malarious intermittent fevers, abound, can easily be explained by the fact that the 5th century is the first period in which we encounter substantial literary works, such as the Hippocratic writings, likely to mention issues of public health. It does not prove that the disease was new.

Now Jones seems to anticipate this objection by giving prominence to mentions of the disease in non-medical literature such as historiography, tragedy and comedy (especially Aristophanes' *Wasps*). Here, however, his textual interpretations are at least open to question; especially dubious is his view that all references to fever in non-medical literature refer to malaria – it is a presupposition which Jones mentions several times but which he nowhere substantiates. Of course, it would have suited Jones' theory if there was evidence of a fairly large-scale malarial epidemic in the second half of the 5th century. Yet in this regard Jones' dealing with the famous Athenian 'plague' of 430/429 is remarkable. On the one hand, he does not go as far as to identify the plague with malaria, presumably because Thucydides' description clearly does not fit the malarial symptoms. On the other hand, he does at some point say that 'It is hard to believe that any other disease except malaria could produce so much sickness in so short a time' (Jones 1909a, 29). And in relation to Sophocles' description of the plague of Thebes in the *Oedipus Tyrannus*, which according to Jones does show some malarial symptoms (especially infant mortality), Jones similarly wants to have it both ways by arguing that although this play was clearly inspired by the Athenians' experience of the great plague, 'the truth seems to be that Sophocles has united in one picture the symptoms of three different diseases, one of which was remembered as a tradition, while the other two formed part of the personal experience of his audience' (Jones 1909a, 27). This is of course not impossible, but it cannot be used as evidence that his audience was familiar with malaria.

Something comparable can be observed in Jones' handling of Diodorus of Sicily's account of the plague, which according to Jones is the product of similar confusion of two diseases and which allows of the conclusion that 'either malaria was the most common type of pestilence in later times, so that writers were tempted to confuse it with other diseases, or else there was in Attica during the early years of the Peloponnesian War a serious epidemic of malaria, which was afterwards identified with the Plague' (Jones 1909a, 37). Jones tries to support his assumption that when an Athenian layman says 'fever', he means malaria, by the observation that Thucydides never uses the word *puretos* at all, not even in talking about the plague: 'He employs instead *kauma* or *therme*, just as though he were afraid of causing misapprehension if he used an expression which, in the common speech, was in his day of a peculiar and limited application' (Jones 1909a, 41). Again, this is not impossible – though highly unlikely if malaria was a *new* disease – but Jones fails to test his own theory by considering alternative explanations, e.g. by studying Thucydides' use of medical terminology in general. This lack of self-criticism is a weakness that inheres in Jones' theory on a number of points; the most striking example is when he refers to the apathy as one of the characteristic deleterious effects of malaria: 'I have found no expression of this apathy among the ancient Greeks, but it may be that references to the serious consequences of malaria would be more numerous if the very presence of the disease had not blinded the eyes of those who lived under its influence' (Jones 1909a, 86).

To be sure, Jones shows himself explicitly aware of the limits to which literary evidence can be used; but it seems that he fails to apply this awareness with the required extent of rigour. Even if literary evidence might be capable of proving the occurrence of malaria in a certain time and a certain place, it is very unlikely to allow of quantitative conclusions about the extent to which the disease was present in different periods. Apart from this, there is the question of whether a particular piece of information is based on autopsy or hearsay, whether it simply copies from other writers or reflects the author's own observations (a question that arises, for example, with the Roman author Celsus). Jones is aware of these methodological *caveats*, but he seems to pay lip service to them, for his realisation of the problems posed by the lack of evidence of the later Hellenistic and Imperial period does not prevent him from making very selective and peculiar usage of it. Thus he analyses at considerable length a treatise by Plutarch on the preservation of health. Now Plutarch is not a doctor or medical writer; his treatise reflects the general concern with dietetics and disease prevention prevalent in the period of the Second Sophistic, and presents a good example of popularisation of medical theory. Yet Jones concludes from Plutarch's obsession with health that the times in which he lived must have been particularly unhealthy, and that everything points in the direction of malaria. The only concession Jones is prepared to make here is that 'the writer does not seem to be referring to infectious sickness, for he nowhere mentions either contagion or infection' (Jones 1909a, 51–2). But this is, of course, hardly to be expected from an ancient author, because the notions of contagion or infection did not exist in antiquity. This confusion between ancient and modern understanding affects Jones' argument on a number of occasions, e.g. when he distinguishes between remittent and intermittent fevers but fails to acknowledge that a determination of this distinction in antiquity would have been very difficult to carry out, or when claiming that the ancient notions of *phrenitis* and *melancholia* in fact refer to malaria, which completely ignores the great diversity of ancient conceptions corresponding to these disease names.

Jones' reason for using diseases like these is that they show the influence of disease on character; and here we come to the fundamentals of Jones' theory, viz. the influence of malaria on race and character. For this connection between the physical and the spiritual is essential to Jones' theory of the cultural decline that set in as a result of the onset of malaria in the Greek world. Malaria, Jones argues, affects character and spirit, and has a degenerating effect on the human race. Here, Jones does not shy away from using language which nowadays would be regarded as politically completely incorrect. Thus when discussing the possibility that the Persian invasions brought malaria into Greece, he suggests in a footnote that 'the malarious low-lying districts of Western Asia possibly contributed to the degeneration of the Persians themselves' (Jones 1909a, 29 n. 3). Among the Greeks, malaria caused the worst vices to come to the surface: 'barbarity, want of good faith, insincerity, fickleness, incapability of united efforts ... laziness, cowardice and apathy' (Jones 1909b, 41). This happened in the 4th and 3rd century BC, periods in which:

> 'the Greeks gradually lost their brilliance ... their initiative vanished; they ceased to create and began to comment. Patriotism ... became an empty name, for few had the high spirit and energy to translate into action man's duty to the state. Vacillation, indecision, fitful outbursts of unhealthy activity followed by cowardly depression, selfish cruelty and criminal weakness are characteristic of the public life of Greece from the struggle with Macedonia ... Philosophy also suffered, and became deeply pessimistic even in the hands of its best and noblest exponents' (Jones 1909a, 102).

Even developments in religion and superstition, e.g. the cult of the *Dea Febris*, were explained by Jones by reference to the spread of malaria (for a critical assessment see Burke 1998, 2266–71).

In his negative evaluation of the post-classical period in Greek history, that is everything that happened after the Golden Age of Greek civilisation, Jones echoes a judgement that was typical of 19th century classical scholarship but which, during the 20th century, has been subject to revolutionary revision. In this prejudice about what is called the Hellenistic period, Jones was certainly not alone, although his explanation for this cultural decline by reference to malaria is certainly remarkable – it is almost as if one reads the author of the Hippocratic work *Airs Waters Places*, or Aristotle's comments in the *Politics* (VII, 6) on the various peculiarities of character of the peoples that surrounded Greece.

Yet one of the most peculiar aspects of his theory is his view that the spread of malaria enhanced the role of women, evidence for which Jones perceives in the role of women in New Comedy:

> 'Ignorant and superstitious, the women of Greece often had recourse to charms and amulets, and flocked in large numbers to the dream-oracles to find out the means of curing their loved ones who were sick. But in spite of this, the Greek wife must have been trained in sympathy and tact by her work as nurse, and in this way happier relations were established between her and her husband, who possibly learnt, when prostrated year after year by a lingering disease, to appreciate those virtues which belong, in a peculiar way, to women, and especially to a mother and a wife. It will probably never be known how much the human race owes to disease for the development of the kindlier virtues of mercy, sympathy, and tenderness' (Jones 1909a, 126).

Depending on one's personal background (and perhaps gender), passages like this may make one either smile or feel outraged. From a methodological point of view, however, the weaknesses of Jones' theory become painfully clear. It is based on arguments from silence in a situation where the demonstrable loss of most primary material makes it particularly questionable to use these. Furthermore, the theory cannot be subject to falsification, as every piece of counter-evidence can be accommodated within it. It makes selective use of the evidence; and its interpretation of the evidence is biased and uncritical, unashamedly guided by overt moral judgements and by a lack of appreciation for the cultural significance of the Hellenistic and Imperial periods of Greco-Roman antiquity.

Acknowledgements

I am very grateful to Professor Demetrios Michaelides for the invitation to speak at the Nicosia conference, and to the other participants for their comments. An earlier version of this paper was presented at a symposium on Malaria in the Ancient World held at Green College, Oxford, in May 2000, and I am grateful to the organisers (Mary Dobson and Robert Arnott) and to the other participants for their comments. I should like to acknowledge the support of the Wellcome Trust for my research.

Notes

1 Editor's note: I would like to thank Mrs Elizabeth Ennion-Smith, Archivist of St Catharine's College, Cambridge, for her assistance in obtaining this photograph of W. H. S Jones.

2 I should stress that I lay no claim to expertise in the history of malaria, nor to comprehensive coverage of the very large body of literature on the topic. My main sources of information have been: Grmek 1989; 1994; Sallares 1991; 2002; Dunn 1993; de Zulueta 1973; Burke 1998; Roberts *et al.* 2005. See also Corvisier 1994 and Collin-Bouffier 1994

3 Grmek, 1989, 279–83, e.g. 281: 'Most of Jones's conclusions still evoke our assent, but on condition that his hypothesis of the first introduction of malaria into Greece can be replaced by that of the reintroduction of falciparum malaria'.

Bibliography

Brunt, P. 1971: *Italian Manpower 225 BC–AD 14*, Oxford.

Burke, P. F. 1998: 'Malaria in the Greco-Roman World: a historical and epidemiological survey', 2252-81 in W. Haase (ed.), *Aufstieg und Niedergang der römischen Welt* II.37.3.

Cartwright, F. F. 1972: *Disease and History*, New York.

Collin-Bouffier, S. 1994: 'Marais et paludisme en Occident grec', 321–36 in R. Ginouvès, A. M. Guimier-Sorbets, J. Jouanna and L. Villard (eds), *L'eau, la santé et la maladie dans le monde grec*, Athens.

Corvisier, J. N. 1994: 'Eau, paludisme et démographie en Grèce péninsulaire', 297–319 in R. Ginouvès, A. M. Guimier-Sorbets, J. Jouanna and L. Villard (eds), *L'eau, la santé et la maladie dans le monde grec*, Athens.

Dunn, F. L. 1993: 'Malaria', 855–62 in K. F. Kiple (ed.), *The Cambridge World History of Human Disease*, Cambridge.

Grmek, M. D. 1989: *Diseases in the Ancient Greek World*, Baltimore.

Grmek, M. D. 1994: 'Bibliographie chronologique des études originales sur la malaria dans la Méditerranée orientale préhistorique et antique (depuis la découverte des agents pathogènes et des vecteurs)', in *Université Jean Monnet, Saint Etienne, Centre Jean-Palerne, Lettre d'Informations* 24 (mai 1994), 1–7.

Jones, W. H. S. 1907: *Malaria, a Neglected Factor in the History of Greece and Rome*, Cambridge.

Jones, W. H. S. 1909a: *Malaria and Greek History*, Manchester.

Jones, W. H. S. 1909b: 'Disease and history', *Annals of Archaeology and Anthropology* 2, 33–41.

Jones, W. H. S. 1909c: 'Dea Febris', *Annals of Archaeology and Anthropology* 2, 97–124.

Jones, W. H. S. 1924: *The Doctor's Oath. An Essay in the History of Medicine*, Cambridge.

Jones, W. H. S. 1946: *Philosophy and Medicine in Ancient Greece*, Baltimore.

Jones, W. H. S. 1947: *The Medical Writings of Anonymus Londinensis*, Cambridge.

Jones, W. H. S. 1953: 'Ancient documents and contemporary life with Special Reference to the Hippocratic Corpus, Celsus and Pliny', 100–10 in E. Ashworth Underwood (ed.), *Science, Medicine and History. Essays on the Evolution of Scientific Thought and Medical Practice written in honour of Charles Singer*, vol. 1, London and New York.

Roberts, C. A., Lagia, A., Triantaphyllou, S., Bourbou, C. and Tsaliki, A. 2005: 'Health and disease in Greece: past, present and future', 32–58 in H. King (ed.), *Health in Antiquity*, London.

Sallares, R. 1991: *The Ecology of the Ancient Greek World*, London.

Sallares, R. 2002: *Malaria and Rome*, Oxford.

Zulueta, J. de 1973: 'Malaria and Mediterranean history', *Parassitologia* 1–15.

16. Medical Dialogue in the Books on Dietetics in the *De medicina*: Celsus Taking Account of the Patient as a Friend and Individual

Aurélien Gautherie

In books 1–4 on dietetics of his De medicina, *Celsus, a Roman encyclopaedist from the 1st century AD, highlights from time to time the importance of the medical dialogue between the doctor and his patient. By analysing in detail examples from the text, I shall demonstrate that the attention paid to the patient and the role he might play at each stage of the medical process differ from what they were in the* Corpus Hippocraticum *and that they are indeed greater than one might have expected. I will try to argue that Celsus' original presentation of the medical dialogue comes within the general context of the emergence, in the Roman medical literature of the first century AD, of the idea of the patient as a 'medical self'.*

Introduction

As summarised by Jouanna in his *Hippocrate* (Jouanna 1992, 192–4), the *Corpus Hippocraticum* emphasises the importance of the medical dialogue between the doctor and his patient. But, although scholars have quite rightly drawn many parallels between Celsus' *De medicina* and this Greek corpus, in which the Roman encyclopaedist found plentiful material for his own writing (see for example Mudry 1985), surprisingly little, if any attention has been paid so far to the medical dialogue in Celsus' work.

I would, therefore, like to analyse this practice as described in the *De medicina*, concentrating on the first four books on dietetics, as this aspect of medicine played a major part in the ancient Mediterranean world. The medical dialogue appears only four times in these books, but its analysis, if one looks closely at the texts, proves most valuable. Not only do the grounds and motivations differ from those in the Hippocratic corpus, but these differences reveal a deeper evolution in the Roman medical literature of the 1st century AD: the emergence of the idea of the patient as a *medical self*.

The medical dialogue in the establishment of a diagnosis

In the Hippocratic corpus, the establishment of a diagnosis was mostly based on the observation of symptoms. This clinical observation still plays a great part in Celsus, but one can also detect, from time to time, the importance of dialogue to make a diagnosis. It is, for example, presented by Celsus as a necessary preliminary to the pulse taking:

> '*Ob quam causam, periti medici est, non protinus ut uenit, apprehendere manu brachium, sed primum residere hilari uultu percunctarique, quemadmodum se habeat, et si quis eius metus est, eum probabili sermone lenire, tum deinde eius corpori manum admouere*' (Celsus, *De medicina* III.6.6).[1]
>
> 'On this account a practitioner of experience does not seize the patient's forearm with his hand, as soon as he comes, but first sits down and with a cheerful countenance asks how the patient finds himself; and if the patient has any fear, he calms him with convincing talk, and only after that moves his hand to touch the patient'.

Just before this text, Celsus says that the patient's pulse can be altered by the fear that the doctor may hide information from him concerning his condition. Using the genitive *periti medici*, Celsus gives a definition of the experienced doctor.

He should ask the patient about his feelings, *percunctarique quemadmodum se habeat*: unambiguously, the reflexive pronoun *se* shows that the patient himself is the source of the physician's information. The doctor's answer, in the tone of an informal conversation (*sermo*), is designed to calm his patient's potential fears (*si quis eius metus est, eum probabili sermone lenire*). I will return later to the therapeutic virtue of the dialogue. What I would like to emphasise now is that dialogue here is clearly an essential step towards the establishment of a proper diagnosis. In this case, it has to precede any act performed by the doctor, as revealed by the structure of the sentence: *non protinus... sed primum... tum deinde*.

If the medical dialogue can yield valuable conditions for the establishment of a good diagnosis, it can also function as an additional diagnostic tool:

> '*Longioris [morbis] uero, ubi suppuratio in iocinore est, dolorque modo finitur, modo intenditur, dextra parte praecordia dura sunt et tument; post cibum maior spiritus difficultas est; accedit maxillarum quaedam resolutio*' (Celsus, *De medicina* IV.15.1).
>
> 'But in a more chronic [disease], when there is suppuration within the liver, and the pain at times ceases, at times is intensified, the praecordia on the right side become hard and swollen; after a meal there is greater difficulty in breathing; then supervenes a sort of paralysis of the lower jaws.'

This passage raises the question of the source of the doctor's information; that he is aware of the alternation of the pain, *dolorque modo finitur, modo intenditur*, as a symptom of a chronic liver disease can imply one of two things. In the first, this alternation would be observed by the practitioner himself, who would attend the patient's bedside. But this explanation seems rather unlikely. Our knowledge of everyday medical practice is that, except when they were at the exclusive service of high-class Roman citizens, most ancient physicians were itinerant, and visiting a patient at the exact time of a crisis was most unlikely.[2] The other alternative would be to admit, reading between the lines, that Celsus may consider, in some cases, the patient himself (or, at least, the members of his *familia*) as competent to give information about the symptoms to the doctor. In the case of chronic diseases, the importance of such a medical dialogue seems to be greater than ever and a valid means of establishing a diagnosis.

The medical dialogue in the choice of therapeutics

The medical dialogue also appears once in the *De medicina* when Celsus writes on the treatment of lientery. He indicates that the doctor has to take into consideration the will of his patient:

> '*Alterum quoque, quod aeque ad omnes similes affectus pertinet, in hoc maxime seruandum est, ut, cum pleraque utilia insuauia sunt, qualis est plantago, et rubi et quidquid malicorio mixtum est, ea potissimum ex his dentur, quae maxime aeger uolet. Deinde, si omnia ista fastidit, ad excitandam cibi cupiditatem interponatur aliquid minus utile, sed magis gratum*' (Celsus, *De medicina* IV.23.2–3).
>
> 'There is another thing which, whilst applicable equally to all similar affections, is to be specially observed in this, that as many beneficial medicaments are disagreeable to the taste, such as the mixture containing plantain and blackberries and any mixture containing pomegranate bark, that shall be chosen which the patient likes most. Moreover, if he loathes all of them, something to excite his appetite should be interposed, less useful, perhaps, but more pleasant.'

Celsus considers the patient's potential aversions to the treatments in two ways. Either it is based on the general feature of the medication, *pleraque... insuauia sunt*, or on a personal dislike, *si omnia ista fastidit* (whether the dislike is expressed by the patient himself, or a relative, does not matter; the pertinent fact is that it is taken into account). In each case the patient's will and feelings, *uolet* and *gratum*, are crucial and even take precedence over the treatment's efficacy.

Also, Celsus establishes a clear opposition between the concept of *utile* and the concept of *gratum* (announced already by the idea of *suauitas* conveyed by the negative adjective *insuauia*). It is true that a passage very close to this one can be found already in the Hippocratic *Aphorisms* II.38. But in that text as in the *Corpus Hippocraticum* in general, such a consideration is motivated only by the physician's will to establish or increase his good reputation (see Mudry 1986). In the *De medicina* on the contrary, it looks as though Celsus believes that the patient's contentment is an aim in itself, independent of the doctor's repute. The patient, who seems to be judged as a person more than as the 'container of a disease' able to back up a doctor's prestige, is here almost on the same level as the practitioner, a fact illustrated by the echo between *maxime seruandum est* and *maxime aeger uolet*.

The medical dialogue as therapeutics

The closeness between the doctor and his patient is to be found on another level. The prologue of the *De medicina* advocates that they should be engaged in a relationship based on *amicitia*, in order to make the treatment more useful (*utiliorem tamen medicum esse amicum quam extraneum* – *Prooemium* 73). In this context, the medical dialogue is to be analysed as a dialogue between *amici* and can sometimes be seen in itself as therapeutic. I would like to come back to the first text we have studied, and now pay attention to this aspect of the dialogue:

> '*Ob quam causam, periti medici est, non protinus ut uenit, apprehendere manu brachium, sed primum residere hilari uultu percunctarique, quemadmodum se habeat, et si quis eius metus est, eum probabili sermone lenire, tum deinde eius corpori manum admouere*' (Celsus, *De medicina* III.6.6).
>
> 'On this account a practitioner of experience does not seize the patient's forearm with his hand, as soon as he comes, but first sits down and with a cheerful countenance asks how the patients finds himself; and if the patient has any fear, he calms him with convincing talk, and only after that moves his hand to touch the patient.'

The practitioner's attitude is described with words usually applied to a speaker. First, he needs to adopt a specific approach and *actio* with regard to both the situation and his addressee: *hilari uultu*. Above all, he has to use *probabili sermone*, 'convincing talk'.[3] It is remarkable that Celsus uses here an adjective referring to the rhetorical category of the *probatio*. In the *oratoris officia*, *probare*, 'to prove', is synonymous with *docere*, 'to teach' (Pernot 2000, 283). This means that the physician has to calm (*lenire*) his patient's reluctance by setting out his medical knowledge in order to reassure him.

Within the medical dialogue as envisioned by Celsus, the doctor does not seem to care about how he appears to others by using grandiloquent sentences; Celsus' physician's psychotherapeutic words have more than a practical virtue, as they had in the *Corpus Hippocraticum* (see, for example, Lain Entralgo 1970, 163). On the contrary, his words, because they are addressed to an *amicus*, are purposely combined with a friendly face and tone (*hilari, lenire*). Not only, as we have seen above, do they help create the best conditions for the establishment of a diagnosis, but they can also be seen, in a way, as a kind of therapeutics and a first step on the road to recovery.

Celsus, earlier in the *De medicina*, indicates how a 'good practicioner', a *bonus medicus*, should convince his patient to endure a bloodletting:

> '*Sed si nullum tamen appareat aliud auxilium, periturusque sit qui laborat, nisi temeraria quoque uia fuerit adiutus, in hoc statu boni medici est ostendere, quam nulla spes sit sine sanguinis detractione, faterique, quantus in hac ipsa metus sit, et tum demum, si exigetur, sanguinem mitter*' (Celsus, *De medicina* II.10.7).
>
> 'If, however, there appears to be no other remedy, and if the patient is likely to die unless he be helped even at some risk – that being the position, it is the part of a good practitioner to show that without the withdrawal of blood there is no hope, and to confess how much fear there may be in that step, and then at length, if the attempt is demanded, to let blood.'

The verbs used here by Celsus mirror the process of the dialogue in both a logical and chronological order. First, the doctor has to demonstrate (*ostendere*) that the bloodletting is the only solution. Then, he has to confess, *fateri,* indicating how frank the dialogue must be, that such a treatment does not go without risks. In the last place only (*tum demum*), and at the patient's request (the conditional clause *si exigetur* proving that the patient – or, again, at least his relatives – does express his will), the bloodletting will be performed. We see clearly here that the ability of the doctor to start a dialogue with his patient and to justify a demanding therapy are, in Celsus' eyes, major criteria to judge a doctor as a good practitioner. One can measure how far we stand here from, for example, the very beginning of the Hippocratic *Prognostics*, where a *iatros agathos* is so judged based only on how well he foresees the outcome of a disease.

Conclusion

Concerning medical dialogue, the Hippocratic heritage of the *De medicina* is clear: one can find the same attention to his patient asked from the practitioner and the same demands to act usefully. But the Roman context of the 1st century AD leads Celsus to go far beyond this heritage and, in the end, to deeply modify it.

In the establishment of a diagnosis, the medical dialogue is now a conceivable alternative to clinical observation. In the choice of therapeutics, the doctor should not only take into consideration the usefulness of a treatment, but must sometimes recognise and incorporate his patient's likes and dislikes. Above all, the concept of *amicitia*, to be found in the *Prologue* of the *De medicina*, influences the relationship between the practitioner and his patient throughout the whole book. The closeness of the two makes the medical dialogue therapeutic in itself.

There may be only a few samples of medical dialogues in the books on dietetics in the *De medicina*. But these, nonetheless, reveal an underlying but crucial change taking place at the time when Celsus' encyclopedia was written.[4] In the *De medicina*, the doctor does not talk with an entity affected by a disease, who can possibly provide him with a valid indication, but about whom he is still wary, as would be the case in general within the Hippocratic corpus (Lain Entralgo 1970, 153). In the *De medicina*, the doctor truly talks with another self, with whom he strikes up a genuinely Roman relationship based on *amicitia*. The attention paid to the patient and the role he might potentially play at each stage of the medical process are, therefore, greater than one might have expected. In Celsus' work, one can discover, by reading between the lines, the birth of the original concept of a medical self, and, within a larger trend in the 1st century AD, towards the consideration of the individual as an independent and worthy value.

Notes

1 Ancient sources and their translations (with pinpoint modifications) in this article are all from the Loeb Classical Library.

2 Celsus does indicate that a good physician *non multum ab aegro recedit* (*De medicina* III.4.9). But even such an expression does not imply a constant presence. On this well-debated passage, see in particular Mudry 1980.

3 And not, in my opinion, 'entertaining talk', as in Spencer's Loeb translation.

4 See Mudry 1997, 320–31 : 'Nous pourrions dire, de façon imagée, que le fameux triangle hippocratique, cher à D. Gourévitch, "maladie, malade, médecin", perd une de ses composantes pour se restreindre au couple "médecin-malade", puisque déontologiquement il ne s'agit plus tant de vaincre la maladie que de secourir le malade.'

Bibliography

Jouanna, J. 1992: *Hippocrate*, Paris.

Lain Entralgo, P. 1970: *The therapy of the word in Classical Antiquity*, New York and London.

Mudry, P. 1980: '*Medicus amicus*. Un trait romain de la médecine antique', *Gesnerus* 37, 17–20.

Mudry, P. 1985: 'Le premier livre de *La Médecine* de Celse. Tradition et nouveauté', 141–50 in I. Mazzini and F. Fusco (eds), *I testi di medicina latini antichi. Problemi filologici e storici. Atti del 1° Convegno Internazionale, Macerata S. Severino M., 26–28 aprile 1984*, (Università di Macerata, Pubblicazioni della Facoltà di Lettere e Filosofia 28), Rome.

Mudry, P. 1986: 'La déontologie médicale dans l'antiquité grecque et romaine : mythe et réalité', *Revue médicale de la Suisse romande* 106, 3–8.

Mudry, P. 1997: 'Ethique et médecine à Rome : la préface de Scribonius Largus ou l'affirmation d'une singularité', 297–337 in *Médecine et morale dans l'Antiquité* (Entretiens de la Fondation Hardt 43), Vandœuvres, Genève.

Pernot, L. 2000: *La rhétorique dans l'Antiquité*, Paris.

17. The Contribution of the 4th Century North African Physician, Helvius Vindicianus

Louise Cilliers

North Africa, and in particular re-founded Carthage, experienced a blossoming of economic, cultural and scientific activities in the 4th and 5th centuries AD, and also proceeded to produce some physicians of excellence. Quite a number of the medical texts produced in the Roman Empire at large during this period originated in North Africa, in particular from physicians and/or medical authors such as Helvius Vindicianus, Theodorus Priscianus, Cassius Felix and Caelius Aurelianus. In this paper the emphasis will be on the contribution of Vindicianus, whose three short works were among the most widely excerpted medical works throughout the Middle Ages. The popularity of his works and the high regard in which he was held by his contemporaries and after his death give rise to the question what made him stand out among his contemporaries. The only clue that we have are his works and a few remarks by students or later authors. I therefore intend to investigate his works in order to find information about his background and especially his prowess as physician – an aspect to which no attention has been paid as yet.

Introduction

Helvius Vindicianus[1] was in many respects a pioneer. His works, written in the late 4th century AD, are among the earliest Latin medical writings to have come from Africa,[2] and are also the first of a number of Latin medical compilations to be produced by practicing doctors in Northern Africa in the period AD 370–450 (Langslow 2000, 63). Vindicianus' works are also unusual in that they were not limited to compilations of medical recipes such as those of most of his contemporaries,[3] but also treated aspects such as the humoural theory, anatomy and embryology. He was a product of his times: in the late 4th and early 5th century the emphasis in the province of Africa Proconsularis was on the preservation of the extensive Graeco-Roman medical tradition and the dissemination of existing knowledge rather than on original research (which in fact ended with Galen some two centuries before). The medical writers of this era were on the whole summarisers and encyclopaedists, producing translations and adaptations of earlier Greek works and referred to as the 'medical refrigerators' of antiquity (Nutton 1984, 2); they were, however, not just compilers and dumb copyists, but they also selected, abbreviated, translated and added new material.

The works of Vindicianus that have been transmitted are:

i the *Gynaecia* (a short work on anatomy and embryology),
ii a letter to his nephew Pentadius (on the humoural theory), and
iii a letter to the emperor Valentinian (which served as an introduction to a now lost collection of medical recipes).

Vindicianus as physician

Testimonia

The high regard in which Vindicianus as physician[4] was held by contemporaries and also after his death is confirmed by various *testimonia*. In *c.* AD 400 St Augustine, one of his students who later became famous, left the following testimonial of the mentor of his youth: 'There was at that time a man of deep understanding, who had an excellent reputation for his great skill as a doctor…' (*Confessiones* IV.3). Elsewhere he refers to Vindicianus as 'that great physician of our time' (*Epistula* 138). Another testimonial is from Vindicianus's student Theodorus Priscianus who stated that Vindicianus' fame after his death was even greater than during his lifetime (*Physica* 3). Then the mere fact that he was Proconsul of Africa[5] and had the high rank of *comes archiatrorum* or Count in charge of the Roman College of Physicians (newly established by the emperor Valentinian I in 368),[6] speaks for itself.

Pathologies: diagnoses and prognoses

The Gynaecia

This short treatise on anatomy[7] contains an overview of the different organs and their function and place in the body, followed by a section on reproduction and embryology.[8] It is a short work and the description of the parts of the body and their functions does not go into any detail, but the aim and the target group of the work must be taken into account. It was most probably written as a textbook for medical students for whom the information would have been sufficient and very useful, or as an invaluable *vademecum* for doctors when travelling,[9] or even as a self-help book for the common man[10] – in short, a kind of 'Idiot's Guide' on basic anatomy, reproduction and embryology.

The *Gynaecia* contains various passages on pathological conditions. In some cases the mere description of an (abnormal) organ indicates the disease (not unusual since a doctor normally sees only diseased organs), at other times there is an attempt to identify the disease.

i A passage on the perforation of the teeth due to a noxious fluid constantly dripping onto them from the head.[11] The problem is attributed to excessive moisture which gathers in the head, from where it flows downwards and causes diseases in other parts of the body.[12]

ii The uvula is referred to as an *uva* or 'grape'.[13] This organ is normally a small fleshy finger-like flap of tissue that hangs in the back of the throat and is an extension of the soft palate, but if it is called a 'grape' it is obviously swollen and refers to a pathological condition. In the Hippocratic treatise *Prognostic* c.23 an infected uvula is also called a 'grape' (*staphulê*).[14]

iii Then there is a reference to an exudation from the ears,[15] which is obviously a morbid condition – once again based on the Hippocratic view that excessive moisture gathers in the head (see above (i)) and that the only chance of recovery was if it could break out through an orifice such as the ears or nose.[16]

The Epistula ad Pentadium nepotem suum de quattuor umoribus in corpore humano

Two letters[17] of Vindicianus have been transmitted, the first to his nephew Pentadius, who had just started his medical studies. This didactic letter[18] which purports to be a translation of 'the core of the medical works of Hippocrates'[19] is in fact a medical treatise in its own right, and gives an account of the theory of the four humours as it was interpreted in the late 4th century AD – the first systematic exposition of the humoural theory in Latin.[20] The varying predominance of each of the humours is shown to be linked to a season of the year, and also to specific hours of day and night as well as to the stages in the life of man. Its influence on man's character and on the pulse rate is also sketched; finally, the diseases caused by an immoderate increase in one of the humours are mentioned with the relevant therapies. It was an authoritative work throughout the Middle Ages, and according to a doctoral thesis of Schoch (1996, 123) who traced the development and application of the humoural theory to the modern day, this 'Roman' version of the theory of the four humours played a role until the late 19th century with practically no change in content.

In relating the humours to diseases, Vindicianus follows the Hippocratic principle that health depends on the equilibrium and right mixture of the four humours (*Nature of Man* c. 4). However, during a specific season of the year one of the humours will increase,[21] which can then make man predisposed to diseases associated with this humour: blood increases in spring, red bile in summer, black bile in autumn, and phlegm in winter.[22] And when that particular humour has increased immoderately, then disease sets in, which will last long if, according to Vindicianus, an inexperienced or negligent doctor does not recognise from which humour it has originated. Treatment is based on the Hippocratic principle of *contraria contrariis*,[23] e.g. a disease of the blood which is sweet and wet and hot must be counteracted by something which is cold and bitter and dry.

The Epistula Vindiciani comitis archiatrorum ad Valentinianum imperatorem

Vindicianus' letter to the emperor Valentinian I (364–375) served as a preface to a (lost[24]) collection of pharmaceutical recipes. The letter has not yet been discussed in detail by anybody.

In the light of a remark by Nutton that medical texts in antiquity 'have a bias towards theory rather than the realities of day-to-day practice' (1988c, viii.24), this letter of Vindicianus is unusual. It is to my knowledge the only Latin medical text which contains a complete case history, describing the symptoms, the diagnosis, the prognosis, the therapy and the outcome. It resembles the case histories in the Hippocratic *Epidemics* but is much more detailed (however, it lacks auscultation, the urine test and the critical days often referred to in the Hippocratic case histories).

The tone of self-recommendation in the letter in which

Vindicianus shows his superior knowledge as physician as compared with the foremost doctors of his day, could be seen to reflect his high position as Count of the Roman College of Physicians in Rome. It was also clearly written for a wider audience than the emperor Valentinian and his family, in fact for posterity, as Vindicianus himself states in the last paragraph.

In the letter Vindicianus illustrates the success of his remedies and his therapy by describing two case histories, one of which he took over after the treatment of the other doctors had failed, and in the other he intervened to stop their treatment.

(I) The patient with constipation

The patient has developed a fever after having been constipated for 12 days.[25] The doctors advised giving him an enema, which did not help. Then Vindicianus steps in and, after first observing the appearance of the patient like a good Hippocratic doctor,[26] deduces from his colour that the man is totally dehydrated and exhausted. His therapy then basically consists in giving the patient three potions and sending him to the baths to rehydrate his body: at first a potion of cold water with salt in 'for his fever' – to the horror of the other doctors who obviously believed that cold water should not be taken when one is hot[27] (a belief still going strong today). However, Vindicianus used his common sense – a feverish person is dehydrated and thirsty and will consequently feel better when drinking the cold water, which will also to some extent cool his feverish body; and, furthermore, if enough salt had been added in the water, it will have had the same effect as magnesium sulphate, namely to clean the bowels (an enema only cleans the colon, whereas a salty potion will also clean the small intestine). After having imbibed the cold water it is reported that the patient did indeed feel better, that he fell asleep, and then started to perspire heavily when the fever broke. When he woke up, there was a drastic evacuation of the bowels.

Now only follows the diagnosis/prognosis.[28] One should keep in mind that Vindicianus has not been told anything, he only knows that the patient has been constipated for 12 days and is feverish, and he deduced from his appearance that he is dehydrated. He diagnoses the patient's problem as excessive eating and drinking. Then he gives a prognosis and predicts the course the disease will take.[29] Due to the congestion of undigested food or too great a mixture of different wines, the fluid in the bowels becomes bitter, insomnia occurs, followed by a disease which presents itself as a latent fever, together with a throbbing headache and constipation causing inflammation (believed until quite recently). Then even worse symptoms will follow: the lungs will inflate, and the spleen and the lobes of the liver distend, which causes gall to be forced out, resulting in the body becoming yellow. Fortunately for the patient, Vindicianus intervened at the right moment!

(II) The patient with the eye problem

The second case history is that of a patient who had a continuous flux of tears (par. 8).[30] Vindicianus' eminent colleagues prescribed as therapy that his eyelids be cut, that the side of his head be cauterised,[31] and that after his head had been shaved, incisions be made in the veins, and that tinder be put on it (presumably to cauterise the wounds).[32] And when all this did not help, they ordered that his veins be cut[33] (the right arm when the right eye has a flux, and the left arm for the left eye). At this stage, when this treatment too was unsuccessful, Vindicianus writes that he intervened and stopped the phlebotomy because he regarded it as utterly senseless under the circumstances.

This kind of treatment seems to have been practiced widely in the ancient world[34] and was apparently used even up to modern times among the Libyans in Northern Africa.[35] The theory underlying it was that the flux or discharge originated within the head beneath the skull, either superficially or deeper down,[36] and that the peccant fluid was carried down to the eyes by the superficial veins, or by veins from within the skull to the back of the eyes. An operation in which incisions were made, was supposed to withdraw the fluid by way of the wounds which were then cauterised. The cutting of the eyelids would probably refer to scarification, still practiced today for trachoma.[37]

We do not know what the success rate of this treatment was in antiquity, but it is in any case clear that Vindicianus had no faith in it, and reprimanded his colleagues for subjecting the patient to such torments, and, capping everything, in their ignorance (*indocte*) inflicting phlebotomy on a man who is already half dead. In this case Vindicianus does not propose an alternative treatment (there was no alternative – his learned colleagues had tried all known treatments), but uses the opportunity to parade his knowledge with his diagnosis (a blockage of fluid in the brain) and his prognosis (par. 9).

The procedures followed by Vindicianus's colleagues were thus deficient since they lacked the knowledge to discern that the patient was suffering from a flux that originated in the brain below the skull and was intractable; to inflict phlebotomy on him after all the previous painful treatments had failed would, according to Vindicianus, have killed the patient rather than cured him. The letter thus ends with the cautionary remark that not all doctors and therapies should be trusted, and the plea that the sick should not be given remedies which are worse than the disease[38] – surgery and cautery should in any case not be applied in the very sensitive area of the eyes (par. 10).

Conclusion

Vindicianus' views on the causes of diseases and his suggested therapies as they came to the fore in the discussion of his works, would leave a modern reader grateful for not being one of his patients, but should be seen in context. Much of the knowledge that he lacked only came to light in the 19th and 20th century. He must, therefore, have had some qualities which led to the high esteem in which he was held in his own time and the century thereafter. His common sense – even in opposition to traditional treatments and beliefs – and his acute observance of symptoms have already been pointed out. Furthermore, his sound knowledge of the Hippocratic treatises comes to the fore in all three of his works. Probably under the influence of the Hippocratics too, was his preference for a gentle and mild approach rather than dramatic surgical intervention, as it appears in his letter to the emperor. His suggested remedies too are far removed from the 'Dreckapotheke', which was part of the folk medicine still in use in his day. Vindicianus' treatment consisted of medicaments (natural potions made of salt water and plant and animal extracts) and hydrotherapy (a recommendation of baths and ointments). In short, Nature played an important role in his attempt at healing. With the benefit of hindsight and in the light of the limited knowledge of anatomy and physiology in antiquity, one can only commend this approach.

Notes

1 There is some confusion regarding the person of Vindicianus: Jones, Martindale and Morris (1971, 967–8) record four persons by the name of Vindicianus: (i) Vindicianus: *Vicarius* (in West) 378; (ii) (Helvius) Vindicianus: *comes archiatrorum* around 379 (?), *proconsul Africae* around 379–382; (iii) Astius Vindicianus: *flamen perpetuus*; (iv) Avianus Vindicianus: *V(ir) C(larissimus), Consularis Campaniae*. It is Helvius Vindicianus (ii) who is in my opinion the well-known doctor and friend of St Augustine. Deichgräber (1961, *RE* IX.29), Jones (1973, Vol. II, 1012 and 1045) and Schoch (1996, 5–9) conflate him with Avianus Vindicianus (iv), but Beschaouch (1968, 17–9), supported by Vásquez Buján (1982, 26 and n. 3), firmly state that Helvius Vindicianus (ii) the physician should not be confused with his namesakes.

2 Caelius Aurelianus could possibly have been earlier, but it is impossible to know. Gargilius Martialis wrote in the early 3rd century, but was not a doctor.

3 With the exception of Caelius Aurelianus who translated works of Greek authors such as Soranus' *Gynaecology*.

4 Nutton (1984, 12) has, without any reference to Vindicianus, commented on a reason for the high status of doctors in late antiquity: '... the doctor ... has a much greater public profile beyond the confines of his city and civic life. He becomes a bishop, a church leader, even a saint; an ambassador, a provincial governor, even the Master of Offices'. As a possible reason for this situation Nutton mentions their abilities as 'bilingual men of culture, able to cross political frontiers ...'.

5 Dated by Beschaouch (1968, 135) in either 1 July 379–30 June 380, or 1 July 380–30 June 381.

6 Cf. Codex Theodosianus XIII.3.12 in which Vindicianus is ordered by the emperors Valens, Gratian and Valentinian to guard the privileges of the chief physicians (*archiatrorum*) and those presented with the rank of count (*qui comitivae honore donati sunt*). They were a highly privileged group, enjoying special exemption from all the normal burdens of their elevated rank, including the *gleba senatoria* (= a tax on the land of senators). According to Korpela (1987, 140), the *comes archiatrorum* had in the 4th century the highest position in the inner hierarchy of the privileged group; Below (1953, 47) adds that those who were *comitivae primi ordinis* had the same status as chief commanders of provincial armies. Cf. too Nutton 1988c, VIII.27 and 1984, 11 note 92.

7 This treatise was transmitted in at least 13 manuscripts, in texts which are very divergent in scope and even content. In the introductory chapter of two of the manuscripts it is stated that the work is 'a rendering of Greek books into Latin for the sake of those who no longer understand Greek' (Codex Parisinus 4883: *Hanc epistolam disponere ex libris Graecis in latinum sermonem*... and Codex Laurentianus 73.1: *placuit propter quondam huius modi sermone ignorantiae in latinitatem interpretare*).

8 The title '*Gynaecia*' is a misnomer – the subject of Vindicianus' work is basically human anatomy; only about a quarter of the chapters in the texts contain a discussion of or a reference to the female reproductive system. Furthermore, in only two of the 13 manuscripts do the texts have the title *Gynaecia*, and in both cases the text in that particular manuscript is flanked by gynaecological treatises, which might have influenced a subsequent copyist to give this misleading title to a nameless medical document.

9 For the necessity to a traveller of taking along a good medical handbook (failing which, having a doctor as companion, as e.g. St Paul who had the evangelist Luke as companion, *Colossians* 4.14), cf Dio Crysostomos, *Orations* 9.4; Galen V.18 K (=Kühn) and XI.357 K.

10 Cf Nutton (1988c, VIII.38): 'The boundary between the self-acknowledged doctor and the educated layman was very narrow'.

11 This occurs in the texts in five of the manuscripts (Codex Monacensis (M) cc. 5 and 24, and c. 24 in the Codices Casinensis (C), Sangallensis (G), Parisinus 11218 (D) and Parisinus (P); the texts in the latter three manuscripts then have additional information on a multitude of other diseases pertaining to teeth (in a very badly transmitted section of the text): sores on the head and skin seemingly associated with alopecia, pains in the body, dizziness, inflammation of the eyes and ulcers under the eyelids, a polyp in the nostrils, inflammation of the jaw-bones, an ulcer under the tongue, uncovering of the gums, a swelling of the throat etc.

12 Two kinds of fluxes seem to have been distinguished by the Hippocratics, namely that of noxious stuff flowing from the scalp above the skull which can readily be healed, and that flowing from the brain below the skull which is serious and intractable. Cf. also note 30.

13 M c. 7, and c. 9 of the Codex Laurentianus 73.1 (L 73.1), D, P and C, and the Codices Lipsiensis (L) line 106 and Bambergensis (L III.9) line 107.

14 Aristotle too referred to the uvula as 'a bunch of grapes' (*staphulê*) when it gets 'unduly moistened and inflamed' and tends to cause suffocation, *Historia Animalium* 493a3–5. Cf. too Hippocrates, *Diseases* I.29 where this term is used to describe a swollen uvula. M c.8 and the fragments in the Codex Hunterianus (T) and the Copenhagen excerpt Gamle Kongelige Samling 1653 (H) add that the Greeks called the uvula *cionula* or *gargareon*. The latter transliterated Greek word is found in Hippocrates, *Prognosis* c. 23 where it indicates a morbid condition of the uvula ('it is dangerous to cut away or lance the uvula when it is red and enlarged …'). Cf. too Hippocrates, *Affections* c. 4 and *Diseases* II c. 10.

15 'The ears are the passages of hearing inasmuch as Nature has connected them to the cerebrum, and when coming from the cerebrum, they cause an exudation…' (C c. 9, M c. 9, L lines 117–21 and L III 9 lines 117–21. Cf. too the comments on pathological conditions of the ears in Vindicianus' letter to Valentinian par. 9.

16 *Diseases* II c. 14 and 16; III c. 2; *Glands* c. 13.

17 Langslow (2000, 74) points out that letters feature 'quite prominently in the Latin medical corpus', either as prefaces (e.g. to Scribonius Largus' and Vindicianus' respective collections of recipes) or as theoretical treatises in their own right (e.g. Vindicianus' letter to Pentadius).

18 Cf Schoch (1996, 123) who also regards it as a 'typischer Lehrbrief'.

19 *ex libris medicinalibus Hippocratis intima latinavi* (Rose 1894, 485).

20 Passing remarks on individual humours are found in Celsus (*passim*) and a few paragraphs in the two pseudo-Hippocratic letters serving as introduction to Marcellus's *De Medicamentis* (Niedermann and Liechtenhan 1968, 18–33 *passim*), but nothing resembling this systematic discussion of the humours.

21 Vindicianus' exposition resembles in some respects the dietetic calendar given in the pseudo-Hippocratic letter to king Antiochus (in Niedermann and Liechentenhan 1968, 24), where the author also links the increase of the various humours to certain periods in the year (6 periods are distinguished, differing greatly from those given in Vindicianus' letter); the emphasis in the pseudo-Hippocratic letter is however on the right food to be taken at that time, and not as in Vindicianus' letter on the diseases caused by the increase of the humours and the relevant therapy.

22 Hippocrates is more specific than Vindicianus about which diseases develop from the particular humour and during which season: in *Nature of Man* cc. 7 and 15 it is e.g. stated that in autumn jaundice can occur, in summer diseases of the spleen, and in a cold spring coughs, pneumonia and angina.

23 *Nature of Man* c. 9; *Epidemics* I.11; *Breaths* c. 1. This principle of allopathy is the basis of Hippocratic healing, but in *Places in Man* c. 42 there is also a reference to what is clearly homeopathy. Cf. in this regard Jouanna (1999, 342–3).

24 Of the collection of recipes only four were transmitted, found in Marcellus Empiricus and Cassius Felix:

'Against coughing: fresh, smooth sulphur mixed with very old pork fat, to be taken three pills on the first day, two on the second and one on the third' (Marcellus Empiricus, *De Medicina* XVI.100).

'Against pain in the cheeks: let three medium-sized grains of salt dissolve in the painful area in the mouth in the morning before sunrise, and then rinse it out; if used frequently this will remove damaging stuff and superfluous fluids which could cause pain' (Cassius Felix, *Physica* 32).

'Against vomiting: the resin of the mastic-tree and one ounce pitted raisins with three pinches of lightly roasted cumin, all pounded together, put into a cloth and laid on the stomach like a plaster' (Cassius Felix, *Physica* 42).

Then Cassius Felix reports a recipe against the sting of a scorpion, consisting of a written magic formula which promises an immediate effect (*Physica* 69).

25 Celsus, *Proemium* 55 distinguished between three kinds of diseases: 'one a constriction, another a flux, the third a mixture'. This case would in ancient times have been a classic example of the first: *strictum*, constipation advancing to intestinal obstruction.

26 Cf. *Prognosis* c. 2: 'In acute diseases the physician must conduct his enquiries in the following way. First he must examine the face of the patient, and see whether it is like the faces of healthy people, and especially whether it is like its usual self'.

27 Cf. Hippocrates, *Epidemics* VI.3 6 where we read that 'very cold water will rupture vessels and cause coughs and it causes bulgings, as of the parotid glands, and swellings on the neck'. In *Places in Man* c. 27 too we read that warm water should be given to a patient with fever, 'for if no cold enters the body, the drink, being warm and staying in place, will take something away from the ailing body, whether it passes off in the urine or as a sweat…'. Galen also on one occasion told the family of a patient that 'there was a good chance of healing the patient if he drank nothing cold' (*De consuetudinibus* 11–12, Von Muller). In our letter Vindicianus later explains that hot water would have exacerbated the inflammation.

28 In modern times a distinction is made between diagnosis (the knowledge of what the patient is suffering from) and prognosis (a prognostication of the course the disease will take). The Hippocratic authors, however, and Galen too for that matter, did not make such a distinction. Most important was the prognosis which would, if correct, greatly enhance the reputation of the doctor, and enable him in future to recognise the course of similar diseases and to determine whether the patient will survive or not. Cf. *Prognostic* c. 1–2: 'I hold that it is an excellent thing for a physician to practice forecasting. For if he discovers and declares unaided by the side of his patients the present, the past and the future, and fill in the gaps in the account given by the sick, he will be the more believed to understand the cases, so that men will confidently entrust themselves to him for treatment'. On the importance of the sensory perceptions for diagnosis, cf. Gourevitch (1998, 134–5). Grmek (1998, 254) points out that prognoses were necessary because in antiquity diseases were not regarded as specific nosological entities: the Hippocratic writers of *Prognostic*, *Prorrhetic*, *Praenotiones* and *Epidemics* wanted to dispense with nosological specificity, and to delineate (by

means of prognoses and concrete observations) a set of rules concerning the cause of the symptoms without relying on a specific diagnosis.

29 In the Hippocratic treatise *Regimen* III.73 we find a rather similar description of the results of 'surfeit': 'In certain cases the sufferers from surfeit experience the following symptoms. The head aches and feels heavy; their eyelids close after dinner; they are distressed in their sleep; they appear to be feverish, and occasionally the bowels are constipated'. The recommended cure is a vapour bath and unguents, a purge with hellebore, and light and soft foods and exercise for ten days. In *Affections* c. 53 too a hot bath is recommended which will soften and moisten the body.

30 In Hippocrates *Places in Man* c. 9 there is an explanation of the origin of fluxes: 'Fluxes arise when the tissue is over-chilled, when it is over-heated, or when there is an excess of phlegm ...'. In the latter case, 'the tissues becoming too full are not able to make room for it all, and whatever fluid they are not able to make room for flows wherever it chances to go... until the passages are pinched in'. And then in c. 13: 'If – when fluid has collected between the bone and the flesh – a flux occurs from the flesh and the bone to the eyes ... patients weep from their eyes, but the eyelid does not ulcerate ...'. The treatment is as follows: 'clean the head, reduce swelling with foods and medications that act downwards, so that the flux will be dried out ... if the patient fails to recover with this treatment, make incisions ... in order that whatever collects in them will escape more quickly by flowing off through the wounds'.

31 In order to make sense of this cryptic phrase, one should perhaps understand the Greek word *emicranium* as meaning 'the side of the head/face' (not as 'one side of the head/face'), in which case it could refer to the temples. Cautery of the vessels in the temples was the usual treatment for eye troubles, cf. too Celsus VII.7.15 G. Hippocrates (*Diseases* II.12) also refers to a shaving of the head, and in serious cases incisions made in the head which are then cauterised.

32 The word *esca* is in the German translation given as 'Zunder' (*Thesaurus Linguae Latinae* V.2, 855), i.e. an inflammable substance such as tinder or charcoal.

33 All these procedures are described in the Hippocratic treatise *Sight*: scarification of the eyelids (cc 2 and 4); cautery of the vessels (cc 1 and 3); incisions in the scalp (cc 4 and 8), and phlebotomy (cc 3, 7 and 9).

34 Cf. too Celsus VII.15 who gives much the same advice.

35 Cf. in this regard Spencer (1953, 354): 'Hippocrates (Littré IV.185) mentioned its use among the Libyans, and the practice has prevailed up to recent times in North Africa and the Soudan'.

36 Cf. the discussion in Note 30.

37 In Hippocrates *Prorrhetic* c. 18 we find a reference to what is probably trachoma: 'If.... there is a copious flux of tears over a long period, and there are rheums, predict in the case of men that there will be an eversion of the eyelids, and in the case of women and children, ulceration and an eversion of the eyelids'.

38 What angered Vindicianus was probably that his colleagues had violated the Hippocratic principle of helping, or at least not harming the patient (Hippocrates, *Epidemics* 1.11).

Bibliography

Below, K.-H. 1953: *Der Arzt im römische Recht*, Munich.

Beschaouch, A. 1968: *Mustitana. Recueil des nouvelles inscriptions de Mustis, cité Romaine de Tunisie*, Tome I, Paris.

Deichgräber, K. 1961: 'Vindicianus', 29–36 in *Realencyclopädie der classischen Altertumswissenschaft, hrsg. von Pauly-Wissowa-Kroll-Mittelhaus-Ziegler-John*, Bd. IX.1, Stuttgart.

Gourevitch, D. 1998: 'The paths of knowledge. Medicine in the Roman world', 104–38 in M. D. Grmek, *Western Medical Thought from Antiquity to the Middle Ages*, Cambridge, MA.

Grmek, M. D. 1998a: *Western Medical Thought from Antiquity to the Middle Ages*, Cambridge, MA.

Grmek, M. D. 1998b: 'The concept of disease', 241–58 in M. D. Grmek 1998, *Western Medical Thought from Antiquity to the Middle Ages*, Cambridge, MA.

Jaeger, W. 1963: *Diokles von Karystos. Die griechische Medizin und die Schule des Aristoteles*, Berlin.

Jones, A. H. M. 1973: *The Later Roman Empire 284–602*, Oxford.

Jones, A. H., Martindale, J. R. and Morris, J. (eds) 1971: *The Prosopography of the Later Roman Empire I, AD 260–395*, Cambridge.

Jouanna, J. 1999: *Hippocrates*, Trans. by M. B. DeBevoise, Baltimore and London.

Jouanna, J. 2006: 'La postérité du traité hippocratique de la *Nature de l'homme*: la théorie des quatre humeurs', 117–41 in C. W. Müller, C. Brockmann and C. W. Brunschön, *Ärzte und ihre Interpreten. Medizinische Fachtexte der Antike als Forschungsgegestand der Klassischen Philologie*, Leipzig.

Kollesch, J. 1966: 'Therapeuthische Grundsätze im Werk des Vindician', *NTM. Schriftenreihe für Geschichte der Naturwissenschaften, Technik und Medizin* 3, Heft 7, 27–31.

Korpela, J. 1987: *Das Medizinalpersonal im antiken Rome*, Helsinki.

Kühn, C. G. (ed.) 1964/5: *Claudii Galeni Opera Omnia*, Hildesheim.

Langslow, D. R. 2000: *Medical Latin in the Roman Empire*, Oxford.

Littré, E. (ed.) 1839–1861: *Oeuvres completes d'Hippocrate*, 10 Vols, Paris.

Niedermann, M. and Liechtenhan, E. 1968: *Marcellus. Ueber Heilmittel*, übersetzt von J. Kollesch and D. Nickel (Corpus Medicorum Latinorum V), Berlin.

Nutton, V. 1984: From Galen to Alexander. Aspects of Medicine and Medical Practice in Late Antiquity, 1–14 in J. Scarborough (ed.), *Symposium on Byzantine Medicine, Dumbarton Oaks Papers* 38, Washington, DC.

Nutton, V. 1988a: *From Democedes to Harvey, Studies in the History of Medicine*, London.

Nutton, V. 1988b: 'The perils of patriotism: Pliny and Roman medicine', VII, 30–58 in V. Nutton, *From Democedes to Harvey, Studies in the History of Medicine*, London.

Nutton, V. 1988c: 'Murders and miracles: lay attitudes to medicine in Classical Antiquity', VIII, 23–52 in V. Nutton, *From Democedes to Harvey, Studies in the History of Medicine*, London.

Nutton, V. 2004: *Ancient Medicine*, London, New York.

Rose, V. (ed.) 1894: *Theodori Prisciani Euporiston libri III accedunt Vindiciani Afri quae feruntur reliquae*, Lipsiae.

Schoch, M. 1996: *Die 'Epistula Vindiciani ad Pentadium nepotem' und ihre Einordnung in die Geschichte der Humoraltheorie.*

Inaugural Dissertation, Bayerische Julius-Maximilians-Universität, Würzburg.
Spencer, W. G. (transl.) 1953: *Celsus. De Medicina*. Loeb Classical Library Vol. III, Cambridge, MA.
Vásquez Buján, M. E. 1982: 'Vindiciano y el tratado *De natura generis humani*', *Dynamis* 2, 25–56.
Von Muller, E. (ed.) 1891: *Galeni Scripta Minora*, Vol. II, Leipzig.

Part V

Surgery

18. Back to Basics: Surgeons' Knives in the Roman World

Ralph Jackson

From the reign of Augustus onwards purpose-made medical instruments appear in increasing numbers throughout the Roman Empire. The commonest surviving type of instrument is the scalpel, the surgeon's most basic tool, which usually comprised an iron blade with a copper-alloy handle. Although corrosion has destroyed the vast majority of iron blades a number of exceptional finds have preserved intact scalpels with distinctive blades. Within the context of Roman medical practice and instrument manufacture this paper reviews the intact scalpels (about seventy) and juxtaposes the archaeological, scientific and literary evidence in an attempt to shed new light on the knives used in specific Roman surgical interventions.

Introduction

When Demetrios Michaelides published his comprehensive report on the extensive medical instrumentation found in a rock-cut chamber tomb in excavations at Nea Paphos (Michaelides 1984) he referenced two works in particular. One was Ernst Künzl's ground-breaking and magisterial *Medizinische Instrumente aus Sepulkralfunden der römischen Kaiserzeit*, which had appeared the previous year (Künzl 1983a). The other was an equally seminal, though much earlier, work, John Stuart Milne's *Surgical Instruments in Greek and Roman Times* (Milne 1907). Both were, and continue to be, of fundamental importance in the study of ancient instrumentation, not least that most basic of instruments, the surgeon's knife. Künzl went on to publish extensively on the artefacts and archaeology of ancient medicine, bringing to the subject his deep knowledge of Greek and Roman material culture (see, e.g., Künzl 2002a, with references). Milne was a medical practitioner and surgeon at the cusp of new and old, with first-hand knowledge of the practice of pre-modern medicine. That experience, combined with a classical education, enabled him to write with particular insight into ancient surgery and surgical tools, because some of the ancient procedures, like bloodletting, were still practised and many instruments were little changed. Thus, he combined the evidence of ancient medical writings with that of surviving ancient medical tools, interpreting them within a framework of pre-modern medicine. Not surprisingly, new evidence on all fronts, especially within the last few decades, has caused parts of his work to become obsolete and Larry Bliquez has been working for some time on a replacement embracing the fruits of recent research. Above all, a great increase in the number of well-contexted groups of medical instruments has allowed a better understanding of the practice of medicine in the Roman era, and it is the instruments themselves and the actuality of ancient medicine – how it impacted on daily life at all levels in all parts of the Roman world – that are the focus of this paper.

Roman medical practitioners

The celebrated image of a medical practitioner on a marble tombstone set up in Athens in the first half of the 2nd century AD serves to remind us of the impetus behind the development of medical instruments (Fig. 18.1). It commemorates Jason, a Greek doctor of the Roman era, and vividly illustrates the pressing reality that confronted ancient medical practitioners – patients, sick and injured, in desperate need of care. Like their modern counterparts, therefore, Greek and Roman healers needed to be able to recognise and describe disease, to explain it to their patients and above all to help those patients to get well or to feel better, whether through diet, medication or surgery.

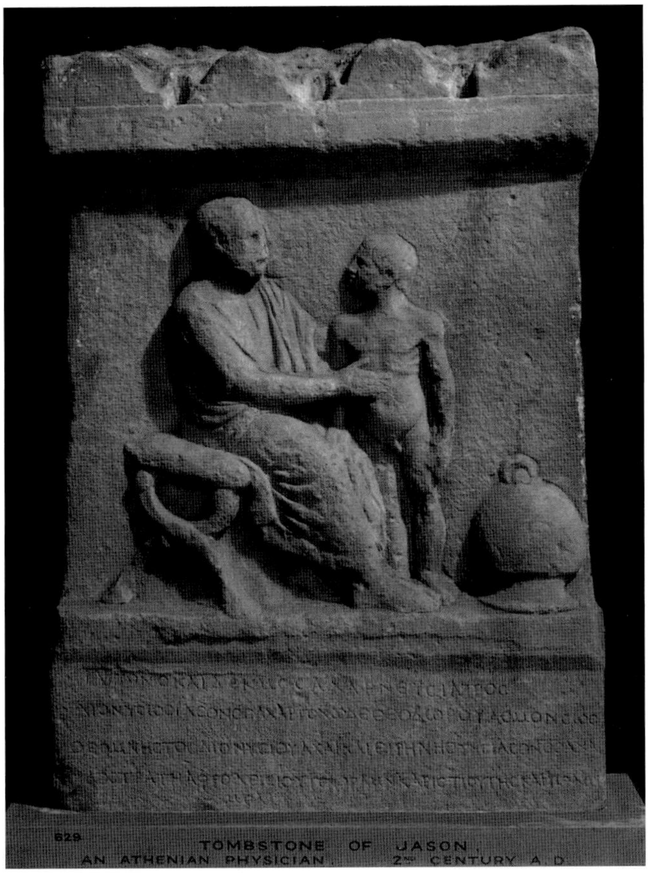

Fig. 18.1. Marble tombstone of Jason, Athens, 2nd century AD (photo: British Museum)

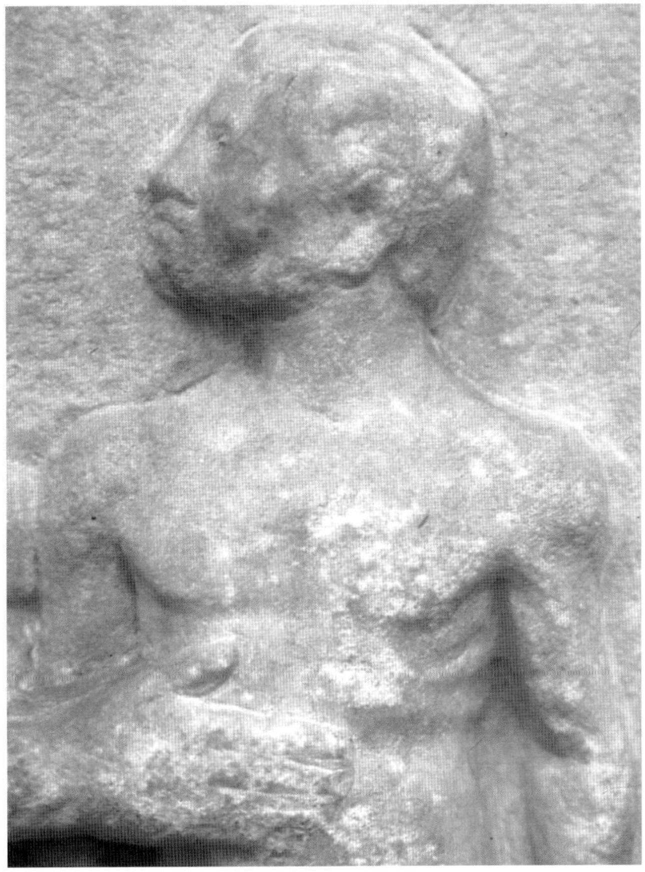

Fig. 18.2. Detail of the tombstone of Jason, showing patient's face and upper torso (photo: author)

The tombstone's central scene shows Jason at work, a seated doctor examining a standing male patient. The doctor, either in accordance with his status or perhaps simply adapted to the available space on the tombstone, is shown disproportionately large in comparison to the patient. He is bearded and draped in the manner of a philosopher and sits on a cushioned stool, while the patient stands naked before him. Because of his relatively diminutive size the patient has often been referred to as a boy or child (e.g. Scarborough 1969, pl. 37). However, close examination reveals that he, also, is bearded and should be regarded as an adult (Fig. 18.2). Questionable, too, is the description of the patient as emaciated or malnourished (e.g. Phillips 1973, pl. 9), for, while his swollen abdomen is evident enough, close examination of the relief reveals that the 'projecting ribs' are more convincingly identified as the fingers of the doctor's left hand, stabilising the side of the patient as he palpates the abdomen with his right hand. This observation is strengthened by the fact that no ribs are visible on the right side of the patient's chest which appears to depict a normal musculature.

In my opinion the scene was carefully chosen and skilfully composed to show, with great clarity, not a patient presenting with a specific disease (though many diseases have been postulated on the strength of the swollen abdomen and perceived emaciation (e.g. Grmek and Gourevitch 1998, 185–6, 355)), but the essential and archetypal image of a doctor at work in that most characteristic of poses, examining his patient. He appears to be doing so in a calm and unhurried manner, in accordance with both Hippocratic and contemporary (1st century AD) medical writings on ethics and etiquette – this is Celsus' dialogue between doctor and patient (e.g. Hippocrates, *In the surgery* 3, 17–21; Celsus, *On medicine* 3, 6, 6; Rufus of Ephesus, *Medical Questions*; Krug 1985, 212; Jackson 1988, 68–9; Hillert 1990, 125–8; Nutton 2004, 209–10; Gautherie in this volume). In particular, the sculptor has very successfully captured the tension in the eye contact between doctor and patient: it is an anxious time for the patient, who looks into the face of the doctor for reassurance; but this is a two-way process, for the doctor, who needed to use all his senses in gathering tell-tale signs and symptoms from which to make a diagnosis and prognosis of the patient's condition, anticipated and sought meaningful signs above all in the face and especially

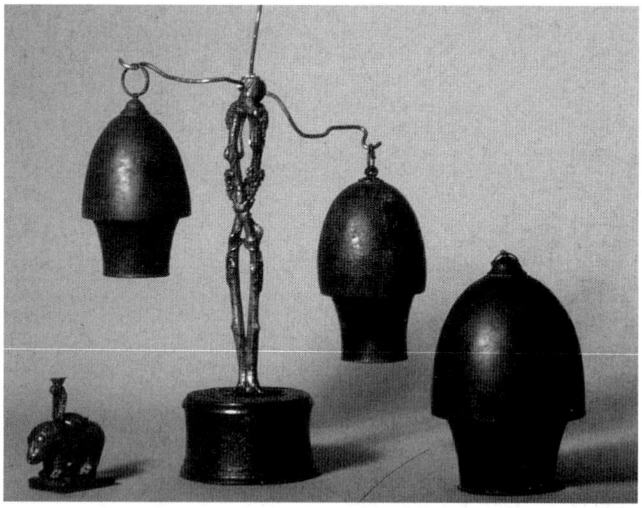

Fig. 18.3. Copper-alloy cupping vessels from the surgeon's grave at Bingen, late 1st–mid-2nd century AD (photo: Römisch-Germanisches Zentralmuseum, Mainz)

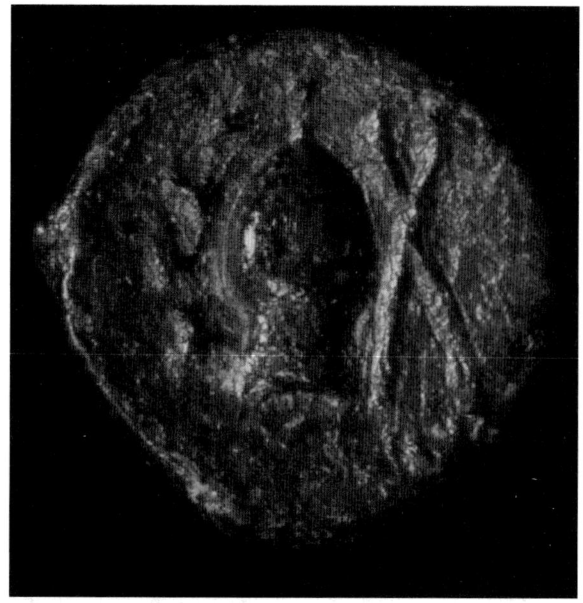

Fig. 18.4. Cupping vessel and dental forceps depicted on the reverse of a coin issued at Atrax, Thessaly, 4th century BC (photo: British Museum)

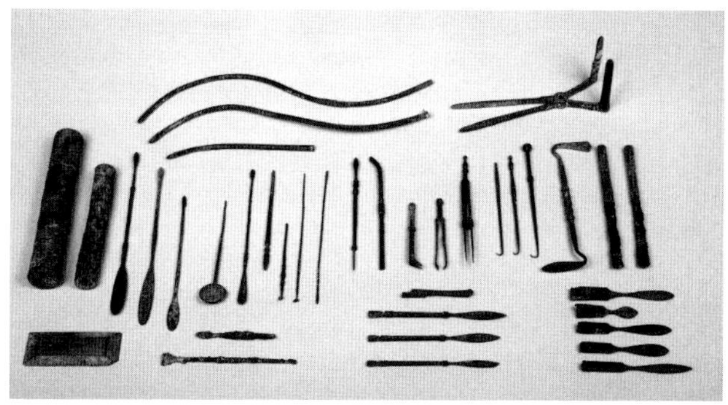

Fig. 18.5. Set of medical instruments, Italy, 1st–2nd century AD. Nine scalpel handles at bottom right (photo: British Museum)

the eyes, at that time regarded as the mirror of the soul and most sensitive indicator of physical and mental health (e.g. Hippocrates, *Prognosis*; Celsus, *On medicine* 2, 6, 1–4; Galen, *On affected parts* 4, 2 (8.223K); *On the method of healing for Glaucon* 1, 2 (11.12K); Garcia-Ballester 1981; 1994).

On the ground next to the patient is a prominent object recognisable as an outsize inverted cupping vessel – a direct allusion to humoral pathology and a clear indication of the ensuing therapy, blood-letting, that very likely awaited the patient. The distinctive domed body, with suspension loop at its apex, carinated shoulder and flared mouth with rolled rim correspond precisely to surviving examples of copper alloy, as in a contemporary surgeon's grave at Bingen, Germany (Fig. 18.3) (Künzl 1983a, 80–5) and in the mid-2nd–early 3rd century AD Nea Paphos assemblage (Michaelides 1984, fig. 2, no. 3). The cupping vessel was the principal instrument of humoral pathology, employed as a suction cup to extract 'vicious humour' through the pores (dry-cupping) or to speed up the letting of blood from an incised vein (wet-cupping). Thus, it was quintessentially the utensil of Graeco-Roman healers and effectively their 'badge of office', as was surely intended by the sculptor who carved this eye-catching example – if any ancient viewer failed to comprehend the medical nature of the main scene and was unable to read the underlying inscription then the image of the cupping vessel was sufficient on its own to characterise Jason as a healer. Images of cupping vessels used to epitomise healing extend as far back as the beginning of the 5th century BC, as on the famous tombstone of a healer, possibly from Bodrum, in the Basle Antikensammlung (Berger 1970), as well as on the coinage of that era, as, for example, with a dental forceps on the reverse of a coin of the 4th century BC issued at Atrax in Thessaly (Fig. 18.4) (*BMC* Greek (Thessaly) VI, 14, no. 3; Jackson 1993, pl. 1a).

Roman medical instruments

With the notable exception of bronze cupping vessels few unequivocal medical instruments have survived in a recognisable form in Greek or Roman contexts before the 1st century BC. But from the reign of Augustus onwards distinctive and recognisable purpose-made medical instruments start to appear in increasing numbers and variety in archaeological contexts throughout the Roman Empire (Jackson 1990; 1994; 1997a; Künzl 1996). Many are identifiable even as single finds without a medical context, while the medical purpose of other, less diagnostic, pieces is disclosed by their presence in sets of medical instruments found in secure dated contexts, principally sepulchral finds (Fig. 18.5) (Künzl 1983a; Bliquez 1994; Jackson 1995; 2003). The high quality of design and manufacture of the instruments is clear evidence of the attention paid to maximising the chance of success in medical and surgical interventions (Longfield-Jones 1978). It is the exact counterpart to the thoughtful and carefully-composed descriptions of operations in the ancient texts and there are a few fragments of evidence to show that it resulted from a fruitful collaboration between medical practitioners and the artisans who made medical equipment. While the technical virtuosity lay principally in the hands of the *fabri*, above all metalsmiths, the stimulus for inventiveness may often have come from the healers themselves.

A number of intriguing papyrus sources from Greco-Roman Egypt shed light on one aspect of manufacture, *organikoi* – literally 'instrumentists'. Their activities as technicians were sometimes the subject of criticism by medical writers at the time, since, on occasion, in their quest to perfect medical equipment they seem to have lost sight of the best overall interest of the patient (Marganne 1998, esp. 157–8). More patient-friendly, we might assume, were the instruments entered for competitions in Ephesus, a city that by the 2nd century AD had become a healing centre of considerable importance, the hub of medical activity in Asia Minor, its residents including, for example, the great physician and medical writer Rufus of Ephesus (*fl.* 98–117). One of the manifestations, perhaps, of this concentration of healing personnel was the organisation of annual medical contests, part of the Great Festival of Asklepios, the results of which were recorded on public inscriptions. A series of these inscriptions of the 2nd 3rd centuries AD has survived and records four categories of competition between doctors, including one – *organa* – which seems to have entailed the design of new medical instruments (Engelmann, Knibbe and Merkelbach 1980, nos 1161–9, 4101b; Nutton 2004, 211).

A remarkable copper-alloy plunger-forceps in the Ashmolean Museum, Oxford is just the sort of instrument we might envisage being entered for that event (Fig. 18.6) (Jackson 1997b). Still in operative condition, it is ostentatious, ingenious and eminently practical, a finely-crafted tool to impress the judges. It comprises a rod-like plunger handle with a precisely-profiled terminal bracket which slides through corresponding slots in the sides of the forceps compressing the jaws as the handle is depressed. Constructed in three pieces, each of an alloy formulation evidently carefully selected for differing required metallurgical properties (British Museum Dept of Conservation and

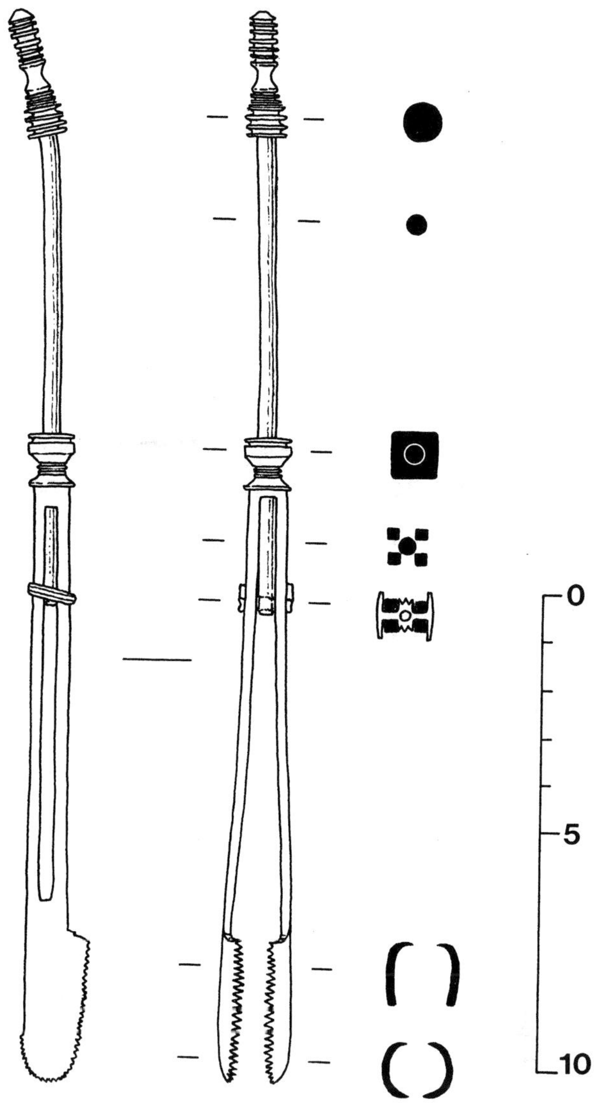

Fig. 18.6. Copper-alloy slot-slide plunger forceps (Drawing: author)

Science File no. 6416/ 44420T), it was manufactured to the highest standard: the mouldings are crisply cut, the functional parts carefully finished, the toothed rims of the jaws (34 teeth per jaw) precisely interlocking and the outer surface of the jaws immaculately smoothed in order to minimise the risk of accidental damage to internal organs and tissue during surgery. The form of the jaws is related to that of the distinctive *staphylagra* type of forceps which Greek and Roman medical writers recommended for use principally in operations on the palatine uvula and on haemorrhoids, but the application of a plunger mechanism is a refinement hitherto unknown (Jackson 1992). The very considerable benefit is that by avoiding encumbrances – the pivot of a cross-legged *staphylagra* or the finger and thumb required to move the sliding lock-ring of a spring-type *staphylagra*

– it enabled the use of the *staphylagra* type jaw in confined spaces deep within the body: it was ideally suited to operate in places beyond the reach of other forceps. While it could have been used to advantage in the operations for anal fistula, piles and amputation of the uvula, it would very likely have served a range of other roles, too, including, perhaps, the fixing and removal of various types of growth and tumour and the extraction of bone fragments and deeply-embedded foreign bodies from wounds.

It is to Galen we turn next for another snippet of evidence on instrumentation, a most illuminating, if brief, section in his *perì alypías* (*De indolentia: On the avoidance of grief*), a formerly lost treatise recently discovered in a monastery in Thessaloniki (Vlatadon 14: Boudon-Millot 2008; Boudon-Millot and Jouanna 2010). The composition of the *perì alypías* was triggered by, and written immediately after, the great fire which devastated Rome's Temple of Peace region in AD 192. Amongst the many public and private buildings, which were destroyed by the fire, including the Temple of Peace and the great libraries of the Palatine, was the warehouse in which Galen had stored many of his books and unpublished drafts, together with his most precious *materia medica*. In *perì alypías*, which includes fascinating details of his everyday life and of life at court under the Emperor Commodus, Galen not only supplies us with additional details of the fire, including the fact that he had believed the stone warehouse, in which he rented storage space, to be fireproof, but also an invaluable comment on his surgical instrumentation. The treatise was a response to a friend's question as to how Galen managed to avoid giving in to sorrow at the loss of his most prized possessions. Galen says:

> '...you were surprised, not that I had felt no sorrow when the fire destroyed part of the silver, gold...and numerous IOU's that were kept there, but rather that I also hadn't when it burned the great quantity of books I had written there, as well as a wide selection of varied medicines, both simple and compound, and instruments of all kinds' (*On the avoidance of grief* 4–5, trans. V. Boudon-Millot).

He goes on to describe the instruments as:

> 'Tools well adapted to medicine, that I had lost but was trying to find, and tools that I had discovered, for which I made wax models that I gave blacksmiths to forge, so that I can't get new ones without much time and effort' (*On the avoidance of grief* 5, trans. V. Boudon-Millot).

Clear evidence, then, that Galen possessed specialised surgical tools that he had acquired, together with those of his own devising for which he had made wax prototypes to give to metalsmiths. As Tucci has observed (Tucci 2008, 141), the 'wax models' are much more appropriate to bronze than iron technology and are better regarded as archetypes for the moulding and casting of bronze instruments by a bronzesmith (*faber aerarius*) than as models for iron instruments to be forged by a blacksmith (*faber ferrarius*). Thus, Tucci translates the passage: 'instruments fit for medicine that obviously I had lost, but I could hope to buy again' and 'instruments that I had created which were part of those for which I myself made the wax models and gave them to the bronze-casters, so that it is not possible to obtain them again without a considerable amount of time and great pain' (*On the avoidance of grief* 5).

We already knew that Galen was particular about his scalpel blades – he demanded Norican steel for the strong two-edged knife he used to dissect the spine – and this additional evidence really bears out the impression of Galen's attentiveness in securing the finest customised surgical instrumentation, just as he ensured himself supplies of the most effective and sought after *materia medica* (Nutton 2004, 245–6). While Galen was undoubtedly exceptional, the information from *perì alypías* might be taken to suggest that other attentive practitioners followed a similar procedure as, for example, the exceptionally well-equipped healer who was practising in Rimini a few decades after the death of Galen (Ortalli 2000; 2008; 2009; Jackson 2003; 2009). It would certainly explain why medical *instrumentaria* in the Roman world often incorporate both standard types of instrument and one or more examples of 'one-off' or adapted instruments, as, for example, the clyster/syringe in the Nea Paphos instrumentation (Michaelides 1984, 327–8; Bliquez and Oleson 1994).

Roman scalpels

Almost invariably the sets of instruments, whether complete or not, include at least one scalpel, the surgeon's tool *par excellence* and the foremost symbol of his craft. Very occasionally scalpels were single-piece instruments, either of copper alloy, as at Pompeii (Bliquez 1994, no. 52), or of iron, as, for example, two scalpels in the idiosyncratic early 1st century AD grave group from Stanway, near Colchester, perhaps following a native British tradition, or two examples of the 3rd century AD from Asia Minor (Fig. 18.12, no. 6) (Jackson 2007; Künzl 2002a, 28, pl. 17, B1, B2). However, most scalpels took a standard form, which maximised utility and economy by combining a robust copper-alloy handle, which incorporated a grip and blunt dissector, with a fine and hard-edged, but less durable, iron blade (Fig. 18.7). In consequence, the great majority of surviving scalpels are represented only by their copper-alloy handle, the vulnerable iron blade having corroded away (Fig. 18.5). That is the case with the British Museum collections which include no intact scalpels. Nevertheless, interesting technical information on the manufacture, decoration and usage of Roman scalpels has been revealed by scientific investigation of the handles (Jackson forthcoming), of which the following is a summary.

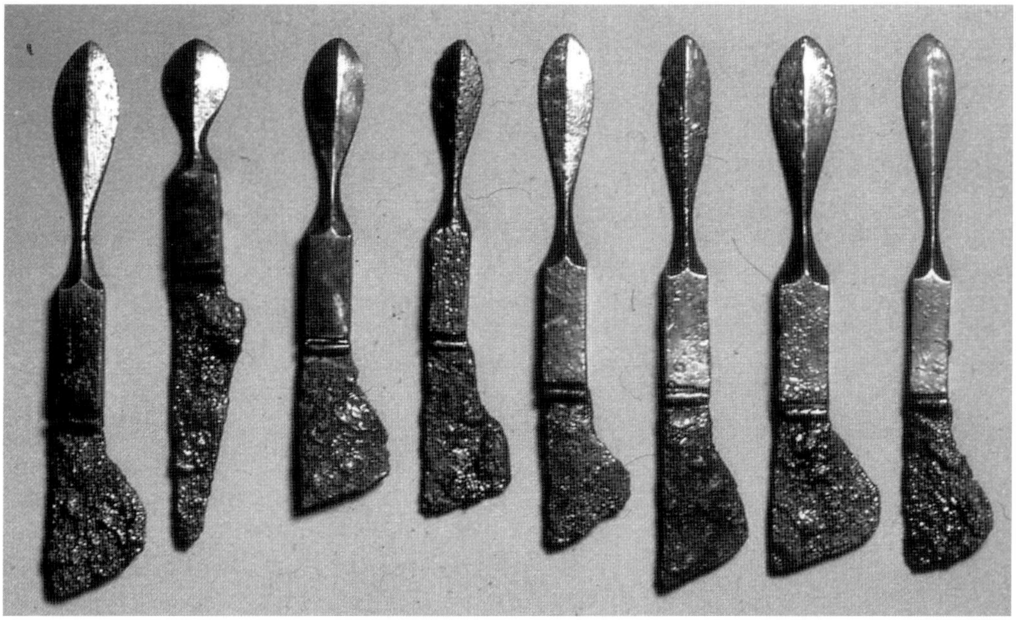

Fig. 18.7. Seven of the intact scalpels from the surgeon's grave at Bingen, late 1st–mid-2nd century AD (photo: Römisch-Germanisches Zentralmuseum, Mainz)

Sockets

There are two principal forms of socket by means of which the tanged iron scalpel blade was secured to its copper-alloy handle, either a simple cut slot or a key-hole type socket distinctive to medical instruments. In both types, where analysis has been possible, traces of tin-lead solder have been detected, demonstrating that blades fixed with solder were the norm (Jackson 1986, 133–4; Krug 1993). Such a bonding medium secured the blade but permitted a straightforward replacement for a broken or worn blade by the localised application of heat together with the use of appropriate tools. So, the blades were permanent but replaceable, meaning that the handle might have a very long life indeed. The additional benefit of the key-hole socket over the simple slotted form was a far greater rigidity of the blade, an important factor where particular force was to be applied to the cutting edge. For the tang of the iron blade, that corresponded with the key-hole socket, terminated in a solid cylinder which fitted snugly in the 'key-hole' when the blade was inserted from the side. This arrangement, clearly revealed by radiography, was evidently designed to prevent movement of the blade in either plane even if the solder failed. While the key hole socket provided a strong and secure seating, it appears sometimes to have proved difficult or impossible to remove an old blade, and several modifications have been found. In some instances a replacement blade with a simpler tang was substituted leaving the terminal cylinder filled only with solder (Fig. 18.8) (British Museum reg. no. 1902,1212.2). Similarly the slot socket, which tended to be the preferred socket for

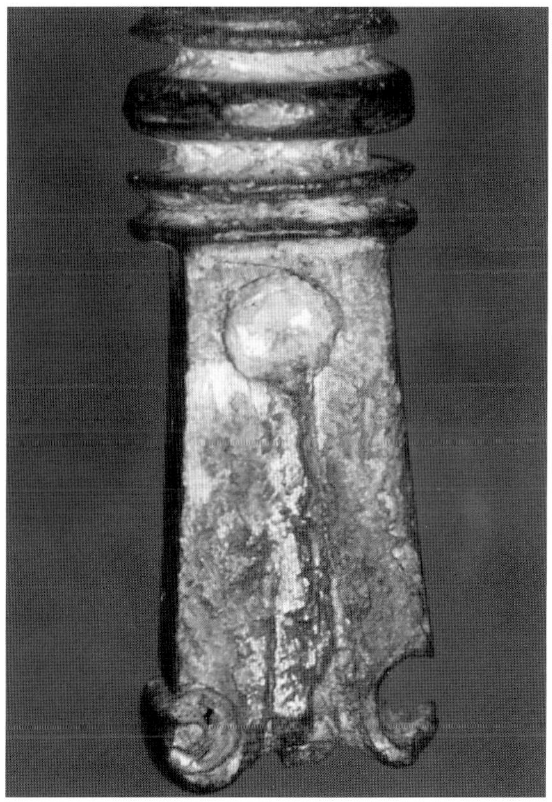

Fig. 18.8. Detail showing the end of the grip of a copper-alloy scalpel handle with key-hole type socket. The simple iron blade tang, probably a replacement, occupies only the slot of the socket, in which it is secured with tin-lead solder (photo: British Museum)

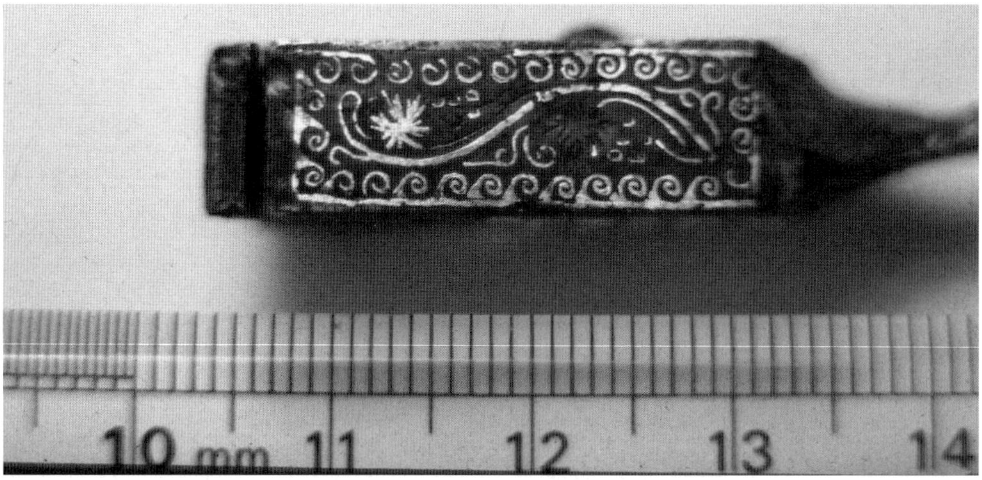

Fig. 18.9. Detail showing silver-inlaid vine-spray and wave-crest motifs on copper-alloy scalpel handle from Cologne (photo: author)

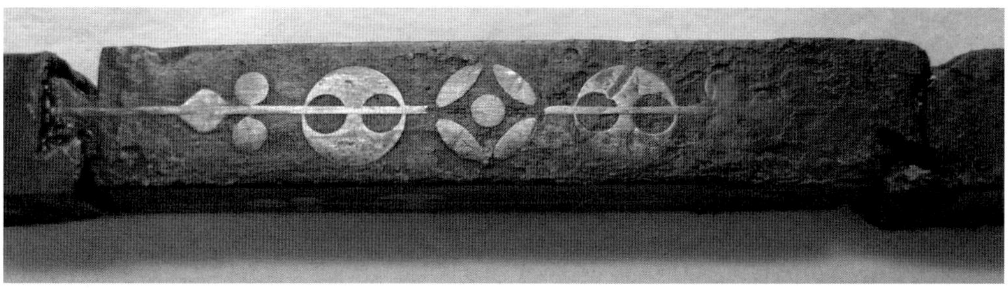

Fig. 18.10. Detail showing silver-inlaid design in Corinthian bronze handle from Rome (photo: author)

slender grips with presumably smaller blades not subject to great pressure, was sometimes modified by the addition of a rivet (British Museum reg. no. 1907,0523.1). A much rarer slender tubular socket into which the blade tang was pegged occurs on a number of 3rd century AD instruments, particularly in the Rimini assemblage (Fig. 18.16, no. 1). It signals a note of caution because the handle on its own would otherwise have been identified as that of a surgical needle: clearly there was sometimes a degree of interchangeability with handles, blades and needles.

Handle decoration

As on other medical instruments decoration was restricted to the non-operative part of the instrument, in the case of the scalpel, to its central grip, and usually took the form of cut mouldings or, less often, inlay. The mouldings are often exquisitely cut and served both to enhance the appearance of the tool and facilitate the practitioner's grip. Inlays are rare in the 1st century AD but become a little more common in the 2nd and 3rd centuries. On scalpel handles with rectangular block-like grips inlaid panels with a vine-spray enclosed by a wave-crest motif were popular (Fig. 18.9) (Künzl 1994; Büsing-Kolbe 2001, Type A). The less common circular-sectioned grips lent themselves well to banded or spiral inlays, often using contrasting coloured alloys such as copper, silver and niello (Künzl 1983a, fig. 26.1). Occasionally the décor is so distinctive that it identifies products of a particular workshop and helps to refine the dating of poorly-contexted instruments. A slender rectangular grip from Rome, once in the Castellani Collection (Fig. 18.10) (British Museum reg. no. 1872,0604.879), is decorated with an elegant symmetrical linear design of pellets, peltas and rosettes. Analysis at the British Museum has shown the inlay to be silver and the body metal to be the even more costly alloy known as Corinthian bronze (British Museum Dept of Conservation and Science File no. 7191-7-W; Craddock and Giumlia-Mair 1993). Other products of this workshop, active, perhaps, in the 1st century AD, since the design is reminiscent of the Third Style of wall-painting at Pompeii (Künzl 1984, 60–1; Büsing-Kolbe 2001, Type B), are known from Gaul, Germany, Britain and Moesia Inferior in 2nd–3rd century AD contexts (Künzl 1983a, figs 26, 53, 68, 87). The implication of a very long working life for the instruments is perhaps not surprising – these were finely-crafted impressive-looking handles representing a degree of wealth, and the operative parts, steel blades and needles, could be repeatedly replaced as necessary.

Scalpels with intact blades

Where scalpel blades have survived they have tended to be large stout examples, the majority of deep, bellied form, which are also the blades most commonly depicted in surviving imagery (Künzl 1983a, 80–5; Jackson 1990, fig. 1; Krug 2008). Of the many other varieties of blades mentioned in Greek and Roman medical texts for specific surgical interventions few remain (Milne 1907, 24–49). The most famous complete scalpels (at least 15) are those from Pompeii, few of which, however, have survived the long and chequered history following their discovery. Fortunately some were drawn in the 1840s and a series of photos was taken at the end of the 19th century preserving important information on the now missing, broken or separated iron blades (Vulpes 1847, pl. vii; Bliquez 1994, pls xiv–xvi). Another valuable source of intact blades (nine) is the cremation grave group from Bingen, excavated in 1924, the extensive instrumentation (over 50 instruments) of a surgeon who appears to have specialised in bone surgery, who was buried at some time between the late 1st and mid-2nd century AD (Como 1925; Künzl 1983a, 80–5; 2002b, 36–8; Jackson 2005).

The small kit of basic surgical tools from a burial of the mid-3rd century AD at Wehringen, near Augsburg (Augusta Vindelicum), excavated in the 1960s, includes just three scalpels, but all are complete with tiny distinctive blades. The set, which was partly covered by a spatula probe and a stone mixing palette, also comprised a sharp hook, a forceps and a bone lever. These six instruments were contained, top-to-tail, in a gilded, leather-bound, folding wooden case placed at the right elbow of the inhumed practitioner, a man aged at least seventy suffering from advanced osteoporosis. Additionally, to the right of his head was a rectangular copper-alloy drug box, with five compartments and a sliding lid. In the central compartment were three silver coins, the latest a scarcely worn antoninianus of Gordian III of AD 238/9. The four flanking compartments contained the remains of *materia medica*, most notably fragments of desiccated *collyria* – two impressed with the stamp of Claudius Ingenuus one with the stamp of Quintus Simplicius Nedo – implying that the Wehringen practitioner's realm of healing included eye diseases (Künzl 1983a, 120–1; Garbsch 1994, 293–4; Nuber 2004).

Most important of all is the remarkable Rimini assemblage, which includes 30 complete scalpels and blades. Discovered in Piazza Ferrari in 1989 and, since the end of 2007, preserved under a cover building, the so-called '*domus* 'del chirurgo'' and the artefacts found within it provide some of the best surviving archaeological evidence for a Roman healer, his equipment and his surgery. The house, built in the second half of the 2nd century AD and destroyed in a fire in the mid-3rd century AD, was a modest-sized two-storey dwelling occupying a triangular plot in the north-east quarter of *Ariminum* overlooking the Adriatic. It comprised six main ground floor rooms, with a communicating corridor and a small courtyard garden. The rooms included a *triclinium* and *cubiculum*, but the principal room has been interpreted as a consulting room and surgery. In here was found a great profusion of surgical instruments and medical paraphernalia in positions suggesting storage on shelves and in cupboards. The fire had destroyed all organic materials and melted the glassware, but about 150 metal instruments were preserved, as well as ceramic medicine pots, stone mortars and pestles and other medical implements. It would appear that the *domus* was the residence, surgery and possibly clinic of an extremely well-equipped healer, a generalist and specialist, of Greek extraction or, at least, Greek-speaking, probably originating in the East Mediterranean, and perhaps with experience of military medicine, who had become a fairly prosperous member of the community in which he lived and practised (Ortalli 2000; 2008; 2009; Jackson 2003; 2005; 2009).

Drawing together the information on intact scalpels from these and other sites (see Appendix) there is evidence for both continuity and change. Most immediately apparent is the unchanging nature – spatial and temporal – of the robust scalpel with distinctive bellied blade. Thus the 1st century examples from Pompeii, Bingen and Cologne are indistinguishable from one found in London and from those in use in Rimini some two hundred years later (Figs 18.11–18.12). Examples are also clearly depicted on stone and terracotta reliefs of the 1st–2nd centuries AD from Athens, Ostia, Palestrina and Kom Ombo (Krug 2008, figs 11, 14–6, 18, 20). It seems reasonable to continue to regard that type of scalpel as the commonest general-purpose surgical knife designed to serve the majority of needs. A similar longevity appears to apply to another robust scalpel type, which has a long triangular blade with straight back and sloping cutting edge. Once more the examples from Pompeii, Bingen and Rimini are undifferentiated (Fig. 18.13, nos 1–3). Ubiquitous, too, is a smaller pointed blade type with convex back and straight cutting edge. It is represented in the 1st century AD finds from Bingen and Cologne (Künzl 1983a, fig. 56, no. 7, fig. 67, no. 7), in a 2nd–3rd century AD context at Sontheim an der Brenz (Künzl 2002b, 42–3, fig. 55) and in a 3rd century AD context at Rimini (Fig. 18.14, nos 1–4) and examples are included in the boxes of instruments depicted on the 2nd century AD tomb reliefs of Publius Aelius Pius Curtianus at Palestrina and Marcus Ulpius Amerimnus at Ostia (Krug 2008, figs 18–21). It is possible that the Rimini scalpels had been handed down

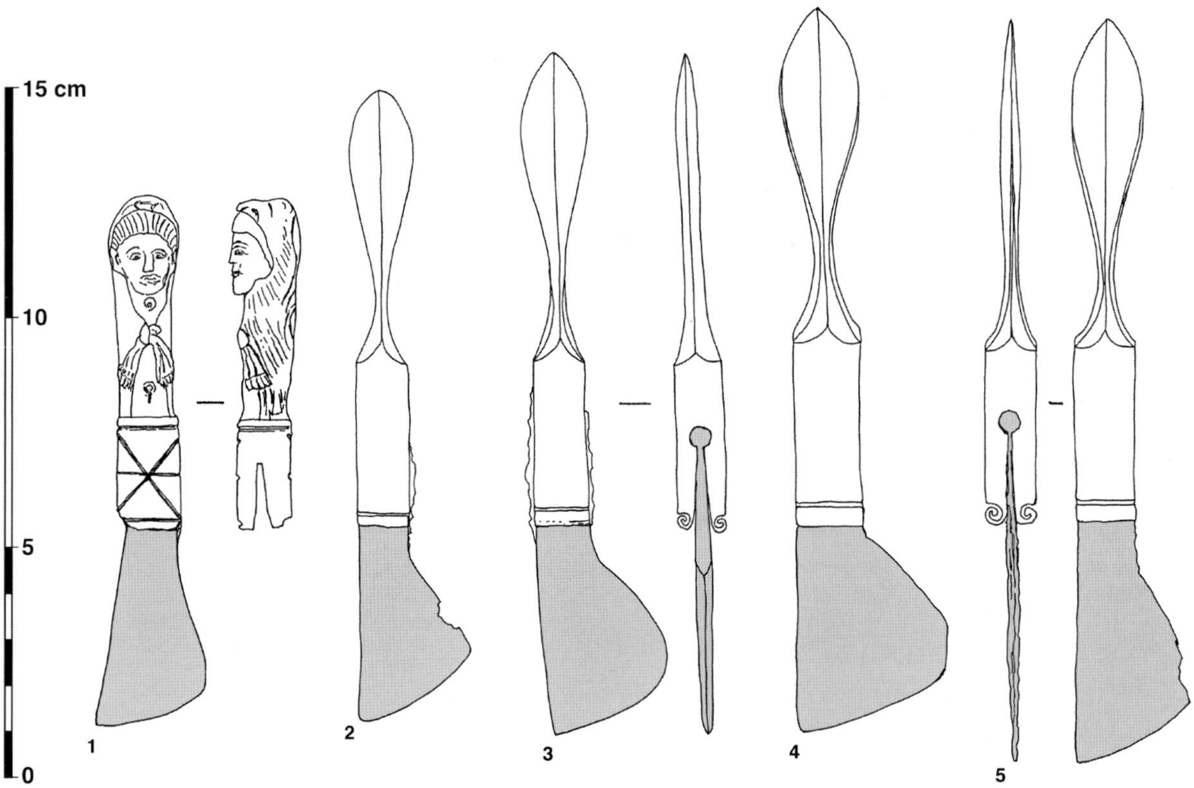

Fig. 18.11. Scalpels from Pompeii (1–3) and Bingen (4–5) (drawing: author)

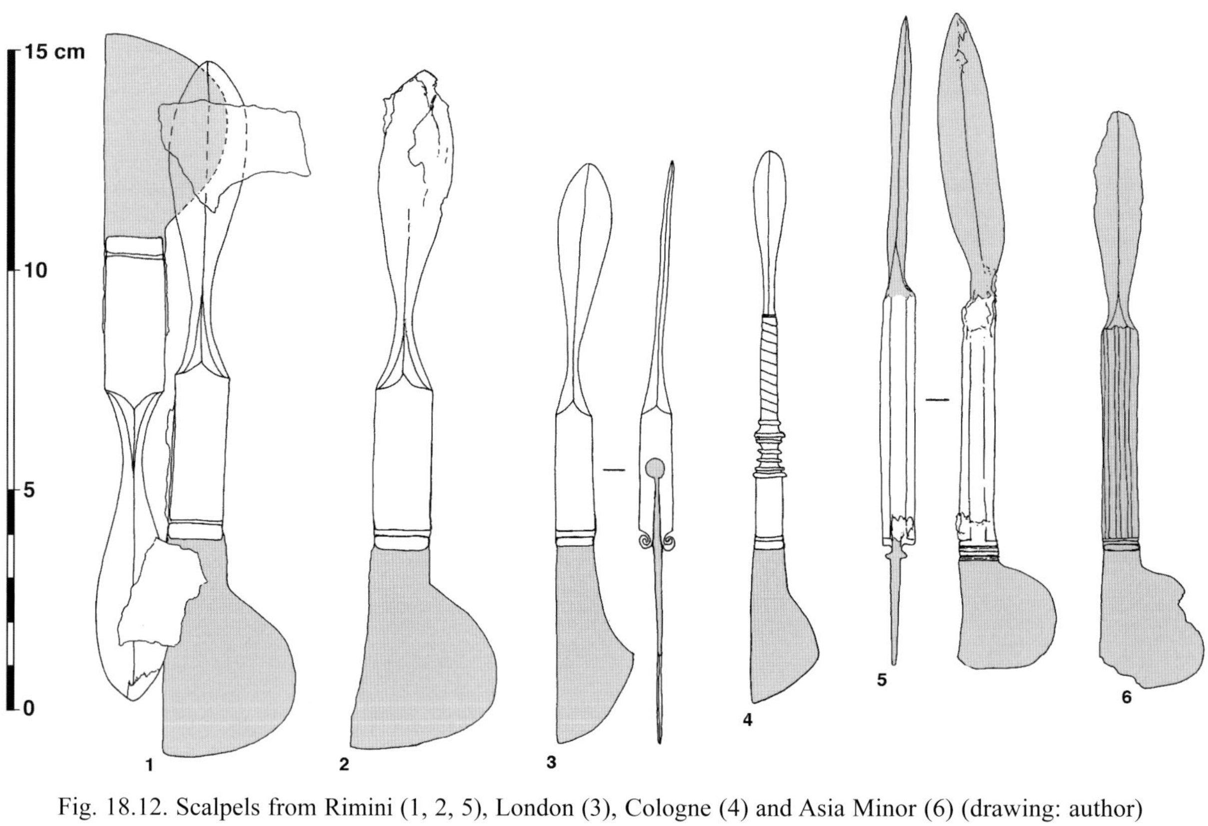

Fig. 18.12. Scalpels from Rimini (1, 2, 5), London (3), Cologne (4) and Asia Minor (6) (drawing: author)

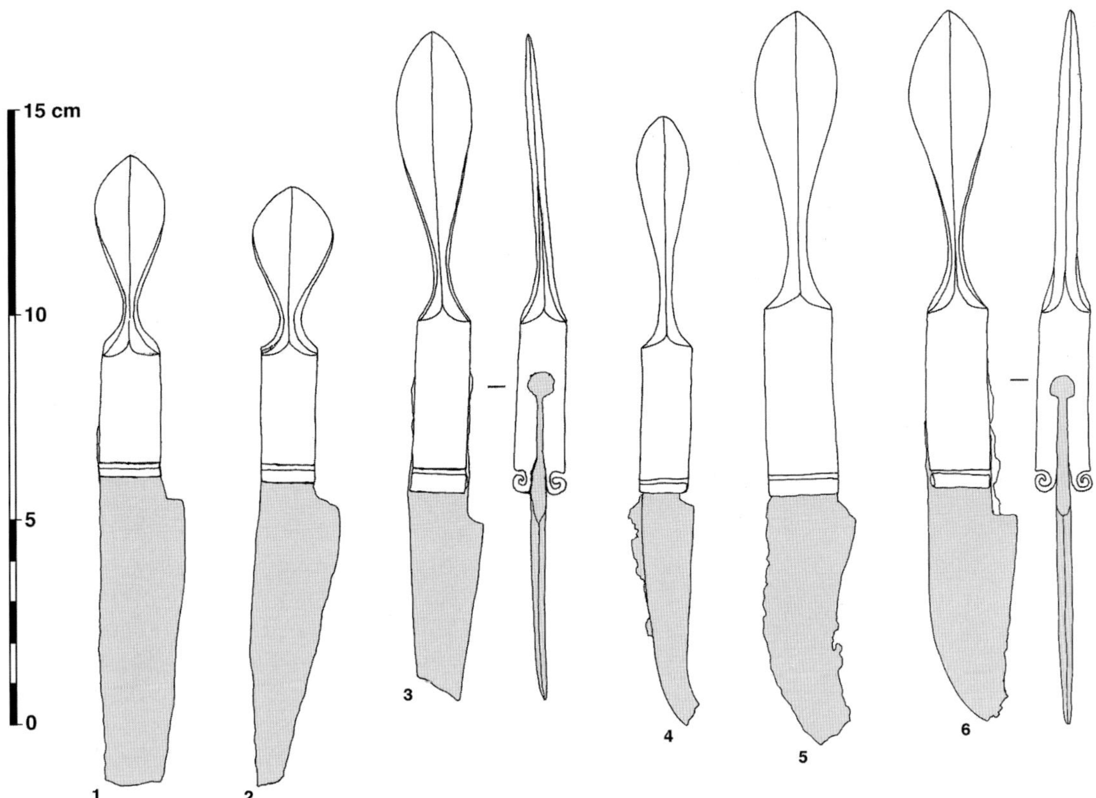

Fig. 18.13. Scalpels from Pompeii (1, 4–6), Bingen (2) and Rimini (3) (drawing: author)

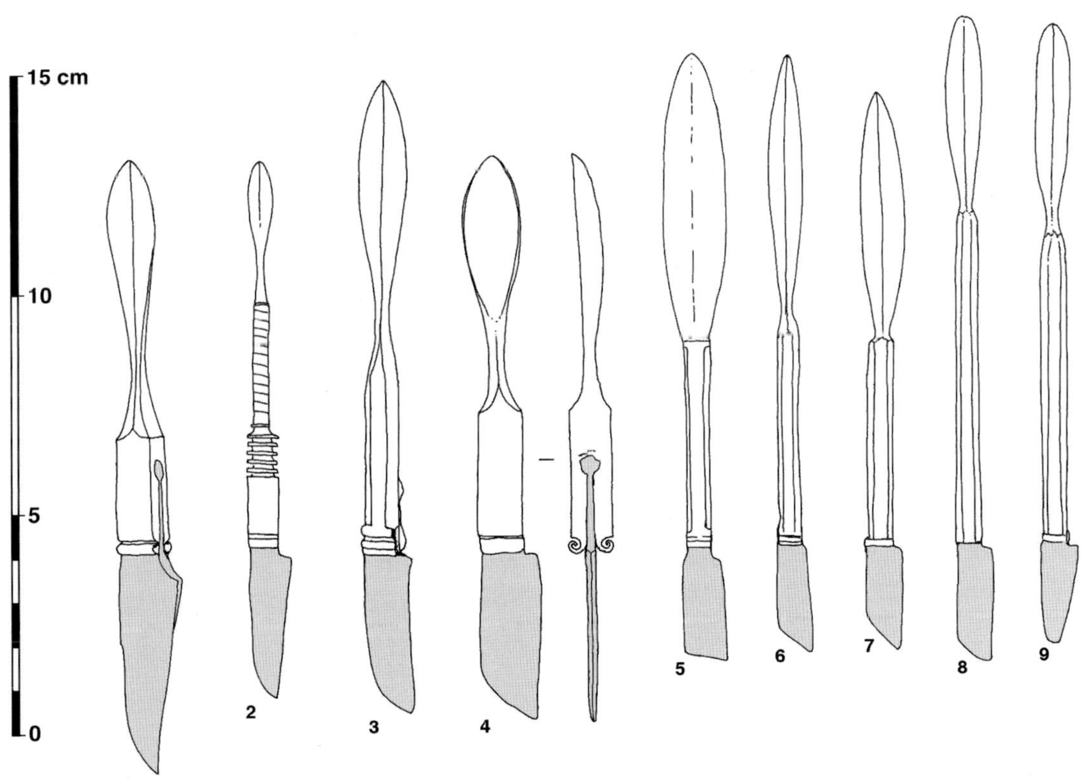

Fig. 18.14. Scalpels from Bingen (1), Cologne (2), Sontheim an der Brenz (3), Rimini (4, 7–9) and Wehringen (5–6) (drawing: author)

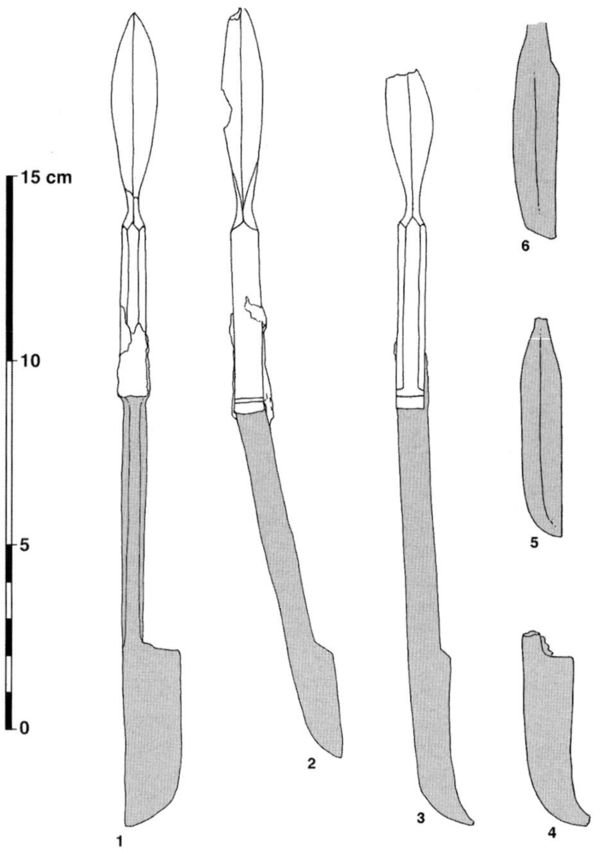

Fig. 18.15. Scalpels (1–3) and blades (4–6) from Rimini (drawing: author)

over the centuries but equally possible that they were freshly manufactured. Moulds were integral to bronze-working, either as part of the craftsman's stock or as a means of replicating an existing object. And, as we have seen from Galen (*On the avoidance of grief* 5), the use of beeswax for modelling or moulding such things was second nature.

However, on present evidence, there also appears to be change in the 3rd century AD, with the increased use of longer and more slender handles and smaller blades. These are seen most strikingly in the kit from Wehringen, the several rolled bundles of portable kits at Rimini and a small kit in the Louvre, in all of which the tiny parallel-sided pointed blade type predominates (Fig. 18.14, nos 5–9). We should anticipate the use of these in a very wide variety of fine surgical interventions, including eye operations, and several of these tiny blades may be identified as the pterygium knife advocated by Aetius (2, 3, 60) and Paul of Aegina (6, 18) for dissecting away the pterygium and by Paul (6, 8) in the operation to remedy trichiasis (Jackson 1996, 2245–6). This identification accords well with the other evidence for eye medicine (desiccated *collyria*) in the Wehringen assemblage. The blades also appear identical to that figured in Albucasis to accompany the passage by Paul on pterygium (Milne 1907, pl. ix, no. 2).

Even more dramatic is the change from the short stout scalpels and blades of the 1st century AD to the slender handled type with very elongated blade stem that is a notable feature of the Rimini assemblage (Fig. 18.15, nos 1–3) and is paralleled by a fragmentary example in the late 2nd to

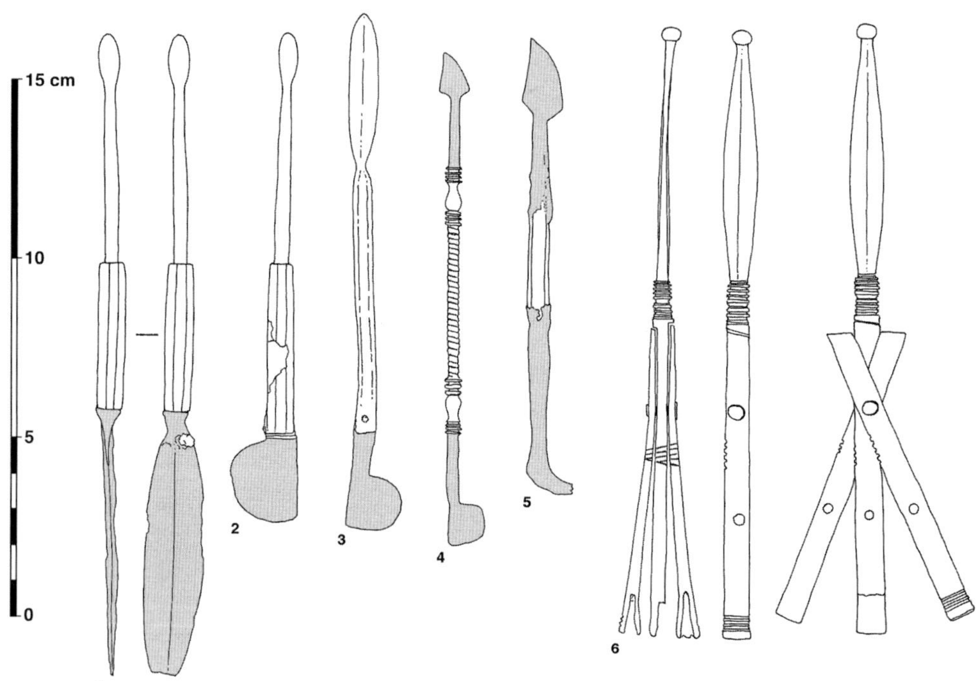

Fig. 18.16. Scalpels from Rimini (1–3, 5), Asia Minor (4) and Rome (6) (drawing: author)

early 3rd century Nea Paphos find (Michaelides 1984, fig. 1, no. 19). The Rimini blades, most of which have not been encountered before, are of very varied form – convex, straight, concave, hooked, combined straight/convex, combined concave/ convex. It is conceivable that one (Fig. 18.15, no. 3) is the 'knife called from its shape "the raven"', the use of which Celsus recommended in the opening of the scrotum for the radical cure of hernia, and/or the 'raven's bill knife' which, some six centuries later, Paul of Aegina advocated for the extirpation of warts (Celsus, *On medicine* 7, 19, 7–8; Paul of Aegina 6, 87). Another pair with blades curved on the flat (Fig. 18.15, no. 1) answer Paul of Aegina's description of knives used in tonsillectomy (Paul of Aegina 6, 30); and two blades (Fig. 18.15, nos 5–6) are of the type discussed by Galen in dissection of the thorax and in fine dissection: 'Use especially the convex part of the double-edged scalpel with both cutting edges curved, but concave on one side, convex on the other' (Galen, *On anatomical procedures* 8.4 (2.673K); Singer 1956, 210).

Another novelty in the Rimini assemblage is a myrtle-leaf-shaped iron blade pegged into the circular socket of a handle with small octagonal grip and slender-stemmed olivary terminal (Fig. 18.16, no. 1). This type of handle, represented in the extensive medical assemblage in a late 2nd–mid-3rd century AD cremation grave from Rheims, was previously thought to have held a surgical needle or fine cautery (Künzl 1983a, fig. 36, no. 31; Künzl and Feugère 2002, fig. 1, no.1e, fig. 6, no. C3). The Rimini blade, which is broken at the tip, is sharp on both edges and, with a central midrib on both faces, it is quite robust. It is conceivably the type of scalpel Galen had in mind for the opening of the vertebral canal. Galen says:

> 'I perform this … with an instrument of my own devising, like the so-called sharp-pointed bistoury. It should be made of the finest steel, like the Norican, that it be not blunted, bent or broken. It must be thicker than a common bistoury, so that, as you press on the junction of the vertebrae, the operation is accomplished with ease' (Galen, *On anatomical procedures* 8.6 (2.682K); Singer 1956, 214).

However, there are other possible applications in descriptions given by Soranus, Galen and Paul of Aegina, including puncturing of the foetal cranium in obstructed labour, opening of the abdomen in ascites, and opening of the thorax in empyema (Milne 1907, 33–4). Additionally, if we restore its broken tip, its appearance is close to that of the lancet used for venesection in Milne's day and, while it is probable that for much bloodletting in antiquity a wide variety of scalpels was used, this blade may correspond to the phlebotome specifically called for in some cases of venesection and for the opening of abscesses (Milne 1907, 32–3).

New, too, is a composite instrument combining a small, strong, ivy-leaf-shaped blade at one end and a broken elevator at the other (Fig. 18.16, no. 5). The blade shape is broadly paralleled by a smaller, thinner example on a double-ended instrument, also of 3rd century AD date, from Asia Minor (Fig. 18.16, no. 4) (Künzl 2002a, A12) and it resembles that of a scalpel in the box of instruments depicted on the well-known 4th century AD sarcophagus of a physician from Ostia (McCann 1978, 138–40, figs 174–5; Jackson 1988, frontispiece; Krug 2008, fig. 25). The Rimini instrument is also similar to a 17th century instrument (Scultetus 1655, pl. ii, no. vii), which combines a blade with a ridged lever and was used at the start of cranial trepanation. As the Rimini instrumentation includes a very wide range of tools for bone surgery, including trepanation, it is possible to suggest that this is another new instrument of bone surgery and represents a further expansion of the known surgical arsenal of Roman practitioners.

Two specialised types of surgical knife from Rome, although lacking their blades, complete this brief survey. One is a unique triple instrument of copper alloy (Fig. 18.16, no. 6). Restoring three blades (probably of the common bellied type) to the now empty sockets I believe we may have the triple-bladed scalpel which Paul of Aegina tells us was used by some practitioners to make three scarifications at one stroke before wet-cupping (Paul of Aegina 6, 41; Milne 1907, 28). The other knife is a distinctive double-ended tool in a set of ten instruments used by a Roman specialist to cut for stone in the urinary bladder (Fig. 18.17). The set, donated to the Cambridge Museum of Classical Archaeology in 1921–2, was found in Italy in the late 19th century and is believed to have come from a tomb in the vicinity of Rome (Jackson 1986, 142 n. 80; 2010, 401–12). As Künzl (1983b) pointed out, the combination of a roughened scoop with an iron-stained socket for the now missing blade allow the identification of two of these tools (Fig. 18.17, 2nd and 3rd from left) as the lithotome (lithotomy knife) used in that most perilous of ancient operations and clearly described by Celsus and Rufus of Ephesus (Celsus, *On medicine* 7, 26, 2H-L; Rufus, *On diseases of the kidneys and bladder* 9, 9–10; Sideras 1977). Celsus' account continued with a description of the procedure for a less straightforward operation in which the stone had a very irregular or spinous surface. While noting that 'many use a scalpel here also', by which we may take him to mean the scalpel end of a combined scoop and blade, Celsus warned that the blade might not be strong enough to completely divide the tissue above projections or spines. To avoid the potentially fatal consequences that might follow a failed operation a more robust customised instrument was developed for the removal of this type of stone, an invention that Celsus attributed to Meges (of Sidon), a Greek surgeon practising in Rome in the 1st century BC (Celsus, *On medicine* 7, 26, 2M-O). Despite Celsus' quite detailed description of Meges' knife, and several attempts to identify or picture it (Milne 1907, 41–3, pl. viii, nos 4–6), it has remained stubbornly elusive, but an ingenious and closely-

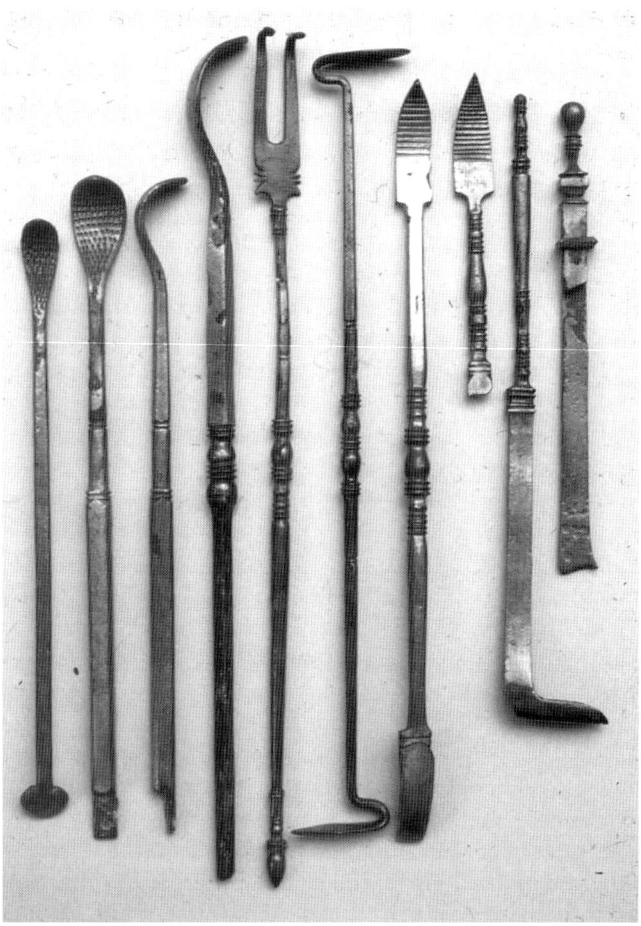

Fig. 18.17. Set of lithotomy instruments, believed to have come from a tomb in the vicinity of Rome (photo: author)

argued case has recently been made for the idiosyncratic knife with curved blade and sinuous handle depicted on the Berlin relief (Krug 2008, 42–3, fig. 26).

To conclude, new light may be shed on ancient surgical practice by integrating archaeological and scientific evidence with that gleaned from medical texts and ancient images of instruments. The comparison of scalpels with complete blades (however few) to descriptions in medical texts (however meagre) occasionally allows the identification of a surgeon's knife intended for a specific operation but more often raises the potential for a wider range of surgery. Certainly we should beware of over-identification and avoid exclusivity, since it is clear that in antiquity one instrument often served numerous roles, but we can at least discern the many different types of knife and blade potentially available to Roman practitioners, while study of their instruments also advances our understanding of the *modus operandi* and surgical finesse of those practitioners.

Bibliography

Berger, E. 1970: *Das Basler Arztrelief. Studien zum griechischen Grab- und Votivrelief um 500 v. Chr. und zur vorhippokratischen Medizin*, Basel.

Bliquez, L. J. 1994: *Roman Surgical Instruments and Other Minor Objects in the National Museum of Naples*, Mainz.

Bliquez, L. and Oleson, J. P. 1994: 'The origins, early history, and applications of the *pyoulkos* (syringe)', 83–119 in G. Argoud (ed.), *Science et vie intellectuelle à Alexandrie (Ier–IIIe siècle après J.-C.)*. (Centre Jean-Palerne Mémoires XIV), Saint-Étienne.

Boudon-Millot, V. 2008: 'Un traité perdu de Galien miraculeusement retrouvé, le *Sur l'inutilité de se chagriner*: texte grec et traduction française', 67–118 in V. Boudon-Millot, A. Guardasole and C. Magdelaine (eds), *La science médicale antique: nouveaux regards. Études en l'honneur de J. Jouanna*, Paris.

Boudon-Millot, V. and Jouanna, J. 2010: *Galien. Tome IV. Ne pas se chagriner*, Paris.

Büsing-Kolbe, A. 2001: 'Ein römischer silbertauschierter Skalpellgriff aus Ficarolo', *Archäologisches Korrespondenzblatt* 31, 107–16.

Como, J. 1925: 'Das Grab eines römischen Arztes in Bingen', *Germania* 9, 152–62.

Craddock, P. and Giumlia-Mair, A. 1993: '*Hśmn-Km*, Corinthian bronze, *shakudo*: black-patinated bronze in the ancient world', 101–27 in S. La Niece and P. Craddock (eds), *Metal Plating and Patination. Cultural, Technical and Historical Developments*, London.

De Carolis, S. (ed.) 2009: *Ars medica. I ferri del mestiere. La* domus *'del chirurgo' di Rimini e la chirurgia nell'antica Roma*, Rimini.

Engelmann, H., Knibbe, D. and Merkelbach, R. 1980: *Die Inschriften von Ephesos*. Teil 4. (Inschriften aus griechischer Städte Kleinasiens, Band 14), Bonn.

Garbsch, J. 1994: *Römischer Alltag in Bayern: das Leben vor 2000 Jahren*, Munich.

Garcia-Ballester, L. 1981: 'Galen as a medical practitioner: problems in diagnosis', 13–46 in V. Nutton (ed.), *Galen: Problems and Prospects*, London.

Garcia-Ballester, L., 1994: 'Galen as a clinician: his methods in diagnosis', 1636–71 in W. Haase and H. Temporini (eds), *Aufstieg und Niedergang der römischen Welt (ANRW)* II, 37.2, Berlin, New York.

Grmek, M. and Gourevitch, D. 1998: *Les maladies dans l'art antique*, Paris.

Hillert, A. 1990: *Antike Ärztedarstellungen* (Marburger Schriften zur Medizingeschichte 25), Frankfurt am Main.

Jackson, R. 1986: 'A set of Roman medical instruments from Italy', *Britannia* 17, 119–67.

Jackson, R. 1988: *Doctors and Diseases in the Roman Empire*, London.

Jackson, R. 1990: 'Roman doctors and their instruments: recent research into ancient practice', *Journal of Roman Archaeology* 3, 5–27.

Jackson, R. 1992: '*Staphylagra, staphylocaustes,* uvulectomy and haemorrhoidectomy: the Roman instruments and operations',

167–85 in A. Krug (ed.), *From Epidauros to Salerno* (Symposium held at the European University Centre for Cultural Heritage, Ravello, April, 1990), *Journal of the European Study Group on Physical, Chemical, Biological and Mathematical Techniques Applied to Archaeology (PACT)* 34, 1992 (1994).

Jackson, R. 1993: 'Roman medicine: the practitioners and their practices', 79–101 in W. Haase and H. Temporini (eds), *Aufstieg und Niedergang der römischen Welt (ANRW)* II, 37.1, Berlin, New York.

Jackson, R. 1994: 'The surgical instruments, appliances and equipment in Celsus' *De medicina*', 167–209 in G. Sabbah and P. Mudry (eds), *La medicine de Celse: aspects historiques, scientifiques et littéraires* (Centre Jean-Palerne Mémoires XIII), Saint-Étienne.

Jackson, R. 1995: 'The composition of Roman medical *instrumentaria* as an indicator of medical practice: a provisional assessment', 189–207 in P. J. van der Eijk, H. F. J. Horstmanshoff and P. H. Schrijvers (eds), *Ancient Medicine in its Socio-cultural Context* Vol. 1. Amsterdam, (= *Clio Medica* 27), Atlanta.

Jackson, R. 1996: 'Eye medicine in the Roman Empire', 2228–51 in W. Haase and H. Temporini (eds), *Aufstieg und Niedergang der römischen Welt (ANRW)* II, 37.3, Berlin, New York.

Jackson, R. 1997a: 'Medical instruments in the Roman world', *Medicina nei Secoli* 9(2), 223–48.

Jackson, R. 1997b: 'A novel Roman forceps', *The Ashmolean* 33, 15–6.

Jackson, R. 2003: 'The Domus 'del chirurgo' at Rimini: an interim account of the medical assemblage', *Journal of Roman Archaeology* 16, 312–21.

Jackson, R. 2005: 'Holding on to health? Bone surgery and instrumentation in the Roman Empire', 97–119 in H. King (ed.), *Health in Antiquity*, London.

Jackson, R. 2007: 'The surgical instruments', 236–52 in P. Crummy *et al.*, *Stanway: an Elite Burial Site at Camulodunum* (*Britannia* Monograph 24), London.

Jackson, R. 2009: 'Lo strumentario chirurgico della *domus* riminese'/ 'The surgical instrumentation of the Rimini *domus*', 73–91 in De Carolis 2009.

Jackson, R. 2010: 'Cutting for stone: Roman lithotomy instruments in the Museo Nazionale Romano', *Medicina nei Secoli* 22.1–3, 393–418.

Jackson, R. forthcoming: *Greek and Roman Surgical Instruments and Medical Objects in the British Museum*, London.

Krug, A. 1985: *Heilkunst und Heilkult: Medizin in der Antike*, Munich.

Krug, A. 1993: 'Römische Skalpelle: Herstellungstechnische Anmerkungen', *Medizinhistorisches Journal* 28(1), 93–100.

Krug, A. 2008: *Das Berliner Arztrelief*, Berlin.

Künzl, E. 1983a: *Medizinische Instrumente aus Sepulkralfunden der römischen Kaiserzeit.* (Kunst und Altertum am Rhein 115), Cologne, Bonn.

Künzl, E. 1983b: 'Eine Spezialität römischer Chirurgen: die Lithotomie', *Archäologisches Korrespondenzblatt* 13, 487–93.

Künzl, E. 1984: 'Einige Bemerkungen zu den Herstellern der römischen medizinischen Instrumente', *Alba Regia* 21, 59–65.

Künzl, E. 1994: 'Ein dekoriertes römisches Skalpell des 1. Jahrhunderts n. Chr. aus Vetera I', 211–7 in G. Precht (ed.), *Xantener Berichte: Grabung – Forschung – Präsentation*, Cologne, Bonn.

Künzl, E. 1996: 'Forschungsbericht zu den antiken medizinischen Instrumenten', 2434–639 in W. Haase and H. Temporini (eds), *Aufstieg und Niedergang der römischen Welt (ANRW)* II, 37.3, Berlin, New York.

Künzl, E. 2002a: *Medizinische Instrumente der römischen Kaiserzeit im Römisch-Germanischen Zentralmuseum* (Kataloge vor- und frühgeschichtlicher Altertümer 28), Mainz, Bonn.

Künzl, E. 2002b: *Medizin in der Antike. Aus einer Welt ohne Narkose und Aspirin*, Stuttgart.

Künzl, E. and Feugère, M. 2002: 'Les instruments ophtalmologiques romains. Essai de synthèse', 115–26 in *Autour de l'oeil dans l'Antiquité. Approche pluridisciplinaire* (Table ronde de Lons-le-Saunier, Jura, 11–12 Février 1994), Lons-le-Saunier.

Leemans, C., 1842: *Romeinse steenen Doodskisten*, Arnhem.

Longfield-Jones, G. M. 1978: 'Surgical instruments', 246–51 in J. F. Healy, *Mining and Metallurgy in the Greek and Roman World*, London.

Marganne, M.-H. 1998: *La chirurgie dans l'Égypte gréco-romaine d'après les papyrus littéraires grecs* (Studies in Ancient Medicine 17), Leiden.

McCann, A. M. 1978: *Roman Sarcophagi in the Metropolitan Museum of Art*, New York.

Michaelides, D. 1984: 'A Roman surgeon's tomb from Nea Paphos', *Report of the Department of Antiquities Cyprus*, 315–32.

Milne, J. S. 1907: *Surgical Instruments in Greek and Roman Times*, Oxford (repr. Chicago, 1976).

Nuber, H. U. 2004: 'Eine Grablege reicher Landbesitzer in Wehringen', 168–70 in L. Wamser, C. Flügel and B. Ziegaus (eds), *Die Römer zwischen Alpen und Nordmeer. Zivilisatorisches Erbe einer europäischen Militärmacht* (Katalog-Handbuch zur Landesausstellung des Freistaates Bayern, Rosenheim, 2000), Mainz am Rhein.

Nutton, V. 2004: *Ancient Medicine*, London, New York.

Ortalli, J. 2000: 'Rimini: la *domus* "del chirurgo"', 513–26 in M. M. Calvani (ed.), *Aemilia. La cultura romana in Emilia Romagna dal III secolo a. C. all'età costantiniana*, Venice.

Ortalli, J. 2008: 'Il *medicus* di *Ariminium*: una contestualizzazione archeologica dalla *domus* "del chirurgo"', *Rivista storica dell'antichità* 37 (2007), 101–18.

Ortalli, J. 2009: 'Archeologia e medicina: la casa del "chirurgo" riminese', 21–45 in De Carolis 2009.

Phillips, E. D. 1973: *Greek Medicine*, London.

Scarborough, J. 1969: *Roman Medicine*, London.

Scultetus, J. 1655: *Armamentarium chirurgicum*, Ulm.

Sideras, A. 1977: *Rufus von Ephesos, über die Nieren- und Blasenleiden. Corpus Medicorum Graecorum* 3.1, Berlin.

Singer, C. 1956: *Galen On Anatomical Procedures*, Oxford.

Tucci, P. L. 2008: 'Galen's storeroom, Rome's libraries, and the fire of A.D. 192', *Journal of Roman Archaeology* 21, 133–49.

Vulpes, B. 1847: *Illustrazione di tutti gli strumenti chirurgici scavati in Ercolano e in Pompej e che ora conservansi nel Real Museo Borbonico di Napoli compresa in sette memorie lette all'Academia Ercolanese*, Naples.

Appendix: Blade forms of intact Roman scalpels (about 70 examples)

1 A short, deep, bellied or sub-triangular blade, with a short stem, a straight back in line with the handle and a convex cutting edge of lunate, elliptical or angular form (Figs 18.11–18.12).
[Pompeii (Bliquez 1994, nos 14–15, pls xiv–xvi – two in Hercules handles; one in knob finial handle; two in Type I handles); Bingen (Como 1925, nos 1–5 = seven complete bellied blades); Asia Minor (Künzl 2002a, B9, B1–B2 – both one-piece iron scalpels); Rimini 184324(2); 184477/8(1) and (2)]
Variants have a longer stem (Fig. 18.12, no. 4)
[Pompeii (Vulpes 1847, pl. VII, vi); London (Jackson 1990, fig. 1, no. 7); Morlungo (Künzl 1983a, fig. 84); Stanway (Jackson 2007, fig. 121, nos 26–7) – one-piece iron scalpels]
and/ or a small or very small blade (Fig. 18.12, nos 4–5, Fig. 18.16, nos 2–4).
[Luzzi (Künzl 1983a, fig. 85, no. 3); Pompeii (Bliquez 1994, A24; Bliquez 1994, no. 52 – one-piece bronze scalpel); Cologne (Künzl 1983a, fig. 67, no. 9); Asia Minor (Künzl 2002a, B10, A12); Louvre kit; Rimini 184370–1 – three blades; 184465A; A1, A2 and B3; 184460]

2 A slender myrtle-leaf-shaped blade, apparently sharp on both convex edges, with a midrib on both faces and a pointed tip (Fig. 18.16, no. 1).
[Rimini 184465B; 184363/ 184370; 184330-1 – two blades]
Some examples combine a myrtle-leaf- shaped blade with a bellied blade.
[Rimini 184370/ 184356/ 184329; 184370/ 184331; possibly A1, A2 and B3; Nijmegen – two examples (Leemans 1842, nos 16, 17); possibly Sontheim an der Brenz – two examples (Künzl 2002b, fig. 55)]

3 A long, apparently parallel-sided blade, with a ?pointed tip.
[Strée (Künzl 1983a, fig. 44, no. 2); Pompeii (Bliquez 1994, pl. XIV – in Hercules handle)]

4 A long triangular blade, with a straight back in line with the handle, a distinct heel and a straight cutting edge which slopes up to the blade tip (Fig. 18.13, nos 1–3).
[Pompeii (Bliquez 1994, no. 30 = Vulpes 1847, pl. VII, i); Bingen (Como 1925, no. 6); Rimini 184314]

5 A long triangular blade, with a straight back in line with the handle and a very lightly convex cutting edge which slopes up to the blade tip.
[Rimini 184479(1); 184477/8(8) – blade]

6 A parallel-sided blade, with a profiled heel and a lightly convex cutting edge, strongly-curved at the end as it slopes up to meet the straight back, which is in line with the very long, slender, octagonal-sectioned stem, itself in line with the handle (Fig. 18.15, no. 1).
[Rimini 184477/8(6) and (7)]

7 A sub-triangular blade, with a convex back in line with the handle, a distinct heel and a straight cutting edge which slopes up to the blade tip (Fig. 18.14, nos 1–4).
[Bingen (Como 1925, no. 7); Cologne (Künzl 1983a, fig. 67, no. 7); Rimini 184477/8(3) with 184335 (blade); Sontheim an der Brenz (Künzl 2002b, fig. 55); Pompeii (Vulpes 1847, pl. vii, v)]

8 A small, sub-triangular blade, with an angled heel, a straight cutting edge and a convex back in line with the very long rectangular-sectioned stem, which is set at an angle to the handle (Fig. 18.15, no. 2).
[Rimini 184324(1)]

9 A hooked blade, with a convex back, a distinct heel and a concave cutting edge (Fig. 18.13, nos 4–6).
[Pompeii (Bliquez 1994, no. 28 = Vulpes 1847, pl. vii, iv; Vulpes 1847, pl. vii, iii; Vulpes 1847, pl. vii, ii?)]

10 A slender, hooked blade, with an angled heel, a concave cutting edge, a strongly-curved tip and a convex back in line with the very long rectangular-sectioned stem, which is in line with the slender handle (Fig. 18.15, nos 3–4).
[Rimini 184321; 184334 – blade]

11 A slender, narrow-stemmed blade, with a midrib on both faces, combining a lightly concave cutting edge with a convex cutting edge with strongly curved tip (Fig. 18.15, nos 5–6).
[Rimini 184336–7 – blades, only]

12 A tiny, parallel-sided blade, with a distinct heel and a straight back which slopes down to the short straight cutting edge at the tip (Fig. 18.14, nos 5–8).
[Wehringen – two examples (Künzl 1983a, fig. 96, nos 4 and 6); Rimini C8 and B1]
Variants have a lightly concave cutting edge.
[Louvre kit, four examples]

13 A tiny, triangular blade, with a distinct heel, a straight back and a short straight cutting edge which slopes up to the rounded tip (Fig. 18.14, no. 9).
[Rimini A3]

14 A tiny, sub-triangular ('ivy leaf shaped') blade with a thick lightly concave back and a convex cutting edge (Fig. 18.16, no. 5).
[Rimini C9]
A variant is much thinner and sharp on both the convex and concave edges and is combined with a tiny bellied blade (Fig. 18.16, no. 4).
[Asia Minor (Künzl 2002a, A12)]

19. Alexander's Wounds as a Paradigm for War Surgery

Alfredo Musajo Somma

Historians and biography writers have pointed out the problems connected with the wounds which afflicted Alexander the Great during his long military service. Since the 19th century medical historians have analysed the wounds which affected epic heroes as described in the Homeric works and they have also discussed Alexander's wounds. The weapons, wounds and the clinical follow-up of a prominent individual in history like Alexander the Great are paradigmatic of knowledge of ballistic evolution of thrown stones, arrows and darts. Moreover surgical instruments found at archaeological sites in the Mediterranean area help to detail the operative procedure that war surgeons, like Kritodemos of Kos, were asked to cope with even on the battlefield. The Macedonian king's empire eventually stretched from Greece to India; wars became much more extensive than before and thousands of trained soldiers marching across Europe, Africa and Asia were wounded on the battlefields. Dedicated medical teams and innovative field hospitals offered through the centuries better means of surgical assistance which would not have been thought of in civilian practice.

Conflict between cities was the norm during the Classical Greek era. Trauma care was delivered on the ancient battlefields, using techniques developed and refined in both military and civilian trauma settings.

For nearly 2500 years, Alexander represented a central vision of mankind. His life has the flavour of a fairy story, in part because it inspired so many. Physically beautiful, a fine warrior, educated by Aristotle, born to a royal court, he chose to risk his inheritance confronting the greatest empire in Europe and Asia. He defeated the Persians in every battle and conquered their territory to the very edge of the known world. At the banks of the last river of the Punjab he wept because he had no more lands to conquer. The empire he established over a million square miles survived in various forms for 300 years. He introduced a coinage, a legal system, a form of philosophy and a style of art that transformed culture across Asia. All this he achieved before he died at the age of 32. His life was magnificent in scope, scale and conviction. Ancient commentators were prepared to accept this without concealing his flaws. Classical historians attacked him for massacring populations and destroying ancient cities, for murdering his senior staff and for leading his troops on dangerous and pointless desert crossings. Conservative Athenians saw him as a half-barbarian, capricious Macedonian despot prone to indecent excesses of intemperance and ostentatious displays of vanity. His Macedonian followers were shocked by the respect he showed to local customs after his conquest of the Persian city of Babylon, in modern Iraq. Compared with his drunken father, Philip, or the Persian king Darius, who kept 365 concubines and went to battle with a platoon of pastry chefs, Alexander seems relatively ascetic and level-headed. Most importantly, ancient writers were prepared to allow that, for all his faults, Alexander was still indubitably a hero.

The legendary biography of Alexander, known as the Pseudo-Callisthenes, was written by a native of Alexandria before the 3rd century BC. Primary sources are unavailable because papers by contemporary *epistolographoi* like Onesicritus, Nearchus, Ptolemy, Aristoboulos, Kleitarchos, Ephippos, Callisthenes, Anaximenes are missing; however, secondary literary sources, such as the histories written by Diodorus, Plutarch, Strabo and Arrian are milestones in the interpretation of Alexander the Great's life.

'You may wonder', said Arrian in the introduction to his *Alexandrou Anabasis* 'why I am writing another book on Alexander the Great when there have been so many already' (Arrian, *Alexandrou Anabasis* I, 12, 1–5). Arrian wrote at the end of the 1st century AD. Indeed Arrian's and Plutarch's biographies of the *cosmocrator* offer the opportunity for a systematic record and interpretation of the major wounds suffered by the king on the battlefield (Table 19.1).

Two wounds inflicted while the king was in Maracanda are worthy of mention:

1 during the night invasion in that area, a stone hit Alexander on the neck and the king suffered a transient confusional status with no complications at all;
2 an arrow pierced Alexander's leg and a bone was broken. According to Plutarch (*Life of Alexander* 45, 5–6) it was the tibia, while according to Arrian's version (*Alexandrou Anabasis*, III, 30,11) it was the fibula, which suffered a compound fracture.

Alexander suffered another dangerous wound during the Mallian campaign, in the Indian subcontinent, when a high energy arrow was driven towards his chest from a short distance, hitting the sternal bone. 'Air and blood were spitting out from the wound and Alexander fainted' (Arrian, *Alexandrou Anabasis*, VI, 10–11). Kritodemos from Kos, a doctor from the clan of the Asklepiades, operated on Alexander and removed the arrow by breaking the wooden shaft and using proper surgical tools.

Military medical treatment on the battlefield was restricted to external injuries. The physicians would not get involved with the fatally wounded; they recognised these cases empirically. Furthermore, a number of injured warriors did not receive medical attention, if this was not considered necessary. In cases of fainting or concussion, pouring water over the warrior or exposing him to fresh air was considered to be sufficient.

Since the Aegean Bronze Age medical practitioners in the Mediterranean area had been able to cope with broken bones or to manipulate joints when healing was almost impossible without reduction and immobilisation.

The process of the clinical condition that we call war trauma begins at the time of the initial energy exchange between the human body and an object. They are moving at different rates, with a differential energy force. Impact between them transfers energy from the hardest object to the softest one. The soft one is usually the body of the soldier. Because energy can neither be created nor destroyed, this interaction of motion with the human body exchanges the energy and produces living tissue damage. All the weapons that pierced the body had to be extracted. Various methods existed for removing them. The dart was pulled out or, if necessary, was cut out of the body. The warriors seemed to be familiar with these techniques as well as the *periodeutes* physicians.

Few early surgical instruments have been found, but a set made of bronze comes from a Mycenaean chamber tomb at Nauplion excavated in 1971, and dated to 1450 BC. The instruments probably belonged to a palace physician, and were buried with him, indicating the fairly high social status of the occupant. From amongst the instruments found in the grave, of significance are the drills, scalpels, a scoop or spoon and a large pair of denticulate forceps, 34.5 cm long. This suggests that surgery may well have been advanced enough to make proper use of them. Found in the same grave were rasps and grinding stones for the making of medicinal remedies (Protonotariou-Deilaki 1973).

Even if ancient doctors did not know the special injury patterns of aggressive weapons and they had almost no ballistic knowledge, there existed experienced practitioners, like Philip of Acarnania, the doctor who saved Alexander's life in Tarsus in 333 BC. Furthermore, Heraclides of Tarentum, around 70 BC, was the author of a recipe collection, entitled *The Soldier* which may have dealt with military medicine (Heraclides, fr. 7 Gu.).

The treatment of wounds from stones, arrows, lances, *sarissai*, bayonets, gunshot and artillery formed the main repertoire of war surgeons, later emulated by the likes of Ambroise Paré, Baron Larrey and Nikolay Pirogov.

Ambroise Paré (*c.* 1510–1590)

Ambroise Paré was born in France at Bourg Hersent and followed other members of his family in becoming a barber-

Table 19.1 Synoptic view of Alexander the Great's wounds

WOUND AREA	*Head/Neck*	*Thorax*	*Shoulder*	*Thigh*	*Legs*
Weapon	Stone	Arrow	Plutarch: Clod Arrian: Catapult	Plutarch: Darius' sword Arrian: Sword	Arr. Arrow
Geographical area	Maracanda	India (Mallian campaign)	Gaza	Issus	Maracanda
Literary ref.	Plutarch 45, 5 Arrian IV, 3, 3	Plutarch 63, 6–13 Arrian VI, 10–11	Plutarch 25, 5 Arrian II, 27, 2	Plutarch 20, 8-9 Arrian II, 12, 1	Plutarch 45, 5 Arrian III, 30, 11
Outcome	Temporary blindness	Sternum impact	Minor bruise	Minor bruise	Open fracture

surgeon. He gained experience in surgical ingenuity as assistant surgeon first at the Hotel-Dieu, a public hospital in Paris, and then as war surgeon attached to Maréchal de Montejan. The challenge posed by gunshot wounds on the battlefield prompted Paré to practice ligature of vessels for haemorrhages instead of performing the application of the traditional hot iron cauteries. The traditional procedure was simple: a piece of metal was heated over fire and applied to the wound. This would cause tissues and blood to heat rapidly to extreme temperatures, in turn causing coagulation of the blood and thus controlling the bleeding, at the cost of extensive soft tissue damage.

Among various artisan classes of healers only a step made a difference between barber-surgeons and surgeons. Paré's contributions to surgical practice were recorded as a cumulative experience gained on the battlefield in his book *Apology and Treatise*. Nevertheless, his procedures made powerful and palpable action statements about the effectiveness of surgical practice, solving health problems that were generally beyond the skill of most lay people. Paré served as a surgeon to four kings and still holds a reputation as the father of military surgery.

Medical and military historians have rightly pointed out the futility of war as well as the apparent inability to learn from past experience. Too often military commanders have placed more value on personal pride and reputation or on weapons and equipment than on human lives.

Dominique-Jean Larrey (1766–1842)

Baron and French military surgeon, born July 8, 1766, Beaudéan, Hautes-Pyrenées. Since he was a teenager, from the age of fifteen, he used to study surgery and therefore served his uncle in his surgical practice. Only six years later, he moved to Paris to study under Antoine Louis (1723–1792) and Pierre Joseph Desault (1744–1795), chief of surgery at the Hôtel-Dieu.

After a short period in the army, Larrey met the commander of an artillery brigade, Napoleon Bonaparte, and in 1792 become *Chirurgien aide-major* of the Army of the North (the army of the Rhine). In this way Larrey gained great clinical experience in the battlefield, evaluating its disorganisation: there was a delay in the clinical assistance and then the victims often died. Therefore he suggested the use of *ambulances volantes* – flying ambulances, as he later described in his report from the Italian Campaign of 1797. Larrey's system of horse-drawn wagons to carry the wounded soldiers from the battlefield to field hospitals was used. The wagons were of two sizes (with the small carrying two patients, and the large, four), and were ventilated and had storage space for medicines and other needed items.

After the Italian Campaign, Larrey was appointed as professor at the École de Médecine Militaire at Val-de-Grâce, but soon after he was in the battlefield again as *Officier de santé en chef* for the Egyptian campaign, where he also used to work with the well known surgeon Baron Réné Nicolas Dufriche Desgenettes (1762–1837). Larrey performed 70 amputations and seven trephinations in Acre in 1799 and wrote about diseases as trachoma, bubonic plague, leprosy and typhus. When he came back to Paris (August 1799) he worked as *Chef-Chirurgien* at the Consular-guard hospital and became medical doctor only in 1803 – even though his dissertation had been ready since 1797!

From 1805 the position of *Inspecteur-genérale du service de santé des armées* allowed Larrey to be in the battlefield again: the War in Spain (1808) was an occasion to study and to perform leg amputations and to treat frostbites. The experience thus gained was really important during the Russian Campaign (winter 1812): soldiers' frozen legs suffered no pain during amputations and the wounds were treated with snow and ice. During the march to Moscow Larrey performed 200 amputations in a day at Borodino, and more than 300 during the retreat at the Berezina River. Moreover, Larrey was among the first surgeons to amputate at the hip. He served during 25 major campaigns including 60 large battles, through the Revolution and the Napoleonic years. Larrey was also a proponent of immediately amputating a damaged limb rather than waiting until it became gangrenous, at which point it was usually far too late to save the limb or the life (Richardson 1974).

Sorting casualties is universally accepted as the best means of coordinating a large number of patients with war injuries. Sorting means classifying casualties by characteristic medical and health features according to three types of criteria, namely diagnosis: gravity of the injury; prognosis: predictable survival; and logistic: evaluation of demand for care and possibilities for evaluation. The sorting process, called '*triage*' by Larrey, was designed to allocate resources to those most in need of urgent care. Today, many of his techniques still prevail in modern medicine (Remba *et al.* 2010).

Nikolay Ivanovich Pirogov (1810–1881)

An expanded humanitarian assistance role for nurses and ancillary personnel was stressed during the Crimean war (1854–6) by Nikolay Pirogov, the surgeon in charge for health services to the Imperial Russian Army. Grand Duchess Helena Pavlovna (1806–73) left St Petersburg with 28 nurses on November 18, 1854 for Simferopol where they arrived almost one month later. They were immediately trained to cope with the triage of casualties under Pirogov's orders.

Thus, during the Crimean War, it was on the Russian side that for the first time in history (November–December 1854) a medical service system of Sisters of Mercy was created, consisting of women working in field conditions for the care of the wounded and sick soldiers. This selfless activity was carried out by the Sisters of Mercy from the Community of the Elevation of the Cross, the Compassionate Widows from the Imperial Widows' Houses and the local women from Sebastopol and other regions of the Crimea. At the same time, on the other side of the front line at the disposition of the allied troops, the first prominent British nursing administrator, Miss Florence Nightingale (1820–1910), began her noble activity, arriving in Scutari on 4 November 1854.

The positive experience of battlefield hospital organisation led Pirogov to become an international representative of the Russian Red Cross during the Franco-Prussian war and, few years later, Chief-surgeon in the Russian-Turkish war for the independence of Bulgaria. He organised the first triage of mass casualties during the Crimean war (McKinnon and Tinker 1997), where ancillary surgical assistance was also offered by Dasha Mikhailova (1836–1910) or Lady Sebastopolskaia, Mary Seacole (1805–1881) or "Lady with a cup" and Florence Nightingale or "Lady with a lamp" (Musajo Somma and Aceto 2008).

Wounds from a lance or bayonet have nowadays been replaced by the potential of irradiation from atomic, hydrogen, and 'dirty' bombs. Managing the injured persons from biological and chemical warfare has become a new challenge. New weapons systems, such as fuel air explosive, can create a devastating number of casualties not yet experienced. Use of the term *modern* is always dangerous unless the appreciation is for 'current' war. Even acknowledging many new challenges and new developments, it still falls to the surgical team to treat patients who have sustained missile wounds, and they labour under less than ideal circumstances, trying to avoid infection. Because we have not been able to eliminate war in the recorded history of the world, we should remain prepared to continue to manage combat casualties to the best of our abilities, based on previous experience and new resources through emerging technologies.

Terrorism is a different form of war and the bomb is its weapon of choice. Explosion induces four classes of injury: primary blast injury is induced by the blast itself; secondary blast injury is caused by the projectiles; tertiary blast injury is caused by the thrust of the victim against stationary objects and by wind disruption; and quaternary blast injury results from fire and heat generated by the explosion. In addition, a mechanism induced by the toxicity of the explosive material has been recognised. This last mechanism is the result of toxic materials from the explosive absorbed by the human body, leading to different haemodynamic alterations. It is the combination of these simultaneously acting mechanisms that causes the unique clinical entity observed among victims of bomb explosion.

The interrelationship between war and advances in medicine is both fascinating and paradoxical. It is an irony of the highest order that war, arguably the most destructive societal force in the cause of suffering and loss of human life, has been the most effective agent in the advancement of medicine, the discipline most dedicated to preserving life and relieving pain. The intimate connection between these two apparently contradictory and dissimilar domains dates back to ancient times.

Although it is somewhat difficult to reconcile the fact that the organisational, therapeutic and procedural advances we have come to enjoy were conceived by the horrible events of war that cause so much human pain, suffering, and loss of life, we realise that war is only the milieu in which these advances take place. War concentrates injuries and disease in such overwhelming numbers into specific points in time, thus challenging creative minds to find unique solutions to seemingly unsolvable problems.

Bibliography

Arrian, *The Campaigns of Alexander*, trans. A. De Selincourt (rev. J. R. Hamilton), Harmondsworth, 1981.

McKinnon, J. G. and Tinker, A. 1997: 'Nikolai Ivanovich Pirogov and the Crimean War', *Clinical and Investigative Medicine*, 20(4), 35.

Musajo Somma, L. and Aceto, G. 2008: 'Oltre Florence Nightingale: l'assistenza ancillare ai soldati in guerra', 355–60 in G. Armocida and I. Gorini (eds), *Storie di Guerra, di Medicina e di Letteratura. 44° Congresso della Società Italiana di Storia della Medicina,* Brescia.

Protonotariou-Deilaki, E.: Πρωτονοταρίου-Δεϊλάκη, Ε. 1973: 'Ακροναυπλία και ανασκαφικαί έρευναι εις περιοχήν Ναυπλίας', *Αρχαιολογικόν Δελτίον*, 28 (B΄1 *Χρονικά*), 90–4.

Remba, S. J., Varon, J., Rivera, A. and Sternbach, G. L. 2010: 'Dominique-Jean Larrey: the effects of therapeutic hypothermia and the first ambulance', *Resuscitation* 81(3), 268–71. Epub 2009 Dec 29.

Richardson, R. G. 1974: *Larrey: Surgeon to Napoleon's Imperial Guard*, London.

Salazar, C. F. 2000: *The Treatment of War Wounds in Graeco-Roman Antiquity*, Leiden.

20. Surgery in Byzantium[1]

Stefanos Geroulanos, Charalambos V. Panaretos and Efterpi Lyberopoulou

Surgery in Byzantium, with respect to the research and results achieved in many other medical fields, has remained more or less impenetrable, despite its major contribution in the conservation, development and transfer of antique knowledge. Byzantine texts provide surprising medical information. Apart from simple surgical procedures, such as incision and drainage of abscesses, they also include fascinating descriptions of severe and very difficult operations. Three of the most important physicians/authors of Byzantium, Oribasius, Aëtios of Amida and Paulus Aegineta, describe and perform amazing operations.

In 1903, Schoene published the names of 54 'Greek-Roman' surgical instruments. For the first time, Milne (1907) attempted to attribute names to the Byzantine instruments and found their Byzantine names; and, since then, with the additions of Maraslis (1983) and Bliquez (1985) the list has increased to 237. Several instruments, however, have different forms, shapes and names, and some were obviously made for particular operations, thus increasing the number of the various known Byzantine instruments to over 500.

The importance of the Byzantine texts in surgery was recognised in France, where, a special decree of July 1607 made them obligatory educational texts for medical students at Sorbonne University in Paris.

Surgery in Byzantium, with respect to the research and results achieved in many other medical fields remained more or less impenetrable, despite its major contribution in the conservation, development and transfer of antique knowledge. Byzantine texts comprise surprising written sources of medical information, which, apart from simple surgical procedures, such as incision and drainage of abscesses, also include descriptions of severe and very difficult operations, thus making their study a fascinating subject. At least three of the most important physicians/authors of Byzantium, Oreibasios (*c.* AD 325–403), Aetios of Amida (6th century AD) and Paulus Aegineta (*c.* AD 625–c. 690) describe and perform amazing operations, like craniotomies, strumectomies, aneurysmectomies, stripping of varices, transvaginal hysterectomies, and others.

In 1903, Schoene published for the first time the names of 54 'Greek-Roman' surgical instruments, and, in 1907, Milne attempted to attribute to the surviving Byzantine instruments their Byzantine names. In 1983, Maraslis was able to broaden the list up to 160 instruments, and Bliquez, in 1985, to 237. However, several instruments have different forms, shapes and names: for example, there are 18 names for cautery, 25 for *mele* and 24 for scalpel. These were obviously made for special operations, thus increasing the number of the various Byzantine instruments known to over 500. Out of these, 207 can be classified according to their special use to one or several surgical specialties.

In this study we have tried to collect the most commonly performed operations and classify them according to modern surgical specialties. In order to illustrate their precise description we have added the exact Byzantine descriptions of three operative procedures. They beautifully illustrate the anatomical knowledge of the Byzantine physicians and their endeavour to transfer their experience to the next generations.

To each specialty we have added the instruments that can be attributed to the specific group. However, instruments such as scalpels, probes or others that can be placed under different surgical procedures are mentioned – with the exception of two or three of them – only once. For the surgical instruments no citations are given since they are all cited by Maraslis (1983) and Bliquez (1985).

General surgery2

Operations: Strumectomy (with reference to the importance of the recurrent nerve) (P.A. II, 76), herniotomy and herniorrhaphy (P.A. II, 106–7; and A.A. 16, 151), hydro- and varicocele operations (P.A. II, 102 and A.A. 16, 150; P.A. II, 105 and A.A. 16, 151 respectively) . Entero- and omphalocele (P.A. II, 106 and 88 respectively), laparocentesis (P.A. II, 87), gastrorrhaphy (P.A. II, 89, 129), lymph node and ganglion excision (P.A. II, 76), hexadactily operation (P.A. II, 84), abscess incision and drainage (P.A. II, 71; Or. B. & D. 3, 568), liver and 'spleen' abscess drainage (P.A. II, 86–7; Or. B. & D. 3, 586; 5, 506), scrofulosis (P.A. II, 76), panaritium incision (P.A. II, 126; Or. B. & D. 5, 351), ingrown nail operation (P.A. II, 126), removal of foreign bodies (P.A. II, 129), finger, arm and leg amputation (P.A. II, 126).

Instruments: *Akis* (fine needle), *belone* (needle), *raphis* (thick needle), *ramma* (suture), *kochliarion* (spoon), *kyathiscos* (spoon-like instrument), *xyster* (raspatorium), *angistron* (skin retractor), *angter* (wound adapter), *psallis* (scissors), *lavis* (forceps), *oxylabidion* (fine forceps), *spathion* (lancet), *spathistes* (spatula), *hypospathistes* (spatula), *beloulkos* (arrow extractor), *dioster* (arrow pusher), *diocleios* (arrow extractor of Diocles), *grammister* (stylus), *grapheion* (stylus), *kauterion* (cauter), *drepanon* (sickle), *parakenterion* (trocar), *doidyx* (pestle), *igdion* (mortar), *thyia* (mortar), *mydion* (forceps), *sarkolavos* (flesh or tumour forceps), *akone* (sharpener), *solen* (tube). *Mele* (probe), *spathe* (spatula), *spathomele* (spatula probe), *amphimelon* (double probe), *pyren* (olivary end of probe), *apyrenomele* (probe without olivary end), *dipyrenon* (double olivery probe), *elasma* (flat part of instrument), *koparion* (probe or scalpel).

Dermatology

Operations: Excisions of steatomas or atheromas (P.A. II, 74), corns, styes and warts (P.A. II, 128), surgical removal of scrofula (P.A. II, 76), incision of furuncles (P.A. II, 71 and Or. B. & D. 3, 664), excision of lipomas (P.A. II, 74), opening of fistulas (P.A. II, 118–9). Wound care of ulcers (P.A. II, 160, 182; A.A. 16, 59; Or. B. & D. 5, 325–39), bites with special emphasis on rabies (A.A.13, 266–8). Therapy of erysipelas (P.A. IV, 21).

Instruments: Akanthobolos (thorn removal instrument), *etheirologos* (epilation tweezers), *tricholabis* (tweezers for hair removal), *pyoulkos* (pus extractor), *xyraphion* (razor), *xystra* (dermabrasion instrument or hair scraper).

Neurosurgery

Operation: Trepanation, craniotomy, elevation of impressed bone segments, several operations in cranial fractures (P.A. II, 136–42).

Instruments: *Meningophylax* (meningeal protector), *trypane* or *trypanion* or *trypanon* (drill), *kephalotrypanon* (trepanation drill), *choinikes* (hollow drill or crown trepan), *abaptiston* (drill that cannot be baptised, e.g. traumatise the meninges), *aris* (bow drill), *kephalikon sphyrion* (surgical hammer), *kouphister* (ring pad around trephine opening), *pilarion* (cap of bandage for hydrocephalus).

Angiology

Operations: Ligation of arteries (P.A. II, 48), arteriotomy (P.A. II, 47; Or. B. & D. 5, 19), arterial resection in temporal arteritis (P.A. II, 48), aneurysmectomy (P.A. II, 75; Or. B. & D. 4, 51), varicectomy (various methods including stripping) (P.A. II, 125; Or. B. & D. 4, 31–43), haemostasis by compression (Or. B. & D. 5, 354), ligation (P.A. II, 74, 48; Or. B. & D. 4, 495), cauterisation (P.A. II, 84; A.A. 16, 62) and haemostyptics (Or. B. & D. 4, 495).

Instruments: *Sikya* (bleeding cup), *phlebotomos* (phlebotome), *epikroustikon* (hammer-like phlebotome), *kirsoulkos* (varix retractor), *exymenister* (membrane cutter), *menoides kauter* (semilunar cauter), *katias* (a type of phlebotome).

Ophthalmology

Operations: Blepharotomy (P.A. II, 56–7), blepharoplasty of distichiasis (P.A. II, 51), lagophthalmus operation (P.A. II, 54), ektropion operation (P.A. II, 55), anabronchismus (P.A. II, 55), hydatic cyst removal (P.A. II, 56), chalazion (P.A. II, 58), pterygion (P.A. II, 58), cataract operations (P.A. II, 60), eyelid-sty treatment (P.A. II, 347; Or. B. & D. 4, 58).

Instruments: *Blepharokatochon* (eyelid retractor), *blepharodiastoleus* (eyelid opener), *blepharotomon* (eyelid scalpel), *blepharoxyston* (fine raspatorium), *anarrhaphikon smilion* (eyelid knife), *melotes* (perforated probe), *ophthalmostates* (instrument for the fixation of the eye), *pterygotomos* (pterygion remover), *ptilon* (hair remover), *belone kataraktou* (cataract needle), *parakenterios belone* (couching needle).

Ear-nose-throat

Operations: Rhinoplasty after nose accident (P.A. II, 62), resection of nosepolyps (P.A. II, 64). retroauricular acoustic pore opening (P.A. II, 62), plastic ear reconstruction (Or. B. & D. 4, 58), reposition of mandibular luxation (P.A. II, 163; Or. B. & D. 4, 142), maxilla and mandibular fixation (P.A.

II, 145; Or. B. & D. 4, 142), tooth extraction (P.A. II, 66), sialolithiasis operation (Or. B. & D. 4, 11), uvulectomy (P.A. II, 68), tonsillectomy (P.A. II, 67), tracheostomy (P.A. II, 70).

Instruments used in Otology: *Melotes* or *melotres* (ear probe), *otike iris* (ear syringe), *otenchytes* (ear rinser), *otikos klyster* (ear clyster), *otoglyphis* (ear scoop), *lavis leptotate* (extra fine forceps), *rhin-oto-rhinion* (small file).

Instruments used in Rhinology: *Polypikon spathion* (semilunar nose polyp knife), *polyposphaktes* (polyp cutter), *polypotomos* (polyp knife), *polypoxystes* (nose polyp remover), *rhinenchytes* (nasal syringe), *rhinotorhinion* (small file), *rhinospathion* (nose knife), *smilarion stenon* (nose polyp lancet).

Instruments used in Laryngology: *Akanthobolos* (pharyngeal forceps), *angylotomos* (curved tonsil knife), *antiotomon* (tonsil knife), *antoptra* (pharyngeal mirror), *mydion* (shell-like forceps), *staphylagra* (uvula remover), *staphylepartes* (uvula lifter), *staphylokaustes* (uvula cauter), *staphylolabis* (uvula forceps), *staphylotomos* (uvula knife).

Instruments used in Stomatology: *Bouglosson* (tongue scraper or depressor), *dactylethra* (finger stall), *lithanaboleus* (parotid duct stone hauler), *stomatodiastoleus* (mouth opening instrument), *sphenarion* (wedge to keep mouth open), *sarkolavis* (flesh pincer).

Instruments used in Odontology: *Odontagra* (tooth extractor), *odontoxyster* (tooth scaler), *smyris* (emery), *rizagra* (tooth root forceps).

Breast and thoracic surgery

Operations: Resection of breast tumours (P.A. II, 84), mastectomy (P.A. II, 85; A.A. 16, 60–4), combined mamma preserving tumour resection and cauterisation (A.A. 16, 61, 40–4), incision of breast abscess (Or. B. & D. 3, 564–8; A.A.13, 39), removal of milk stones (Or. B. & D. 4, 19), excision of necrosis and fistulas (Or. B. & D. 3, 591, 631–5; A.A. 16, 58), gynaecomasty operation (P.A. II, 86), rib resection (Or. B. & D. 3, 582), drainage of empyema (Or. B. & D. 3, 579; P.A. II, 84), separation of Siamese twins (the first in the world) (Joannes Skylitzes: Thurm 1973, 232).

Instruments: *Ekkopeus* (bone cutting instrument), *parakenterion* (trocar), *platymele* (flat probe), *pleurokopos* (rib cutter), *pleuroprister* (rib saw), *rhine* (file).

Visceral surgery

Operations: There are several unclear abdominal and other operations mentioned under 'general surgery' (P.A. II, 129). *Instruments: Enterophylax* (intestinal spatula), *parastoleus* (stomach instrument), *hydrokelikon koparion* (hydrocele dissector), *pyalos* (bathing tub for treatment of enterocele), *siphon* (drainage tube for hydrocele).

Gynaecology and obstetrics

Operations: Transvaginal hysterectomy (A.A. 16, 109), drainage of a pyometra or uterus empyema (P.A. II, 113; A.A. 16, 134–6), operation of cervix varices (A.A. 16, 147), nymphectomy (A.A. 16, 152), operation of hymenal, vaginal and uterus atresia (A.A. 16, 146), resection of pudendal, vaginal and cervical condylomas (P.A. II, 124), major improvements in irregular birth, use of forceps, embryotomy, support of genitals during birth (P.A. II, 114–5), manual extraction of placentar remains (P.A. II, 118), manual cleansing of uterus in postpartal infection, abortion, operation on hermaphrodites (P.A. II, 112).

Instruments: Chytra (fumigation apparatus), *dactylethra* (finger stall), *dioptra*, *dioptrion*, *dioptron* (vaginal specula), *diphros paredros* (gynecological chair), *diphros maioticos* (chair for births and fumigation), *metranyktes* (uterus dilatator), *metrenchytes* (uterus lavage instrument), *metroskopion* (speculum), *pessos* (pessary), *physarion* (syringe), *kephaloklastes* (cranioclast), *katiadion*, *katias* (dead embryo chisel), *embryoulkos* (midwife forceps), *embryotomos* (embryotome), *embryothlastes* (spike for dispatching a foetus), *onyx* (fish-hook-like instrument for extraction of dead foetus).

Urology

Operations: Circumcision and phimosis operation (P.A. II, 95; Or. B. & D. 4, 466–9), hypospadias operation (building neourethra) (P.A. II, 94; Or. B. & D. 4, 463), resection and cauterisation of condylomas (P.A. II, 97; Or. B. & D. 4, 470), catheterisation of bladder and lavage (P.A. II, 98; A.A. 16, 149), transurethral and transvaginal cystolithotrypsy (P.A. II, 99; A.A. 16, 149), transvaginal and transperineal cystolithiasis removal, castratio (P.A. II, 111; A.A. 16, 149), operation of hermaphrodites (P.A. II, 112).

Instruments: Avliskos (small tube, reed), *kalamis pterou* (shaft of bird's feather), *kalamiskos* (drainage tube), *katheter* (catheter), *kauloklyster* (urethra clyster), *syringion* (small tube, fistula), *lithanaboleus* (stone extractor), *lithokopos* (stone cutter, scalpel), *lithotomos* (scalpel for lithotomy), *lithoulkos* (stone extractor), *skenorrhaphion* (frenulum preputii needle), *skolops* (urethra lancet).

Proctology

Operations: Haemorrhoidectomy (including ligation and cauterisation) (P.A. II, 173), fistulotomy and fistulectomy

(P.A. II, 118–20; Or. B. & D. 3, 591, 611, 615), seton technique (P.A. II, 120; Or. B. & D. 3, 635), perianal abscess drainage (Or. B. & D. 3, 587), anal atresia operation (P.A. II, 124).

Instruments: Dioptra (speculum), *dioptron micron* (small speculum), *diastoleus* (dilatator), *hedroskopion* (anal speculum), *eneter* (enema syringe), *keras* (tube of clyster), *klyster* (clyster), *ascoma* (wine skin bellows), *avliskos* (small tube, reed), *brochos* (ligature), *drepanoides organon* (fistula knife), *haemorrhoidokaustes* (heamorrhoidal cautery), *hemispathion* (half-sword, lancet), *ipoterion* (small tube from papyrus), *syringotomon* (fistula knife).

Traumatology and orthopedics

Operations: All possible reductions of simple and complicated bone fractures (P.A. II, 129, 136, 142, 146, 148–63; Or. B. & D. 4,142–68, 211–3) and repositions of luxations (P.A. II, 163–81; Or. B. & D. 4, 142–67), extractions of arrows, spears etc. including gastro-, duodeno-, jejuno-, colono- and vesicorrhaphy (P.A. II, 129).

Instruments: *Anaboleus* (elevator), *antiboladion* (bone lever), *beloulkos* (arrow forceps), *dioster* (impellent), *ekkopeus* (bone cutting forceps), *plakotos ekkopeus* (lens-like ekkopeus), *epikroustion* (hammer), *gamphoter* (chisel), *ostagra* (bone forceps), *ostanaboleus* (bone lever), *ostenchytes* (bone irrigator), *osteokopos* (bone cutting instrument), *perilabeus* (bone reduction instrument), *perixyster*, *perixystes* (raspatorium), *prion* (saw), *rizagra* (bone remover), *narthex* (splint), *mochliskos* (bone lever), *rhine* (rasp), *spathe ipotris* (reduction instrument), *sphenarion* (cuneolus), *spheniskoi* (small cuneoli), *sphyra*, *sphyrion* (hammer), *traumatike mele* (specillum vulnearium), *xystron* (scraper), *xyster* (raspatorium).

Wound care

Operations: Wound cleansing, wound cauterising, wound excision, with several plastic corrections of the wound (P.A. IV, V).

Instruments: atherologion (remover of foreign bodies), *angter* (pincer and/or bandage), *desmos* (bonds of surgical bed), *epidesmos* (bandage), *iska* (sponge-like fungus growing on trees), *lemniskos* (woolen thread), *likonymos* (ligature?), *pessos* (wick or pessary), *motos* (wound powder and/or gauze, etc.), *motophylax* (bandage to keep *motos* in place), *ptygmation* (gauze), *spongos* (sponge), *taenia* (strap, ribbon), *tiltos* (lint), *telamon* (bandage and/or tourniquet), *xanton* (lint).

Unclassified

Operations: Several operations cannot be clearly classified as designed for one or other specialty (e.g. cauterisation, cupping, burning over the spleen or the stomach for different disorders). They have, therefore, been omitted from this list. There are, however, several instruments that we feel are of importance. They could have been used in several specialties.

Instruments: Cherniboxeston chalkoun (copper wash basin), *deltarion* (deltashape instrument, cautery?), *deltos* (tablet or medical box), *diedrion* (twin chairs), *encheiridion* (instruments case), *ipoterion* (papyrus stent to hold *solenarion*), *kyrtis* (strainer), *charaktes* (stylus?, trephine?), *skythomyle* (a sort of probe), *kyathos* (spoon-like instrument ?), *louterion* (bath), *lekanis* (washing bowl), *physiter* (air bellows), *prasia* (?).

These lists are definitely incomplete. However, they reflect the variety of the operations that the Byzantine surgeon was confronted with and should be able to perform. All these operations are extensively described, mainly by Paulus Aegineta. Their indications and contra-indications are accurately described. As it would be impossible to describe all above operations, we would like to cite only three of the most impressive texts:

Tracheotomy (laryngotomy)

> 'When, therefore, we engage in the operation we split open a part of the arteria aspera (for it is dangerous to divide the whole) below the top of the windpipe, about the third or fourth ring. For this is a convenient situation, as being free of flesh, and because the vessels are placed at a distance from the part which is divided. Wherefore, bending the patient's head backwards, so as to bring the windpipe better into view, we are to make a transverse incision between two of the rings, so as that it may not be the cartilage which is divided, but the membrane connecting the cartilages. If one be more timid in operating, one may first stretch the skin with a hook and divide it, and then, removing the vessels aside, if they come in the way, make the incision'.

These are the words of Antyllus, cited by Paulus Aegineta (VI, 34) and translated by Adams (1846). Despite this unique description, tracheotomy was more or less forgotten because Asklepiades (2nd century BC), who first performed it, Antyllus (1st century AD), who first described it accurately and Paulus Aegineta (6th century AD), who at least saved the text of Antyllus, are speaking of laryngotomy and not of tracheotomy. However, laryngotomy was performed by all three authors (Asklepiades, Antyllos and Paulus) between the 3rd and the 4th ring of the trachea and not through the larynx. The operation was rediscovered in the 19th century and then correctly named tracheotomy. However, up to the end of the 20th century the technique was identical with the Byzantine method of 'laryngotomy'.

Strumectomy

'The strumae are formed either on the anterior part of the neck, or on either side of it, or on both, and they consist of one, two, or more, all contained in their proper membranes… Those that are of a malignant nature, are to be considered as carcinomatous and it is obvious that they do not readily yield to a surgical operation. But such as are mild to the touch and the seasonable application of medicines, may be operated upon in this manner. To such as are superficial and incline towards the skin, we use a simple section, and free them from the surrounding bodies, and stretching the skin with hooks we flay the lips of the incision, as we said in describing the operation of angiology, and by degrees remove them entirely. But such as are mild to the touch and the seasonable application of medicines, may be operated upon in this manner. But such as are larger, having transfixed them with hooks, we raise up, and dissecting away the skin from them in like manner, we must free them entirely from the surrounding bodies, avoiding in particular the carotid arteries and recurrent nerves. If any divided vessel obscures the operation, we may include it in a ligature, or cut it asunder, if not large. And when the base of the scrofulous tumour runs out into a narrow point, we may cut it away readily, and introducing the index finger search if there be any other strumae lying there, and remove them in the same manner. But if we suspect that a large vessel or vessels are situated at the bottom of the scrofulous tumour, we need not cut it out from the base, but include it in a ligature, so that it may fall off spontaneously in pieces without danger, when we may effect the cure by the application of lint; but if cut away at once we may unite the lips of the incisions' (Paulus Aegineta, VI, 35, transl. Adams 1846).

Five centuries earlier, Galen recommends incision or septic applications (Galen, *De methodo med*endi XVI and *De locis affectis* I, 6: Adams 1846, II, 308). He is against operation, as he relates an unfortunate case in which an ignorant surgeon occasioned loss of speech by cutting both recurrent nerves. In contrast to Galen, Paulus suggests operation.

Aetius, who lived 100 years before Paulus, cites a long extract from Leonidas on the treatment of scrofula often mentioned together with strumae (Aetius XV, 5: see Maraslis 1983). His directions for dissecting tumours in the neck are again such as experience alone could have dictated. In operating on the neck, he cautions us to avoid the jugular veins, carotid arteries, and the nerves of speech, and with this intention he recommends us to make the incisions longitudinal rather than transverse, a practice that is followed till our times. However, in contrast to Paulus, he does not make any mention of ligature. When there is a discharge of blood he recommends styptics (Adams 1846, 308).

Aneurysmectomy

'But those (aneurysms) which occur in the extremities, the limbs, or the head, we operate upon thus. We make a straight longitudinal incision in the skin, and then having separated the lips with hooks, as we mentioned in the operation of angiology, and having dissected away the skin, and separated it with instruments used for operations on membranes, we lay bare the artery, and passing a needle under it, and tying it with two ligatures, and having first divided the intermediate part of the artery with a lancet used for bleeding, and evacuated its contents, we have recourse to the suppurative treatment until the falling off of the ligatures. If the aneurysm be occasioned by rupture of the artery, we must seize in the fingers along with the skin as much as possible of the aneurysm, and then below what we hold in our hand we push a needle having a double thread, and after it has passed through we cut the double, and thus with the two threads we bind the tumour on this side and on that, as we mentioned for staphyloma. If any apprehension be entertained from the falling off of the ligatures, we must push another needle entirely through, in the course of the first, having in like manner a double thread and cutting the noose into four pieces, we may bind the tumour' (Paulus Aegineta, VI, 37, transl. Adams 1846).

Paulus is not the first to treat the aneurysm. Antyllus, Galen and others had successfully treated them as well. However, he is the one that, contrary to Galen's recommendations, has conserved the knowledge of Antyllus, propagated his practice and passed this experience on to the Arabs and to the West. The same is valid for several other texts.

The lists of instruments mentioned above are also indicative of the need for specialised medical instruments and of their wide use. They also enlighten our knowledge as to the quality of medicine practiced. Most of these types of instruments are still in use and 30% of them still today bear the same name in Greek. This is also valid for many surgical instruments of today, that have kept the same name even in English (approx. 10%), such as *kauter*/cautery, *trypanon*/trepan, *embryotomos*/embryotome, *katheter*/catheter, *pessos*/pessary etc. Other instruments' names in English have retained the Latin derivative of the original name, e.g. raspatorium, forceps, spatula, cuneolus, etc., proving the great influence of Byzantine medicine on Western medicine.

The importance of the Byzantine texts in surgery was recognised very early in the Arab world. Albucasis produced their exact translations and added his personal experiences. Rhazes, Haly Abbas, Avicenna and Albucasis describe many of the operations performed in Byzantium; they cite, however, more Albucasis than the original texts.

In the West the experience of the Byzantine physicians was perfectly known in Sicily and southern Italy (Salerno) up to the end of the 11th century (Lyons and Petrucelli 1987, 294–6).

However, this amount of knowledge was more or less lost in the years that followed, as most of the physicians of the West spoke mainly Latin and not Greek. An exception was France, where the Greek texts of Paulus Aegineta became by a special decree (of 1 July 1607) obligatory for the medical students of Sorbonne University in Paris. This continued to be so up to the end of the 18th century; and, being the golden standard for these two centuries, Paulus Aegineta's texts have greatly influenced the development of surgical praxis that followed for a 1000 years after their conception. Most of his directives are still valid today.

Notes

1 This paper was published in part in M. Grünbart, E. Kislinger, A. Muthesius and D. C. Stathakopoulos (eds), *Material Culture and Well-being in Byzantium (400–1453): Proceedings of the International Conference, Cambridge 8–10 September 2001* (Veröffentlichungen zur Byzanzforschung Band XI), Vienna 2007, 129–34; and presented also in part at *The 8th International Conference on Anticancer Research*, Kos, 17 October 2008: see Geroulanos 2008.

2 The following abbreviations are used in the lists that follow:
A.A. 13: Aetios of Amida, *Logos XIII,* ed. Sk. Zervos, Athens 1905
A.A. 16: Aetios of Amida, *Logos XVI,* ed. Sk. Zervos, Leipzig 1907
Or. B.& D. Vols 3–5: U. C. Bussemaker and C. Daremberg, *Oeuvres d'Oribase,* Vols 1–6, Paris 1851–1876.
P.A. Vol. II: Paulus Aegineta in J. L. Heiberg, *Corpus Medicorum Graecorum,* vol. II, 1924.

Bibliography

Adams, F. 1844–7: *The Seven Books of Paulus Aegineta*, Sydenham Society, London.

Aetios of Amida: *Editio princeps,* Books I–VIII, Aldus Manutius, Venice 1534.

Aetios of Amida: *Logos XIII*, ed. Sk. Zervos, Athens 1905.

Aetios of Amida: *Logos XVI*, ed. Sk. Zervos, Leipzig 1907.

Bliquez, L. J. 1984: 'Two lists of Greek surgical instruments and the state of surgery in Byzantine times', 187–204 in J. Scarborough (ed.) *Symposium on Byzantine Medicine. Dumbarton Oaks Papers* 38, Washington.

Bussemaker, U. C. and Daremberg, C. 1851–1876: *Oeuvres d'Oribase,* Vols 1–6, Paris.

Geroulanos, S. 2008: 'Byzantine surgery', in "Abstracts of Proceedings of the 8th International Conference of Anticancer Research, Kos, October 17–22", in *Anticancer Research* 28, no 3157-35562008.

Lascaratos, J., Cohen, M. and Voros, D. 1998: 'Plastic surgery of the face in Byzantium in the fourth century', *Plastic and Reconstructive Surgery* 102, 1274–80.

Lyons, A. S. and Petrucelli, R. J. 1987: *Medicine: an illustrated history*, New York.

Maraslis 1983: Μαρασλής, A. 1983: *Η Χειρουργική στο Βυζάντιο* (*Surgery in Byzantium* in Greek), Athens.

Milne, J. S. 1907: *Surgical Instruments in Greek and Roman Times*, Oxford.

Paulus Aegineta: *Epitomes Iatrikes*. *Editio princeps*, Aldus Manutius, Venice 1528.

Paulus Aegineta: in J. L. Heiberg (ed.), *Corpus Medicorum Graecorum*, Vol. II, Leipzig 1924.

Schoene, H. 1903: 'Zwei Listen chirurgischer Instrumente', *Hermes* 38, 280–4.

Thurn. I. (ed.) 1973: *Ioannis Skylitzae Synopsis Historiarum, editio princeps* (Corpus Fontium Historiae Byzantinae V), Berlin and New York.

21. Plastic Surgery of the Face in Byzantine Times

Marios Papadakis, Evangelos Sfakiotakis, Marios Fragakis, Constantinos Trompoukis, Maria Fragaki, Moschoula Leivadara and Andreas Manios

The aim of this work is to present the facial reconstructive procedures performed by physicians (mainly Oribasius of Pergamum, Aëtius of Amida and Paul of Aegina) during the Byzantine period. These procedures include operations upon the lips, nose, forehead, cheeks, eyebrows, eyelids and auricles for the reconstruction of skin defects. The surgical management of the nasal fractures was also a part of everyday surgical practice. We conclude that the principles of reconstruction in the Byzantine period followed the same patterns of mobilisation and preparation of local flaps as those used today.

Introduction

During the Byzantine period there was a continuous series of physicians whose inspiration was largely derived from ancient Greek sources. Most of these preserved in their writings the knowledge of the ancient Greek physicians, many of whose works are now lost, enriched with their own personal experience. As a result, Byzantine medicine had a significant influence on Islamic medicine and the Western rebirth of medicine during the Renaissance. In this paper we chose to present the evidence for the facial reconstructive procedures performed by physicians during the Byzantine period.

Material – Methods

A study and analysis of the original texts of Byzantine physicians, including Oribasius (4th century AD), Aëtius (6th century AD) and Paul of Aegina (7th century AD), was undertaken (Dumont and Smith 1992). As previously mentioned, these works are very valuable on account of the fact that they preserve numerous extracts from writers whose works are no longer extant. The references concerning reconstruction of facial deformities were analysed, and the removal of Justinian II's nose and the nose of a porphyry head, which is believed to represent a case of reconstructive rhinoplasty, were also examined.

Oribasius of Pergamum (4th century AD)

Oribasius, Julian the Apostate's physician, was born in Pergamum in the beginning of the 4th century and studied at the school of Zenon the Cypriot at Alexandria in Egypt. It is not known exactly how he became acquainted with Julian, the emperor, but he was soon honoured with his confidence and friendship. He accompanied Julian on his expedition against Persia, and was present at the time of his death in AD 363.[1]

On Julian's order, Oribasius started to compile the most important written medical works of early times in an anthology. Oribasius collected this medical material in seventy or (according to the Souda) in 72 books, under the title *Συναγωγαὶ Ἰατρικαί* (*Collectiones Medicae*). Of this large work, also known as *Ἑβδομηκοντάβιβλος* (*Hebdomecontabiblos*), rather more than one-third is still extant.

Aëtius of Amida (6th century AD)

Aëtius, was born in Amida, a city on the banks of the Tigris in Mesopotamia, and studied medicine in Alexandria, and probably lived at the beginning of the 6th century. The work for which he is now known is his *Tetrabiblos*, a compilation from all the physicians who preceded him, particularly Galen, Archigenes and Dioscorides, and appears to have originally consisted of sixteen books, the first eight of which were printed in Greek by Aldus Manutius at Venice in 1534.

Paul of Aegina (7th century AD)

Paul of Aegina was an eminent Byzantine physician who lived in the 7th century AD. He was born on the island of Aegina, a small island in the Saronic Gulf, but he studied and practised medicine in Alexandria, up to his death in AD 690. He wrote a medical encyclopaedia (*Epitome of Medicine*) divided into seven books, a monumental work which brought him international fame. The sixth book is dedicated exclusively to surgery. The first edition of the *Epitome* was also published by Aldus Manutius in Venice, in 1528. Latin translations were printed in 1551 and 1567. The *Epitome* was also translated into English in 1844 by Francis Adams, who added a commentary after each chapter comparing Paul's opinions with those of his predecessors. A French translation of the sixth book was published in 1855 by René Briau.

Discussion of results

We discovered the existence of several types of facial plastic surgery operations during the Byzantine period, including operations upon the lips, nose, forehead, cheeks, eyebrows, eyelids and auricles for the reconstruction of skin defects (*colobomas*). Ancient physicians used the term *coloboma*, to describe skin defects in general. The word *coloboma* (*κολόβωμα*) comes from the Greek verb *κολοβόω* which means to mutilate.

Lips and auricles

Paul refers to colobomas of auricles and lips, noting that 'the lips of the wounds should be united and sutured after the dissection of the skin and the removal of the lesion (the 'callous' parts)'. Oribasius notes that the H-shaped flap can also be used for the reconstruction of aural deficiencies (see below).

Eyelids

Oribasius, Aëtius and especially Paul describe the surgical management of palpebral deficiencies in detail.

Colobomas of the Eyelid

Oribasius includes in his work Antyllus' description for the management of colobomas of the eyebrow with the creation of an H-shaped flap (Fig. 21.1):

> 'When there is a skin defect by the eyebrow we first create a square defect around the original one. We extend the horizontal sides (the one over the forehead and the one over the brow) towards the nose medially and the ear laterally. This way an H-shaped design is created. We then undermine the skin, join together the two flaps and suture without tension' (Lascaratos, Cohen and Voros 1998, 1276).

Ectropion

Ectropion (ἐκτρόπιον) is the turning out of the eyelid so that the inner surface is exposed. In ancient medicine, the term was used only for the lower eyelid.[2] Paul of Aegina gives a thorough description of the surgical correction of this defect (Fig. 21.2):

> 'Taking a needle, armed with a double thread, we perforate the fleshy mass, pushing it through from the left canthus to the right. Then by means of the thread fastened to both of its extremities, we stretch the skin with the needle, and cut down upon it with a scalpel, removing the needle at the same time. If the eversion continues, we apply the back of the specillum to the divided eyelid and on the inside of the eyelid, having made two incisions, beginning at the two angles of the incision formerly made, and terminating in an acute point, and meeting together like the Greek Λ. We then remove it, so that its acute point may be below at the eye, and the broad above at what is called the tarsus. Afterwards we unite the separated parts with a needle containing a woollen thread, being satisfied with two sutures' (Adams 1844–1847, vol. ii, 267).

Lagophthalmos

Lagophthalmos (λαγώφθαλμος) is defined as the inability to fully close the upper eyelid. The term *lagophthalmos* derives from the Greek words *lagos*, meaning a hare, and *ophthalmos*, meaning the eye, since the hare was believed to sleep with its eyes open (Van de Graaf, Ijpma and Nicolai 2008, 573).[3] Paul explains its surgical correction (Fig. 21.3):

> 'Lagophthalmos arises either naturally or from the cicatrix of a wound or from the operations of the suture or burning having been improperly performed; moderate relief can only be accomplished when the eyelid is sufficiently thick. We must divide the cicatrix and having separated the lips with a tent, use bandages until the cure is completed, avoiding very desiccative substances, and having recourse to those which are fatty and relaxing' (Adams 1844–1847, vol. ii, 265).

Aëtius, adopting Celsus' technique directs us to make a lunated incision below the eyebrows and turn downwards the horns of the incision, taking care not to wound the muscles (*ibid.*, vol. ii, 266).

Trichiasis

Trichiasis is the ancient Greek word for entropion. Entropion (# ectropion) is the inward turning of the eyelid, causing rubbing of the eyelashes and eyelid skin against the eye surface. Paul describes its surgical management:

> '… we turn the upper eyelid outwards and push a needle having a thread, through the middle of the tarsus from within outwards; then stretching the eyelid with the left hand by means of the thread and having folded out the eyelid and everted it behind the thread, with the point of a scalpel held in the right hand, we make the under-incision within the hairs which irritate the eye, extending from the larger canthus to the smaller, along the

56 ORIBASE. COLLECT. MÉD. XLV, 25.

Mai 58-59.

ριαιρεῖν, καταλιπόντας ἐκεῖνο ὅπερ ὑπὸ τῶν ῥαμμάτων ἐσφίγγετο· οὕτω γὰρ ἀναιμοῤῥάγητος ἡ χειρουργία γίνεται.

κε'. Περὶ κολοβωμάτων. Ἐκ τῶν Ἀντύλλου.

Ἔσλι μὲν τὸ κολόβωμα ἔλλειψις μορίου, ἢ τινος δέρματος κα- 1
λύπλοντος τὰ σώματα. Εἰ μὲν οὖν ἐν ὀφρύϊ γένοιτο τὸ κολόβωμα, 2
οὕτω χειρουργήσομεν· τετράγωνον ἐκκοπὴν ποιησόμεθα, εἰ μή πως αὐτὸ κατὰ συντυχίαν τετράγωνον εἶναι τύχοι, ὥσ7ε ἐν τῇ τετραγώνῳ ἐκκοπῇ περιειλῆφθαι τὸ κολόβωμα, ἔπειτα τὴν ἄνω πλευρὰν τοῦ τετραγωνίσματος, λέγω δὲ τὴν γενομένην ἐπὶ τῷ μετώπῳ, ἐπὶ ἑκάτερα ἐκβαλοῦμεν, διαιροῦντες καὶ ὡς πρὸς τὴν ῥῖνα καὶ ὡς πρὸς τὸ οὖς, ὥσ7ε πολὺ ἐπιμηκεσ7έρας τῆς τοῦ τετραγώνου πλευρᾶς γενέσθαι τὰς ἑκατέρωθεν ἐκτεταμένας διαιρέσεις. Παραπλη- 3
σίως δὲ καὶ τὴν ἀντικειμένην πλευρὰν τὴν ἐπὶ τῇ ὀφρύϊ ἐπιδιελοῦμεν ἐπὶ ἑκά]τερα, ὥσ7ε τὸ σχῆμα γενέσθαι συμπάσης τῆς διαιρέσεως 57

prise dans les fils : par ce procédé, l'opération a lieu sans qu'il survienne d'hémorragie.

25. DU COLOBOME (PERTE DE SUBSTANCE ET ARRÊT DE DÉVELOPPEMENT). — TIRÉ D'ANTYLLUS.

Le colobome est un manque de substance intéressant une partie dans 1
toute son épaisseur, ou seulement la peau qui la recouvre. Si donc le 2
colobome existe au sourcil, nous pratiquons l'opération suivante : nous faisons quatre incisions qui se réunissent à angle droit (à moins que par hasard la mutilation elle même ne constitue un rectangle), de telle sorte que nous circonscrivons la mutilation dans un rectangle; ensuite nous prolongeons à droite et à gauche le côté supérieur du rectangle, je veux dire celui qui est sur le front, en dirigeant les incisions d'un côté vers le nez, et de l'autre vers l'oreille, d'où il résulte que les incisions prolongées de part et d'autre deviennent beaucoup plus longues que le côté du rectangle (d'où elles partent). De même, nous prolongeons 3
aussi de part et d'autre le côté opposé, celui qui occupe le sourcil; ainsi, la figure de l'ensemble de toutes les incisions, y compris le

1. ἐπὶ R.

Fig. 21.1. Antyllus' description for the management of the colobomas of the eyebrow with the creation of an H-shaped flap (Bussemaker and Daremberg 1851–1876: BIUM Collection Medica)

tarsus. Then, we make the first incision, shaped like a short dart, a little above the hairs, extending from canthus to canthus, and penetrating only the depth of the skin; and afterwards we perform the incision called the lunated, beginning at the same place as the former, and carrying it upwards to such a height as to comprehend the whole redundant skin, and ending in like manner. Thus the whole skin comprehended within the incisions will have the shape of a myrtle leaf, of which portion, having perforated the angle on the right hand with a hook we dissect away the whole skin: then we unite the lips of the incision by three or four sutures, beginning at the middle and passing the needle itself through the under-section. Having cut away the superfluity of the thread, not close to the sutures, but so as to leave a superfluity of three fingers breadth, we stretch this remainder along the forehead and fasten it by means of any of the agglutinative plasters...' (Adams 1844–1847, vol. ii, 259).

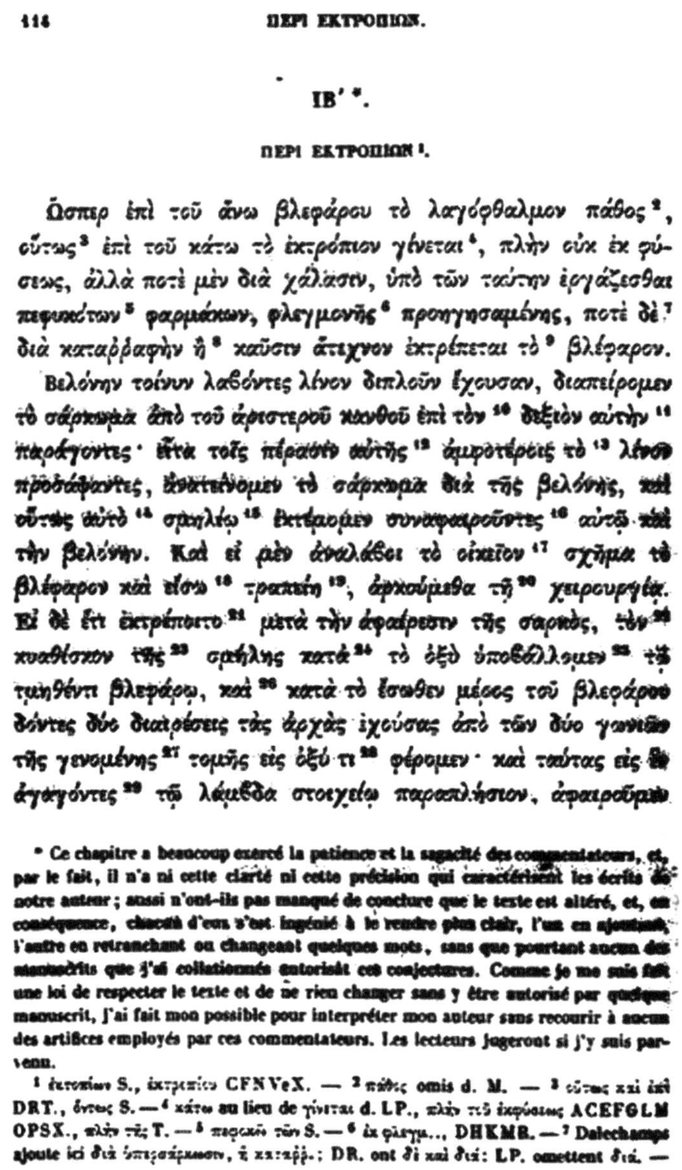

114 ΠΕΡΙ ΕΚΤΡΟΠΙΩΝ.

ΙΒʹ *.

ΠΕΡΙ ΕΚΤΡΟΠΙΩΝ [1].

Ὥσπερ ἐπὶ τοῦ ἄνω βλεφάρου τὸ λαγόφθαλμον πάθος [2], οὕτως [3] ἐπὶ τοῦ κάτω τὸ ἐκτρόπιον γίνεται [4], πλὴν οὐκ ἐκ φύσεως, ἀλλὰ ποτὲ μὲν διὰ χάλασιν, ὑπὸ τῶν ταύτην ἐργάζεσθαι πεφυκότων [5] φαρμάκων, φλεγμονῆς [6] προηγησαμένης, ποτὲ δὲ [7] διὰ καταῤῥαφὴν ἢ [8] καῦσιν ἄτεχνον ἐκτρέπεται τὸ [9] βλέφαρον.

Βελόνην τοίνυν λαβόντες λίνον διπλοῦν ἔχουσαν, διαπείρομεν τὸ σάρκωμα ἀπὸ τοῦ ἀριστεροῦ κανθοῦ ἐπὶ τὸν [10] δεξιὸν αὐτὴν [11] παράγοντες· εἶτα τοῖς πέρασιν αὐτῆς [12] ἀμφοτέροις τὸ [13] λίνον προσάψαντες, ἀνατείνομεν τὸ σάρκωμα διὰ τῆς βελόνης, καὶ οὕτως αὐτὸ [14] σμιλίῳ [15] ἐκτέμνομεν συναφαιροῦντες [16] αὐτῷ καὶ τὴν βελόνην. Καὶ εἰ μὲν ἀναλάβοι τὸ οἰκεῖον [17] σχῆμα τὸ βλέφαρον καὶ εἴσω [18] τραπείη [19], ἀρκούμεθα τῇ [20] χειρουργίᾳ. Εἰ δὲ ἔτι ἐκτρέποιτο [21] μετὰ τὴν ἀφαίρεσιν τῆς σαρκὸς, τὸν [22] κυαθίσκον τῆς [23] σμίλης κατὰ [24] τὸ ὀξὺ ὑποβάλλομεν [25] τῷ τμηθέντι βλεφάρῳ, καὶ [26] κατὰ τὸ ἔσωθεν μέρος τοῦ βλεφάρου δόντες δύο διαιρέσεις τὰς ἀρχὰς ἐχούσας ἀπὸ τῶν δύο γωνιῶν τῆς γενομένης [27] τομῆς εἰς ὀξύ τι [28] φέρομεν· καὶ ταύτας εἰς ἓν ἀγαγόντες [29] τῷ λάμβδα στοιχείῳ παραπλήσιον, ἀφαιροῦμεν

* Ce chapitre a beaucoup exercé la patience et la sagacité des commentateurs, et, par le fait, il n'a ni cette clarté ni cette précision qui caractérisent les écrits de notre auteur; aussi n'ont-ils pas manqué de conclure que le texte est altéré, et, en conséquence, chacun d'eux s'est ingénié à le rendre plus clair, l'un en ajoutant, l'autre en retranchant ou changeant quelques mots, sans que pourtant aucun des manuscrits que j'ai collationnés autorisât ces conjectures. Comme je me suis fait une loi de respecter le texte et de ne rien changer sans y être autorisé par quelque manuscrit, j'ai fait mon possible pour interpréter mon auteur sans recourir à aucun des artifices employés par ces commentateurs. Les lecteurs jugeront si j'y suis parvenu.

[1] ἐκτροπίων S., ἐκτροπίου CFNVeX. — [2] πάθος omis d. M. — [3] οὕτως καὶ ἐπὶ DRT., ὄντως S. — [4] κάτω au lieu de γίνεται d. LP., πλὴν τοῦ ἐκφύσεως ACEFGLMOPSX., πλὴν τῆς T. — [5] παρακειμένων S. — [6] ἐκ φλεγμ.., DHKMR. — [7] Dalechamps ajoute ici διὰ ὑπερσάρκωσιν, ἢ καταῤῥ.; DR. ont δὲ καὶ διά: LP. omettent διά. —

Fig. 21.2. Paul's description of the operation for ectropion (French translation of the *Epitome*: BIUM Collection Medica)

On adhesion of the eyelids

The adhesions of the upper eyelid represent a distinct chapter in the sixth book of the *Epitome*. Paul writes:

> 'The upper eyelid undergoes adhesion sometimes to the lower tarsus, sometimes to the conjunctiva, and sometimes to the cornea itself, obstructing the motions of the eye. Applying an ear-specillum to the broad margin of the eyelid, or stretching it with a hook-like instrument, we free the adhesion with the scalpel used in the operation for pterygia (pterygotomos), taking care that the cornea is not wounded. After the incision and after having bathed the eye, we separate the eyelids with tents, to avoid the recreation of the adhesion' (Adams 1844–1847, vol. ii, 272).

Nose

In the 26th chapter of his work, Oribasius describes the operation for the defects of the nose, again with the creation of an H-shaped flap (Lascaratos, Cohen and Voros 1998, 1275–6):

> 'The defects on the tip of the nose are treated in the same way as a defect on the eyebrow. We create a square defect and extend the horizontal sides of the square towards the alae. We undermine the two flaps and bring them together towards the nasal tip. The same stands for defects in the columella but in this case the flaps are vertical' (Fig. 21.4a–c).
>
> 'If there is a defect on the ala, we create a square defect around the original one and extend the vertical lines of the square towards the medical canthus medially and the eyelid

I′.

ΠΕΡΙ ΛΑΓΟΦΘΑΛΜΩΝ.

Λαγοφθάλμους καλοῦσι τοὺς τὸ[1] ἄνω βλέφαρον ἀνεσπασμένον[2] ἔχοντας. Τοῦτο δὲ γίνεται τὸ[3] πάθος ἢ φυσικῶς, ἢ ἐξ οὐλῆς τραύματος· καὶ τούτου[4] ἢ αὐτομάτως, ἢ ὑπὸ[5] ἀναῤῥαφῆς[6], ἢ καύσεως, ὡς ἀρτίως ἐλέγομεν, ἀφυῶς γεγενημένης. Ἐφ' ἧς καὶ μόνου[7] μετρία δύναται γενέσθαι διόρθωσις, πάχος ἱκανὸν ἔχοντος[8] τοῦ βλεφάρου· οὐ[9] δεῖ γὰρ αὐτὴν τὴν οὐλὴν ἐπιδιελόντα[10] καὶ διαστήσαντα τὰ[11] χείλη διὰ μοτοῦ[12], καὶ δεσμῷ[13] πάντως ἄχρι τελείας ἀποθέσεως[14] χρῆσθαι, μὴ τοῖς ἄγαν[15] ξηραίνουσι χρώμενον[16], ἀλλὰ τοῖς χαλαστικωτέροις[17]

[1] τὸ omis d. F. — [2] ἐσπασμένον LP., ἔχοντα LP. — [3] τὸ omis d. R. — [4] ταύτης DHKR., τοῦτο E. — [5] ἀπὸ LP. — [6] φαρμάκου au lieu de ἀναῤῥαφῆς M.; ἢ est omis dans ABCDFGHJKLMOPRT. — [7] μόνης P. — [8] ἔχον τὸ βλέφαρον ABCDFGHJKLNOPTRSVeBa. — [9] οὐ δεῖ Ve., εἰ δεῖ ABCFMOT., εἰδῇ S., οὐδὴ L... XEBa., d'accord avec Cornarius et d'autres commentateurs, rejettent οὐ; cependant, j'ai cru devoir conserver ce mot, parce qu'il est dans les meilleurs manuscrits,

Fig. 21.3. Paul's description of the surgical management of lagophthalmos (French translation of the *Epitome*: BIUM Collection Medica)

laterally, and after undermining we suture them. We do not agree with surgeons who use flaps from the nasal tip to correct such a defect' (Fig. 21.5a & b).

As mentioned above the square defect technique can also be used for the correction of aural deficiencies.

Nasal fractures

Oribasius follows exactly the Hippocratic treatment in cases of contusion of the nose avoiding the application of complicated bandaging and recommending a simple bandage with a poultice (Lascaratos *et al.* 2003, 161).

According to Paul, the three steps in the management of nasal fractures are restoration, packing and bandaging. In addition, the problem of nasal respiration after packing had been solved by the use of quills made from goose feathers wrapped into rags. Special packing nasal attachments with tubes helping nasal respiration have only been introduced in the last two decades (Skoulakis *et al.* 2008, 280–1).

The Carmagnola head

The Carmagnola head (Fig. 21.6) is placed on the balustrade of the exterior balcony of the Basilica of San Marco in Venice. The porphyry head is believed to be a sculpture of the Early Byzantine period, looted by the Venetians during the capture of Constantinople in 1204.

The statue's name

The origin of the statue's name is much in doubt. 'Carmagnola' was the nickname of Francesco Bussone, a Venetian traitorous condottiere who was found guilty of betrayal and connivance with the enemy and beheaded in Piazzetta in 1432. The reason why this particular name was chosen from the thousands of similar cases of this period remains a mystery (Breckenridge 1981, 1).

The sculpted nose

The most outstanding feature of the sculpture is definitely its nose, which has an extremely flat profile: a gouge in the front section and a furrow cut transversely across the base of the missing nostrils. These irregularities seem to have been made intentionally and not as a result of damage.

Identification

The historical identification of the person represented is

controversial. It was taken for granted that the person was a sovereign of the Late Empire, not only because of the crown but also because red porphyry was considered a very special stone, reserved almost exclusively for imperial portraits. Various suggestions about the emperor's name have been put forward, the most probable being Justinian II (the Rhinotmetus) or Justinian I.

Justinian II, Rhinotmetus

Justinian II was first deposed in AD 695 by Leontios. He had his nose cut off (hence his nickname Rhinotmetus i.e. the split-nosed) with the intent of forever preventing him from returning to power, since an unblemished appearance

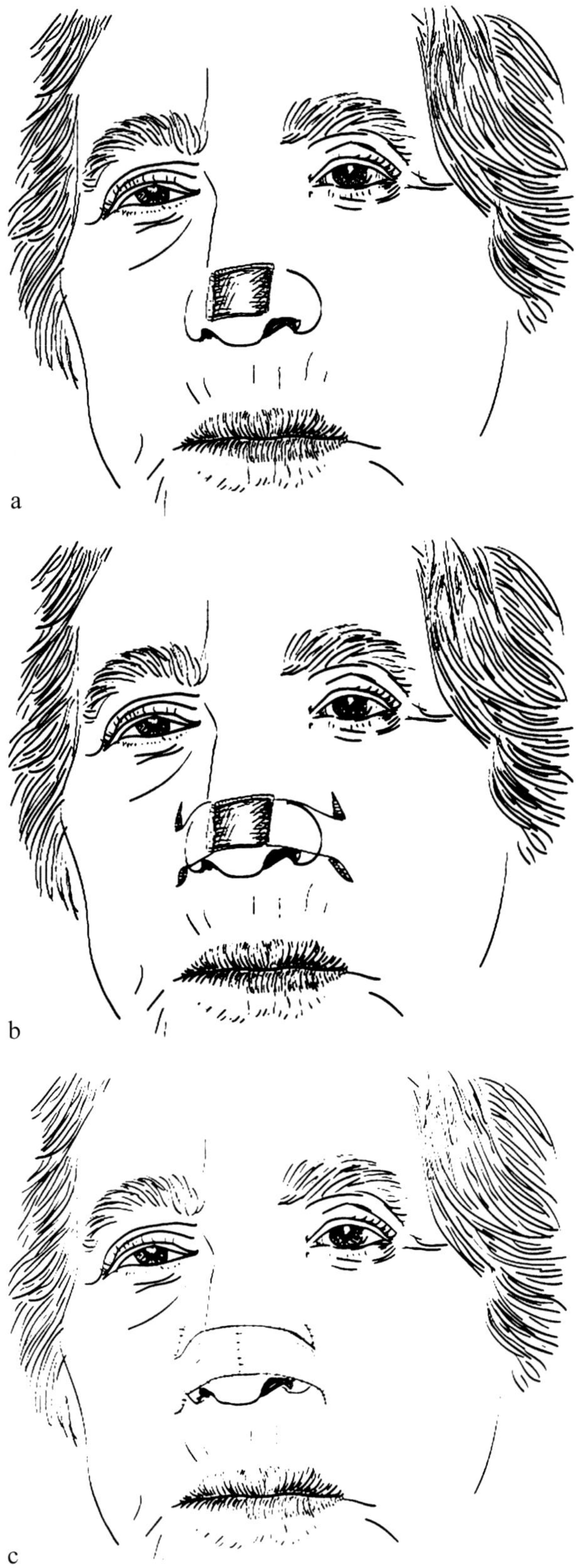

Figs 21.4a–c. Correction of defects on the tip of the nose according to Oribasius' technique (created by the plastic surgeon Dr A. Manios)

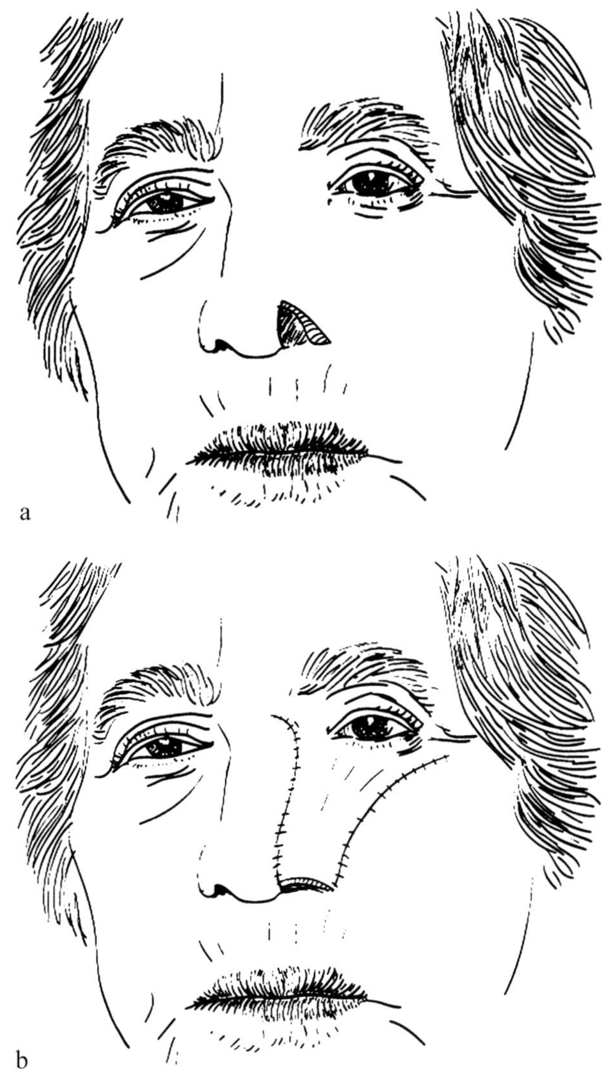

Figs 21.5a–b. Correction of defects on the ala according to Oribasius' technique (created by the plastic surgeon Dr A. Manios)

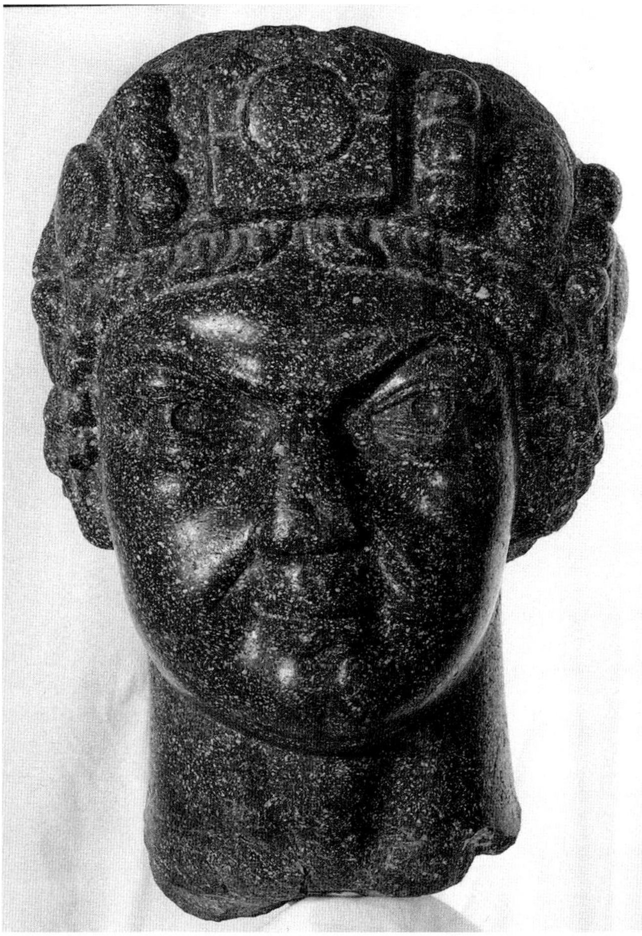

Fig. 21.6. The Carmagnola head, Basilica of San Marco in Venice (http://www.museosanmarco.it/WAI/images/potere/carmagnola.jpg).

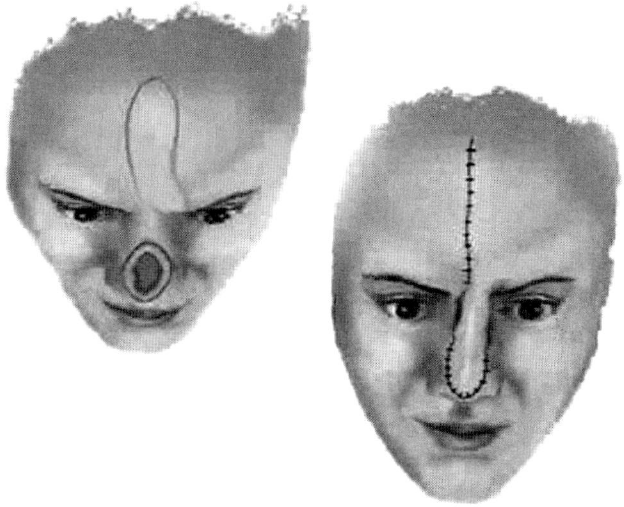

Fig. 21.7. Nasal reconstruction using an Indian flap (created by the plastic surgeon Dr A. Manios)

was a requirement of imperial rule. He was banished to Cherson on the Crimean peninsula but he reclaimed his throne in 705 before his permanent removal in 711.

The art historian Richard Delbrück suggested in 1914 that the Carmagnola head depicts Justinian II Rhinotmetus, noting that the nasal abnormalities represent a nasal reconstruction with an Indian forehead flap, carried out to help him regain the throne (Delbrück 1914, 71–89). In the Indian method, skin is taken from the forehead and brought down from the root of the nose toward the nostrils to cover the defect (Fig. 21.7). In 1979, three plastic surgeons (Remensnyder, Bigelow and Goldwyn) examined the statue and found 'definite irregularities (scars?) in the nose and forehead, suggesting a donor area and a recipient site of an Indian forehead flap'. But they wonder 'If Justinian the Rhinotmetus did have a nasal reconstruction, how was the knowledge of the technique transmitted from northern India to the Byzantine Empire by the end of the 7th century?'. Furthermore, the Indian flap cannot sufficiently explain all the nasal irregularities and this cannot be attributed only to poor surgical technique. The forehead, too, does not seem to us to give the impression of a scarred and re-stitched skin.

For all these reasons, our opinion is that a nasal reconstruction with the Indian method is impossible. Nevertheless, the curious nasal conformation could be the result of a reconstructive rhinoplasty according to Oribasius' technique. The H-shaped flap described above can explain the gouge in the frontal section (compare with Fig. 21.4c). In this case, the mild forehead abnormalities can be considered as highlighted normal wrinkles.

Justinian I

Another theory, given more credit today, is that the sculpture represents Justinian I, last emperor of the Eastern Roman Empire, who reigned from AD 527 to 565. This theory is based on the portrait of this sovereign's gold coins minted at Constantinople in the 530s. Justinian I, unlike Justinian II, did not have his nose cut off but, according to Körbler's theory, he contracted syphilis from his wife Theodora (Körbler 1974). Syphilis can cause destructive lesions of the nasal septum and therefore alter the nasal appearance (saddle nose), but this complication is more common in patients suffering from the congenital form of the disease.

Conclusions

The principles of reconstruction in the Byzantine period followed the same patterns of mobilisation and preparation of local flaps as those used today. Although the applied flaps were different, they seemed to suit their basic purpose, which was the correction of skin deficiencies.

Notes

1 The succeeding emperors, Valentinian and Valens, were not favourably disposed towards Oribasius. They confiscated his property and banished him, but, in the end, recognising the magnitude of his professional skills, they recalled him from banishment, restored his confiscated fortune, and loaded him with honours.

2 Ectropion is usually caused by the aging process and the weakening of the connective tissue of the eyelid. It can also be caused by contraction of the scar tissue from burns or from facial palsy and may occur as a congenital defect.

3 We now know that hares are able to close their eyes when sleeping. For this reason, the term lagophthalmos nowadays is not very common and has been replaced by the term 'ectropion of the upper eyelid'.

Bibliography

Adams, F. 1844–1847: *The Seven Books of Paulus Aegineta*, London.

Breckenridge, J. 1981: 'Again the "Carmagnola"', *Gesta* 20, 1–7.

Briau, R. 1855: *Chirurgie de Paul d'Égine*, Paris.

Bussemaker, U. C. and Daremberg, C. 1851–1876: *Oeuvres d'Oribase*, Vols 1–6, Paris.

Delbrück, R. 1914: 'Carmagnola: porträt eines byzantinischen Kaisers', *Römischen Mitteilungen des Kaiserlich Deutschen Archäologischen Instituts* 29, 71–89.

Dumont, D. S. and Smith, R. M. (eds) 1992: *Thesaurus Linguae Graecae*: CD ROM Musaios, Version 10d-32, California.

Körbler, J. 1974: 'Die Krebswerkrankung der byzantinischen Kaiserin Theodora (Ein Betrag zur Geschichte der Syphilis)', *Janus* 61, 15–22.

Lascaratos, J., Cohen, M. and Voros, D. 1998: 'Plastic surgery of the face in Byzantium in the fourth century', *Plastic and Reconstructive Surgery* 102, 1274–80.

Lascaratos, J., Segas, J., Trompoukis, C. and Assimakopoulos, D. 2003: 'From the roots of rhinology: the reconstruction of nasal injuries by Hippocrates', *Annals of Otolology, Rhinology and Laryngology* 112, 159–62.

Remensnyder, J., Bigelow, M. and Goldwyn, R. 1979: 'Justinian II and Carmagnola: a Byzantine rhinoplasty?', *Plastic and Reconstructive Surgery* 63(1), 19–25.

Skoulakis, C., Manios, A., Theos, E., Papadakis, C. and Stavroulaki, P. 2008: 'Treatment of nasal fractures by Paul of Aegina', *Otolaryngology – Head and Neck Surgery* 138, 279–82.

Van de Graaf, R., Ijpma, F. and Nicolai, J. P. 2008: 'Lagophthalmos or hare eye: an etymologic eye opener', *Aesthetic Plastic Surgery* 32(3), 573–4.

Part VI

Medicaments and Cures

22. The Headache Remedies of the *Pseudo-Apuleius*. A Modern Reappraisal

Giorgio Zanchin

The Codex Vindobonensis *93 is a manuscript on vellum, presumably copied in the first half of the 13th century, which is preserved in the National Library in Vienna (Talbot and Unterkirchen 1972). Among the collection of late classical works on* Materia Medica *it contains, we examined, under the profile of headache treatment and of the related iconography, the so-called* Pseudo-Apuleius. *One of the most used herbals of the late classical period, it lists 127 illuminated plants, along with their therapeutic qualities. Thirteen plants are indicated for headache, although in generic terms (ten* 'ad capitis dolorem'*, two* 'ad capitem deplendum'*), except in one case (*'ad imicraniam'*). In seven cases the illuminated herb is accompanied by a representation of the headache sufferer. Both from the herb recommended* 'ad imicraniam'*, i.e. the opium-containing* 'papaver silvaticum'*, and the peculiar assistance given to the patient, it is evident that the anonymous illuminator makes a net distinction between a migrainous attack in comparison to a more generic headache. The interest of the author in headaches is clearly demonstrated: indeed, about ten per cent of the herbs considered are indicative of this ailment. We are at present completing a search of modern pharmaceutical studies showing, at least in some of the plants of these series, the presence of substances potentially effective against headache.*

Introduction

The name *Codex Vindobonensis 93* identifies a manuscript on vellum, presumably copied in the first half of the 13th century, which is preserved in the National Library in Vienna (*Codex Vindobonensis 93*, Facsimile vol. xxvii, 1972). Compiled from different Greek and Roman sources, mainly Pliny and Dioscorides, it consists of a richly illuminated codex of Latin works on the therapeutic use of plants and animals. The fine, full colour pictures include the representation of patients, doctors and nurses. Among the collection of the classical works on *Materia Medica* it contains, we examined, under the profile of the headache treatment and of the related iconography, the so-called *Pseudo-Apuleius*.

This manuscript brings us one of the most commonly used herbals of later classical times. The original was written in Latin, some time before the 5th century by an unknown author who was not a professional physician. This accounts for his negative presentation of doctors, whom he describes as professionally inadequate and more interested in profit than the patient's care; and for his magic, superstitious beliefs, evidenced by the use of herbs as amulets (e.g. *'plantago'*, that we will consider soon) and by the rituals prescribed in the gathering of the plants which, if in some instances (e.g. plucking them before the rising or setting of the sun, or at a special time of the year) they are in keeping with the principles of the official medicine of the time, reveal also the acceptance of magic beliefs (e.g. walking away without looking back).

Results and discussion

Precious manuscripts were already adorned with illuminated pictures from the Hellenistic period. In herbals, however, the iconography was not merely exornative, but particularly relevant in integrating the written description, since it was from the illumination that the reader would learn the morphological features of the plant, which would allow its precise identification in the field for practical, therapeutic uses.

When, at the end of the 1st century AD, the vellum codex was added to the papyrus roll as a new writing support, the

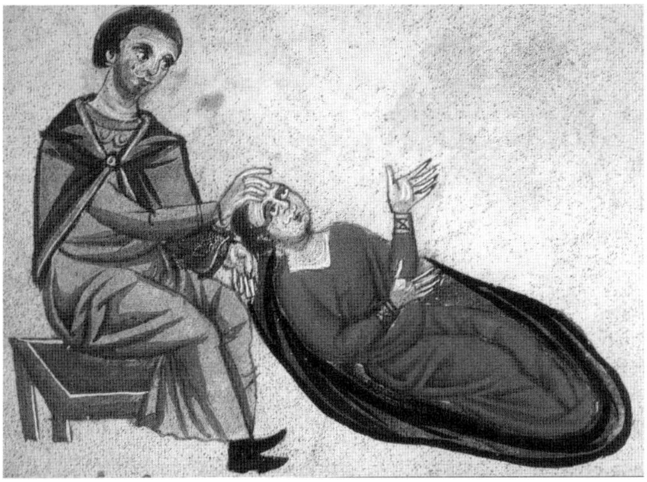

Fig. 22.1. Assistance given '*ad capitis dolorem*' (*Codex Vindobonensis* 93, f. 14 v. Facsimile vol. XXVII. Reproduced courtesy of Akademische Druck, u. Verlanganstalt, Graz, 1972).

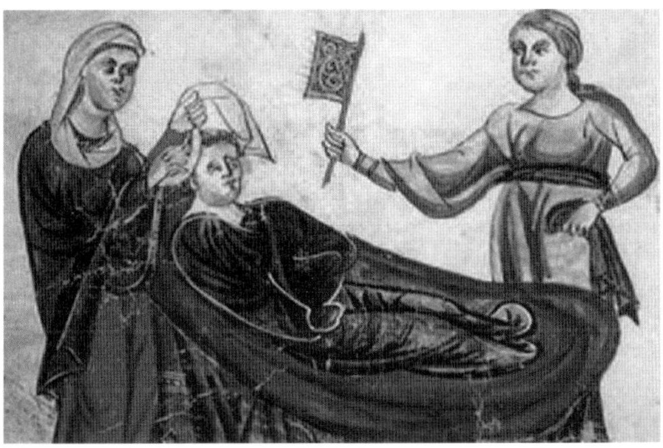

Fig. 22.2. Assistance given '*ad imicraniam*'. In this illuminated scene the intensity and the accompanying symptoms of a migraine attack are well represented (*Codex Vindobonensis* 93, f. 65 v).

iconography continued to embellish and enrich the text. Although the plant representations were probably originally based on naturalistic models, being repeatedly copied they could be expected to become less and less recognisable. However, a comparative study of this version of the *Pseudo-Apuleius* shows that in many cases the illustrations of plants are fairly faithful, despite about seven hundred years having elapsed between the Codex and its ancestor manuscript.

The *Pseudo-Apuleius* lists 127 illuminated plants, together with their therapeutic qualities. Thirteen plants were found to bear the therapeutic indication for headache, although in generic terms (ten '*ad capitis dolorem*'; two '*ad capitem deplendum*'), except in one case ('*ad imicraniam*'). Therefore, we can clearly realise the interest of the author in headaches: indeed, about ten per cent of the herbs considered are indicated for this ailment.

In seven cases the illuminated herb is accompanied by a representation of the headache sufferer, usually attended by one or two characters: these are giving a massage or spreading the remedy on the patient's head (Fig. 22.1).

The sole case bearing a specific indication for migraine therapy shows a visibly very suffering patient, lying down in bed. Two women are assisting him: one is holding a handkerchief to be put on his forehead, the other is refreshing him with a fan (Fig. 22.2). The scene describes with evident emphasis the incapacitating intensity of the pain and the presence of accompanying symptoms typical of a migraine attack. This peculiar assistance, requiring two persons, and the herb prescribed, the opium-containing '*papaver silvaticum*', underlines the distinction made by the anonymous illuminator between migraine and a more generic, milder headache (Zanchin *et al.* 2010). Indeed, in this latter condition (Fig. 22.1), a more limited assistance, with the nursing of just one person, is offered; moreover, an evidently less suffering patient is represented and a much lighter therapy, '*anethum*' (Fig. 22.3), is suggested.

We will now consider the herbs recommended in the *Pseudo-Apuleius* for the aches of the head in the light of present knowledge, and examine their possible therapeutic action. In other words, what is the efficacy of these plants from a modern pharmacological perspective? Bearing in mind their active components and their present indications, the therapeutic utility on headache of some of them seems to be very mild or nil (Zanchin 2010). For instance, today *anethum* is regarded as a good stomachic for children, but finds no indication for the therapy of headache.

It is probable that in most cases the success of these herbs was founded on the well known placebo effect (Macedo, Farre and Banos 2006; Diener *et al.* 2008), which also today constitutes an ever present problem in the evaluation of the effectiveness of anticephalalgic drugs, able to influence the result obtained with a weight of about 40%. A particular example given is the ritual used to cure the headache with *plantago*. A therapeutic action was supposedly obtained wearing it as a necklace (Fig. 22.4). If, for obvious reasons, we discard the possibility of an absorption by nasal route, in a sense anticipating the modern way of administering anti-migraine drugs as a nasal spray formulation (Treves *et al.* 1998; Dahlöf 1999), we have to admit adherence to a magic belief behind this peculiar method of application, and a placebo effect as the explanation of possible positive results. Even more so, when we assess that the contemporary analysis of the plantago's active components, identified as the mucilage and the fixed oil it contains, shows an action which finds no room in headache therapy, being instead indicated, as demulcent, for bronchitis and diarrhoea.

However, still today, in addition to the opium-containing

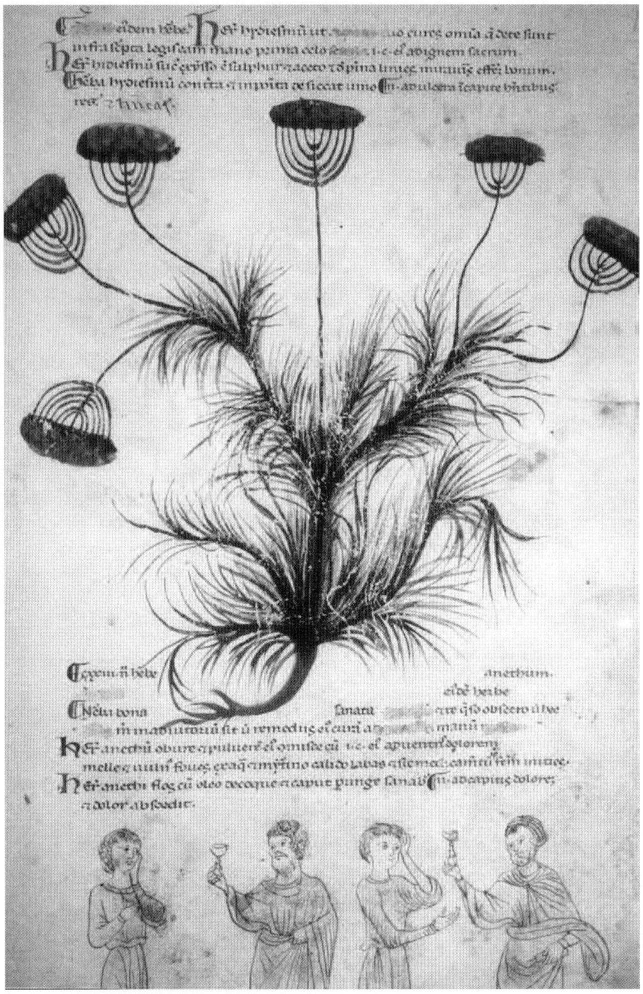

Fig. 22.3. *Anethum* (*Codex Vindobonensis* 93, f. 112 r).

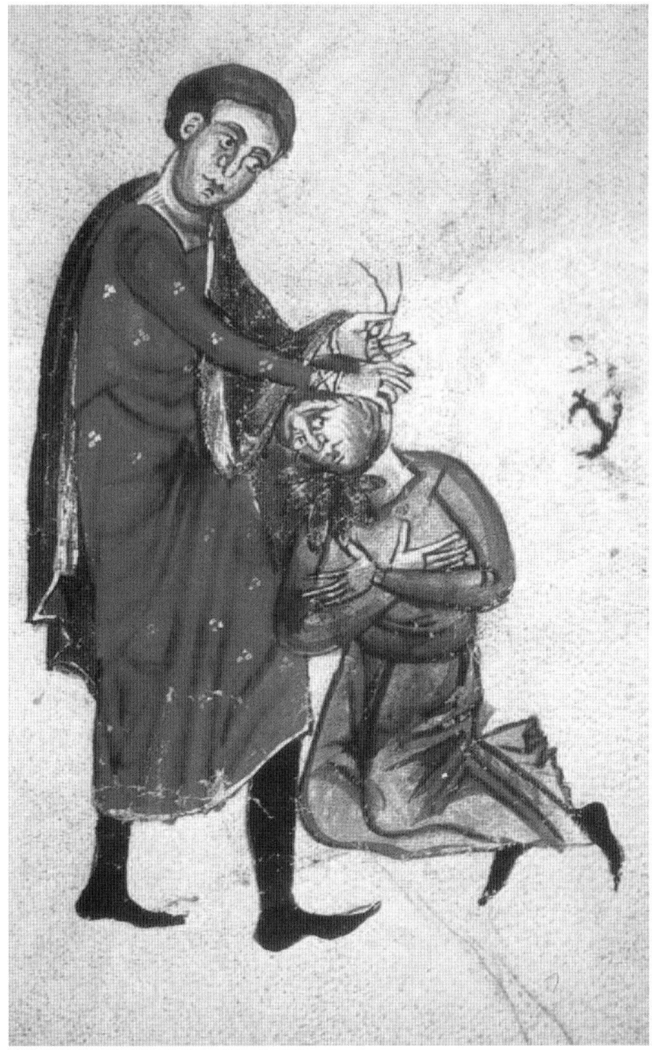

Fig. 22.4. The *plantago* effect was supposedly obtained wearing this plant as a necklace (*Codex Vindobonensis* 93, f. 10 v).

poppy (*Papaver silvaticum*), with its recognised strong analgesic and sedative actions, we can find a suggestion as a remedy indicated for the headache at least for some of these herbs, although there are no double blind clinical studies confirming their effectiveness. We are at present carrying out a detailed analysis of the contemporary pharmaceutical literature, which in some instances assesses in the plants of this series the presence of active principles potentially useful against headache.

Bibliography

Dahlöf, C. 1999: 'Sumatriptan nasal spray in the acute treatment of migraine: a review of clinical studies', *Cephalalgia* 19, 769–78.

Diener, H.-C., Schorn, C. F., Bingel, U. and Dodick, D. W. 2008: 'The importance of placebo in headache research', *Cephalalgia* 28, 1003–11.

Macedo, A., Farre, M. and Banos, J. E. 2006: 'A meta-analysis of the placebo response in acute migraine and how this response may be influenced by some of the characteristics of clinical trials', *European Journal of Clinical Pharmacology* 62, 161–72.

Talbot, C. H. and Unterkirchen, F. (eds): *Medicina Antiqua. Libri quatuor Medicinae, codex Vindobonensis 93 der Österreichische National Bibliothek* (Facsimile vol. xxvii), Graz.

Treves, T. A., Kuritzky, A., Hering, R. and Korczyn, A. D. 1998: 'Dihydroergotamine nasal spray in the treatment of acute migraine', *Headache* 38, 614–7.

Zanchin, G. 2010: 'Headache: an historical outline', 375–86 in S. Finger, F. Boller and K. L. Tyler (eds), *History of Neurology* (Handbook of Clinical Neurology, Vol. I, 95, 3rd series), London.

Zanchin, G., Mainardi, F., Dainese, F. and Maggioni F. 2010: 'La cefalea: introduzione storica, 1–13 in L. A. Pini, P. Sarchielli and G. Zanchin (eds), *Trattato italiano delle cefalee*, Turin.

23. Compound Medicines in Antiquity: a First Approach

Alain Touwaide

Therapeutic literature in Classical Greece, from the Corpus Hippocraticum *(mainly 5th and 4th centuries BC) to Dioscorides'* De Materia Medica *(1st century AD) and to Galen (AD 129 – after [?] 216), contains numerous formulas for the preparation of medicines that have not been the object of much scholarly attention, apart from repeated studies of the* Materia Medica, *particularly the plants. In the context of the research programme 'Medicinal plants of Antiquity' aimed to sum up the information on the plants used as medicines in the Classical World, these formulas are submitted to a rigorous scientific analysis: not only the* Materia Medica *of the three kingdoms (vegetal, mineral and animal), but also the excipients, ligands and other substances, and the formulas themselves. This paper presents the first data of this research, with a special emphasis on the* Corpus Hippocraticum.

For a long time medicines in classical antiquity were made of a single ingredient with the addition of an excipient[1] and possibly one or more other substances aimed to alter – or compensate for – any undesired quality or effect of the medicine, such as a bitter taste in the case of a medicine to be taken internally, or an irritating property in the case of a medicine applied externally (Touwaide 2007a). Such strategy, which certainly dates back to the origin of the art of healing, was surveyed in the 1st century AD by Dioscorides (Touwaide 2007b; Scarborough 2007) in his work *Περὶ ὕλης ἰατρικῆς* (Wellmann 1906–1914; Beck 2005) according to its Greek title and *De Materia Medica* in an exact Latin translation, which is an encyclopaedia of the natural products of vegetal, animal and mineral origin used to prepare medicines and known to its author.

According to a historiography that is now traditional,[2] another therapeutic strategy developed from a period that is not exactly known but usually identified as the 1st century BC/1st century AD (although its origin has been pushed back to *c.* 300 BC: Watson 1966, 11): compound medicines, that is, medicines made of more than one active ingredient. Such supposedly new approach to pharmaceutical therapy is considered to have reached its zenith with the Cretan physician Andromachos (Nutton 2008; Touwaide 2008), archiater to the Roman emperor Nero (emp. AD 54–68), who composed a formula for a drug made of more than 80 ingredients (edition of the Greek text in Heitsch 1963–4, vol. 2, 8–15). Whatever its novelty and origin, this strategy was largely echoed in the therapeutic treatises by Galen (AD 129 – after [?] 216) (Nutton 2004, with extensive bibliography; Hankinson 2008), principally *De Antidotis* (*On Antidotes*) (Kuhn 1827, 1–105 [Book 1] and 106–209 [Book 2]) and *De Theriaca ad Pisonem* (*On Theriac, to Piso*) (Kuhn 1827, 210–94; Latin text with Italian translation in Coturri 1959). I exclude the booklet *De Theriaca ad Pamphilianum* (*On Theriac, to Pamphilianus*), as it is most probably inauthentic (see Nutton 1997). Also, it greatly developed later on, be it in the Arabic world, the medieval west, or the Renaissance,[3] and has been the object of intense theoretical and philosophical speculation – particularly in the Arabic world – aimed to evaluate the final therapeutic property of the medicines resulting from such strategy: was it equal to, higher than, or different from the sum of the properties of the components (including a new property resulting from the interaction of the components between them)?[4]

Whatever their background and interests, modern historians of health sciences have paid only little attention to this change in therapeutics, whenever it occurred and however important it might have been.[5] Generally speaking, they locate its major development in the field of toxicology (venoms and poisons) – and not in therapeutics – and attribute the idea of mixing together a whole range of bio-

Table 23.1. The most ancient physicians credited with the preparation of formulas for compound medicines

Author	*Period*	*Number in Appendix*
Aristogenes of Knidos	260–240 BC	40
Dositheos of Pelousion	250–210 BC	77
Andreas of Karustos	*c.* 250–217 BC	13
Apollophanes of Seleukia 'Pieria'	223–187 BC	34
Arkhagathos of Lakonika	fl. 219 BC	43
Diagoras of Cyprus	220–180 BC?	68

Table 23.2. Vaginal applications

Ingredients							*Form*	**D.W.**[1]	*Littré 1853*
cumin	laurel				incense	honey	tampon	1.75	8.170.1-5
		cypress	pumpkin		incense	honey	tampon	1.75	8.176.6-8
		cypress		rose	incense	honey	tampon	1.75	8.176.2-3

1 *D.W.* for *Diseases of Women*

active components to the king of Pontos Mithridates VI Eupator (b. 132; king 120; d. 63 BC) (Olshausen 2006), renowned for having absorbed increasing doses of poisons (starting with sub-lethal doses) so as to generate a reaction of tolerance (now called *mithridatism*, precisely because of Mithridates) and to become immune to possible criminal intoxications.[6] The historiographical tradition built on these premises analyses the subsequent history of compound medicines as a development of Mithridates' formula, however problematic the evidence is (Totelin 2004), and focuses on one such compound medicine: the theriac created by Andromachos by modifying (actually expanding) Mithridates' formula. Such tradition also studies the place of theriac and such supposedly new strategy in Galen's therapeutics (see e.g. Stein 1997; Jacques 1997), and the continuity in the use of theriac and similar compounds through history (actually until the early 20th century) (see e.g. such a general study on theriac in the Germanic world as Holste (1976), and later a study of a document (primary source) illustrating a moment in the history of theriac: Holste and Keil (1982)). Regarding the therapeutic efficacy of theriac, which has not been explored by any pharmaco-chemical laboratory analysis, works often dismiss the claims of ancient texts by considering that, if theriac had any efficacy, it owed it to only one of its components: opium.

Although fresh work has shed new light on some aspects of theriac, its creation and its epiphenomena,[7] no research has tackled so far the history of compound medicines. The question is complex, as it involves a great multiplicity of aspects and disciplinary fields that need to be brought together and studied in a cross-disciplinary perspective, from botany to therapeutics, including pathology, pharmacology and pharmaceutical technique. It is not my objective here to venture into such study, but only to suggest directions for research. This is all the more necessary because the place of compound medicines in ancient therapeutics was much more important than stated so far in medical history. They were not limited to theriac and its epiphenomena, and were not restricted to toxicological uses, but included a large range of products, and were administered to treat a great variety of pathologies.

As a sign of the quantitative importance and frequency of compound medicines, one could take the number of physicians who are known to have used, developed, or created formulas for such medicines. In the recent *Encyclopedia of Ancient Natural Scientists* (Keyser and Irby-Massie 2008), which includes, for example and among many others, the several authors of compound medicines quoted by Galen in *De antidotis*, as many as half of the pharmacists are credited with a place in the history of compound medicines (see Appendix).[8]

Furthermore, the practice of compound medicines probably started much earlier than the traditional historiography evoked above postulates by focusing on Mithridates. Based on the list in our Appendix,[9] the most ancient physicians credited with the preparation of formulas for compound medicines are listed in Table 23.1, in probable chronological order. On this basis and although the textual

Table 23.3. Wounds in the womb

Ingredients						*Form*	D.W.	*Littré 1853*
celery	perfume			myrrh	incense	injection	1.78	8.194.1-2

Table 23.4. Wounds in the womb with stranguria

Ingredients						*Form*	D.W.	*Littré 1853*
celery	leek	anis	myrrh	incense	wine	injection	1.90	8.216.11-14
							2.209	8.404.7-9

body currently preserved reflects without any doubt only a part of the historical phenomenon under consideration here, it seems safe to consider that the strategy of compound medicines started well before Mithridates, that is, at least around the mid-3rd century BC, if not earlier.

As a first contribution to an analysis of this therapeutic strategy, I present here (Table 23.2) some formulas for compound medicines extracted from the *Corpus Hippocraticum*, specifically the work *Diseases of Women I* (one of the formulas is duplicated in *Diseases of Women II* (see Table 23.4)) dated to the late 5th/early 4th century BC by modern philologico-historical research.[10] The formulas under scrutiny here are relatively simple when compared with those of a later period, and may seem to proceed from a different system of reasoning. However, precisely thanks to their simple nature, they contribute to the understanding of the origin of the strategy of compound medicines, not so much in terms of author(s), place(s), and historical circumstances, but rather as a system aimed to offer the best possible response (that is, the most practical) to requests for health care.

The formulas analysed here are all for gynaecological disorders and can be divided into two major groups: the first group (Table 23.2) includes formulas for vaginal tampons, and the second (Tables 23.3 and 24.4) formulas for two main cases of pathologies in the womb.

The three formulas in the first group contain four ingredients, two of which are present in all four: honey and incense. While honey may be seen as an excipient aimed to amalgamate the other ingredients in a viscous compound – a role that it certainly had – it probably was also an active ingredient, thanks to its antifungal and bactericidal properties (Macdonald Hocking 1997, 378). The second component of all formulas, incense, was not included as a costly, fashionable ingredient according to a recent interpretation of Hippocratic pharmacology (Totelin 2009), but as an anti-inflammatory (Langenheim 2003, 363–8.). The other components added to this basis in the three formulas are cumin and laurel in the first, cypress and pumpkin in the second, and cypress and rose in the third. Apart from the first, which is isolated in the group here, the other two formulas create gradual variations on their common basis, with differentiations probably based on local and/or seasonal availability, and were diuretic, analgesic, or cleaning substances (for the properties of the medicinal plants mentioned in this essay, see e.g. van Wyk and Wink 2004, *passim*).

The formulas in the second group (Tables 23.3–23.4) are all for injections, and were aimed to treat two different cases of womb pathologies: wounds and wounds with stranguria. They contain a minimum of four ingredients and a maximum of six. On a common basis (celery, incense and myrrh), they differ by other components, each of which is a response to the specific condition to be treated.

The common basis includes an anti-inflammatory (incense), an antiseptic agent (myrrh) (Langenheim 2003, 368–73) and a diuretic (celery) (van Wyk and Wink 2004, 399). It was probably aimed at preparing the field for more specific actions by eliminating possible secondary infections (thanks to the action of incense and myrrh) and the possible mechanic action of peripheral organs on the womb, that is, a pressure on the womb in the case the bladder were full (thanks to the diuretic action of celery).

The presence of myrrh and incense should not necessarily be considered as redundant, and favour the idea that these substances have been included in order to create the impression that the medicines were efficacious because they contained exotic, rare and costly substances. Recent scientific research has demonstrated, indeed, that two waves of therapeutic action may be needed, preferably with different agents (so as to avoid the drug-resistance reaction), in order to eliminate pathogens out of the body. The second therapeutic action is, in a certain way, a control, aiming not to leave any pathogen untreated, and to eliminate as much as possible a later relapse.

In the treatment of the wounds in the womb (Table 23.3),

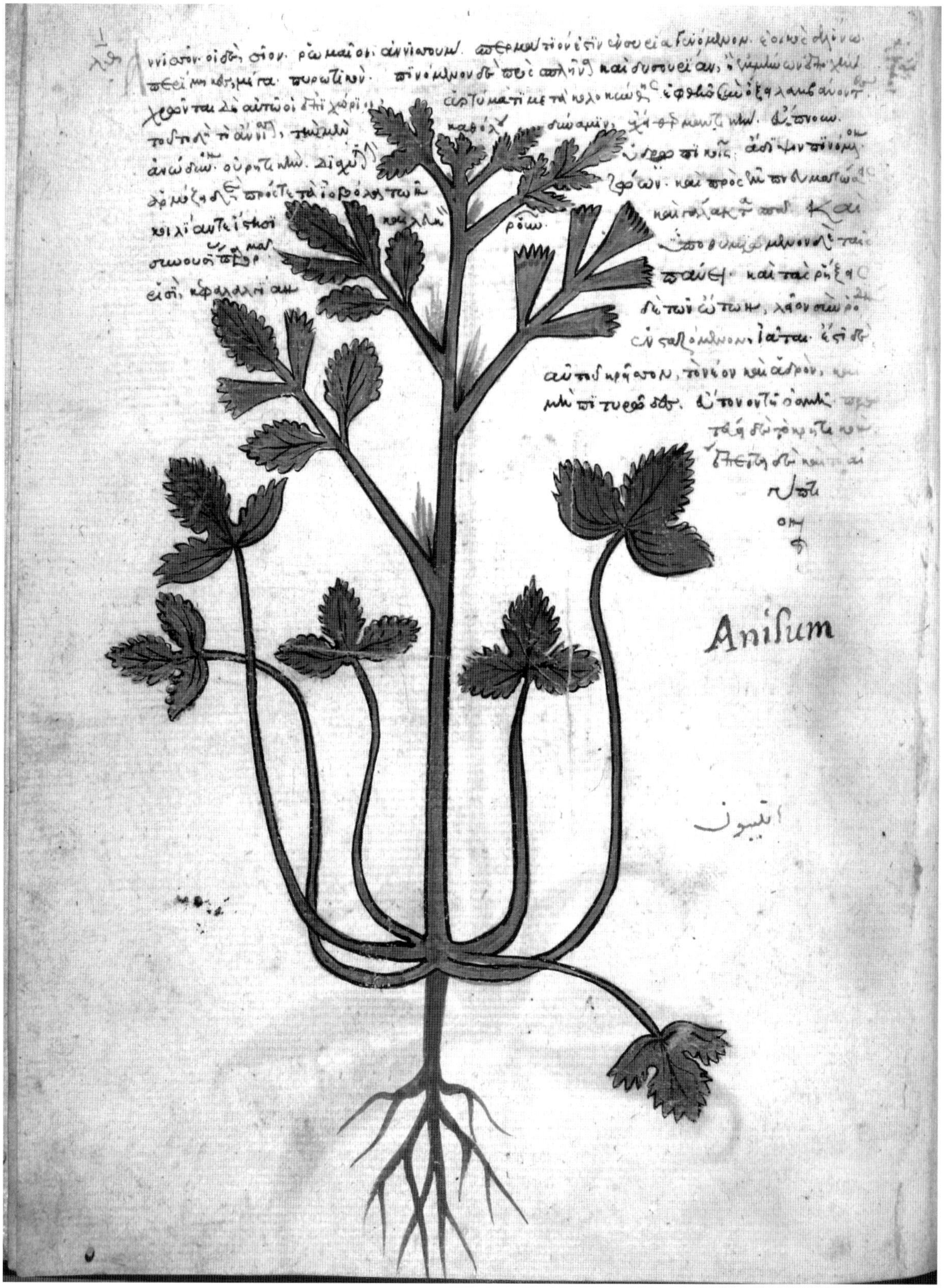

Fig. 23.1. *Anison*, illumination from mid-14th century manuscript (Padua, Biblioteca del Seminario, 194, f. 17v). Padua, Biblioteca del Seminario, 194 is a mid-14th century manuscript written in Constantinople, attributed to (but not necessarily by) Neophytos Prodromênos. It contains extracts (so-called alphabetical herbal) and illustrations from Dioscorides, *De Materia Medica*

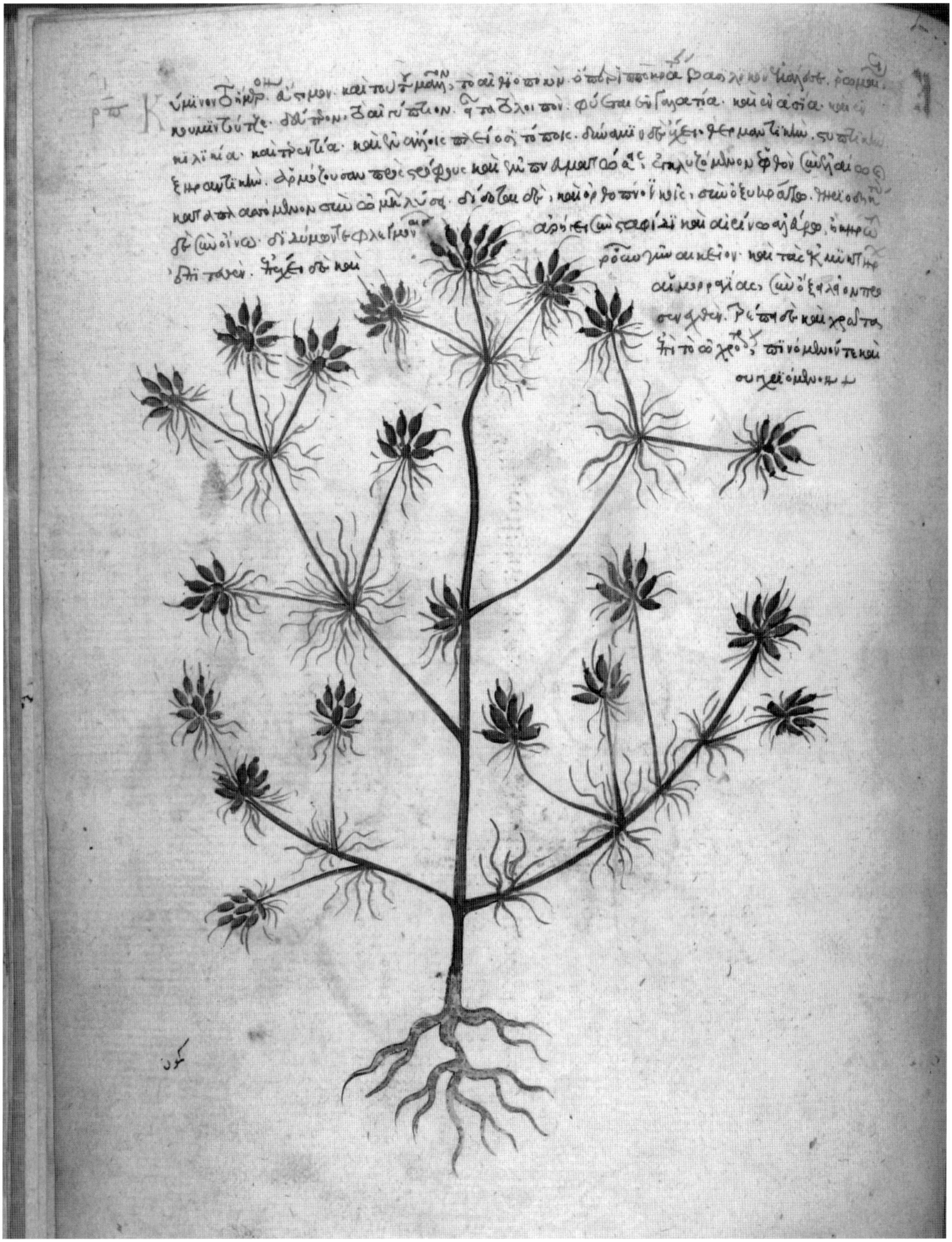

Fig. 23.2. *Kuminon to makron*, illumination from mid-14th century manuscript (Padua, Biblioteca del Seminario, 194, f. 82v)

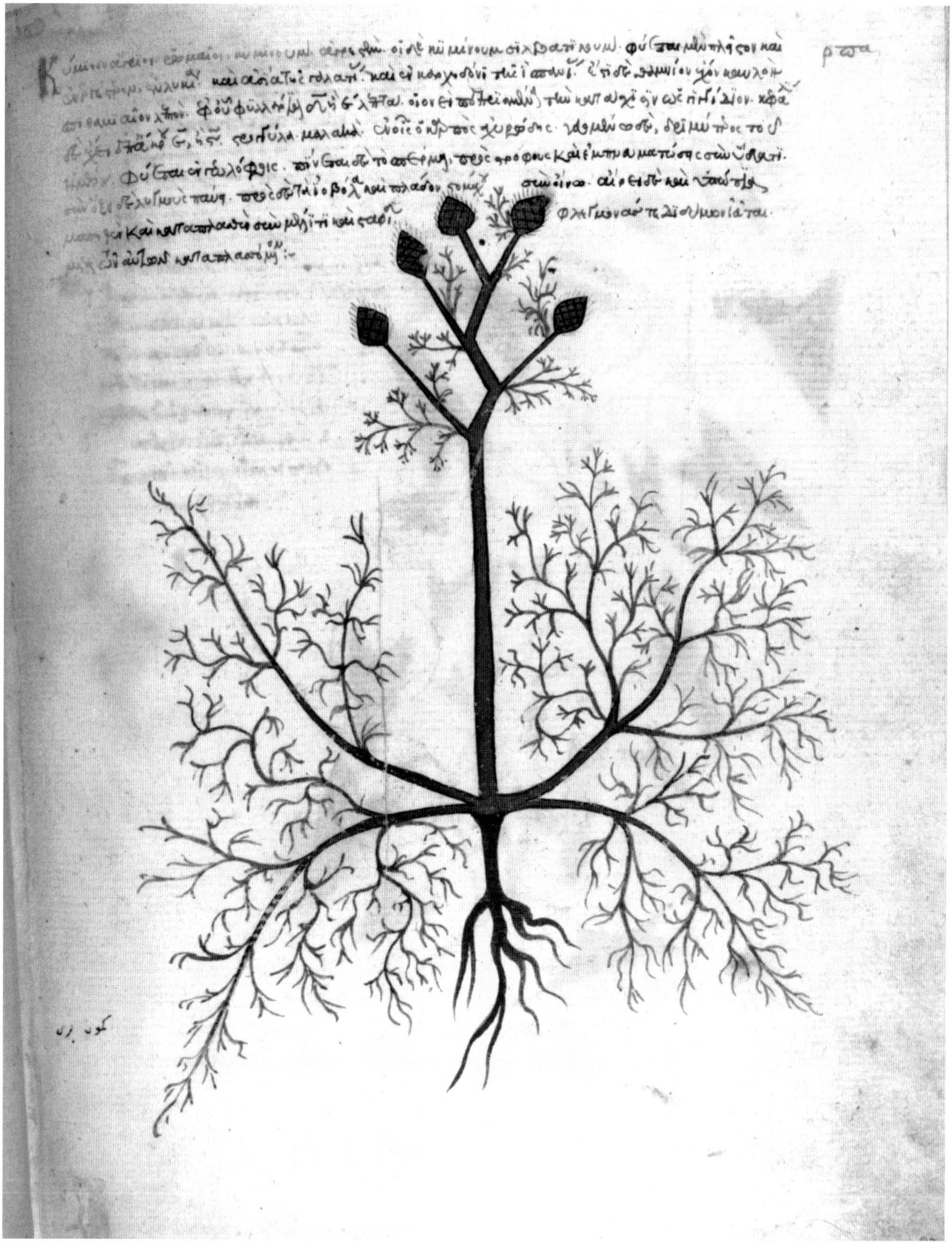

Fig. 23.3 *Kuminon agrion*, illumination from mid-14th century manuscript (Padua, Biblioteca del Seminario, 194, f. 83r)

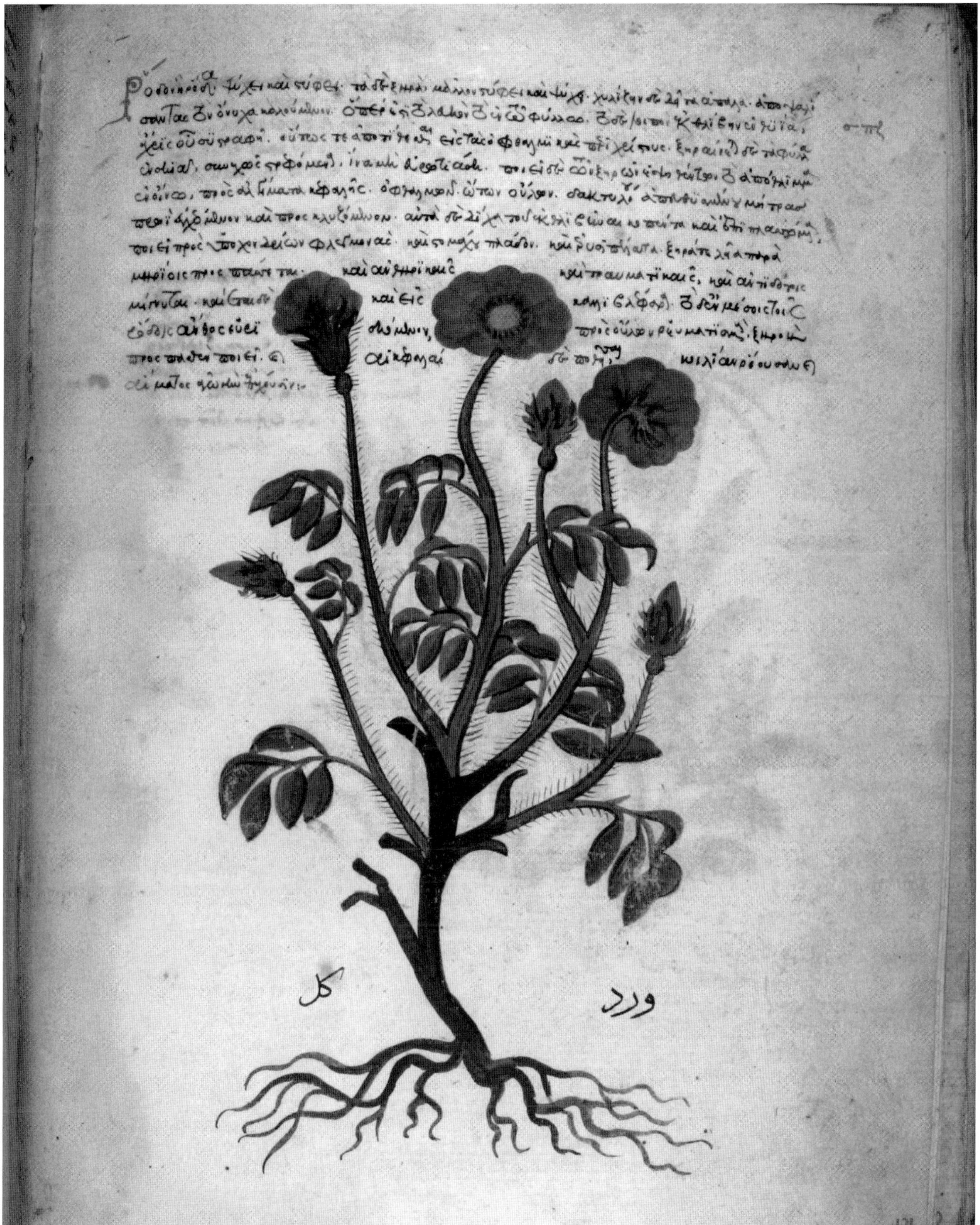

Fig. 23.4. *Rodon*, illumination from mid-14th century manuscript (Padua, Biblioteca del Seminario, 194, f.134 r)

perfume only is added to this basis in the first formula. However strange it may seem, this ingredient was close to what is now called an *essential oil*. It was mainly oil, which probably smoothed the womb thanks to its emollient action (due to its fatty nature), mixed with one or more active principles from plants soaked in the oil.[11] Usually, plants used for perfumes in antiquity were credited with warming properties, that is, were cathartic, stimulant and/or astringent for example.[12] As such, their active principle would certainly have contributed to the treatment of wounds.

The formula for the second infection (Table 23.4) is built on the same basis as the first formula. It cleans the womb, avoids possible secondary infections, provokes a diuresis (leek) and stimulates the organism (anis), probably in order to further increase diuresis.

However limited it is, the analysis above aims to open new avenues for the study of compound medicines. It certainly suggests that the use of compound medicines did not start with Mithridates, did not stem from toxicology, and was not limited to the antecedents of theriac, to theriac or to similar products. It proposes, instead, that compound medicines resulted from a strategy theoretically well-defined and aimed to create medicines with a double nature: general, and appropriate to specific pathologies. To this end, compound medicines mixed two or more groups of components: general ones, which opened the way to the specific therapy by eliminating possible secondary infections and could have been identical in an entire class of medicines, and specific ones, which treated specific pathologies (probably their effects rather than their causes) and varied according to such pathologies. From one group of components to another and within the same group of therapeutic agents, there might have been agents credited with similar if not identical properties and action. This duplication, apparently seeming redundant, may, instead, have been intentional, in order to guarantee the success of the therapy: in some cases, patients may have not responded to one of the two therapeutic agents, and in others two different agents may have been necessary to eliminate the pathogens that could have resisted one of the therapeutic agents.

On this basis, compound medicines seem to have resulted from a well-designed strategy based, on the one hand, on a good, though most probably empirical, knowledge of the pathologies to be treated, and, on the other hand, on an equally good knowledge – and also a skilful mastery – of the therapeutic action(s) and mixture of the natural products used as ingredients of medicines, including non-native substances imported from afar. Contrary to a widely diffused opinion, they do not seem to result from the addition of each of the agents supposedly aimed to treat a specific pathology so as to be efficacious against a broad spectrum of medical conditions.

Also, this analysis suggests that a certain strategy of compound medicines was already familiar at least to the physicians who, in the late 5th and/or early 4th century, authored gynaecological treatises further circulated as part of the *Corpus Hippocraticum*, and that this form of compounding may have resulted from a therapeutic tradition dating far back in time, well before the Hippocratics.

Notes

1 According to *Webster's Encyclopedic Unabridged Dictionary of the English Language* (new revised edition 1989), an excipient is 'a pharmacologically inert, adhesive substance, as honey, syrup, or gum arabic used to bind the contents of a pill or tablet'.

2 The current standard historiography of this question has been largely shaped by the study (still not replaced) by Watson (1966). The existence of formulas for compound medicines in medieval pharmaceutical literature had already been pointed out, however, by Sigerist (1958, especially p. 144), with no other definition than 'recipes that have many ingredients and sometimes have pompous names'.

3 For an overview of the history of pharmacology from Antiquity to the Renaissance, see, for example, Touwaide 2009.

4 For a general presentation of this issue in the Arabic world, see, for example, Touwaide 1996. For an analysis of the reception in the West of the theories generated on this question in the Arabic world, see McVaugh 1975.

5 See, for example, over the past two decades such monographs as (in chronological order of publication): Lorenz 1990; Stille 1994; Schmitz 1998; Schulze 2002; and Gil 2004. Nor was the topic treated in scientific symposia specifically devoted to therapeutics: see mainly Kawakita, Sakai and Otsuka 1990; Bynum and Nutton 1994; and, more recently, Collard and Samama 2006. Finally, even in a specific study devoted to medicines (Guardasole 2001), the question was not raised.

6 This historical tradition is represented, for example, by such works as Loria 1960 and Watson 1966. Its approach can still be found in such a recent work as Radici Colace *et al.* 2009, particularly in entries like: 'Andromaco di Creata', p. 124 (P. Tempone); 'Contravveleni composti', pp 309–11 (L. Radici); 'Farmacologia. 1. Introduzione', pp 469–71 (S. Sconocchia); 'Farmacologia. 3. Alcuni tipi di medicamenti composti', pp 496–500 (S. Sconocchia); 'Terapeutica', pp 955–6 (S. Sconocchia); 'Veleni e contravveleni', pp 974–7 (L. Radici).

7 See e.g. Touwaide 1994a, (especially pp 1900–5 and 1975–81 for *De Antidotis* and *De Theriaca ad Pisonem* and *De Theriaca ad Pamphilianum*); Bénezet 1999, 546–635 (analysis of the several types of compound medicines); Ciaraldi, 2000 (for the analysis of archaeological remains in a jar that seem to have been the ingredients of theriac); Totelin 2004 (for the identification of Mithridates' formula).

8 According to the list of authors by topics contained in Keyser and Irby-Massie 2008, 991–1020, the pharmacists (p. 1013–9) total 500, of whom 255 (see Appendix) have been identified in the primary sources as involved in some way in the history of compound medicines.

9 Chronological data in Keyser and Irby-Massie 2008 are problematic in several entries under consideration here, with

such time periods as 300 BC–AD 400 (corresponding to 700 years) (see number 163), 250 BC–AD 95 (corresponding to 345 years) (see number 066), or 250 BC–AD 540 (corresponding to 790 years) (see number 027). I have taken into consideration only precise dates/time periods. Also, I reproduce the names as they appear in this *Encyclopedia*, although the spelling adopted in it may diverge from earlier scholarly tradition.

10 For this date and localisation, see Jouanna 1992, 547–8 for a synthesis of recent research (English translation pp 385–6). See also Hanson 1971, 25–9. I read the Greek text in the edition of Littré (1853), 1–233. For an unpublished English translation, see Whiteley 2003.

11 On the production of perfumes in antiquity, see Touwaide 1994b, 393–413.

12 See, for example, Dioscorides, *De materia medica*, in Book 1, chapters 1–29 for the plants used in the production of perfumes; 30–42 for the several oils (essential oils) produced by soaking plants in oil; and 43–63 for the perfumes.

13 On the dates and periodisation system of the authors listed here, see note 9 above.

Bibliography

Beck, L. Y. 2005: *Pedanius Dioscorides of Anazarbus, De Materia Medica* (translation) (Altertumswissenschaftliche Texte und Studien 38), Hildesheim.

Bénezet, J.-P. 1999: *Pharmacie et médicament en Méditerranée occidentale (XIIIe–XVIe siècles)* (Sciences, techniques et civilisations du moyen âge à l'aube des Lumières 3), Paris.

Bynum, W. F. and Nutton, V. (eds) 1994: *Essays in the History of Therapeutics*, Amsterdam and Atlanta.

Ciaraldi, M. 2000: 'Drug preparation in evidence? An unusual plant and bone assemblage from the Pompeian countryside, Italy', *Vegetation History and Archaeobotany* 9, 91–8.

Collard, F. and Samama, E. (eds) 2006: *Pharmacopoles et apothicaires. Les «pharmaciens» de l'Antiquité au Grand Siècle*, Paris.

Coturri, E. 1959: *Claudio Galeno, De theriaca ad Pisonem. Testo latino, traduzione italiana ed introduzione* (Biblioteca della 'Rivista di storia delle scienze mediche e naturali' 8), Florence.

Gil, L. 2004: *Therapeia. La medicina popular en el mundo clásico*, Madrid.

Guardasole, A. 2001: 'La médecine hellénistique et la pharmacologie: les remèdes «mains des dieux»', *Lalies* 21, 97–112.

Hankinson, R. J. 2008: 'Galen of Pergamon', 335–9 in P. T. Keyser and G. L. Irby-Massie (eds), *Encyclopedia of Ancient Natural Scientists: The Greek Tradition and its Many Heirs*, London and New York.

Hanson, A. E. 1971: *Studies in the Textual Tradition and the Transmission of the Gynecological Treatises of the Hippocratic Corpus*, Ph.D. Thesis, University of Pennsylvania,

Heitsch, E. 1963–4: *Die griechischen Dichterfragmente der römischen Kaiserzeit*, 2 vols (Abhandlungen der Akademie der Wissenschaften in Göttingen, Philologisch-historische Klasse, Dritte Folge, Nr. 58), Göttingen.

Holste, T. 1976: *Der Theriakkrämer. Ein Beitrag zur Frühgeschichte der Arzneimittelwerbung* (Würzburger medizinhistorische Forschungen 5), Pattensen.

Holste, T. and Keil, G. 1982: 'Ein Strassburger altdeutscherr Theriaktraktat', 511–22 in G. Keil (ed.), *„gelêrter der arzenîe, ouch apotêker": Beiträge zur Wissenschaftgeschichte. Festschrift zum 70. Geburtstag von Willem F. Daems* (Würzburger medizinhistorische Forschungen 24), Pattensen.

Jacques, J.-M. 1997: 'La méthode de Galien pharmacologue dans les traités sur les médicaments composés (Peri suntheseôs farmakôn)', 103–29 in A. Debru (ed.), *Galen on Pharmacology: Philosophy, History and Medicine. Proceedings of the Vth International Galen Colloquium, Lille, 16–18 March 1995* (Studies in Ancient Medicine 16), Leiden, New York, Köln.

Jouanna, J. 1999: *Hippocrate*, Paris (English translation: *Hippocrates*, Baltimore and London, 1999).

Kawakita, Y., Sakai, S. and Otsuka, Y. (eds) 1990: *History of Therapy: Proceedings of the 10th International Symposium on the Comparative History of Medicine – East and West, September 8-September15, 1985, Susono-shi, Shizuoka, Japan*, Tokyo.

Keyser P. T. and Irby-Massie, G. L. (eds), *Encyclopedia of Ancient Natural Scientists: The Greek Tradition and its Many Heirs*, London and New York.

Kühn, K. G. 1827: *Claudii Galeni Opera omnia*, vol. 14, Leipzig.

Langenheim, J. H. 2003, *Plant Resins: Chemistry, Evolution, Ecology, Ethnobotany*, Portland (OR) and Cambridge.

Littré, E. 1853: *Œuvres complètes d'Hippocrate, traduction nouvelle avec le texte grec en regard collationné sur les manuscrits et toutes les éditions accompagné d'une introduction, de commentaires médicaux, de variantes et de notes philologiques, suivie d'une table générale des matières*, vol. 8, Paris.

Loria, L. 1960: 'Il Mitridatismo e Mitridate', *Pagine di storia della medicina* 4 (1960), 27–32.

Lorenz, G. 1990: *Antike Krankenbehandlung in historisch-vergleichender Sicht. Studien zum konkret-anschaulichen Denken* (Bibliothek der klassischen Altertumswissenschaft, Neue Folge, 2. Reihe, 81), Heidelberg.

Macdonald Hocking, G. 1997: *A Dictionary of Natural Products: Terms in the Field of Pharmacognosy Relating to Natural Medicinal and Pharmaceutical Materials and the Plants, Animals and Minerals from which they are derived*, Medford (NJ).

McVaugh, M. R. 1975: *Arnaldi de Villanova, Opera medica omnia*, vol. 2: *Aphorismi de gradibus*, Granada and Barcelona.

Nutton, V, 1997: 'Galen on Theriac: Problems of Authenticity', 133–51 in A. Debru (ed.), *Galen on Pharmacology: Philosophy, History and Medicine. Proceedings of the Vth International Galen Colloquium, Lille, 16–18 March 1995* (Studies in Ancient Medicine 16), Leiden, New York, Köln.

Nutton, V. 2002: 'Andromachus [4] the Elder', col. 686 in H. Cancik and H. Schneider (eds), *Brill's New Pauly: Encyclopaedia of the Ancient World*, vol. 1, Leiden and Boston.

Nutton, V. 2004: 'Galen of Pergamum', cols 654–61 in H. Cancik and H. Schneider (eds), *Brill's New Pauly: Encyclopaedia of the Ancient World*, vol. 5, Leiden and Boston.

Olshausen, E. 2006: 'Mithridates [6] VI. Eupator Dionysius', cols 80–82 in H. Cancik and H. Schneider (eds), *Brill's New Pauly: Encyclopaedia of the Ancient World*, vol. 9, Leiden and Boston.

Radici Colace, P., Medaglia, S., Rosetti, L. and Sconocchia, S. (eds) 2009: *Dizionario delle scienze e delle tecniche di Grecia e Roma*, 2 vols (Biblioteca di «Technai» 1), Pisa and Rome.

Scarborough, J. 2008: 'Dioskouridēs of Anazarbos', 271–3 in P. T. Keyser and G. L. Irby-Massie (eds), *Encyclopedia of Ancient Natural Scientists: The Greek Tradition and its Many Heirs*, London and New York.

Schmitz, R. 1998: *Geschichte der Pharmazie*, I: *Von den Anfängen bis zum Ausgang des Mittelalters*, Eschborn.

Schulze, C. 2002: *Die pharmazeutische Fachliteratur in der Antike. Eine Einführung* (Göttinger Forum für Altertumswissenschaft, Beihefte, 10), Göttingen.

Sigerist, H. E. 1958: 'The Latin Medical Literature of the Early Middle Ages', *Journal of the History of Medicine and Allied Sciences*, 13, 127–46.

Stein, M. 1997: 'La thériaque chez Galien: sa préparation et son usage thérapeutique', 199–209 in A. Debru (ed.), *Galen on Pharmacology: Philosophy, History and Medicine. Proceedings of the Vth International Galen Colloquium, Lille, 16–18 March 1995* (Studies in Ancient Medicine 16), Leiden, New York, Köln.

Stille, G. 1994: *Der Weg der Arznei von der Materia Medica zur Pharmakologie. Der Weg von Arzneimittelforschung und Arzneitherapie*, Karlsruhe.

Totelin, L. M. V. 2004: 'Mithradates' Antidote: A Pharmacological Ghost', *Early Science and Medicine* 9/1, 1–19.

Totelin, L. 2009: *Hippocratic Recipes: Oral and Written Transmission of Pharmacological Knowledge in Fifth- and Fourth-Century Greece* (Studies in Ancient Medicine 34), Leiden and Boston.

Touwaide, A. 1994a: 'Galien et la toxicologie', 1887–1986 in W. Haase (ed.), *Aufstieg und Niedergang der römischen Welt: Geschichte und Kultur Roms im Speigel der neueren Forschung*, Teil II: *Principat*, Band 37: *Philosophie, Wissenschaften, Technik*, 2. Teilband: Wissenschaften (Medizin und Biologie), Berlin and New York.

Touwaide, A. 1994b: 'Les techniques antiques de préparation de l'huile en vue de la confection des parfums', 393–413 in C. Kircher-Durand (ed.), *Nomina rerum: Hommages à J. Mannessy-Guiton*, Nice.

Touwaide, A. 1996: 'Theoretical Concepts and Problems of Greek Pharmacology in Arabic Medicine: Reception and Re-elaboration', *Forum* 6, 327–44.

Touwaide, A. 2007a: 'Pharmacology', cols 927–32 in H. Cancik and H. Schneider (eds), *Brill's New Pauly: Encyclopaedia of the Ancient World*, vol. 10, Leiden and Boston.

Touwaide, A. 2007b: 'Pedanius [1]: Pedanius Dioskorides', cols 670–2 in H. Cancik and H. Schneider (eds), *Brill's New Pauly: Encyclopaedia of the Ancient World*, vol. 10, Leiden and Boston.

Touwaide, A. 2008: 'Andromakhos of Crete (Elder)', 79 in P. T. Keyser and G. L. Irby-Massie (eds), *Encyclopedia of Ancient Natural Scientists: The Greek Tradition and its Many Heirs*, London and New York.

Touwaide, A. 2009: 'Pharmacology', cols 357–66 in M. Landfester (ed.) in collaboration with H. Cancik and H. Schneider, *Brill's New Pauly: Encyclopaedia of the Ancient World. Classical Tradition*, vol. 4, Leiden and Boston.

Watson, G. 1966: *Theriac and Mithridatum: A Study in Therapeutics* (Publications of the Wellcome Historical Medical Library, New Series 9), London.

Wellmann, M. (ed.) 1906–1914: *Pedanii Dioscuridis Anazarbei, De materia medica libri quinque*, 3 vols, Berlin.

Whiteley, K. 2003: *Hippocrates' 'Diseases of Women' Book 1: Greek Text with English Translation and Footnotes*, M.A. Thesis, University of South Africa.

van Wyk, B.-E. and Wink, M. 2004: *Medicinal Plants of the World: An Illustrated Scientific Guide to Important Medicinal Plants and their Uses*, Portland (OR).

Appendix

List of physicians known in ancient medical literature to have used, developed or created formulas for compound medicines, based on Keyser Irby-Massie 2008.[1]

Authors of more than one entry are identified by means of the following abbreviations:

AT	Alain Touwaide
GLIM	Georgia L. Irby-Massie
JMJ	Jean-Marie Jacques
JS	John Scarborough
PTK	Paul T. Keyser

1 On the dates and periodisation system of the authors listed here, see note 9 above.

Num.	*Name*	*Dates/Period*	*Page(s)*	*Author*
001	Abaskantos of Lugdunum	10 BC–80 CE	29	PTK
002	L. Aelius Gallus praefect Aegypti	45–5 BC	34–35	JS
003	Aineios (of Kos?)	10 BC–110 AD	49	PTK
004	Akhaios	200 BC–80 AD	51	GLIM
005	Akhillas	120 BC–80 AD	51	PTK
006	Akholios	400–500 AD?	52	PTK
007	Alkimion	120 BC–25 AD	60	PTK
008	Ambrosios of Puteoli Rusticus	40–80 AD	64	PTK
009	Ammonios of Alexandria	50–10 BC	66	PTK
010	Amphion	250 BC–95 AD	68	PTK
011	Amuthaon	120 BC–80 AD?	69	PTK
012	Anastasios	200?–540 AD	71–72	PTK
013	Andreas of Karustos	*ca* 250–217 BC	77–78	GLIM
014	Andromakhos of Crete (Elder)	50–65 AD	79	AT
015	Andromakhos of Crete (Younger)	70–90 AD	79–80	AT
016	Andron (Pharm.)	225?–75 BC	80	JMJ
017	Andronikos (Pharm.)	250 BC–80 AD	81	PTK
018	Anthaios Sextilius	25–75 AD	89	PTK
019	Antimakhos	30 BC–80 AD	94	PTK
020	Antiokhos Paccius	20 BC–14 AD	95	JS
021	Antiokhos VIII Philometor	141–96 BC	95–96	JMJ
022	Antipatros (Pharm.)	30 BC–80 AD	96–97	AT
023	Antonius Musa	40–20 BC	101	JS
024	Antonius "root-cutter"	100 BC–95 AD	101	PTK
025	Aphrodas	90 BC–80 AD	103	PTK
026	Aphrodisis	50 BC–95 AD	104	PTK
027	Aphros	250 BC–540 AD	104	PTK
028	Aphthonios of Rome	250–350 AD	104	PTK
029	Apion of Oasis Egypt	20–50 AD	104	PTK
030	Apios Phaskos	100 BC–110 AD	104–105	PTK
031	Apollinarios (Pharm.)	*ca* 160–260 AD?	105	GLIM
032	Apollonios Claudius	40?–80 AD	110	PTK

Num.	*Name*	*Dates/Period*	*Page(s)*	*Author*
033	Apollonios of Tarsos	250 BC–80 AD	116	PTK
034	Apollophanes of Seleukeia "Pieria"	223–187 BC	117–118	JS
035	Apuleius Celsus of Centauripae	*ca* 20–40 CE	119	JS
036	Aquila Secundilla	10 BC–95 AD	121	PTK
037	Arbians of Indos (Lukia)	120 BC–80 AD	124	PTK
038	Areios of Tarsus Laecanius	54–77 AD	128–129	JS
039	Aristarkhos of Tarsos	30–70 AD?	133	JMJ
040	Aristogenes of Knidos	260–240 BC	137	PTK
041	Aristokles	120 BC–80 AD	137	GLIM
042	Aristolaos	250 BC–80 AD	138	PTK
043	Arkhabathos of Lakonika	*fl.* 219 BC	156	PTK
044	Arkhelaos (of Herakleia Salbake?)	40–95 AD	158	GLIM
045	Arrabaios (of Macedon?)	250 BC–25 AD	162–163	PTK
046	Artemidoros of Perge, Cornelius	75–70 BC	165	PTK & GLIM
047	Artemon (Med.)	20 BC–25 AD	166	PTK
048	Asklepiades Pharmakion	*ca* 90–100 AD	169–170	AT
049	Aspasios (Pharm.)	250 BC–90 AD	174	PTK
050	Athenion (of Athens?)	50–10 BC	178	PTK
051	Athenippos	120 BC–40 AD	178	PTK
052	Atimetos	10–40 AD	179	PTK
053	Attalos III of Pergamon, Philometo	138–133 BC	179–180	P. Thibodeau
054	Aurelius	*ca* 155–200 AD?	182	GLIM
055	Axios	45 BC–100 AD	184	PTK
056	Bathullos (?)	100 BC?–10 AD	191	PTK
057	Bithus of Kurrakhion	80 BC?–75 AD	193	PTK
058	Blastos	30 BC–80 AD	194	PTK
059	Boupha(n)tos	120 BC–565 AD	199	PTK
060	Brenitus	120 BC–*ca* 90 AD	199	PTK
061	Candidus	30 BC–80 AD	205	PTK
062	Castus	50–80 AD	211	PTK
063	Celer the Centurion	10 BC–95 AD	211	PTK
064	Cornelius	120 BC–80 AD	216	PTK
065	Damokrates, Servilius	*ca* 70–80 AD	226	S. Vogt
066	Deileon	250 BC–95 AD	229	PTK
067	Dexios	120 BC–25 AD	243	GLIM
068	Diagoras of Cyprus	220–180 BC?	244	PTK
069	Diogenes (Pharm.)	10 BC–30 AD	251	PTK
070	Diokles of Khalkedon	250 BC–95 AD	257	PTK
071	Diomedes	250 BC–95 AD	257–258	GLIM
072	Dion (Med.)	120 BC–120 AD	258	PTK
073	Dionusios of Samos	250 BC–95 AD	265	GLIM
074	Diophantos of Lukia	40–10 BC	268–269	GLIM
075	Dioskoros (Pharm.)	120 BC–80 AD	269	PTK
076	Domitius Nigrinus	*ca* 20 BC–*ca* 90 AD	274	PTK
077	Dositheos of Pelousion	250–210 BC	277	PTK

Num.	*Name*	*Dates/Period*	*Page(s)*	*Author*
078	Eirenaios	250 BC–25 AD	280	GLIM
079	Emboularkhos (?)	30 BC–540 AD	282	PTK
080	Epaphroditos of Carthage	25–80 AD	286	PTK
081	Epidauros (?)	120 BC–80 AD	290	PTK
082	Epigonos	250 BC–10 AD	291	PTK
083	Epikouros	250 BC–80 AD	292	F. Stok
084	Erasistratos of Sikuon	250 BC–95 AD	297	PTK
085	Eruthrios	*ca* 350?–640 AD	301–302	PTK
086	Esdras	100–500 AD?	302	AT
087	Euangeus (?)	250 BC–80 AD	303	PTK
088	Euboulos (Pharm.)	250 BC?–80 AD	304	AT
089	Euelpides	15–35 AD	314–315	AT
090	Eugamios	250 BC–300 AD?	316	PTK
091	Eugeneia	120 BC–80 AD	316	PTK
092	Eugrasia	120 BC–90 AD	316	PTK
093	Euhemeros	200 BC–925 AD	316	PTK
094	Euphemios of Sicily	1000–2000 AD	319	AT
095	Euphramor (Pharm.)	200 BC–95 AD	320	PTK
096	Euskhemos the Eunuch	100 BC?–90 AD	323	PTK
097	Eutonios	250 BC–365 AD	325	GLIM
098	Faustinus	*ca* 100 BC–*ca* 80 AD	328	PTK
099	Flauianus of Crete	60 BC–80 AD	329	PTK
100	Flauius "the boxer"	30 BC–80 AD	330	PTK
101	Florus	20 BC–20 AD?	331	PTK
102	Gennadios	250 BC–95 AD	345	PTK
103	Glaukon/Glaukos (Med.)	120 BC–77 AD	349	PTK
104	Harpalos (Pharm.)	120 BC–80 AD	356	GLIM
105	Harpokras of Alexandria	250 BC?–80 AD	356	AT
106	Harpokration	80 BC–80 AD	357	GLIM
107	Heirodotos (of Boiotia?)	205–185 BC?	360	PTK
108	Hekataios (Pharm.)	250 BC–25 AD	360	GLIM
109	Heliades	250 BC–540 AD	362	PTK
110	Heras of Kappadokia	20 BC–20 AD	374	AT
111	Hermeias (Ophthalm.)	250 BC–95 AD	376	PTK
112	Hermolaos (Pharm.)	120 BC–450 AD	380	PTK
113	Hermon of Egypt	120 BC–10 AD	380	PTK
114	Hermophilos	120 BC–95 AD	380	PTK
115	Herodotos (Pneum., of Tarsos?)	70–100 AD	383–384	AT
116	Heron (Med.)	100–50 BC	384	PTK
117	Hieras of Thebai	250 BC–25 AD	392	GLIM
118	Hikesios of Smurna	120–80 BC?	396	JS
119	Hubristes of Oxyrhynchos	120–100? BC	423	PTK
120	Ianuarius	*ca* 250–400 AD	431	PTK
121	Idios	250 BC–80 AD	432	PTK
122	Ioannes of Antioch, arkhiatros	1200–1500 AD?	437–438	AT

Num.	*Name*	*Dates/Period*	*Page(s)*	*Author*
123	Ioudaios	250 BC–25 AD	442	GLIM
124	Irion (?)	250 BC–80 AD	442	PTK
125	Isidoros of Antioch	50?–80 AD	443	AT
126	Isidoros of Memphis	250 BC–540 AD	444	PTK
127	Iulianus (Pharm.)	520–540 AD	447–448	PTK
128	Iulius Agrippa	10 BC–90 AD	450	PTK
129	Iulius Bassus	*ca* 10–40 AD	451	JS
130	Iulius Secundus	*ca* 10 BC–*ca* 90 AD	455	PTK
131	Iunia/Iounias	30 BC?–80 AD	456	PTK
132	Iustinus (Pharm.)	30 BC–115 AD	458	PTK
133	Iustus the Pharmacologist	30 BC–*ca* 150 AD	458–459	JS
134	Kallinikos (Pharm.)	20?–90 AD	464	PTK
135	Khaldikeus	250 BC–95 AD	470	PTK
136	Kharikles	120 BC–80 AD	470–471	PTK
137	Kharixenes	30 BC?–95 AD	471	AT
138	Khrusermos of Alexandria	*ca* 70–30 BC?	473	GLIM
139	Kimon	250 BC–30 AD	476	GLIM
140	Kleoboulos (Pharm.)	250 BC–95 AD	479	PTK
141	Kleon (of Kuzikos?)	100?–20 BC	481	PTK
142	Kleophantos	80 BC–80 AD	482–483	AT
143	Klutos	200 BC–80 BC	484	PTK
144	Kodios Toukos	250 BC–95 AD	485	PTK
145	Kosmos	80–100 AD	487	PTK
146	Krateros of Antioch	50–25 BC	489	AT
147	Kraton (Pharm.)	120 BC–25 AD	492	PTK
148	Ktesiphon	250 BC–25 AD	496–497	GLIM
149	Kuros of Edessa	50–540 AD	498–499	PTK
150	Lampon of Pelousion	120 BC–80 AD	501	GLIM
151	Laodikos	250 BC–80 AD	501	GLIM
152	Lepidianus	30 BC–360 AD	504–505	PTK
153	Leukios (of Tarsos?), Kathegetes	50–85 AD	505–506	AT
154	Lingon	10 BC–95 AD	508	PTK
155	Logadios	20 BC–450 AD	510	PTK
156	Lukomedes	120 BC–80 AD	513	PTK
157	Lunkeus	250 BC–95 AD	515	PTK
158	Lusias	*ca* 100 BC–35 AD	515	AT
159	Magnus arkhiatros	90–130 AD	519	PTK
160	Magnus of Philadelphia	100 BC–80 AD	520–521	AT
161	Magnus of Tarsos	60 BC–95 AD	521	PTK
162	Makhairon	100 BC–110 AD	522	PTK
163	Manethon (Pharm.)	300 BC–400 AD	523–524	PTK
164	Mantias (Heroph.)	150–100 BC	525–526	JS
165	Marcellinus (Pharm.)	30 BC–80 AD	526	PTK
166	Marcellus (Pharm.)	50–70 AD	527	PTK
167	Marcianus (of Africa?)	10 BC–15 AD	530	PTK

Num.	Name	Dates/Period	Page(s)	Author
168	Meletos	20 BC–25 AD	539–540	PTK
169	Meliton	250 BC–80 AD	542	PTK
170	Menas	350?–540 AD	544	PTK
171	Menemakhos of Aphrodisias	30–90 AD	546–547	GLIM
172	Menenius Rufus	30 BC–90 AD	547	PTK
173	Menoitas/Menoitios	250 BC–10 AD	550	PTK
174	Menophilos	120 BC–25 AD	551	PTK
175	Minucianus	10–80 AD	557	PTK
176	Moskhion (Pharm.)	90 BC–80 AD	563	JS
177	Naukratites medicus	250 BC–25 AD	567	PTK
178	Nearkhos	60 BC–80 AD	568	PTK
179	Neilammon	250 BC–540 AD	569	PTK
180	Niketes (of Athens?)	250 BC–90 AD	576	PTK
181	Nikolaos (Pharm.)	150 BC–95 AD	577	PTK
182	Nikomedes IV of Bithunia	100–74 BC	581	PTK
183	Nikostratos (Pharm.)	50–80 AD	582	PTK
184	Nonnos	200–540 AD	582	PTK
185	Okianos	1000–1400 AD?	587	AT
186	Olumpiakos of Miletos	*ca* 80–150 AD	588	GLIM
187	Olumpionikos (?)	200 BC–90 AD	591	GLIM
188	Olumpos of Alexandria	35–25 BC	591	GLIM
189	Onetides/Onetor	300 BC–80 AD	592	PTK
190	Origeneia	10 BC–90 AD	596	PTK
191	Orion of Bithunia	250 BC–80 AD	596	PTK
192	Oros of Mendes	300 BC–75 AD	597	PTK
193	Pamphilos of Alexandria	60–80 AD	606–607	PTK
194	Pamphilos of Berutos	270–309 AD	607	PTK
195	Pasion	250 BC–10 AD	627	PTK
196	Patroklos	50 BC–10 AD	628	PTK
197	Petronios Musa	*ca* 10–40 AD	639	JS
198	Phaidros	250 BC–90 AD	641	PTK
199	Phanias	250 BC–80 AD	641	PTK
200	Philippos of Macedon	120–10 BC?	647	PTK
201	Philokles	250 BC–80 AD	651	PTK
202	Philokrates	250 BC–25 AD	651	PTK
203	Philon of Tarsos	10–35 AD	657–658	AT
204	Polles (Med.)	120–365 AD	679	PTK
205	Poluarkhos	30 BC–35 AD	680	PTK
206	Polueides	250 BC–25 AD	682	PTK
207	Polustomos	250 BC–80 AD	683–684	PTK
208	Pomponius Bassus	65–95 AD	685	GLIM
209	Primnion	100 BC–80 AD	695	GLIM
210	Proëkhios (?)	120 BC–365 AD	697	PTK
211	Protas of Pelousion	120 BC–80 AD	702	PTK
212	Prothius/Protius (?)	150–378 AD?	702	GLIM

Num.	***Name***	***Dates/Period***	***Page(s)***	***Author***
213	Proxenos	120–30 BC	703	GLIM
214	Prutanis	250 BC–80 AD	703	GLIM
215	Ptolemaios (Pharm.)	70–90 AD	703	PTK
216	Puramos	250 BC–95 AD	710	GLIM
217	Puthion (Pharm.)	50–30 BC	713	PTK
218	Quadratus	*ca* 100 BC–80 AD	716	PTK
219	Ripalus	50 BC–80 AD	719	PTK
220	Romula	180?–400? AD	719	PTK
221	Samithra/Tanitros (?)	100 BC–40 AD	725	PTK
222	Sandarius/Sardacius	550–1300 AD	726	GLIM
223	Sarkeuthites/os	250 BC–80 AD	727	PTK
224	Scribonius Largus	*ca* 25 BC–55 AD	728–729	JS
225	Serenjus (Pharm.)	50–540 AD	733	JS
226	Sergius of Babylon	250 BC–90 AD	735	PTK
227	Sertorius Clemens	30 BC–80 AD	735–736	PTK
228	Silo	*ca* 120 BC–40 AD	741	PTK
229	Sokrates (Med.)	10 BC–100 AD	748	PTK
230	Sokration	250 BC–110 AD	748	GLIM
231	Sosagoras	250 BC–25 AD	751–752	GLIM
232	Sosandros (Pharm.)	250 BC–95 AD	752	GLIM
233	Sosikrates	250 BC–80 AD	753	GLIM
234	Straton of Berutos	90 BC–50 AD	765	AT
235	Suneros (of Campania?)	200 BC–95 AD	769	PTK
236	Telamon	250 BC–90 AD	773	PTK
237	Telephanes	250 BC–80 AD	773	PTK
238	M. Terentius Valens	25–40 AD	773–774	JS
239	Thamuros	200 BC–80 AD	779	PTK
240	Theodoros (of Macedon?)	70–150 AD	786	AT
241	Theokritos	250 BC–80 AD	791	PTK
242	Theophilos (Pharm.)	120 BC–540 AD	797–798	PTK
243	Theopompos	120 BC–300 AD	802	PTK
244	Theosebios	100–300 AD?	803	AT
245	Theotropos	65–90 AD	803	PTK
246	Threptos	100 BC–90 AD	807	PTK
247	Timaios (Pharm.)	250 BC–25 AD	810	GLIM
248	Timokleanos (?)	10 BC–365 AD	813	PTK
249	Timokrates	30 BC–95 AD	813	PTK
250	Truphon of Gortum	*ca* 15 BC–20 AD	817	JS
251	Xanites (?)	250 BC–80 AD	835	PTK
252	Zenon of Laodikeia	250 BC?–80 AD	847	AT
253	Zenophilos	100 BC–360 AD	848	GLIM
254	Zoilos of Macedon	15–75 AD	850	PTK
255	Zozimos (Med.)	10 BC–95 AD	852	PTK

24. Lemnian Earth, Alum and Astringency: a Field-based Approach

Effie Photos-Jones and Allan J. Hall

*Based on Galen's account that Lemnian Earth (*Λημνία γῆ; Λημνία σφραγίς; Terra Lemnia, ayiochoma*) was an astringent medicine because of the occurrence, within, of a 'bit of alum', we present here our evidence to that effect. This evidence is supported by: a) the scrutiny of the classical texts; b) the geological prospection around the area of the alleged location of extraction of the Earth on the island of Lemnos, in the N. Aegean; c) our interpretation of the ritual of its extraction; and, lastly, d) the elucidation of its mineral composition. Lemnian Earth is a complex material consisting of clay minerals and inorganic salts like aluminium sulphate and iron oxide. Its composition may be affected by its possible association with the water from local natural springs. Astringency is the main property of alum and is still relatively little understood. Alum is also a bactericide; we argue that it was perhaps the combination of both properties of alum as an astringent and a bactericide that contributed to the celebrated medicinal attributes of Lemnian Earth. We also present here a brief description of the work undertaken by other researchers, as well as our impending new work on the nature of this intriguing material.*

Introduction

Our research on the earths of the Aegean, mainly clay-based substances which were well-documented by the classical authors (Pliny *Naturalis Historia*, Dioscorides *De Materia Medica*, Galen *De Simplicium Medicamentorum Temperamentis ac Facultatibus*), has led us to believe that they were very versatile materials used for a variety of applications including paints, detergents and medicines (Photos-Jones and Hall 2011); and, furthermore, that the medicinal properties claimed for some earths were likely to be genuine.

Lemnian, Samian and Eretrian Earths were thought to have been particularly useful respectively as antidotes to snake bites (Philumenus *De Venenatis Animalibus eorumqve Remediis*) (*On poisonous animals and their remedies*), inflammation of the eye, and ulcers (Dioscorides *De Materia Medica*); furthermore, belief in the efficacy of the Lemnian Earth, in particular, was sustained from Antiquity into the early 20th century. Deducing exactly what the classical authors understood to be the nature of these substances is certainly problematic, but it is not difficult to appreciate why belief in their efficacy as medicines has gradually faded and eventually totally disappeared. Recently, however, there has been a resurgence in interest in medicinal clays and the field of medical geology in general (Gomes and Silva 2007; Gomes 2013). In attempting to elucidate the nature of the earths we recognised two major problems: first, how and where does one start looking for them in the field, and second, what was/were the active ingredient/s which bestowed the medicinal properties on these clay-based substances.

It was primarily as a medicine that Lemnian Earth acquired its widespread reputation and in particular as an efficient antidote against poisons and snakebites. Pliny describes Lemnian Earth as being an antidote to poisons when poison was already swallowed and even against snake bites (*Naturalis Historia* [henceforth *N.H.*], XXIX.33 and XXXV.14); also, 'in medicine it was used as an ointment around the eyes to relieve pain and inflammation' (Pliny *N.H.* XXXV.14), and as a treatment for dysentery (*N.H.* XXVIII.24, XXIX.33.104, and XXXV.14). Given the richness of the record surrounding the nature, properties and the ritual of extraction of Lemnian Earth we believe we were justified in suggesting that the latter may provide an environmental 'framework' on which geological and anthropogenic events can be pegged and which could underpin our understanding of the healing properties of this Earth.

Since the time of the conference in 2008 we have had the opportunity to publish a number of papers on the topic of alum (Hall and Photos-Jones, 2009; Photos-Jones and Hall 2010) and Lemnian Earth (Hall and Photos-Jones 2008; Photos-Jones *et al.* 2012) as well as one book (Photos-Jones and Hall 2011). This paper shifts attention from the local clay deposits and the local natural springs and the potential association between them and the pit from where the earth was extracted. We, therefore, summarise our attempts to establish the nature, composition, method of processing, and location of extraction, of Lemnian Earth. We have argued that Lemnian Earth the medicine and Lemnian Earth the raw material were two different products; the former resulting from the processing of the latter *via* a proposed ingenious enhancement of the natural geochemistry of the area, under the cover of a ritual, blessed by both ancient gods and Christian clergy. The elucidation of this enhancement led us to provide a theoretical composition for Lemnian Earth consisting of various components each bringing its own properties, e.g. kaolin and montmorillonite its absorbancy, iron oxide its red colour and alum its astringency (Hall and Photos-Jones 2008; Photos-Jones and Hall 2011).

Lemnian Earth – the sources

The earliest reference to the healing properties of Lemnian Earth is firmly embedded within the cycle of poetry associated with the Homeric poems, the Trojan War and its main participants, and in particular the hero Philoctetes who although setting off with the rest of the Greek army to fight at Troy, was left behind on account of having been bitten by a water snake, his wound festering and emanating a malodorous smell (Homer *Iliad* 2, 718–25).

Philostratus Flavius, a Lemnian sophist who lived in the 2nd century AD, in his chapter on Philoctetes (*Heroica* VI, 2), mentions that the priests of Hephaistos cured his wounds with Lemnian bole (βώλου τῆς Λημνίας). However, in the Sophocles version of the Philoctetes myth, the long-suffering hero had used a herb, rather than an earth, only available on the island of Lemnos (Sophocles *Philoctetes*, 659). Furtherme, Philoctetes' wound did not heal until he finally arrived in Troy. Eustathius, Bishop of Thessaloniki, writing in the 12th century AD, in his comments on the *Iliad*, confirms that the priests of Hephaistos were in the habit of healing those who had been bitten by snakes (οἱ τοῦ Ἡφαίστου ἱερεῖς ἐθεράπευον τοὺς ὀφεοδήκτους) with Lemnian Earth (Tourptsoglou-Stephanidou 1986, 84, n. 46).

Up to the middle of the 18th century there appear to have been very few, if any, doubts regarding the curative properties of Lemnian Earth. However, in the late 18th century questions were raised as to whether these attributes may not have rested simply on the belief that it 'does' cure. John Sibthorp, an English doctor and botanist visiting Lemnos in the late 18th century, having been present at the site on the day of its extraction, wrote:

> 'on the 23rd of September … we saw the hole partly filled up and its soil which was a light colored clay … It could not possibly have a therapeutic value. Furthermore in the case of fever, when the stomach is weak, it would aggravate the illness which caused it (the fever) in the first place … this is an example of how superstition and ritual give credit to something which may have little or no value' (Sibthorp in Tourptsoglou-Stephanidou 1986, 292) (all translations from the Greek are by the author).

Earlier travellers, most of them educated men of means, were equally puzzled, but, in their own accounts, each balanced the pros and cons differently. For example, Belon (in Tourptsoglou-Stephanidou 1986, 80) was convinced that it was the ritual that gave the Lemnian Earth its value, rather than the properties of the material itself.

Although there was essentially no scientific evidence regarding the source and nature of Lemnian Earth until the middle of the 19th century, the first contemporary chemical analyses indicated the presence of an aluminum-silicate clay, possibly with sodium and calcium, which would point to the montmorillonite group. It is unfortunate that potash was not mentioned in these early analyses (de Launay in Tourptsoglou-Stephanidou 1986, 505, n. 33), because confirmation of a lack of potash which is present in the common clay illite would be a further indication of montmorillonite. The high iron content reported suggests the presence of a red iron oxide/oxyhydroxide component in keeping with Lemnian Earth often being reported as a red substance. Therefore, at the time, it was concluded that Lemnian Earth was simply a clay. Hence, Louis de Launay's statement below registering his frustration at not being able to pinpoint the active ingredient:

> 'Perhaps the negative results derived from my analyses are one more proof of the risks posed by the application of chemistry to myths, particularly those that are among the oldest or the most vivid' (de Launay in Tourptsoglou-Stephanidou 1986, 505).

There is little doubt that Lemnian Earth of the medicinal variety was fine-grained; the texture was certainly greasy/fatty and it appears to have 'dissolved' in the mouth (Belon in Tourptsoglou-Stephanidou 1986, 57).

Most medicinal Earths are discussed in association with astringency. Galen recognises the astringency in Lemnian Earth (τούτων δ'απασῶν ἡ Λημνία δύναμιν ἰσχυροτέραν ἔχει, προσέστι γαρ αὐτῄ τι καὶ στύψεως – of all the above (earths), Lemnian Earth is the most potent, because in it there is a bit of alum) (Galen *De Simplicium Medicamentorum Temperamentis ac Facultatibus Liber IX* (Chartier edition XIII, 252; authors' translation). The astringent nature of Lemnian Earth is also mentioned by Pierre Pomet in his *Histoire général de Drogues* of 1694, and by Moses Charas, another French author of the late 17th century, in his *Royal Pharmacopoeia, Galenical and Chymical* of 1678 (Thompson 1914, 440).

The ritual of extraction

The ritual of the extraction of Lemnian Earth has fascinated many travellers since Galen's visit to the island because it addresses many issues, practical, technical and religious, such as the exact location of the pit, the actual digging of it, the religious pageantry in the presence of state officials, the industrial process of earth enrichment, the sealing and distribution of the material, to select a few. All of these events are described as having taken place in the space of less than 12 hours and the totality and speed of their execution must have been so well rehearsed as to elude even the most astute of observers.

Regarding the ritual of the extraction we focus on two eyewitness accounts, which provide us with ample detail for the day's activities, that of Galen in the 2nd century AD and that of Belon in the 16th century, who visited the site but not on the day of the extraction. Galen during his visit to the town of Hephaestias, in the north-eastern part of the island, was evidently shown the location of the extraction of Lemnian Earth, and was made aware of its association with the hill on which, according to mythology, Hephaistos fell after having been hurled from Mount Olympus by his own father Zeus.

> '... as to what the poet said about Hephaistos, that he fell in Lemnos, it seems to me that the fable refers to the nature of the hill, which has every appearance of having been burned, both on account of its colour, and from the fact that nothing grows on it. This then was the hill to which at the time I disembarked the priestess came' (Galen in Brock 1929, 193).

The ritual of the preparation of the Lemnian Earth is described by Galen as follows:

> 'The priestess collects this, to the accompaniment of some local ceremony, no animals being sacrificed, but wheat and barley being given back to the land in exchange. She then takes it to the city, mixes it with water so as to make moist mud, shakes this violently and then allows it to stand. Thereafter she removes first the superficial water, and next the greasy part of the earth below this, leaving only the stony and sandy part at the bottom, which is useless. She now dries the greasy mud until it reaches the consistency of soft wax. Of this she takes small portions and imprints upon them the seal of Artemis namely the goat, then again she dries these in the shade till they are absolutely free from moisture' (Galen in Brock 1929, 192).

Galen continues that the priestess, after filling a 'whole wagon with earth, this she took into the town, as I have said, and from it prepared the far-famed Lemnian *sphragis* (seal)' (Galen in Brock 1929, 192).

Belon who visited the same area nearly fourteen centuries later but not necessarily on the day of its collection gives directions to the site of its extraction:

> 'From the corner of the castle [the ruined Byzantine castle of Kotsinas] towards the left, we walked towards the hill which is not more than four arrow-shots away. Between the port and the hill there is a small chapel called St Saviour's, where the monks gather on the 6th of August, the date set for the extraction of the earth from its vein. After leaving the chapel and walking towards the hillock we found two paths, one to the left and one to the right leading to two springs, one about one arrow-shot away from the other' (Belon in Tourptsoglou-Stephanidou 1986, 78).

Later on he adds:

> 'they (priests and monks) walk towards and climb the hill which is not more than two arrow-shots away from the chapel ... the one on our right (the Phthelidia) does not dry up in the summer, however, the one on the left does so completely ... with horses we continued towards the right, towards a place where no trees grow, except of a carob tree, ... and a willow which shadow the spring and where there are stone steps so that one can access the place where they extract the "sealed earth". One climbs uphill and further up towards one's left one can see the place where they extract the earth on the 6th of August. Because they extract it after opening a vein, nothing other than a long trench covered with earth can be seen' (Belon in Tourptsoglou-Stephanidou 1986, 79).

The day's events were preceded by a religious service at the chapel of St Sotiras (St Saviour). The Turkish governor of the island, Turkish and Greek notables, as well as some priests and monks took part in the ceremony. The digging began at or before sunrise and continued for six hours, after which the pit was closed and left undisturbed until the next year. Some Lemnian Earth was given to the officers present and other bystanders, but the bulk of it was sent to the Sultan in Constantinople. A certain amount was sold on the spot by the local magistrate to local merchants.

Two varieties of Lemnian Earth were produced. Belon mentions that the Turks clearly differentiated between two types of earth, *thin – i makhtoum-i ahmer*, i.e. the red earth, and the *thin – i makhtoum-i ebiez,* the white earth (Tourptsoglou-Stephanidou 1986, 111, n. 4), the latter considered of lower quality. It is, therefore, clear, from the accounts of both Galen and Belon, that colour reflected the grade, quality and use of the material. The weight of the sealed earth was *c.* 4 drams (i.e. *c.* 8 gr.).

Is the ritual of the extraction a covert geochemical process?

It is very likely that the extraction of Lemnian Earth witnessed by both Galen and Belon took place in the area of the Phthelidia spring about 1km south of the ruins of the castle of Kotsinas. The spring is now tapped and lies about 150 m. east of the small chapel of St Sotiras. Although most accounts talk about a pit, there are some accounts which discuss a pit in association with either one or two or even three springs; however, what is made clear in these different accounts is that the springs are not linked in any way with the pit (Tourptsoglou-Stephanidou 1986, 161). They merely help locate the pit. There are, however, other accounts, mostly dated to the 16th century, which describe the pit in direct association with a spring. Carlier de Pinon writing in the 1550s and quoted by Tourptsoglou-Stephanidou (1986, 111, n. 4) mentions a spring integrally associated with the pit:

> 'This earth they collect from the mud of a spring which is fenced with a wall and is always guarded by a group of soldiers. There is the custom every year on a particular day for the commander to take a few camel-loads of this earth following a ritual and to stamp it with the seal of the sultan'.

Tourptsoglou-Stephanidou, (1986, 504, n. 32) also refers to de la Vigne and a letter of his dated to February 22nd 1558, with the following information:

> 'They prefer the white (earth) because it is the first one which comes out of the spring when they stir it... They collect it and they stamp it in Lemnos. The red (earth) is the one they prefer in France but it is the one that stays at the opening (mouth) of the spring after they have stirred it.'

In 1581, Jacopo Soranzo, emissary of Venice to the Sultan, gave the following account of the extraction activities:

> 'On a hillock there is a spring; its water is directed through a channel to a pit which has formed naturally (by the accumulating water) ... the pit is covered with planks cut and joined together like the cover for a box which they lock with a key. On the prescribed day (6th of August), they change the course of the water, so that it does not run towards the pit. They lift the cover and remove very carefully all the overlying water (in the pit), which they collect in buckets and (eventually) with sponges. Then they dig the mud and sort the best quality of earth out, first. Then they dig another type of earth, not as good, and then a third. With these three varieties of earth they make three different types of pellets as well as cups for drinking water; they seal them with the stamp of the Grand Efendi, and they fire them all to become hard' (Soranzo in Tourptsoglou-Stephanidou 1986, 119, n. 7).

Finally, another detailed account of the extraction and processing of Lemnian Earth was given by John Covel based on his visit to Lemnos about 1677 (Covel in Tourptsoglou-Stephanidou 1986, 159). He does not specifically talk about a stream but gives a vivid description of the texture of the earth. He writes:

> 'They extract the earth in the following way. Before sunrise they start digging a pit about 1.5 yards wide and a little above a man's height in depth. Then they remove the earth which is soft as butter. The Greeks believe, and I think that the Turks believe it too, that it is the power of the holy liturgy that converted the hard rock to a soft clay; then they remove about 20–30 quintals of this earth, (*one quintal being c.100kg*), they fill up the pit again and leave it like this without any further guarding' (Covel in Tourptsoglou-Stephanidou 1986, 161).

Covel also witnessed the processing of the Lemnian Earth at a large fountain in Hagiapate. Hagiapate or Aghios Ypatios was a Turkish village where the authorities had the right to take some Lemnian Earth and give it to local potters to make pots:

> 'They first dissolve it in water, well working it with their hands; then let the water pass through a sieve and what remains they throw away. They let the water stand till settled, then take of the clear, and when dry enough, they mould in their hands; and most of this we have is shaped from thence. It is all here white, yet I had some given me flesh-coloured. I enquired diligently about it, and they all told me it came out of the same pit; but I expect some of these fellows have found some other place which they conceal' (Covel in Tourptsoglou-Stephanidou 1986, 162).

Based on the above descriptions we suggest that there was a spring in the immediate vicinity of the pit from which the Earth was extracted. The water 'passed over' the pit in the course of a whole year. Sediments within the pit were allowed to settle and clay, silt and sand to separate. It is the fine naturally levigated clay that made up the medicinal Earth and which, when removed at source, required no further treatment. In support of this view, we quote Galen (*De Simplicium Medicamentorum Temperamentis ac Facultatibus Liber IX* (Chartier edition XIII, 249)) who makes it clear that Lemnian Earth should not be washed more than once:

> '... τινὲς δὲ δὶς ἢ τρὶς δέονται πλυθῆναι. τὴν μὲν οὖν Λημνίαν ἕτοιμην λαμβάνεις ἅπαξ πεπλυμένην ὑπὸ τῆς ἱερίας, ἐκ δευτέρου δε πλυθῆναι μὴ δεομένην'
>
> 'Some (earths) are washed twice or three times; but the Lemnian Earth you receive ready washed only once by the priestess; it is not advisable to wash it a second time' (authors' translation).

This comment suggests that the medicinal Lemnian Earth contained a soluble component which was the main ingredient for its efficacy. Further washing would dilute the strength of Lemnian Earth. It is also possible that this soluble component was never associated with the pit but rather was introduced into the pit by the stream itself, in the course of the year. We suggest that the stream, which travelled over the volcanic rock of the area, may have carried a soluble component which may have been dissolved alum.

Field evidence for alum

We did not encounter alum in samples recovered from the Phthelidia spring area but there were several clues that alum could have been produced in this area, given the geological setting. The main clue is that some altered rocks from the Phthelidia spring area which were sampled contain alunite. Rock samples collected from the area are brown to brownish yellow or red with white parts. Petrographic and powder X-ray diffraction analyses indicated that the white parts contain alunite as the main component, with kaolin and cristobalite, whereas the red ochreous material contains alunite and kaolin, with hematite, iron oxyhydroxides and quartz (Hall and Photos-Jones 2008; Photos-Jones *et al.* 2012). Alunite is an insoluble potassium aluminium sulphate mineral similar in composition to alum. It is quite rare and is formed in relatively high temperature hydrothermal acid sulphate alteration of volcanic rocks. Alunite is often found associated with alum group minerals and native sulphur, as on Melos (Hall *et al.* 2003). Its presence in rocks at the Phthelidia spring therefore indicates that the hydrothermal processes in this area had the *potential* to produce alum-group minerals. This alteration process is explained in detail in relation to the origin of Melian *alumen* (Hall *et al.* 2003; Hall and Photos-Jones 2005). Even if it had been produced hydrothermally in abundance, alum is unlikely to be found in surface outcrops near the Phthelidia spring because the geothermal process is no longer active and, being very soluble, alum would have long ago been washed out of surface rocks by rainwater. The samples recovered show pronounced alteration. We infer that the different 'varieties' of Lemnian Earths with various textures (sticky, greasy and granular) and colours (white, yellow and red) that are referred to in the early texts are products of hydrothermal alteration, with various proportions of the alteration products. This is not unexpected in the proximity of a geological fault in a former volcanic area. This fault is inferred from the linear outcrop of crags of volcanic rock at Phthelidia and presumably also constituted the main focus for the former hydrothermal solutions. The existence of alunite in the rock samples collected is therefore only an indicator of the former potential presence of alum, but does provide corroborative evidence in the search for the active ingredient within the Lemnian Earth.

The deposits of altered rock could have been worked as described by Belon in 'vein-like' features, presumably located at geological faults and fracture zones. Over time, soluble sulphates such as alum would have been 'washed' by rain out of the high ground of altered volcanic rocks, into the alluvial sediment of the area of the currently surrounding fields. They could therefore have found their way into man-made traps (pits) set in place and worked by ritual as in the accounts given above. Alum could therefore have been concentrated by absorption by clay minerals as they settled out of the spring water over the period of a year. Altered volcanic rocks would be both exposed and under the spring water. Pivotal to the investigation is the nature of the bedrock over which water flowed. It is possible that more than one pit was used as a trap in any given year. Deciding which pit to excavate at any given time must have been the result of deliberation on the part of the foreman in charge but also of the authorities.

It should be emphasised that although a case is made here for the possible presence of dissolved alum in the spring waters, we cannot exclude the possibility that aluminium may exist in solution as a cation and, as such, be exchanged with the clay minerals that form the main constituents of the earth.

The nature and properties of alum

Alum is currently a mineral group name for a large number of highly soluble hydrated sulphates (usually aluminium-rich sulphates), such as alunogen, $Al_2(SO_4)_3.17H_2O$, and potassium-alum, (K-alum), $KAl(SO_4)_2.12H_2O$. We therefore use the name 'alum' here for alum that is predominantly aluminium sulphate hydrate with or without potassium. Alum was of such commercial importance (as a mordant) in the 19th century that alum nomenclature was the subject of a book (Richardson 1927); it was argued that the word alum should be used only for potassium alum. The main concern seemed to be that K-alum was the standard material in use at that time, and its commercial status was being undermined by calling other minerals alum, in particular alunogen. In any case, alum (Latin: *alumen*; Greek: στυπτηρία, *stypteria*) has long been known for its astringency or styptic/haemostatic property. Although the word 'astringency' is probably best known for meaning a 'sharp' taste sensation, it also implies a 'drawing together', 'shrinkage' and 'drying' of soft body tissues. Astringency, in the latter sense, is a significant property of alum in relation to its medicinal and pharmaceutical uses.

Astringents known as styptics are employed to dry up excessive secretions and to stop oozing of blood. This astringency is a biochemical property, a physical effect involving the shrinking mucous membranes and the drying up of secretions. Astringency is also used to refer to a bitter taste sensation (Lawless *et al.* 1994). The reason for the taste relates to the biochemical properties of the astringents. The 'taste' aspect of 'astringency' is therefore not as 'fundamental' as the biochemical impact but it is understandable that that the word 'astringent' has become associated with the 'quality of taste' of fruit for example (Lawless *et al.* 1994; Eaks 1967).

An investigation of the use of alum as a mouth rinse (Mourughan and Suryakanth 2004) led these authors to consider that the alum acted as a bactericide reducing levels of *Streptococcus mutans* hence decreasing the risk of dental caries. The authors made it clear that the safety of the prolonged use of alum would need to be established before it could be used routinely. An early note by Young (1884) had warned that excessive use of alum can cause disintegration of teeth. Nevertheless, the study by Mourughan and Suryakanth (2004) provides good evidence of the antibacterial properties of alum.

Alum has long been used for large-scale water purification and acts as a flocculating agent, clearing water of microbes, clays as well as phosphorus and heavy metals (Linstedt *et al.* 1974). Martell *et al.* (1996) explain that the purification involves the precipitation of gelatinous aluminium hydroxide around any solid particles present, including bacteria. There is no antibacterial role envisaged in water purification. Yet a special use of alum for purification of contaminated water has been advocated, and in this case the alum is considered to be a bactericide (Ahmad, Jahan and Huq 1984); this study demonstrated that potassium aluminium sulphate (or potash alum) had an antibacterial effect in oral rehydration solution made with waters with a high bacterial count (gram-negative bacteria, *Vibrio cholerae* and *Escherichia coli*). Concentrations of only 500 mg/ml of potash alum per litre were effective within a few hours. The results of this study by Ahmed *et al.* (1984) clearly indicate the efficacy of alum as a bactericide.

In a recently published paper we have argued that minerals like alunite, montmorillonite and colemanite (the suggested active ingredient for the medicinal Samian earth being boron) but also zeolites are active in a biological environment with positive results (Photos-Jones *et al.* 2012, 636). This activity is related to their cation exchange properties. The antibacterial action of these minerals is a complex phenomenon and cannot be predicted on the basis of their mineral structure alone.

In parallel to our own work and that of our colleagues, there have been two separate sets of investigations on the nature of Lemnian Earth (Katsaros 2009, 365; Papoulis *et al.* 2011). These investigators ascribe the medicinal properties of Lemnian earth to the presence of As (and Pb) detected by chemical analysis in the rock/soils extracted at depth from the Kotsinas locality. However, they have also emphasised that in some samples the elevated amount of arsenic may not be beneficial but toxic, particularly under prolonged exposure (Papoulis *et al.* 2011). What is for certain is that the medicinal properties of the Lemnian Earth can not be defined in terms of composition and structure of the constituent parts alone. Studies of Egyptian bentonite for pharmaceutical use have shown that microbial tests are needed to establish the absence of pathogens and that the viable aerobic microorganisms need to be kept within allowed limits. (Abdel-Motelib *et al.* 2011). Although, in Antiquity, Lemnian Earth would not have undergone any quality control tests, it is expected that would have been largely relatively free of pathogens.

Conclusions

It is easy to pose the question 'What was Lemnian Earth?', and from our account so far it should be evident that this is not an easy question to answer. We have argued that the raw material was in itself the product of a man-induced enrichment process on an existing clay deposit. This information derives from documentary evidence, but it is not clear in its details. Yet we argue that it is consistent with many accounts that the earth was 'wet' or 'moist' when it was dug out. We suggest that the clay deposit (a mixture primarily of montmorillonite and kaolin) was being enriched over the course of the year by the waters of streams directed over it. The stream water may have been rich in alum or in aluminium deriving from a number of sources since it passed through what appears to be volcanically, hydrothermally altered rock; we have offered a tentative composition for Lemnian Earth consisting essentially of a clay with approximately 40% montmorillonite, 35% kaolin, 20% alum and 5% hematite (Hall and Photos-Jones 2008). We suggest that Lemnian Earth had alum as its active ingredient and one that might have worked as both an astringent and a bactericide when applied externally and when taken internally. The montmorillonitic clay not only provided the substrate but also could have acted as a poultice to reduce swelling. Its cation exchange capacities would have ensured the efficacy of the alum bearing minerals. One question that needs to be addressed pertains to the analysis of water samples for aluminium content from the surrounding springs. This is an ongoing project supported by field-based research.

Bibliography

Abdel-Motelib, Zainab Abdel Kader, Y.A. Ragab and Maha Mosalamy, 2011: 'Suitability of a Miocene bentonite from North Western Desert of Egypt for pharmaceutical use' *Applied Clay Science* 52, 140–4.

Ahmad, K., Jahan, K. and Huq, I. 1984: 'Decontamination of drinking water by alum for the preparation of oral rehydration solution', *The United Nations University Press: Food and Nutrition Bulletin* 6, 2.

Belon, P. 1588: *Les Observations de Plvsievrs Singvlaritéz et Choses Mémorables Trovvées en Grèce, etc.*, Paris.

Bent, J. T. 1893: *Early Voyages and Travels in the Levant: II. Extracts from the Diaries of Dr. John Covel, 1670–1679.* 1964 edition, New York.

Brock, A. J. 1929: *Greek Medicine, being Extracts Illustrative of Medical Writers from Hippocrates to Galen*, London.

de Launay, L. 1895: 'Notes sur Lemnos', *Revue Archéologique*, Series 3, 27, 318–23.

Eaks, I. L. 1967: 'Ripening and astringency removal in persimmon fruits', *Proceedings of the American Society for Horticultural Science* 91, 868–75.

Gomes, C. S. F. 2013: 'Naturotherapies based on Minerals', *Geomaterials*, 3, 1–14.

Gomes, C. S. F. and Silva, J. B. P. 2007: 'Minerals and clay minerals in medical geology', *Applied Clay Science* 36, 4–21.

Hall, A. J., Fallick, A. E., Perdikatsis, V. and Photos-Jones, E. 2003: 'A model for the origin of Al-rich efflorescences near fumaroles, Melos, Greece: enhanced weathering in a geothermal setting', *Mineralogical Magazine* 67, 363–79.

Hall, A. J. and Photos-Jones, E. 2005: 'The nature of Melian alumen and its potential for exploitation in antiquity', 77–84 in P. Borgard, J.-P. Brun and M. Picon (eds), *L'Alun de Meditérranée. Colloque International, Naples, June 2003. Naples: Centre Jean Bernard* 23.

Hall, A. J. and Photos-Jones, E. 2008: 'Accessing past beliefs and practices: the case of Lemnian Earth', *Archaeometry* 50, 1034–49.

Hall, A. J. and Photos-Jones, E. 2009: 'The juice of the pomegranate: quality control for the processing and distribution of alumen in antiquity and making sense of Pliny's *Phorimon* and *Paraphoron*' 197–206 in A. J. Shortland, I. C. Freestone and T. Rehren (eds), *From Mine to Microscope: Advances in the Study of Ancient Technology*, Oxford.

Katsaros: Κατσαρός, Θ. 2009: *Χρωματολογία Θεοφράστου του Ερεσσίου – Αναλύσεις, Ταυτοποίηση, Συμβολή στην Ανάδειξη Έργων Πολιτιστικής Κληρονομιάς*. Privately published PhD thesis, Rhodes.

Lawless, H. T., Corrigan, C. J. and Lee, C. B. 1994: 'Interactions of astringent substances', *Chemical Senses* 19, 141–54.

Linstedt, K. D., Bennett, E. R., Fox Jr, R. L. and Heaton, R. D. 1974: 'Alum clarification for improving wastewater effluent quality', *Water Research* 8, 753–60.

Martell, A. E., Hancock, R. D., Smith, R. M. and Motekaitis, R. J. 1996: 'Coordination of Al(III) in the environment and in biological systems', *Coordination Chemistry Reviews* 149, 311–28.

Mourughan, K. and Suryakanth, M. P. 2004: 'Evaluation of an alum-containing mouthrinse for inhibition of salivary *streptococcus mutans* levels in children – a controlled clinical trial', *Journal of the Indian Society of Pedodontics and Preventive Dentistry* 22, 100–5.

Papoulis D., Zagana, E., Koutsopoulou, E. and Roumelioti, P. 2011: 'Lemnian Earth: quality and suitability for medicinal uses', Poster paper presented in *GeoMed2011 – 4th International Conference on Medical Geology, Bari, Italy.*

Photos-Jones, E. and Hall, A. J. 2010: '*Stypteria phorime* as alunogen in solution: possible pointer to the gradual cooling of the Melos geothermal system' *Hellenic Journal of Geosciences* 45, 217–26.

Photos-Jones, E. and Hall, A. J. 2011: *Lemnian Earth and the earths of the Aegean: an archaeological guide to medicines, pigments and washing powders*, Glasgow.

Photos-Jones E., Hall, A. J., Περδικάτσης, Β., Δήμου, Ε. and Χιώτης, Ε. 2012: '*Τα όρια μύθου και πραγματικότητας για τις ιαματικές γαίες της αρχαιότητας*', 623–38 in N. Zacharias, M. Georgakopoulou, K. Polykreti, G. Fakorellis and Th. Vakoulis (eds), *Proceedings of the 5th Symposium of the Greek Archaeometry Society 2008*, Athens.

Richardson, W. D. 1927: *The Current Significance of the Word Alum*, Chicago.

Thompson, C. J. S. 1914: 'Terra Sigillata, a famous medicament of ancient times', in *Proceedings of the 17th International Congress of Medicine* 23, London, 433–44.

Tourptsoglou-Stephanidou: Τουρπτσόγλου-Στεφανίδου, Β. 1986: Ταξιδιωτικά καί γεωγραφικά κείμενα γιά τή νήσο Λήμνο (15–20 αιώνας) (Geographic and Travellers' accounts about the island of Lemnos (15th–20th centuries), *University of Thessaloniki, The Polytechnic School*, Vol. IX, Suppl. 33.

Young, M. 1884: 'Effect of alum gargles upon the teeth', *American Journal of Pharmacy* 56, 10.

25. Ancient Desires to Shape Progeny: the Role of Vision and Soul in Greek and Jewish Sources of Late Antiquity

Ohr Y. Margalit and Chariklia Tziraki-Segal

The ancients, like us, desired to influence the characteristics of their progeny. Their writings reveal a number of 'theories' they believed influenced the foetus. This article focuses on the sense of vision and its connection to the soul as a force influencing offspring. Both Jewish and Greek ancient sources are included in our analysis. We conclude that the Aristotelian theories on the vision-soul axis as well as appetite/passion axis appear to be incorporated in the ancient Jewish sources. However, the epistemological nature of Jewish thought requires that both male and female vision play a role in shaping the human foetus.

Introduction

The ancients, like us today, desired to influence the characteristics of progeny they begot. Although they lacked the dazzling technologies that we have at our disposal, their writings reveal a number of 'theories' and notions that impact on the development of offspring. This article focuses on the role of vision in shaping offspring. We present examples of ancient texts that attribute to vision a role in shaping the foetus. What theories of vision (sight) did the ancients generate to express their notions of how visual information enters, interacts and is processed within corporeal living entities? As we shall see, matters related to desire, rational and irrational faculties and the nature of male and female become part of the discourse in the ancient theories of vision (sight).

We focus on extant writings that shaped the development of Western science, and specifically those texts that appear to have provided the fundamental elements for the theories of vision. Aristotle's theories provided the basis of the scientific understanding of vision. Galen made some additions and modifications to Aristotle's theories and observations. The Romans adopted Aristotle's theories with little modification or innovations (Lindberg 1978, 78).

We limit our current study to texts up to the end of the 5th century CE. The scientific additions made by subsequent followers of Aristotle and Galen, the Arabic scientists, such as Ḥunayn Ibn Ishãq and Avicenna, are not included in this article. It is important to mention that the Arabic scientists preserved, translated and re-introduced to Europe ancient Greek thought and science (Conrad *et al.* 1995, 11–2; Green 1985, 73–80; Wade 1998, 17).

In this paper we include both ancient Greek and ancient Jewish sources. These texts are different from one another not only in content, but also in purpose and literary styles. First, Greek texts that are of interest to the issue of vision and reproduction are examined. The focus is on texts reflecting Aristotelian thought.

The nature and composition of the Jewish ancient texts may be less familiar to the reader; therefore, we present an overview of the origins and composition of Jewish sources. We then examine Jewish ancient texts that reflect the possible application of these ancient theories of vision to the reproductive process.

Our aim is to explore how epistemological underpinnings influence 'medical' notions about reproduction and human agency, and how these notions are expressed in the two different kinds of ancient texts. We conclude that the Aristotelian theories regarding vision (sight) appear to be incorporated into the ancient Jewish sources in a manner that reflects the belief that both male and female agency have the potential to influence the human foetus.

With this introduction, we now turn to Greek texts that pertain to our query of how vision (sight), thought and reproduction are related. We present first the Aristotelian texts.

The Aristotelian perspective

An informative text on Aristotle's perspective regarding human agency and reproduction is found in *Problemata*:

> Διὰ τί τοῖς ἄλλοις ζῴοις τὰ ἔκγονα μᾶλλον τὰς φύσεις ὁμοιοῦται ἢ τοῖς ἀνθρώποις; ἢ ὅτι ὁ μὲν ἄνθρωπος πολλαχῶς διατίθεται τὴν ψυχὴν κατὰ τὴν ὁμιλίαν, καθὼς δ' ἂν ὁ πατὴρ καὶ ἡ μήτηρ διατεθῶσιν, οὕτω ποικίλλεται καὶ τὰ τικτόμενα. τὰ δὲ ἄλλα ζῷα τὰ μὲν πλεῖστα πρὸς αὐτὸ τοῦτό εἰσιν. ἔτι δὲ οὐ πληροῦται ὡς ἐπὶ τὸ πολὺ διὰ ταύτην τὴν ἐπιθυμίαν.
>
> 'Why do the offspring of other animals resemble their parents more than is the case with men? Is it because at the time of association, man is variously disposed, and the variations of the offspring depend on the dispositions of the father and mother. The other animals are mostly intent upon the sexual act, whereas human beings are not entirely absorbed in this desire. Further, owing to this avidity impregnation does not usually take place' (*Problemata* X.7, 891^{b}10–11, trans. Hett 1936).

Aristotle, as we discuss further on, has a well-developed 'biological' theory about how foetal conception occurs and how offspring is shaped. His theories on these topics are applicable to human and animal conception. Why then, does Aristotle raise as a problem, the larger phenotypic variations he observes in the human offspring as compared to the animal offspring? We may postulate that Aristotle, being an acute observer, needs some additional theory to explain the phenotypic variants he detects among offspring of humans and their parents. In this text, Aristotle plainly suggests two factors: the fluctuating mental condition of both male and female during sexual intercourse in humans but not in animals; and the variability of 'desire' for coitus in humans. Animals, on the other hand, are wholly absorbed in the act with great desire, and although this may hamper impregnation in some instances, their offspring will resemble them.

Thus, if we wish to know how offspring is shaped to look like the parents, we need to understand how Aristotle perceives these mental fluctuations and the variability in affinity (desire) for coitus among humans.

We argue that for Aristotle, both of these activities involve the soul, ψυχήν. As has been described by classical scholars, Aristotle's views included a hierarchy of souls: the highest being that of the rational soul found uniquely in humans. The lowest is the vegetative, nutritive soul found in plants. In the middle of this hierarchy is the sensitive, animal soul, found in all other living beings. Scholars believe that this hierarchy represents the 'recapitulation' principle of evolution, which suggests that all elements of this hierarchy exist to some degree in humans as well. This type of understanding is crucial to our discussion here.

How do the various kinds of souls come to play such an important role in the biological concerns of our text? The answer to this query, as we shall demonstrate, involves two different sets of processes that interact with each other and the soul.

The first one we discuss, we shall refer to as the process of 'vision-soul' loop. The second we refer to as the 'appetite/passion-soul' loop. We intend to argue that visual input influences the soul and this influence is reflected back to the *conceptus*; a process similar to hormonal or neural biofeedback loops familiar to a modern biology reader. The sentient, rational soul is ultimately involved in both of these loops. However, it is the intermediate level animal soul that connects the rational soul to the corporeal human senses and functions, for example, the reproductive process, which is our focus in this paper.

According to Aristotle, the sensitive soul was made up of three rather distinct faculties: κοινὸν αἰσθητήριον, φανταστικόν, μνημονευτικόν. Aristotle discusses these faculties in his works *De Generatione Animalium*, chapter III, as well as in *De Memoria et Reminiscentia*. We present only key excerpts from these works. In *De Generatione Animalium*, III 414b33–415a3 he describes the κοινὸν αἰσθητήριον (often translated as 'common sense') as related to διανοτικόν. Cognition is perhaps a reasonable translation for what Aristotle wishes to express with the word διανοτικόν, one of the functions of the inner faculty of κοινὸν αἰσθητήριον (see also *De Generatione Animalium*, III, 4–6 as well as his discussions in *On the Soul* 425^{a}14). What does Aristotle signify when he uses the words φαντασία and κοινὸν αἰσθητήριον?

Most scholars are of the opinion that κοινὸν αἰσθητήριον is the place where integrative functions occur. Information arrives from all the five external senses (discussed in *De Generatione Animalium* II 5 12: touch, vision, hearing, smell, taste) as well as input from the other internal faculties. This information is integrated and passed on to the rational soul – νοῦς. This flow of information also happens in the reverse, from the rational soul down to the three inner faculties, creating a loop.

The faculty of φαντασία, *phantasia*, seems to be of central importance in the reproduction of specific kind of offspring. How does Aristotle view the faculty of φαντασία? We argue that Aristotle views the workings of φαντασία in a clearly biological context, similar to the anatomic classification of the other senses generated by the external corporeal organs, such as the eye, ear, skin (Singer 1941, 39–50; Nussbaum 1978, 265–9).

The external organ associated with *phantasia* is the eye and therefore we need to know how Aristotle views the connection between the eye, sight (vision) and the faculty of φαντασία and of course νοῦς, rationality. Aristotle states that 'without presentation (usually translated as imagination) … intellectual activity is impossible' (*De Memoria et Reminiscentia* I 450a30). As a matter of fact, he states that 'to the thinking soul, presentations serve as present sensations' (*De Generatione Animalium* III, 431a, 14–5).

How are these 'presentations' – εἴδωλα, *eidola* – generated? Aristotle evokes the concept of ἀέρας, *aeras*, air, as the medium through which 'presentations' are generated. Aristotle presents his scientific concept of *aeras* as operating as follows: light, movement and colour emanate from the objects and their forms. These emanations are transmitted through the transparent liquid of the eye into the inside of the body to create a presentation (*eidola*) of the object, in the inner faculty of *phantasia* (Wade 1998, 76).[1]

Aristotle's conception of how sight through the medium of air makes the impression from the external environment into the internal faculties is interesting: 'like a seal, it makes an impression without any transfer of material' (*De Generatione Animalium* II, 424a17–22). The impressions created in the faculty of φαντασία, interact both with the faculties of κοινόν αἰσθητήριον [and its διανοτικόν], as well as with μνημονευτικόν, and νοῦς. These impressions – or perhaps more accurately for modern readers – presentations are:

> 'imprinted from an already existing object and could not come from anything non-existent working through the five senses and each sense knows only what it perceives. What remains constant are the visual nature and the associations that this therefore created between perception, thought, and sight, which are all thought to be interactive. Sight in the classical world ... was defined as the most important and reliable of the senses' (Eastmond and James 2003, 61).

Aristotle in his construct of air as the medium of sight, assumes that the eye receives data originating from the object. He differs from his predecessors in this respect. Lindberg (1976, 33–47) discusses the marvellous details between these different theories and points out that extramissionists proposed that light 'with eternal fire' leaves the eye and seeks the object of vision; while the intramissionists viewed the objects as emitting eminences containing 'astral' forces which reach the eye.

Aristotle seems to incorporate elements of both these theories. What both approaches share is the 'astral'/'internal fire' with an almost divine quality to the medium of transmission, air. According to Aristotle, air's nature is to move eternally in a circle, not only in the living beings but also in the universe as a whole. It is a divine substance engulfing the whole of the upper cosmos, stars and planets. The rational soul contains the quintessence of this divine constituent (*De Caelo* 268–9, 289a). Thus, Aristotle theorised that there is a spark of 'heavenly' element in the medium of air. It is this heavenly imbued medium that transports external data from the objects through the sense of sight to the inner faculty of *phantasia*. It is in this faculty that 'presentations' are first imprinted and then become available and interactive to the other inner faculties and *nous*.

As mentioned above, Aristotle locates the faculty of *phatansia* in the animal soul (*De Generatione Animalium* 418a26–424a15). We have to keep in mind that Aristotle's perception of the soul, which he places in the heart, encompasses both his philosophical theories and his biological knowledge and observations (*De Generatione Animalium* 412a6–26). However, Aristotle's biological writings do not often include the words 'common sense' (κοινὸν αἰσθητήριον) in relation to the soul, while his philosophical writings do. Apparently, this difference in the classification and nomenclature of the faculties of the soul appears to be related to the tendency of the ancient Greek physicians to view internal faculties as directly correlated with external organs. Philosophers, on the other hand, tended to define a 'faculty' as something that had an indivisible unique nature (Wolfson 1935, 99).

The line of thought we have presented up to now describes the 'vision-soul' feedback loop. This loop represents the physiological process by which a bridge, so to speak, is created by 'astral' air, for carrying data from the eye, the external organ of the sense of vision, to the internal senses. These data are transmitted to the φανταστικὸν section of the animal soul, present in humans as well as animals. Perhaps this connection may explain why Aristotle can comfortably provide an example of a woman who gave birth to twins, one resembling the father and the other the lover. The incident is recorded at the conclusion of the discussion on 'superfoetation' in *De Generatione Animalium* I, 585a, 15. The assumption is that the woman at the time of conception of the first foetus was receiving 'presentations' looking at her lover, and shortly thereafter at her husband! Their respective likeness is 'imprinted' through the sense of vision on the inner faculty of *phantasia* and then through the same medium – air – becomes imprinted on the two foetuses. It may also explain why he recommends that pregnant women be made to take a regular walk in the beautiful temples of ancient Greece:

> καθ' ἡμέραν τινὰ ποιεῖσθαι πορείαν πρὸς θεῶν ἀποθεραπείαν τῶν εἰληχότων τὴν περὶ τῆς γενέσεως τιμήν. τὴν μέντοι διάνοιαν τοὐναντίον τῶν σωμάτων ῥᾳθυμοτέρως ἁρμόττει διάγειν.
>
> '[Women who are with child should be careful of themselves] they shall take a walk daily to some temple, where they can worship the gods who preside over birth. Their minds, however, unlike their bodies, they ought to keep quiet; for the offspring derive their natures from their mothers as plants do from the earth (*Politica*, 1335b, 15–19, trans. Jowett 1921, fol. X)'.

The examples presented so far appear to operate through the 'vision-soul' feedback loop. We now turn our attention to the appetite/passion-soul loop. This loop is also implied in our opening text from *Problemata.* The role of the appetites/passions-soul loop requires that we also understand how desire enters into the interplay between the external sense of vision, and the internal faculties of the animal soul:

διανοτικόν, φαντασία, μνημονευτικόν, and ultimately the higher level of the rational soul, νοῦς.

In a simplified way, Aristotle presents the following theory of how this interaction takes place: he assumes that appetite, desire – ὄρεξις – evokes the sense of ἐπιθυμία, a sensation that is influenced in both humans and animals by μνημονευτικόν (*De Generatione Animalium* II, 3, 414b 1–2; *De Memoria et Reminiscentia* 2, 453a 9–14). We have already seen that this sense is influenced by vision through the faculty of *phantasia*, φανταστικόν. Desire and wanting – ὄρεξις and ἐπιθυμία – are in turn modulated by other sensations such as irritability and anger (*Nicomachean Ethics* VI, 7, 114a28). In turn, these sensations are modulated by the inner power of ψυχικὴ δύναμις (will-power) which Aristotle appears to view as existing within the domain of the faculty of διανοτικὸν in humans, and in animals by σύνεσις.

The whole idea of movement initiated and modulated by the various faculties is of course to influence the choice of action to be made in the process of movement. We would suggest, following Nussbaum's analysis, that Aristotle is of the opinion that the power of the living being influences what choice of action is made following the input of the external senses as synthesised and modulated by the inner faculties and the *nous* (rational soul) (Nussbaum 1978, 381–2). We need to be mindful of the fact that, that 'intellect, imagination and other internal senses did not always harmonize with each other or with the external senses' (MacCormack 1991, 26).

We can now see a general picture emerging. On the one hand, the vision-soul feedback loop interacts and influences the three internal faculties: διανοτικόν, φανταστικόν (*phantasia*) μνημονευτικόν (memory). This loop in turn intersects with the appetite/passion-soul loop that connects the sense of appetite – ὄρεξις, desire – ἐπιθυμία, and διανοτικόν. Both loops interact with *nous*.

As Nussbaum suggests, it is in the sphere of the appetite/passion soul loop where issues of moral control come into play, as we can see in the following text:

> ἀλλ εἴ τις πρὸς ἃς οἱ πολλοὶ δύνανται ἀντέχειν, τούτων ἡττᾶται καὶ μὴ δύναται ἀντιτείνειν, μὴ διὰ φύσιν τοῦ γένους ἢ διὰ νόσον, οἷον ἐν τοῖς Σκυθῶν βασιλεῦσιν ἡ μαλακία διὰ τὸ γένος, καὶ ὡς τὸ θῆλυ πρὸς τὸ ἄρρεν διέστηκεν. ἀκρασίας δὲ τὸ μὲν προπέτεια τὸ δ' ἀσθένεια. οἳ μὲν γὰρ βουλευσάμενοι οὐκ ἐμμένουσιν οἷς ἐβουλεύσαντο διὰ τὸ πάθος, οἳ δὲ διὰ τὸ μὴ βουλεύσασθαι ἄγονται ὑπὸ τοῦ πάθους· ἔνιοι γάρ, ὥσπερ προγαργαλίσαντες οὐ γαργαλίζονται, οὕτω καὶ προαισθόμενοι καὶ προϊδόντες καὶ προεγείραντες ἑαυτοὺς καὶ τὸν λογισμὸν οὐχ ἡττῶνται ὑπὸ τοῦ πάθους, οὔτ' ἂν ἡδὺ ᾖ οὔτ' ἂν λυπηρόν. μάλιστα δ' οἱ ὀξεῖς καὶ μελαγχολικοὶ τὴν προπετῆ ἀκρασίαν εἰσὶν ἀκρατεῖς· οἳ μὲν γὰρ διὰ τὴν ταχυτῆτα οἳ δὲ διὰ τὴν σφοδρότητα οὐκ ἀναμένουσι τὸν λόγον, διὰ τὸ ἀκολουθητικοὶ εἶναι τῇ φαντασίᾳ.

> 'But it is surprising if a man is defeated by and cannot resist pleasures or pains which most men can hold out against, when this is not due to heredity or disease, like the softness that is hereditary with the kings of the Scythians, or that which distinguishes the female sex from the male. Of incontinence one kind is impetuosity, another weakness. For some men after deliberating fail, owing to their emotion, to stand by the conclusions of their deliberation, others because they have not deliberated are led by their emotion; since some men (just as people who first tickle others are not tickled themselves), if they have first perceived and seen what is coming and have first roused themselves and their calculative faculty, are not defeated by their emotion, whether it be pleasant or painful. It is keen and excitable people that suffer especially from the impetuous form of incontinence; for the former by reason of their quickness and the latter by reason of the violence of their passions do not await the argument, because they are apt to follow their imagination' (*Nicomachean Ethics* 1150b 14–18; 20–33, trans. Irwin 1999).

Now, it is perhaps a bit easier to understand our opening text in *Problemata* regarding the easily distracted humans during coitus and the consequences of this distraction. In addition, however, our text informs us of possible hereditary defects in these two loops. More significantly, for our current argument, Aristotle informs us that there are gender related defects on how these two loops operate. The female has a weaker appetite/passion-soul loop, thus her rationality does not take charge of her passions.

In the *Problemata* text cited above, Aristotle implicates both the male's and female's fluctuating mental status, the vision-soul loop, and the appetite/passion loop. In the above text, the gender difference of these two loops becomes quite apparent. In the female, the appetite/passion-soul axis is weaker and not so well developed by Nature! While the vision-soul loop is considered to be 'constantly disrupted by menstruation' (*On Dreams* 460, 7–46). Thus, female vision and *phantasia* are not 'stable' due to the menstruation cycle and the weaker ψυχικὴ δύναμις (will-power) in Nature's design of the female. Therefore, the female must be made to focus during coitus. It is her desires that must be channelled and controlled, in order to influence the foetus in a specific manner.

Galen's views of the female and his notion of the medium involved in vision are somewhat different. We would like to briefly consider his adaptations of Aristotelian notions, since Galen's books and style of writing 'scientific' treatises was most appealing to the Arabic scientists. Greek scientific knowledge was revived, expanded and transmitted back to the West through the Arabic scholars (Green 1985, 71).

Galen adapted the Aristotelian model of the five external senses and the three internal faculties (Wolfson 1935, 72). However, Galen included some important modifications. The anatomical knowledge generated by Herophilus at the Alexandrian school of medicine, was incorporated by Galen in his understanding of vision (Von Staden 1989, 73). Galen introduced the term *pneuma* instead of the Aristotelian *aeras*, air. This new scientific term refers to an ethereal substance present throughout the body and the universe, an unseeing and unfelt medium, through which light reflected from objects and forms is carried through the lenses of the eye to the optic nerve, a previously unidentified organ, existing behind the pupil of the eye. The optic nerve carries this *pneuma* to the brain, another new anatomical piece of knowledge (Wade 1998, 73). Specifically, Galen locates the διανοτικόν, φαντασία, μνημονευτικὸν in the anterior, middle and posterior brain ventricles respectively. Avicena (10th century CE) adopted and refined the system of external organs and inner senses further while retaining the meaning and functions as defined by Aristotle, although adding new vocabulary and subcategories to the inner senses and the composition of the animal soul (Siegel 1970, 216).

In the view of most scholars of the history of science, Aristotelian thought was crucial to the western scientific enterprise (Magner 2005, 40). Yet his theories were interpreted and construed to serve a variety of purposes and political agendas.

> 'Although Aristotle had many disciples, he completely overshadows them. His ideas dominated biology as well as other aspects of theories of the phenomena of live being. The great tragedy is that while Aristotle's own approach to the study of nature called for a close and accurate observation, respect for facts, systematic collection of evidence, and deductions from facts, this part of his teachings was almost completely neglected. Later scholars tended to become slavish followers of the words, rather than the spirit of Aristotle.... Indeed the biology of antiquity and the Middle Ages never really got beyond Aristotle' (Magner 2005, 40).

It is for this reason that throughout this paper we prefer the terms of maternal or female *phantasia*. This phraseology maintains, in our opinion, a closer approximation of the Aristotelian thought as found in his texts. The term *phantasia* is often translated as 'imagination' a term that is not entirely consistent with what Aristotle means, for there is a difference between 'imagination' and 'fancy' in the English language (Schofield 1978, 100). The terms of 'maternal imprinting' that recent scholars are using in connection to *phantasia*, masks the connection of the sense of vision (sight) to the faculty of *phantasia*. This connection allows for a reading of the ancient texts relating to the use and understanding of *phantasia* in a way that brings into focus the vision-soul loop in a scientific context. Moreover, the term 'maternal imprinting' appears first in Mediaeval texts and then not in a well-defined manner (Boucé 1982, 88). How the Aristotelian concepts were re-interpreted within the religious environment of Christianity and Islam is beyond the scope of this paper.

However, within the historic period under consideration here (up to the 5th century CE) there are several examples of texts that demonstrate how these concepts of the vision-soul and the appetite/passion-soul loops come into play in both human and animal foetal development.

Other Greek examples of the influence of *phantasia*

Aristotle's beliefs regarding maternal thoughts during coitus and gestation are also reflected in the works of other major ancient writers who followed him. A selected few are presented next.

Soranus, a physician who lived in the 1st–2nd century CE, writes:

> τί δεῖ λέγειν, ὅτι καὶ τὸ ποιὸν τῆς ψυχῆς κατάστημα φέρει τινὰς περὶ τοὺς τύπους τῶν συλλαμβανομένων μεταβολάς; οὕτως ἐν τῷ συνουσιάζειν πιθήκους ἰδοῦσαί τινες πιθηκομόρφους ἐκύησαν· ὁ δὲ τῶν Κυπρίων τύραννος κακόμορφος ὢν εἰς ἀγάλματα περικαλλῆ κατὰ τοὺς πλησιασμοὺς τὴν γυναῖκα βλέπειν ἀναγκάζων [ὁ] πατὴρ εὐμόρφων ἐγένετο παίδων..... οὖν μήτε ἄμορφον ἀποτελεσθῇ τὸ γεννώμενον ἀλλοκότους φαντασίας ἐν τῷ μεθύειν τῆς ψυχῆς ὑπομενούσης, νηφέτωσαν αἱ γυναῖκες ἐν τοῖς πλησιασμοῖς, εἶθ' ὅτι καὶ πρὸς τὰς μητέρας ὁμοιότης τις οὐ κατὰ σῶμα μόνον, ἀλλὰ καὶ κατὰ ψυχὴν ἀναφέρεται τῶν γεννωμένων. καλὸν οὖν εὐσταθούσῃ τῇ ψυχῇ καὶ μὴ παρακόπῳ διὰ μέθην ὅμοιον ἀποτελεσθῆναι τὸ γεννώμενον.
>
> 'What is one to say concerning the fact that various states of the soul also produce certain changes in the mold of the fetus? For instance, some women, seeing monkeys during intercourse, have borne children resembling monkeys. The tyrant of the Cyprians, who was misshapen, compelled his wife to look at beautiful statues during intercourse and became the father of well-shaped children; and horse-breeders, during covering, place noble horses in front of the mares ... Thus in order that the offspring may not be rendered misshapen, women must be sober during coitus because in drunkenness the soul becomes the victim of strange fantasies; this furthermore, because the offspring bears some resemblance to the mother as well, not only in body but in soul' (Soranus, *Gynecology*, I, 39, trans. Tempkin 1956).

Soranus reflects the Aristotelian thought regarding breeding of beautiful animals. The process of human and animal reproduction in this respect appears to be the same. He emphasises the important influence of the female state of mind and body. He clearly demonstrates that both the vision-soul and appetite/passion-soul feedback loops of the female during coitus need to be brought under control to have a properly formed offspring. He, like Aristotle, does not provide examples of the male vision-soul feedback loop and its role in human or animal reproduction.

This same story is also found in the writing of Galen but with some significant information of how vision works:

> ἐμοὶ δὲ καὶ λόγος τὶς ἀρχαῖος ἐμήνυσεν ὅτι τῶν ἀμόρφων τὶς δυνατὸς εὔμορφον θέλων γεννῆσαι παῖδα, ἐποίησε γράψαι ἐν

πλατεῖ ξύλῳ εὐειδὲς ἄλλο παιδίον, καὶ ἔλεγε τῇ γυναικὶ συμπλεκόμενος ἐκείνῳ τῷ τύπῳ τῆς γραφῆς ἐμβλέπειν. ἡ δὲ ἀτενὲς βλέπουσα καὶ ὡς ἔστιν εἰπεῖν ὅλον τὸν νοῦν ἔχουσα οὐχὶ τῷ γεννήσαντι, ἀλλὰ τῷ γεγραμμένῳ ὁμοίως ἀπέτεκε τὸ παιδίον, τῆς ὄψεως, οἶμαι, διαπεμπούσης τῇ φύσει, ἀλλ' οὐκ ὄγκοις τισὶ τοῦ γεγραμμένου τοὺς τύπους.

'Some old story informed me that a powerful man, ugly, wishing to beget a beautiful child, had made a painting of another good-looking baby, and he told his wife to watch that painted image while embracing him, she then, continually looking and, so to say, having her entire mind [on it], delivered the baby, not similar to the begetter but to the painted one; I am of the opinion that her vision transmitted the features of the painted one by nature, not by some particles' (Galenus, *De theriaca ad Pisonem* IX, 449; Kuhn (1821–33) 449).

This story has the amazing detail of a child painting. We can hypothesise that, based on the discussion so far, the sight of the woman, seeing the beautiful painting created a 'presentation' through the mediation of *pneuma*, not of particles (Democritus' opinion was that particles were involved). This 'presentation' is transferred through the optic nerve to the middle ventricle, where the inner faculty of *phantasia* is located and from there to the foetus through the *pneuma* who travelled along the nerves to all the parts of the body. The transfer, we are led to believe, is enhanced by the concentration of mind, an undisturbed intension focused on the desired painting. It is interesting that Galen is the only one that actually mentions that the painting was that of a child, as opposed to an adult representation.

Yet despite Galen's advanced anatomical knowledge, including the optic nerve, brain ventricles and female ovaries and 'seed', he also sees that the female 'appetite/passion-soul' and the 'vision-soul' loops had a manipulability at the hands of the male. Thus, a male, ugly as he may be, can beget a beautiful offspring not resembling his ugly male maker.

Gourevitch (1987, 561) includes this technique, also referred to occasionally as *eupaideia* by Dionysius of Halicarnassus (Kuchler, 446), in her thorough review of Greco-Roman sources and the use of statues during procreative intercourse.[2]

An illustrative example of female vision influencing the offspring is found in the work of Oppian of Apamea (or Pella) in Syria. He wrote a poem on hunting, *Cynegetica,* which is dedicated to the emperor Caracalla (thus possibly placing the text *c.* 211 CE). In this text, Oppian gives numerous examples of how to breed horses and birds of different colours by putting varied coloured cloths in front of the copulating animals. He calls this a 'glorious device' used by animal breeders (*Cynegetica,* I. 330–57). This technique was apparently equally effective when used by husbands on their wives to produce beautiful sons:

ναὶ μὴν ὧδε Λάκωνες ἐπίφρονα μητίσαντο αἶσι φίλαις ἀλόχοις, ὅτε γαστέρα κυμαίνουσι· γράψαντες πινάκεσσι πέλας θέσαν ἀγλαὰ κάλλη, τοὺς πάρος ἀστράψαντας ἐν ἡμερίοισιν ἐφήβους, Νιρέα καὶ Νάρκισσον ἐϋμμελίην θ' Ὑάκινθον, Κάστορά τ' εὐκόρυθον καὶ Ἀμυκοφόνον Πολυδεύκην, ἠϊθέους τε νέους, τοί τ' ἐν μακάρεσσιν ἀγητοί, Φοῖβον δαφνοκόμην καὶ κισσοφόρον Διόνυσον· αἱ δ' ἐπιτέρπονται πολυήρατον εἶδος ἰδοῦσαι, τίκτουσίν τε καλοὺς ἐπὶ κάλλεϊ πεπτηυῖαι.

'Nay, even so also the Laconians contrived a subtle device for their dear wives when they are pregnant. Near them they put pictures of beautiful forms, even the youths that afortime were resplendent among mortal men, Nireus and Narcisssus and Hyacinthus of the goodly ashen spear, and Castor with his helmet, and Polydeuces that slew Amyeus, and the youthful twains who are admired among the blessed gods, laurel-crowned Phoebus and Dionysus of the ivy wreath. And the women rejoice to behold their lovely form and, fluttered by their beauty, bear beautiful sons' (*Cynegetica* 1.358–367; Papathomopoulos (ed.) 2003, 17)

This text demonstrates how statues of specific admired male heroes are used to produce beautiful sons, much like the Cypriot tyrant and his use of a child painting. The child painting does appear more appropriate, at first glance. However, as we show below in relation to the Jewish sources, the statues of brave and beautiful heroes used by Spartans may have had the additional advantage of creating and transmitting presentations of characteristics other than physical beauty. Here we also note that the woman's vision-soul loop is operating during gestation, not just during conception.

The male ensures that the beautiful male statues are in the visual field of their pregnant female. This story, told amidst a hunting poem, clearly *en passant*, without any conscious religious or philosophical propaganda, suggests that the reproduction of certain types of animals and children by manipulation of the female vision-soul loop was a widespread belief among all kinds of writers, not just doctors and philosophers/scientists.

The underlying assumptions of the examples we have presented so far, suggest that the prevailing theory of reproduction is that the offspring is expected to resemble the father. Some scholars rightly assert that this need for paternal resemblance of the offspring is a reflection of the male's anxiety about who the father is. Motherhood is of course a social and biological given (Doniger and Spinner 1998, 101; Shildrick 2000, 24). Aristotelian conception of the ancient belief that paternity implies paternal resemblance of the offspring would be helpful in our elucidating the intertwining of science and social constructs, such as gender.

Aristotle was a strong proponent of the 'hematogenetic' principle of sperm generation where the male sperm, having been cold and more 'concocted', was the prime mover in the shaping of the foetus (*Historia Animalium* 3.2, 511^{b}31–512^{b}10). The maternal contribution was only of nutritive support (ὕλη). De *Generatione Animalium*, book I, discusses these notions in detail. This axiom, along with the concept of *epikrateia,* where the stronger of the two sperms, male or female, becomes the primary influencing force on the foetus, do present challenges in understanding Aristotle's human generation theories. This issue is addressed by numerous scholars (for example, Morsink 1979; Witt 1985).

For Aristotle, therefore, the perfect offspring would be a male resembling the father, a belief common also in ancient Near East societies (Tigay 1977, 146). Aristotle, however, was a true observer of nature and could not, therefore, explain the numerous phenotypical variations of offspring. We may suggest that in addition to the concept of strife resulting from the notion of *epikrateia* of the strongest sperm, female *phantasia*, unbridled by the weaker will-power, ψυχικὴ δύναμις, of the female, offers an attractive alternative to phenotypic variations observed in offspring. The alternative would be to admit that paternity can never be ascertained or that impregnation occurred by another male not the husband/father. The alternative explanation would have been neither suitable nor socially viable for an ancient patriarchal Mediterranean society. Aristotle, therefore, invented theories of generation and heredity that were compatible with the social constructs of the society of which he was a member (Caston 1996, 55).

We would like to suggest that the texts cited so far demonstrate that Aristotle and his followers positioned female vision-soul loop as well as appetite/passion-soul loop in the contexts of social constructs that allow male control of these faculties, partly in order to ensure control over anxieties about paternity and thus the continuation of self. This may explain why we do not encounter any examples in the Greek texts where male *phantasia* is manipulated in the service of reproduction.

Perhaps one could suggest that Aristototle believed that males having a higher level of control of their will-power, ψυχικὴ δύναμις, over their appetites did not allow their vision or their passions to dictate their actions.

However, his hypothesis is not entirely satisfactory. Let us demonstrate using the ugly Cypriot tyrant story (real or myth is not crucial). The tyrant had the option, given his stronger will-power to force himself to look at a beautiful child statue. He was the ugly one, who desired a beautiful offspring – not one resembling him. The tyrant himself, we must conclude, believed both in the theory of *epikrateia* and in the weak female vision-soul loop. For he obviously accepted as his own, this beautiful son, believing it was his seed, and only the child's outer appearance was changed through the manipulation of his wife's vision-soul feedback loop.

Notions related to the vision-soul loop and the appetite/passion loop in the reproductive process, are also found in the works of early Christian writers. We present here an example given by Hieronymus (Saint Jerome, Ευσέβιος Σωφρόνιος Ιερώνυμος, *c.* 347–420 CE). He is a good bridge to the Jewish sources that follow, because he was believed to be trained as a doctor who lived in Palestine during the historical time we are considering in this article. Moreover, his example is taken from a shared ancient Jewish text, the biblical book of *Genesis*. In his Christian commentary to *Genesis* 30: 32–47, he describes in detail the process by which Jacob used rods in the drinking troughs of the sheep which resulted in the generation of the spotted sheep that Jacob desired. He then adds the following commentary in relation to verse 33 which is directly relevant to our subject:

> 'Now it is not astonishing that this is the nature of female creatures in the act of conception: the offspring they produce are of such a kind as the things they observe or perceive in their minds during the most intense heat of sexual pleasure. For this very thing is reported by the Spaniards to happen even among herds of horses; and Quintilian, in that lawsuit in which a married woman was accused of having given birth to an Ethiopian, brought as evidence in her defense that what we have been describing above is a natural process in the conception of offspring' (Jerome, trans. Hayward 1995, 67–8).

Here again we note that animal reproduction and human reproduction techniques are mentioned as if equivalent processes from a 'biological' perspective. Hieronymus, does not even bother to give an explanation of why the *phantasia* of the female specifically, is believed to have influenced the offspring either by direct sight or by a stored vision 'presentation' in the memory of the animal soul. He just states that this occurrence is not surprising!

We could hypothesise that Hieronymus, knowledgeable in the classics, expresses his view of the female nature in a way reminiscent of the views of Aristotle. That is to say, as we have explained previously, females are colder, therefore weaker, not just bodily, but in their rational faculties as well. Their vision-soul loop is in flux due to the constant fluctuations caused by menstruation. Their appetite/passion-soul loop is weaker due to their nature (they were born weak).

Hieronymus' story is also significant for it inserts an example where the above-given explanation of the female vision-soul loop impact on the foetus is not only a theoretical suggestion but a 'fact', with evidence admissible in court in the event that the offspring did not resemble the father.[3]

Background on the ancient Jewish sources

As we now turn our attention to ancient Jewish sources, we first present a brief introduction of their literary characteristics and historicity.

Greek scientific writings have been widely studied. The nature of these sources is well documented in studies of the history of medicine as attested by the voluminous literature even on the subject of reproduction (see, for example, Stol and Wiggermann 1997; Wilson 1991; Kottek and Baader 2000; Findley 1933; Preuss 1970; Nussbaum 1978). Less has been written on the topic as it appears in ancient Jewish sources, and the discourse is usually limited within Jewish scholarship, rather than being a discourse on the literature about the history of science and medicine (see, for example, Fonrobert 2006, 128–54). The nature of the ancient Jewish sources may, therefore, be less familiar to a broader audience. Thus, we would like to introduce the nature of the Jewish texts we include in our analysis.

Greek sources are in general well-defined treatises, analysing and criticising previous scientific thought and presenting those of the author as more rational. They include in their composition, what we would define today as 'scientific' terms and vocabulary. The Jewish sources are of a different dialectic and structure. We will be drawing primarily from two different texts: the midrashic text of the *Midrash Rabbah Genesis* (*Genesis MR*) and the *Babylonian Talmud* (*BT*). The *Genesis MR* is extant in various manuscript versions and is believed to be a reduction of teachings of various sages living in Palestine, most likely between the 2nd–3rd century CE. Its parables, moral teachings and homilies are a commentary on the biblical book of *Genesis*. The redactor(s) of this collection is(are) not known, although specific names of sages are associated with the midrashic text.

The second source, the *Babylonian Talmud*, is the compilation of teachings from sages living in Palestine as well as Mesopotamia, where there has been a continuous active and productive Jewish presence since the destruction of the first Temple of Jerusalem in 567 BCE well into the 7th century CE. This voluminous collection covers all aspects of Jewish life and history (Hasan-Rokem 2000). It is primarily a discourse of religious law, and is used as such to this day. Most scholars are of the opinion that this corpus of material was 'canonised', redacted, *c.* CE 520, although it clearly incorporates and reworks material from much earlier Palestinian sources of *c.* CE 220.

The *BT* is considered a primarily legal text and as such covers all aspects of life, consistent with the fact that Jewish Law is relevant to all human experiences and activities. The *BT* is in that sense, an ethnographic study spanning more than 1000 years of cultural experience (Hasan-Rokem 2003, 111). These texts, however, also incorporate the scientific knowledge of the time, especially in medicine, astronomy and mathematics (Fisch 1997; Efron 2007, 39–65).

Both of the Jewish sources include a wealth of medical information on anatomy, embryology, birth and heredity. Preuss created a compendium of this knowledge in 1911 in German, with a later English translation by Rosen (Preuss 1978). The hermeneutics of the Jewish texts demonstrate that the sages utilised a 'rational' and 'scientific' paradigm of thought in their discourse. Moreover, these sources have much to reveal about the epistemology of the culture that produced them.

> 'It is a common assumption that important religious books tend to speak from authority that demand to be taken at their word. The Talmud is not this sort of holy book ... In the Talmud, theories about the working of nature are often coupled with different or competing theories, and the apparent conflict between them is only sometimes adjudicated and only rarely adjudicated with any finality. In contrast to, say, pre-Socratic or later Greek natural philosophy in which advocation of one theory sought logically to demonstrate the superiority of their approach, in Talmudic arguments one finds little attempt to reach finality' (Efron 2007, 42).

The midrashic texts, such as the *Midrash Rabbah Genesis* quoted in this paper, also follow a similar paradigm of discourse. David Stern, a well-recognised authority on *Midrash* writes:

> 'the presentation of multiple interpretations (often, though not always, prefaced by the formula 'davar aḥer', 'another interpretation') is probably its most ubiquitous feature, almost a kind of stereotype or common place' (Stern 1988, 137).

In the Jewish sources, therefore, unlike the comprehensive and definitive treatises of ancient Greek texts, we find a dialectic that is 'in principle, like science, a continuing, open-ended inquiry' (Fisch 1997, xii).

Thus, although Talmudic literature does not include a treatise on reproduction or *phantasia*, we argue that rabbinic literature contains information, reflecting the rabbis' understanding of how vision and *phantasia* influence both animal and human reproduction. We do not attempt in this paper to establish the basis of their knowledge, but find the recent work of Montgomery relevant to the transmission of 'scientific' knowledge, as he states that:

> 'Knowledge, whatever its contents, has always been a mobile form of culture. However one cares to define it – as a body of facts and hypotheses the product of a specific labor, or an instrument of domination – human understanding, literary or scientific, has undergone enormous passages between peoples and places over the span of history. Its movement has come on the heels of war and conquest, commerce and trade, religious conversion, immigration, discovery' (Montgomery 2000, 2).

With this background information on the Jewish sources, we now present some illustrative and poignant examples of *phantasia* in action within these sources. First, we present examples that relate to animal reproduction, followed by those relating to human reproduction.

Ancient Jewish texts

Perhaps the most familiar example is the biblical text mentioned above as discussed by Hieronymus. The *Genesis MR* discussed the biblical text of *Genesis* 30: 35–43 and 31: 7–12. The biblical text describes the technique Jacob used to produce spotted sheep. The midrashic discussion of these biblical verses including the following:

> ״ויקח לו יעקב מקל לבנה לח ולוז וערמון״, חוטר חוור הטיב ודלוז ודדלוב, כך היה אבינו יעקב נותן את המקלות בתוך הבריכות שלמים והיתה הבהמה באה לשתות ורואה את המקלות ונרתעת לאחוריה והזכר רובעה והיתה יולדת כיוצא בו, א״ר [אמר רבי] הושעיה נעשו המים זרע בתוך מעיהם ולא היו חסירות אלא צורת הולד בלבד... [4]

> 'And Jacob took rods of fresh poplar, and of the almond and of the plane-tree" (*Genesis* 30: 37); he took a white rod, and rods of the almond and the plane-tree. This is what the patriarch Jacob did: He set the rods in the watering troughs. When an animal came to drink, it saw the rod and started back, and the male copulated with it, after which it bore [young marked] like the rod. R' Hoshayah said: The water turned to semen within them, so that they merely required the image of the young' [i.e. its particular markings which Jacob supplied with the rods] (*Midrash Rabbah Genesis* 73:10, based on the 1939 trans. of Freedman and Simon, with slight modifications).

The *Midrash* describes a technique that involved a physical intervention by Jacob, placing rods of different colours in the troughs, which he must have thought would result in a particular kind of offspring.[5] The discussion of the biblical passage suggests that the female sheep, which must have been black, came to drink while the rods were in the watering gutters. The colour of the rods startled the female animals. As they moved backwards away from the water troughs the males mounted them in their retreat. Thus, the implication is that the females saw the rods of different colours during copulation and those colours became 'bound' to the *conceptus* during coitus (Etkin 1965, 7). Rabbi Hoshayah presents a different explanation. He states that insemination happened miraculously. However, he also states that the vision of the female generated the desired colour in the offspring. The rabbis thought Jacob got his spotted animals by manipulating the vision of the female animal.

The next text is also from husbandry and concerns the (re)production of the red heifer, the cultic red-haired cow used in purification rights. This animal is ritually acceptable only if its hair is entirely red, evidently a naturally rather uncommon occurrence.

> אמר מר: ישראל היו משמרין אותה משעה שנוצרה. מנא ידעינן? אמר רב כהנא : כוס אדום מעבירין לפניה בשעה שעולה עליה זכר. א״ה [אי הכי] אמאי דמיה יקרין? הואיל ושתי שערות פוסלות בה. ומאי שנא דידהו? אמר רב כהנא: במוחזקת.

> 'The master said: Israelites had been guarding it [the cow] from the moment it was formed. How can we know [that the fetus would indeed be a red hiefer]? R' Kahana said: They pass a red cup before [the mother] at the time that a male mounts her. If so, why is [a red heifer] expensive? [It is] because [even] two [black or white] hairs disqualify it [ritually as a red heifer]. And why are their [cows] different [from ours that do not breed red cows]? R' Kahana said: [They did it] with [a cow] established [as having a tendency to produce red offspring when this procedure was done]' (*BT* Avodah Zarah 24a).[6]

This text is found in the middle of a discourse concerning the production of a red heifer free from idolatrous practices and any hairs of a colour other than red. The technique of achieving the desired red colour is simple: place a red cup (most likely red wine) in front of the female while copulation takes place. This technique is not unlike the method used by Jacob: a visual image placed in front of the female during copulation. This is not magic, miracle nor cultic ritual. Rather, we would argue it represents an application of the knowledge available to the rabbis on how the visual-soul loop operates.

In the text there appears to be an exchange of rational scientific theories among the various sages. Rabbi Kahana (died *c.* CE 414 in Babylonia) had spent considerable time learning in Palestinian academies. He offers an additional suggestion of how to get a red heifer. He hints that the technique is most likely to work better if the female cow came from a family where red offspring are found. Although this text does not offer enough information on heredity, it does indicate that the rabbis were aware of both hereditary aspects of generation as well as the use of *phantasia.* Both could be manipulated to produce a specific kind of offspring both in animals and in humans. We now present an example involving human reproduction.

> מעשה בכושי אחד שנשא לכושית אחת, והוליד ממנה בן לבן. תפס האב לבן ובא לו אצל רבי. אמר לו: שמא אינו בני? אמר לו: היה לך מראות בתוך ביתך? אמר לו: הין. אמר לו: שחורה או לבנה? אמר לו: לבנה. אמר לו: מיכן שהיה לך בן לבן.

> 'It once happened that an Ethiopian, married to an Ethiopian, begot a white-skinned son by her. Thereupon the father took the child and went to Rabbi [Judah the patriarch], asking him: Perhaps he is not my son. Did you have any pictures in your house, he asked. Yes, he replied. Black or white? [asked Rabbi]. White, he answered. This accounts for your white-skinned son, he assured him'[7] (*Midrash Rabbah Genesis* 70:10, trans. Freedman and Simon 1939).

This story is very reminiscent of that found in Heliodore, *The Ethiopean*, IV, 8, 3–5 (3rd century CE). Rabbi Judah associated with this text lived in Palestine during the 2nd century CE and reportedly knew Greek and was friendly with the Hellenic elite of his time. It could be argued that he was merely trying to keep the peace in the Ethiopian family. However, the use of the visual stimulus (a picture) during coitus influencing the mother to produce a 'white' child (different from that of the dark father) is good evidence that the rabbis were familiar with the notion of vision-soul loop.

The following text also demonstrates that the rabbis were familiar with the impact of female vision on the *conceptus* as practised by the Romans:

"בני ציון היקרים המסולאים בפז" - מאי מסולאים בפז? אילימא דהוו מחפי בפיזא, והאמרי דבי רבי שילא: תרתי מתקלי איסתירי פיזא נחות בעלמא, חדא ברומי וחדא בכולי עלמא! אלא שהיו מגנין את הפז ביופיין. מעיקרא, חשיבי דרומאי הוו נקטי בליונא דגושפנקא ומשמשי ערסייהו, מכאן ואילך מייתו בני ישראל ואסרי בכרעי דפורייהו ומשמשי.

'The precious children of Zion who are weighed with [the precious stone] *piza* (Lamentations 4: 2). What does 'weighed with *piza*' mean? If you say that they were covered with *piza*; but they taught in the school of R' Sheila: Two astir-weights of *piza* were bestowed upon the world: one was given to Rome and one to the entire world [and hence Zion cannot be said to be particularly abundant in *piza*]. Rather they put *piza* to shame with their beauty [the beauty of the children of Zion was more 'weighty' than *piza*, i.e. surpassed that of *piza*]. Originally, the aristocrats of Rome used to take the figures on signet rings when they engaged in conjugal relations. But from then on [after the conquest of Israel] they took Jewish boys and tied them to the legs of their beds when they engaged in conjugal relations' (*BT* Gittin 58a).

It could be that the rings and the beautiful boys were simple erotic devices. However, the text could also be interpreted to mean that the beautiful boys served much the same function as the statue of the Cypriot tyrant discussed above. We take this approach in our discussion here. Danielle Gourevitch discusses the Greek and Latin texts regarding this '*en trois*'. She states it was a common Roman custom to place beautiful statues in the chamber where sexual procreative intercourse took place, in order to influence the visual images of the female. She leaves open, as does our *Midrash*, the issue of whether the male or only the female or both, looked at the statues (Gourevitch 1987, 567). The rabbis, it appears, knew that the Romans used the vision-soul loop for reproduction purposes. The vision of a beautiful or desired image seen by the female and perhaps the male during coitus appear to directly impact on the appearance of the *conceptus*.

We now introduce a clear example of how the vision of the female can directly influence not only the physical characteristics of the offspring, but also its non-physical characteristics. This text involves Rabbi Yohanan, a famous, good looking and brilliant, 2nd century CE Palestinian rabbi apparently knowledgeable in Greek.

רבי יוחנן הוה אזיל ויתיב אשערי טבילה, אמר: כי סלקן בנות ישראל מטבילת מצוה לפגעו בי, כי היכי דלהוו להו בני שפירי כוותי, גמירי אורייתא כוותי.

'Rabbi Yohanan was accustomed to sit next to the entrance to the *miqvah* (ritual purification bath chamber). He explained: When the Jewish women emerge from the required immersion, let them encounter me so that they will have children as beautiful as I and as learned of the Torah as I' (*BT* Baba Metzi'a 84a).[8]

According to Jewish Law, following the cessation of menstrual blood flow, women must purify themselves prior to intercourse with their husband. This is achieved by immersion in the waters of the *miqvah*, a ritual bath chamber. Our text describes a scene in the proximity of this ritual bath.

Upon exiting the ritual bath, the women in the story would look at the physically handsome and learned Rabbi Yohanan, go home and have sexual intercourse with their husbands, presumably with the 'presentation'/*phantasia* of Rabbi Yohanan in their minds and thus beget children in his likeness, beautiful physically and mentally.

We now see a new parameter that could be transmitted in the 'presentation' that vision generates: 'acquired characteristics', such as love of scholarship and learning. The profound effect of the 'desired' on the *conceptus*, is perhaps best demonstrated in the story of the woman in the market place:

"וגם אחרי כן אשר יבאו בני האלהים אל בנות האדם" (בראשית ו:ד) אמר רבי ברכיה היתה אשה יוצאת לשוק ורואה בחור, מתאוה לו, היתה הולכת ומשמשת מטתה והיתה מעמדת בחור כיוצא בו.

'And also after that, when the sons of God came unto the daughters of men" (Gen. 6: 4). Rabbi Berekhiah said: A woman would go out to the market place, see a young man, and conceive a passion for him, whereupon she would go, cohabit [with her husband], and give birth to a young man like him [resembling]' (*Midrash Rabbah Genesis* 26,7, trans. Freedman and Simon, London 1939).

This midrashic story, we may suggest, includes the workings of the various elements of *phantasia,* both the vision-soul and the appetites/passion loops. The vision is the crucial first step in the process. A young woman eyes a young male while in the market. She finds him pleasing, and develops a passion for him. Later, while having intercourse with her husband, the desire for this pleasing young man evokes the *phantasia* of his presentation that gets imprinted in the *conceptus*, 'like a seal'. The child, therefore, resembles the object of desire, the young man from the market, not the husband. The elements of vision, *phantasia* and desire bring about the physical resemblance of the 'desired' on the foetus.

In addition to female vision, desire and *phantasia*, in the Jewish sources there are also examples of what could be interpreted as the equivalent of male desire and *phantasia*.

שאלו את אימא שלום [אשתו של רבי אליעזר][9] מפני מה בניך יפיפין ביותר? אמרה להן: אינו מספר עמי לא בתחלת הלילה ולא בסוף הלילה אלא בחצות הלילה, וכשהוא מספר מגלה טפח ומכסה טפח, ודומה עליו כמי שכפאו שד; ואמרתי לו: מה טעם? ואמר לי: כדי שלא אתן את עיני באשה אחרת, ונמצאו בני[10] באין לידי ממזרות!

'Imma Shalom was asked: Why are your children so exceedingly beautiful? She replied: [Because] he [my husband] 'converses' [euphemism for coitus] with me neither at the beginning nor at the end of the night, but [only] at midnight; and when he 'converses', he uncovers a handbreadth and covers a handbreadth, and is as though he were compelled by a demon. And when I asked him, what is the reason for this, he replied,

So that I may not think of another woman, lest my children be as bastards' (*BT* Nedarim 20b).

R' Eliezer ben Hyrcanos, a 1st/2nd century CE Palestinian sage, is having intercourse with his wife in the middle of the night. He is anxious, the text informs us through the wife, and behaves as if possessed by a demon! Why such anxiety, the wife asks? The answer to this question is most fascinating. The rabbi, a known strict interpreter of Jewish Law, is afraid that he may be tempted to imagine another woman while having coitus with his wife and thus his children born from such a union would be legally bastards (Hebrew *mamzer)*! He, therefore, chose to have intercourse during the time when there would be the least amount of distraction, in the middle of the night. Paternity, in the Talmudic writings, is of equal importance as that found in the Greco-Roman world. Here, however, it is maternity 'in the mind' of the male, that would render the offspring a bastard.

We now present a text where not only the 'legal' status of the offspring is at stake, but also other undesirable non-physical characteristics that can be inflicted on the offspring simply through the thoughts and mental status of the father and, in some cases, the mother.

"ולא תתורו אחרי לבבכם" - מכאן אמר רבי: אל ישתה אדם בכוס זה ויתן עיניו בכוס אחר. אמר רבינא: לא נצרכא אלא דאפילו ב' נשיו. "וברותי מכם המורדים והפושעים בי" - אמר רבי לוי: אלו בני תשע מדות, בני אסנ"ת משגע"ח: בני אימה, בני אנוסה, בני שנואה,[11] בני נידוי, בני תמורה, בני מריבה, בני שכרות, בני גרושת הלב, בני ערבוביא, בני חצופה.

'And you shall not follow your heart' (*Numbers* 15: 19). Based on this, Rabbi said: A man should not drink from this cup, while setting his eyes on another cup [That is, he may not think of another woman while cohabiting with this one]'. Ravina said: This is not needed except to [teach] that [this is forbidden] even [where both of the] two are his wives'.

'I will select from among you those who rebel and those who transgress against me' (Ezekiel 20: 38). R' Levi said [in explanation of this verse]: These [the rebels and transgressors] are the children of nine characteristics: children of fear [the husband forces his wife to cohabit with him], children of a forced [raped] woman, children of a hated woman, children of an excommunicated man, children of an exchanged woman [that is a man is cohabiting with one woman while thinking of another], children of strife [husband and wife are in discord], children of drunkenness [either one of the partners is intoxicated], children of a woman who has been divorced in the mind [the husband had decided to divorce his wife but had not yet given her the divorce papers], children of the mingling [sperm from a previous husband], children of a brazen woman [one that demands marital relations from her husband]' (*BT* Nedarim 20b).

One possibility suggested by our text is that the rabbis saw the birth of rebels and transgressors as divine punishment. However, as we read the text 'against the grain' so to speak, we may find the following hypothesis equally tenable. Thoughts in the mind of the male during intercourse with each specific female can influence the *conceptus*. Such thought could include, for example, desire for another woman other than the one that he was having intercourse with, or even intercourse with a woman that he had decided in his mind to divorce. Although paternity may be the underlying anxiety here, we could, based on the arguments we have developed, suggest that this text is dealing with issues of the male appetite/passion-soul loop.

Certain undesirable states of mind of the male or female during coitus are thus operating like *phantasia.* Although no vision is evoked by the text, thoughts (in the Aristotelian model the inner sense of κοινὸν αἰσθητήριον and φανταστικόν, *phantasia*) appear to have an impact on the kind of offspring generated not in the physical, corporeal sense but in what we would describe as 'acquired' characteristics or personality.

How can we explain the presence of male *phantasia* in the Jewish sources? As Doniger points out, male *phantasia* is found only in the Jewish sources. She does not, however, offer a possible explanation for this unique phenomenon (Doniger and Spinner 1998, 102). Of course, the absence of male *phantasia* in the Greek texts does not, by itself, imply that there were no such cases. However, we would like to suggest that in *praxis*, the Aristotelian model of cosmology does not encourage the conceptualisation of an active role for male *phantasia* in the reproductive process. In order to place this cosmology in context, a brief outline of the reproductive process according to Aristotle would be useful.

Aristotle's (and Galen's) paradigm of creation and the natural world at large is based like much of his epistemology, on dichotomy, polarity (like: hot/cold, wet/dry, water/fire, earth/air), as a prevailing principle in the natural order of the world among ancient Greek philosophers (Lloyd 1966, 65). His basic assumption about the generation of both animals and humans reflects a similar dialect. As mentioned previously, there is 'strife' between the male seed which possesses the 'vital energy' for shaping the foetus and the female menstrual blood – which Aristotle considers as the counterpart to male seed, which usually provides only nourishment for the foetus. It is only when the male seed is weak that the female 'seed' takes the pivotal role in shaping the offspring.

ἀρχὴ δὲ πρώτη τὸ θῆλυ γίγνεσθαι καὶ μὴ ἄρρεν – ἀλλ' αὕτη μὲν ἀναγκαία τῇ φύσει· δεῖ γὰρ σώζεσθαι τὸ γένος τῶν κεχωρισμένων κατὰ τὸ θῆλυ καὶ τὸ ἄρρεν …

'The first beginning of this deviation is when a female is formed instead of a male, though this indeed is a necessity required by Nature, since the race of creatures which are separated into male and female has got to keep in being' (*De Generatione Animalium* IV, 3, 767b8–10).

Thus, according to Aristotle, the perfect offspring is not only male, but resembles the father, and any deviation from this natural order leads to the generation of a monstrosity. Galen disputes this view in numerous places in his works and states that the female seed also contributes to the foetus (Lloyd 1966, 51–2), but the 'strife' principle remains (Galen 633, Book 614 303, trans. Tallmadge 1968).

A female offspring is thus viewed by Aristotle as a necessity for the survival of the species. This is not a 'sexist statement' but rather reflects a very important cosmological premise of both Aristotle and Galen. It is a view that accurately reflects Aristotelian teleological thought, where Nature does nothing that is not useful. Nature is the ultimate source for designing and functioning of all things in our world. Any theories about the functioning of our world had to be consistent with this worldview (Morsink 1979).

What is the comparable ancient Jewish thought on these issues of human reproduction and underlying cosmology? Before we present specific texts on this topic, it should be noted that the ancient Jewish sources created by the androcentric and patriarchal rabbinic culture, express significant male anxiety about paternity not dissimilar to that found in Greco-Roman literature (Fonrobert 2000; Katz 1992; Satlow 2001).

However, the epistemological assumptions about generation of a human, offer a different epistemological view, as our next text demonstrates.

> תנו רבנן: שלשה שותפין יש באדם, הקב"ה ואביו ואמו. אביו מזריע הלובן, שממנו עצמות וגידים וצפרנים, ומוח שבראשו, ולובן שבעין. אמו מזרעת אודם, שממנו עור ובשר [ודם][12] ושערות, ושחור שבעין. והקב"ה נותן בו רוח ונשמה וקלסתר פנים, וראיית העין, ושמיעת האוזן, ודבור פה, והלוך רגלים, ובינה והשכל[13].

> 'Our Rabbis taught: There are three partners in man, the Holy One, blessed be He, and his father, and his mother. His father supplies the seed [semen, the white substance] out of which are formed the child's bones, sinews, nails, the brain in his head and the white in the eye; his mother supplies the red [substance] out of which is formed his skin, flesh [and blood], hair, and the black of the eye; and the Holy One, blessed be He, gives him the spirit and the breath, beauty of features, eyesight, the power of hearing [of the ear] and the ability [of the mouth] to speak and to walk [walking of the feet], understanding and discernment' (*BT* Niddah 31b).

The origin of this text, based on its linguistic formulation, תנו רבנן, is most likely Palestinian of the Tannaitic period (*c.* 2nd century CE). This would be roughly the time when Soranus and Galen were refining and reformulating the ancient Greek notions of generation and gynaecological conditions (see Green 1985, 71). It is likely that this text reflects a biological notion consistent with the two seed theory of reproduction as advocated by Galen and also found in the biblical text. The two seed theory as found in the biblical text is thoroughly discussed by Van der Horst (1966, 112–34).

In addition to the two seed theory implied by the text, there are two other notions worthy of further discussion since they contribute to our understanding of the rabbis' world view as it relates to human reproduction. One is the issue of the partnership between male, female and God; the second relates to the specific contribution of each partner and the cultural significance with which the partner's bodily contribution is imbued.

The specific contributions of God in the partnership in human reproduction have important theological implications, not central to our focus here[14]. What is important to our argument is the partnership term – שותפין – that in the language of the sages has legal implications of cooperation and mutual obligations. In fact, this partnership in the creation of the human foetus, forms the basis for the Jewish law that demands a child to honour his mother, father and God (see, for example, *BT* Kiddushin 30b).

We suggest that the Palestinian rabbis of our text are basing this 'partnership' notion in part on the biblical first story of Creation (*Genesis* 1, 27). In this version, God created an androgynous being, male and female both equal. Schremer (2007; 2003, 320–9) suggests that this Palestinian adaptation of the first Creation story is what gives rise to the Palestinian rabbis' positive views regarding marriage and love. Just as in the original story of the godly creation of humans, male and female are equal (first story of creation of Adam and Eve in *Genesis* 1, 27), the male and female remain partners in creating a foetus. The physical attributes of the substances secreted by both parents, according to our text, result in the generation of specific body parts and fluids in the foetus. A viable foetus needs the male and female 'seed' (Heb. *zera'*) as well as God's contribution. Perhaps, we should note here that embryological concepts as found in rabbinic sources are very similar to the theories of the Greeks (Kottek and Baader 2000).

Through his seed, the male contributes all the parts of the body that are hard and or white: bones, nails, brains and the white of the eye. The female seed contributes more soft and earthy coloured parts, like blood, skin and hair, as well as the pupil of the eye. God's contributions to the foetus include the human attributes we are likely to consider more ethereal, the essence of being human, the sense of vision, the ability to talk, understand and discern, and, of course, the immortal soul.

Theology and biology are bound together in a more direct way than the 'astral' forces of Aristotelian theories. The sense and the inner faculties are reminiscent of Aristotelian notions, provided not by Nature but God. It is interesting that even in the male foetus, the pupil through which the sense of vision enters the inner part of the corporeal body, is a maternal contribution. In the theoretical framework of the Galenic vision theory, that we have referred to as the vision-soul loop, it is the pupil of the eye that serves as the portal, through which movement initiated by the sense of vision is transmitted by the *pneuma,* to the optic nerve and reaches the inner faculty of *phantasia* located in the middle ventricle of the brain.

We cannot claim, based on this text alone, that the Galenic vision theory is reflected in the ancient Jewish sources. However, we would like to suggest that based on the other textual ancient Jewish examples presented above, the rabbis appear to be informed of the essential working of the vision-soul and appetite-soul loops. The lack of the specific 'scientific' terminology is perhaps a reflection of the legal rather than the medical/biological nature of the text. Development of medical terminology is a function of the text and the culture creating it, and usually involves physical metaphors (Langslow 2000, 161).

Let us now examine how these anatomical contributions are interpreted in our two different texts. Male and female contributions to the foetus, from an anthropological perspective, suggest a representation of 'soft' = female contribution; and 'hard' = male contribution; hard being strong and 'good/right'. This opposition of male/female; right/left; hard/soft, is seen also in many other cultures, as discussed by several scholars (Needham 1934, 78; Sassi 2001, 82; Lloyd 1962).

Aristotle, for example, also assigns to the female similar biologically-based contributions to the foetus (*De Generatione Animalium* II, 6 745b1). Bones and sinews are male contributions to the foetus (*De Generatione Animalium* II, 6 744b20–25). Therefore, from an anatomical classification, the foetal contribution of male and female are similar in Aristotelian and Jewish writings. From an epistemological point of view, the classification reveals an underlying world view that is different in the two cultures. The difference lies in the symbolic value of the male and female anatomical contributions and in the general cosmology within which male and female agency is placed in relation to the reproductive process.

Let us examine first the female contribution of blood to the foetus, in the Hebrew text presented above. Blood plays a very significant symbolic role in Jewish thought.[15] Blood is the source of life in Jewish thought (Kottek 2005).[16] It is central to the anthropological/theological concepts of purity and defilement in relation to the Temple rituals. In addition, most relevant to our discussion here, it governs male/female sexual intercourse and timing. Biblical commandments regulate the handling of animal and human blood. Menstrual blood is also regulated by biblical commandments, which are reworked by the male rabbis into elaborate Laws governing daily life of male and female alike. It is these Laws, not Nature, that occupy the rabbis' thoughts.

Blood is also fundamentally central in Aristotelian thought. Blood is considered the 'ultimate nourishment' which maintains and keeps the body and its parts. Both male and female have blood, from which they contribute to the foetal generation and growth. The only difference between male and female is a matter of the degree of 'concoction'. The female being colder achieves less concoction than the hotter male. Therefore, menstrual blood, which Aristotle states is the female contribution to the foetal formation, is a 'residue' of lower purity than the highly purified blood from which male sperm is formed. Female contribution although of a similar kind in physiological terms, is less pure, not as 'good' as the male pure contribution. Aristotle provides a specific reason for this lesser 'good':

> τὸ γὰρ θῆλυ ὥσπερ ἄρρεν ἐστὶ πεπηρωμένον καὶ τὰ καταμήνια σπέρμα, οὐ καθαρὸν δέ· ἓν γὰρ οὐκ ἔχει μόνον· τὴν τῆς ψυχῆς ἀρχήν.
>
> 'The reason is that the female is as it were a deformed male; and the menstrual discharge is semen, though in an impure condition; i.e., it lacks one constituent, and one only, the principle of the Soul' (*De Generatione Animalium* II 737a33–5, trans. Peck 1953).

Aristotle does present somewhat contradictory views of what is the female and male contribution to foetal formation, or, for that matter, what are male and what are female 'principles' in the generation process. For example, he states that:

> καθάπερ γὰρ εἴπομεν τῆς γενέσεως ἀρχὰς ἄν τις οὐχ ἥκιστα θείη τὸ θῆλυ καὶ τὸ ἄρρεν, τὸ μὲν ἄρρεν ὡς τῆς κινήσεως καὶ τῆς γενέσεως ἔχον τὴν ἀρχήν, τὸ δὲ θῆλυ ὡς ὕλης. [....] τῷ γὰρ ἀποκρίνεσθαι τὸ τοιοῦτον μόριον ἀπὸ τοῦ θήλεος καὶ τοῦ ἄρρενος καὶ ἐν τούτοις τὴν ἀπόκρισιν εἶναι καὶ ἐκ τούτων, διὰ τοῦτο τὸ θῆλυ καὶ τὸ ἄρρεν ἀρχαὶ τῆς γενέσεώς εἰσιν. ἄρρεν μὲν γὰρ λέγομεν ζῷον τὸ εἰς ἄλλο γεννῶν, θῆλυ δὲ τὸ εἰς αὑτό· διὸ καὶ ἐν τῷ ὅλῳ τὴν τῆς γῆς φύσιν ὡς θῆλυ καὶ μητέρα νομίζουσιν, οὐρανὸν δὲ καὶ ἥλιον ἤ τι τῶν ἄλλων τῶν τοιούτων ὡς γεννῶντας καὶ πατέρας προσαγορεύουσιν.
>
> 'As we mentioned we may safely set down as the chief principles of generation the male and the female (factor); the male as possessing the principle of movement and of generation, the female as possession of that of matter ... We must not fail to notice how the semen itself is formed from the male and the female, since it is because this part is secreted from the male and female and because its secretion takes place in them and out of them, that the male and female are the principles of generation: By male animal we mean one which generates in another, by "female" one which generates in itself. This is why in cosmology too they speak of the nature of the Earth as something female and call it 'mother,' while they give to the heaven and the sun and anything else of that kind the title of 'generator' and father' (*De Generatione Animalium* I, 716a 5–6 and 11–18, trans. Peck 1953).

Let us, for the sake of our argument here, suggest that the female principle and its contribution to the process of generation in Aristotelian cosmology is essential but not equal to that of the male. This is compatible with the Aristotelian position that Nature has a 'generator', a Maker so to speak, and he is embodied in the male principle.

In the Jewish source presented above, we may argue, there is a different epistemology. There is a Maker, God, who in partnership with humans participates in the generation of the human foetus. This partnership involves three principles: God, male, and female. Certain Laws that are God's, not Nature's, govern this partnership. These Laws are detailed in minutiae in rabbinic literature covering all aspects of daily life and the cosmos (which we are not discussing here). These Laws govern human agency, both male and female. Within these Laws, in the creation of a human foetus, the male and female principle are viewed as equals not as a polarity. There is, therefore, an opportunity to create a biological role for male phantasia without endangering the social construct of the rabbis' patriarchal society. It is not surprising, therefore, to find in the rabbinic writings examples of both paternal and maternal phantasia at work both at coitus and during gestation. Most interesting, the female is depicted as the one that contributes to the foetus the pupil of the eye – the portal through which sight (the outside world) enters into the soul (the inside).

Concluding remarks

Despite the patriarchic nature of both ancient Greco-Roman and Jewish cultures, we would suggest that their cosmologies regarding human reproduction generated different *praxeis* for male and female *phantasia* in the process of human reproduction.

In the Greek sources, the female *phantasia* seems to be instrumental in the shaping of the physical characteristics of the offspring. Maternal *phantasia*, as our examples seem to demonstrate, influences primarily the physicality of the offspring.[17] Women, therefore, it could be argued, played a significant role in shaping the physical characteristics of the offspring, even if theoretically they are not assigned such a role.[18]

Thomas Laqueur (1992, 58) suggests that the prominent role of female *phantasia* reflects not only the androcentric concerns of the texts but also the anxieties about paternity and inheritance. Moreover, issues of controlling female sexuality come into play when we examine female *phantasia* in both Jewish and Greek sources. Doniger rightly suggests that theories of female *phantasia* were:

> '... one way of accounting for divergences from the expected norm without admitting the likelihood of actual impregnation by an alienating male. This sort of mythological embryology involves a kind of pre-scientific cloning: it investigates ways of producing copies of desired stock. But, we must ask, desired by whom? One factor that seems to pervade all variants is the male desire to control female desire' (Doniger and Spinner 1998, 1).

In the Jewish sources, we see that female *phantasia* influences not only the physicality of the foetus, but also its 'acquired characteristics'. Moreover, male *phantasia* influences the foetus' 'legal' status and its 'acquired characteristics'. We suggest that the active role of both male and female *phantasia* is supported by the Jewish notion that reproduction is 'a partnership' process between the female/male and God. For the Hebrew texts, God and his Laws are the driving force in the Universe. The Maker of the world was in the truest sense also its Law.

This is not so for the Aristotelian sources. For Aristotle the driving force was *telos*. Human agency is, therefore, assigned to the service of Nature and governed by *telos* (*Politics* VII 1, 1103a19). The *natura creatrix* of Aristotle creates a Universe that, although impersonal, was harmonious and inventive. It was within this framework that his biological theories are placed, based on empirical observations, which, of course, even for Aristotle, cannot explain the role of social constructs such as moral or political actions of humans (*Nicomachean Ethics* II 1, 1103a1). Thus, in Aristotelian cosmology the relation of law and nature was still seen 'as an irreconcilable antithesis' (Koester 1968, 527). Humans, specifically males, create laws and females are part of Nature, serving a species survival role.

In Jewish sources, God created male and female and the Law. In the patriarchic culture of the male rabbis, the male elaborates and defines the Law. However, when it comes to the reproduction process, the Law does not allow room for the rabbis (despite their attempts) to erase the original divine partnership involved in human reproduction. Male and female *phantasia* is by necessity involved in the reproductive process. It is these epistemological presuppositions that, we are suggesting, explain the presence of both male and female *phantasia* in Jewish texts, as operant in the generation of a 'desired' offspring.

Notes

1 The psychological implications of mental images that are manipulated by other faculties, especially memory, μνημονευτικόν, to create φαντάζματα, are also discussed by Aristotle; however they are not central to our thesis.

2 We are thankful to Prof. Gourevitch for bringing this important paper to our attention in addition to that of B. Maire (2003).

3 Huet, in her 1993 book has suggested that the influence of maternal thoughts and *phantasia* was used throughout ancient times and well into the 19th century as a way of placing responsibility upon women for children born with physical abnormalities. She asserts that the field of teratology, which flourished beginning in the Middle Ages, had its basis on this type of assumption about female *phantasia* (Huet 1993, 162).

4 All Hebrew texts are from the Bar-Ilan University Responsa Project (Version 10.0).

5 Interestingly, R. Shelomo Yitzhaki (Rashi), an 11th century commentator living in France, in his commentary to the biblical text of *Genesis* 30: 39 explains that the word *'aqudim* is connected to the root *'aqad* – to bind, and thus he suggests that differently coloured rods were 'bound' to the ankles, the

forelegs and the hind legs of the animals. Thus, the colours become 'imprinted' on the foetus during conception.

6 All quotations from *BT* are based on the *Soncino Babylonian Talmud*, trans. by Epstein 1935–48.

7 This story does not appear in the manuscript versions of *Genesis MR*. However, a similar version appears in *MR Numbers* 5:19, a somewhat later source. In this version, the man is a king, but the concept remains the same: a black male and female produce a white child, considered more desirable by the ancients.

8 A parallel version of this text occurs in *BT* Berakhot 20a; however, the Torah learning attribute is not mentioned.

9 These words are missing in the printed editions of the *BT*.

10 Although the printed editions have 'his sons', the manuscripts read 'my sons'.

11 Interestingly, instead of listing both the sons of the hated woman and the raped woman, the Moscow Ginzburg 1134 manuscript lists only the sons of the hated woman. This text fits better with R' Levi's statement that speaks of children of nine conditions. In addition, this text spells hated with the letter *samekh* instead of with the letter *sin* and so fits the acronym given in the text more precisely.

12 According to the variant in the Munich Hebrew ms 95.

13 Although there are some minor variations in manuscripts, none is of importance to our discussion here.

14 It raises issues of duality of body/soul, see Urbach 1975, 218–54.

15 The relationship of blood and the sacred is also found in ancient Greco-Roman sources; here we are referring only to blood as the source of life (Branham 2002).

16 We would like to thank Prof. Kottek for raising this important point.

17 Even in our present-day 'gene' culture, the notion that the external environment can significantly influence the offspring is a very active area of current medical research, and it is part of the medical folklore of our times. This is the subject of the book by Janov (2000).

18 The role of women in physically 'shaping' the race is discussed by Schiebinger (1993, 115–34).

Bibliography

Aristotle, *De Generatione Animalium*, trans. A. L. Peck, Cambridge MA, 1953.

Aristotle, *Nicomachean Ethics*, trans. T. Irwin, Indianapolis, 1999.

Aristotle, *Politica*, trans. B. Jowett, Oxford, 1921.

Aristotle, *Problemata*, trans. W. S. Hett, Cambridge, MA, 1936.

Babylonian Talmud, trans. by rabbi I. Epstein, Soncino Press, London 1935–48.

Boucé, P.-G. 1982: *Sexuality in Eighteenth-Century Britain*, Totowa, N.J.

Branham, J. R. 2002: 'Bloody women and bloody spaces: Menses and the Eucharist in Late Antiquity and the Early Middle Ages', *Harvard Divinity Bulletin* 30(4), 15–22.

Caston, V. 1996: 'Why Aristotle needs imagination', *Phronesis* 41, 25–55.

Conrad, L. I., Neve, M., Nutton, V. and Porter, R. (eds) 1995: *The Western Medical Tradition*, Cambridge.

Doniger, W. and Spinner, G. 1998: 'Misconceptions: female imaginations and male fantasies in parental imprinting', *Dedalus* 127/1, 97–103.

Eastmond, A. and James, L. (eds) 2003: *Icon and Word: The Power of Images in Byzantium: Studies Presented to Robin Cormack,* Aldershot.

Efron, N. J. 2007: *Judaism and Science: A Historical Introduction,* Westport, CT.

Etkin, W. 1965: 'Jacob's cattle and modern genetics', *Tradition* 7, 5–15.

Findley, P. 1933: *The Story of Childbirth,* Garden City, N.Y.

Fisch, M. 1997: *Rational Rabbis: Science and Talmudic Culture*, Bloomington.

Fonrobert, C. E. 2000: *Menstrual Purity: Rabbinic and Christian Reconstructions of Biblical Gender*, Stanford.

Fonrobert, C. E. 2006: 'The handmaid, the trickster and the birth of the Messiah: a critical appraisal of the feminist valorization of Midrah Aggada', 245–77 in C. Bakhos (ed.), *Current Trends in the Study of Midrash*, Leiden.

Galen, *On the Usefulness of the Parts of the Body*, trans. by M. Tallmadge, Ithaca, 1968.

Gourevitch, D. 1987: 'Se mettre à trois pour aire un bel enfant, ou l'imprégnation par le regard', *L' Evolution Psychiatrique* 52, 559–63.

Green, M. H. 1985: '*The Transmission of Ancient Theories of Female Physiology and Disease through the Early Middle Ages'*, PhD Dissertation, Princeton University.

Hasan-Rokem, G. 2000: *Web of Life: Folklore and Midrash in Rabbinic Literature*, Stanford.

Hasan-Rokem, G. 2003: *Tales of the Neighborhood: Jewish Narrative Dialogues in Late Antiquity,* Berkeley.

Huet, M. H. 1993: *Monstrous Imagination*, Cambridge, MA.

Janov, A. 2000: *The Biology of Love*, Amherst, New York.

Jerome (Saint), *Saint Jerome's Hebrew Questions on Genesis (Quaestiones Hebraicae in Genesim)*, transl. by C. T. R. Hayward, Oxford and New York, 1995.

Katz, M. 1992: 'Ideology and the status of women in Ancient Greece', *History and Theory* 31, 70–97.

Koester, H. 1968: 'NOMOS ΦΥΣΕΩΣ: The concept of natural law in Greek thought', 521–41 in J. Neusner (ed.), *Religions in Antiquity: Essays in Memory of Erwin Ramsdell Goodenough*, Leiden.

Kottek, S. and Baader, G. 2000: 'Talmudic and Greco-Roman data on pregnancy: a renewed examination', 83–101 in S. Kottek, M. Horstmanshoff, G. Baader and G. Ferngren (eds), *From Athens to Jerusalem: Medicine in Hellenized Jewish Lore and in Early Christian Literature*, Rotterdam.

Kottek, S. S. 2005: 'Blood in ancient Jewish culture', *Medicina nei Secoli: Arte e Scienza* 17, 627–49.

Kuhn, C. G. 1821–33: *Claudii Galeni Opera Omnia*, Leipzig (reprint Hildesheim 1964–5).

Langslow, D. R. 2000: *Medical Latin in the Roman Empire,* Oxford and New York.

Laqueur, T. 1992: *Making Sex: Body and Gender from the Greeks to Freud*, Boston.

Lindberg, D. C. 1976: *Theories of Vision from Al-Kindi to Kepler*, Chicago.

Lindberg, D. C. 1978: *Science in the Middle Ages*, Chicago.

Lloyd, G. E. R. 1962: 'Right and left in Greek philosophy', *Journal of Hellenic Studies* 82, 56–66.

Lloyd, G. E. R. 1966: *Polarity and Analogy; Two Types of Argumentation in Early Greek Thought*, Cambridge.

MacCormack, S. 1991: *Religion in the Andes: Vision and Imagination in Early Colonial Peru*, Princeton.

Magner, L. N. 2005: *A History of Medicine*, Boca Raton.

Maire, B. 2003: 'L'imprégnation par le regard ou l'influence de "simulacres" sur l'embryon', 279–94 in O. Bianchi and O. Thévenaz (eds), Mirabilia *Conceptions et représentations de l'extraordinaire dans le monde antique, Actes du Colloque International, Lausanne, 20–22 Mars 2003*, Lausanne.

Midrash Rabbah Genesis, trans. by H. Freedman and M. Simon, Soncino Press, London 1939.

Montgomery, S. L. 2000: *Science in Translation: Movements of Knowledge through Cultures and Time*, Chicago.

Morsink, J. 1979: 'Was Aristotle's biology sexist'? *Journal of the History of Biology* 12, 83–112.

Needham, J. 1934: *A History of Embryology*, Cambridge.

Nussbaum, M. C. 1978: 'The role of *Phantasia* in Aristotle's Explanation of Action', 221–69 in M. C. Nussbaum, *Aristotle's De Motu Animalium: Text with Translation, Commentary, and Interpretive Essays,* Princeton.

Papathomopoulos, M. E. (ed.) 2003: *Oppianus Apameensis: Cynegetica, Eutecnius Sophistes: Paraphrasis Metro Soluta,* Munich and Leipzig.

Preuss, A. 1970: 'Science and philosophy in Aristotle's Generation of Animals', *Journal of the History of Biology* 3, 1–52.

Preuss, J. 1978: *Biblical and Talmudic Medicine*, Northvale, N.J.

Sassi, M. M. 2001: *The Science of Man in Ancient Greece*, Chicago and London.

Satlow, M. L. 2001: *Jewish Marriage in Antiquity*, Princeton.

Schiebinger, L. 1993: *Nature's Body: Gender in the Making of Modern Science*, Boston.

Schofield, M. 1978: 'Aristotle on the imagination', 99–140 in G. E. R. Lloyd and L. Owen (eds), *Aristotle on Mind and the Senses*, Cambridge.

Schremer, A. 2003: *Male and Female He Created Them: Jewish Marriage in the Late Second Temple, Mishnah and Talmud Period* [in Hebrew], Jerusalem.

Schremer, A. 2007: 'Marriage, sexuality, and holiness: the anti-ascetic legacy of Talmudic Judaism', 35–63 in R. T. Blau (ed.), *Gender Relationships In Marriage and Out* (the Orthodox Forum Series), New York.

Shildrick, M. 2000: 'Maternal imagination: re-conceiving first impressions', *Rethinking History* 4, 243–60.

Siegel, R. E. 1970: *Galen on Sense Perceptions: His Doctrines, Observations and Experiments on Vision, Hearing, Smell, Taste, Touch and Pain, and Their Historical Sources*, Basel.

Singer, C. 1941: *A Short History of Science to the Nineteenth Century,* Oxford.

Soranus' Gynecology, trans. O. Tempkin, Baltimore, MD, 1956.

Stern, D. 1988: 'Midrash and Indeterminacy', *Critical Inquiry* 15, 132–61.

Stol, M. and Wiggermann, F. A. M. 1997: *Birth in Babylonia and the Bible: Its Mediterranean Setting*, Amherst, NY.

Tigay, J. H. 1977: 'He Begot a Son in His Likeness after His Image (Genesis 5:3)', 139–47 in M. Cogan, B. L. Eichler and J. H. Tigay (eds), *Tehilah Le-Moshe: Biblical and Judaic Studies in Honor of Moshe Greenberg*, New York.

Urbach, E. E. 1975: *The Sages: Their Concepts and Beliefs*, Jerusalem.

Van Der Horst, P. W. 1966: 'Sarah's seminal emissions: Hebrews 11.11 in the light of ancient embryology', 112–34 in A. Brenner (ed.), *A Feminist Companion to the Hebrew Bible in the New Testament*, Sheffield.

Von Staden, H. 1989: *Herophilus: The Art of Medicine in Early Alexandria*, Cambridge.

Wade, N. J. 1998: *A Natural History of Vision*, Cambridge, MA.

Wilson, P. K. 1991: 'Out of sight, out of mind?: the Daniel Turner-James Blondel dispute over the power of the maternal imagination', *Annals of Science* 49, 63–85.

Witt, C. 1985: 'Form, reproduction and inherited characteristics in Aristotle's *Generation of Animals*', *Phronesis* 30, 46–57.

Wolfson, H. A. 1935: 'The internal senses in Latin, Arabic, and Hebrew philosophic texts', *The Harvard Theological Review* 28, 69–133.

26. Medicine and Spas in the Roman Period: the Role of Doctors in Establishments with Mineral-Medicinal Waters

Silvia González Soutelo

In our current research project entitled Spas in the Western Empire: the technological and social impact of Rome in the exploitation of mineral-medicinal water,[1] *we attempt to identify the characteristics of Roman spas, in contrast to those baths that used ordinary water, in order to understand their meaning and function. One of the most difficult and interesting topics to develop in our study is the need to recognise the role of medicine in these establishments within the context of health and religion. Therefore, in this paper, we try to show some of the more representative evidence of this duality, starting with the evolution and development of Roman spas.*

1. Baths and spas. The water makes the difference

As is well-known, mineral water has physical characteristics which can be recognised empirically, such as the colour, bad smell, different tastes or high temperature, but what is more important, is that this water also has medicinal properties that were exploited in antiquity. Due to these medicinal properties, mineral waters were highly valued in the ancient world, and were considered, in most cases, as a gift from the gods. So, in order to take advantage of them, a series of infrastructures was built so as to exploit the health-giving properties of this water, in a context of health and religion.

As many authors have noted (e.g. Bonnard 1908; Grènier 1960; Chevallier 1985; Diez de Velasco 1985; 1998; Yegül 1992; Peréx Agorreta 1997), we consider that there is a clear difference between buildings for bathing where mineral-medicinal waters were used, and the *thermae* or *balnea* using ordinary water, that were built wherever they were wanted.

Generally speaking, we can define four main points of difference between healing spas and ordinary baths, based mainly on the nature of the water:

- ***Functionality***: We must distinguish between the religious and healing functions of the baths that use mineral-medicinal water, compared with the hygienic, social and leisure uses of the ordinary baths.
- ***Location:*** Spas were built where mineral waters emerge, in order to make the most of their mineral and calorific properties. In contrast, baths using ordinary water were placed at the most convenient site for the community or wealthy owners, using hydraulic systems to supply ordinary water to a specific location.
- ***Infrastructure:*** When mineral waters were found, the main aim was to use them for health treatments, and, for this reason, these establishments were frequently prepared with structures like, for example, one or more large central pools for bathing in. Nevertheless, in baths using ordinary water, people enjoyed the different pools mainly for leisure, but also for hygienic purposes.
- ***Religiosity:*** Mineral-medicinal waters were always linked to religious contexts. It was believed that one or more divinities resided in or protected these waters and conferred a healthy and sacred character on them. Roman people made dedications and votive offerings to these divinities in the spas and temples in order to obtain their approval; whereas, hygienic baths gradually lost all their religious character (if they indeed had one), and became instead a central attraction in a social context.

In addition to these main ways of differentiating and characterising mineral waters, there are many other aspects that need to be borne in mind in evaluating the archaeological evidence linked to these waters, and in trying to recognise

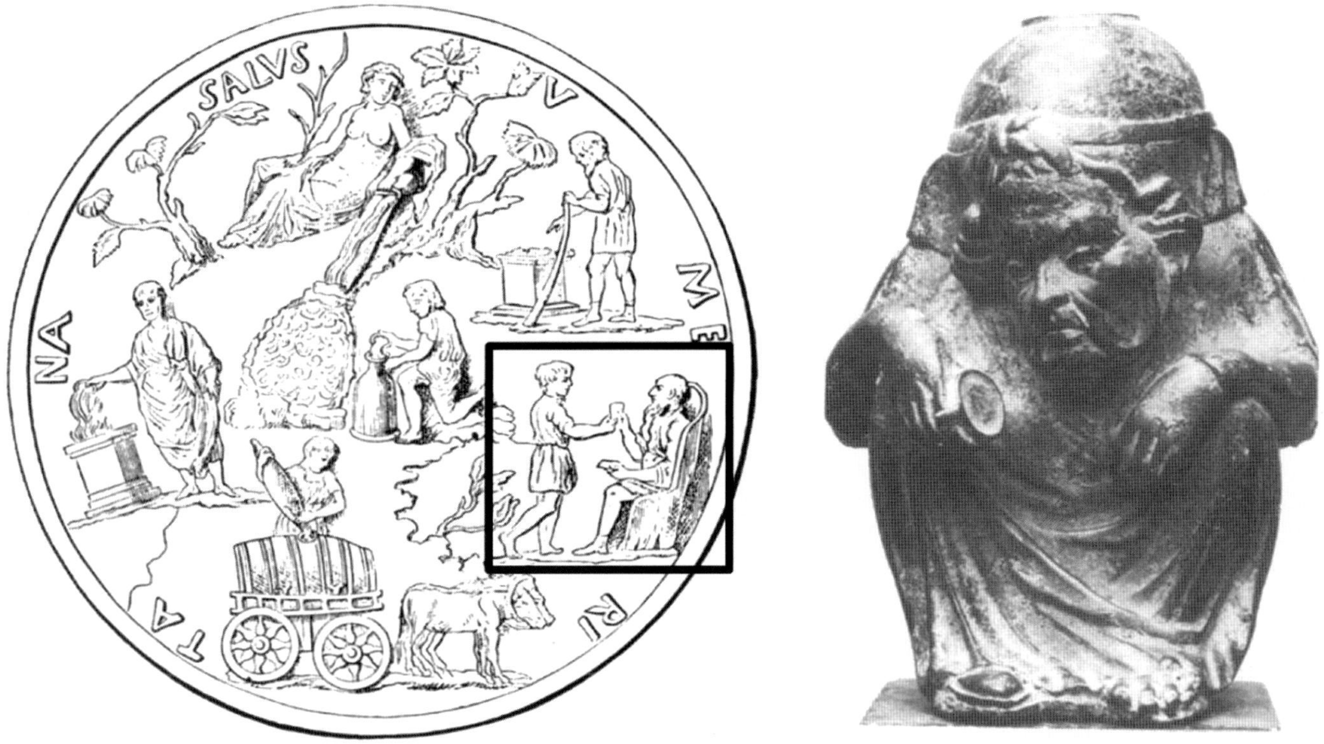

Fig. 26.1. Drawing of the bowl from Otañes (Cantabria, Spain), and photograph of the 'Drinker' from Vichy (France) (from Grènier 1960 and Corrocher 1985 respectively)

a possible building or architectural model for this type of complex.

One of the subjects that has to be revisited in order to better understand the place of spas in the cultural reality of the Roman period is the role that these waters played as treatment in the healing centres where people went to treat their pains and illnesses. Doubts emerge when we try to find the real relationship between scientific treatment and religion, and its reflection in the archaeological evidence. Despite the knowledge that Greek and Roman doctors had about the properties and composition of these waters, it is uncertain if, in the Roman mind, recovery or healing of an illness was considered a result of divine intervention or of the medical treatment.

Although classical medicine developed considerably during the Roman Empire, and the use of these mineral waters was considered in some cases a valuable and 'scientific' treatment, the numerous votive offerings found in these places lead us to believe that a cure was mostly considered a religious miracle.[2] Therefore, in this paper we will make some suggestions about the nature of healing spas in the Roman period and the possible role that physicians played in the configuration and use of these establishments, in order to understand their real meaning and interest.[3]

2. Medicine and mineral water in the ancient world

When we think of mineral-medicinal waters, we should take into account that there was a great variety of them, depending on their physical properties and chemical composition. As a result, each type of mineral water was used in different ways.

We can distinguish two main types of use:

- By drinking it (internal use): as the case is today, some kinds of mineral waters were more suitable for drinking, given their digestive or nutritive properties. In this case, we have no archaeological evidence of special buildings or structures designed specifically for drinking mineral water. However, some references in the works of classical authors,[4] and some evidence coming from anthropology, as well as different objects found around the springs[5] (Fig. 26.1), indicate that these waters were regularly used for drinking.
- By bathing in it (external use[6]). Obviously, this was the most frequent modality in the ancient world, and the one for which more archaeological evidence exists. This is especially the case with thermal springs where the hot water was used in situ as a therapeutic treatment. The hyper-thermal waters were the most valued, and

> we have archaeological evidence that the Romans built many structures in these places in order to help sick people use this thermal water, even installing cooling systems when needed.[7]

It is highly likely that already in the pre-Roman period these springs had some basic structures for the use of the waters, as inferred, for example, from epigraphy. However, direct evidence for these structures is lacking probably due to the perishable materials they were made of. It was, however, above all in the Roman period that these places were provided with monumental buildings equipped for this use.

The mineral steam that emanates from the springs was also recommended in several types of treatments. Initially this steam was used as a treatment in natural caves,[8] but when thermal bath complexes started to be built, rooms were specially prepared to take advantage of these emanations, by building pipes, and drilling structures to create inhalation chambers.[9]

In this way, it is possible to think that some specialisation of the spas in relation to the kind of water and its applications existed (as happens nowadays),[10] although it is difficult to know if the real reason was medical advice or traditional practice. Several authors such as Pliny the Elder insist on this fact:

> '… some (water) has the virtue of sulphur, some of alum, some of salt, some of soda, some of bitumen, some are even acid and salt in combination; of some the mere steam is beneficial, of which the power is so great that it heats baths and even makes cold water boil in the tubs …
>
> To come now to the classes of water: some waters are good for sinews or feet, or for sciatica; others for dislocations or fractures; they purge the bowels; heal wounds; are specific for head, or for ears; while the Ciceronian are so for the eyes.
>
> … Near Rome the waters of Albula heal wounds. These are lukewarm, but those of Cutilia of the Sabines are very cold, penetrating the body with a sort of suction, so that they might seem almost to bite, being very healthful to the stomach, the sinews, and the whole body' (*NH*, XXXI, 2–6, trans. Jones 1975).

This was also stated by Vitruvius when he described the different kinds of waters:

> 'As to the curative power of warm springs, the reason is that the water being thoroughly heated in vitiated soils, takes up an additional and useful quality. For sulphur springs refresh muscular weakness by heating and burning poisonous humours from the body. Alum springs affect parts of the body which are dissolved by paralysis or some stroke of disease; they warm through the open pores and overcome the cold by the opposing power of the heat, and thus forthwith the diseased parts are restored to their ancient health. Bitumen springs furnish draughts which purge and heal interior defects' (VIII, 3, 4, trans. by F. Granger, 1945–1970).

But it was Herodotus who claimed the value of the experience in the use of each type of mineral water:

> 'Comme les eaux minérales présentent chacune en particulier une grande différence dans leurs propriétés, il faut abandonner ce sujet à ceux qui en ont fait l'expérience, car il est impossible de faire une exposition fidèle de chacune de ces eaux, attendu que nous ne faisons pas usage de toutes, et qu'on ne peut pas faire connaître ces eaux en se servant simplement d'étiquettes, comme on le fait pour les médicaments (composés)' (in Oribasius X, 5, trans. Bussemaker and Daremberg 1851–1876).

Therefore, in the case of building medicinal baths, we can ask ourselves on one hand what role was played by the medicinal properties and on the other, what by the ancient doctors in the configuration and organisation of these complexes. According to the nature and characteristics of the mineral water, we ask how much the ancient physicians were involved in the design of these complexes (as happens nowadays, when doctors influence the construction of modern spas). Clearly, this is a question that is not easy to answer, especially because we have no written testimony of the possible link between ancient doctors and the design and construction of these buildings. Nevertheless, from our point of view, some communication between the doctors and the builders was necessary in order to make these bath complexes effective (and useful).

3. The architectural configuration of Roman spas

The great quantity of evidence for spas all around the Roman Empire (Fig. 26.2) shows the importance that these mineral springs had in the ancient world. As mentioned above, the basic element in characterising these buildings was the 'waters', appearing in ancient place names such as *Aquae*,[11] which derived from the value of the springs located in the area[12] (Fig. 26.3). The healing spas were built close to or even over the spring, adapting the topography of each area where the spring emerged, in order to achieve a more suitable structure for the given surroundings. Thus, as healing spas were located only where springs emerged, the sick had to go wherever the waters were (sometimes a long journey) looking for a solution to their health problems.

To allow for the *peregrinatio* made by prospective patients, it was necessary to build infrastructures for accommodation, *tabernae* and other services, which led progressively to the creation of a thermal enclave, and later to the birth of a town or another kind of settlement.[13]

With a concentration of sick people, it would make sense for *medici* and other practitioners to come to such a place looking for new customers, and give advice to the patients on the use of thermal baths, as indicated by some ancient

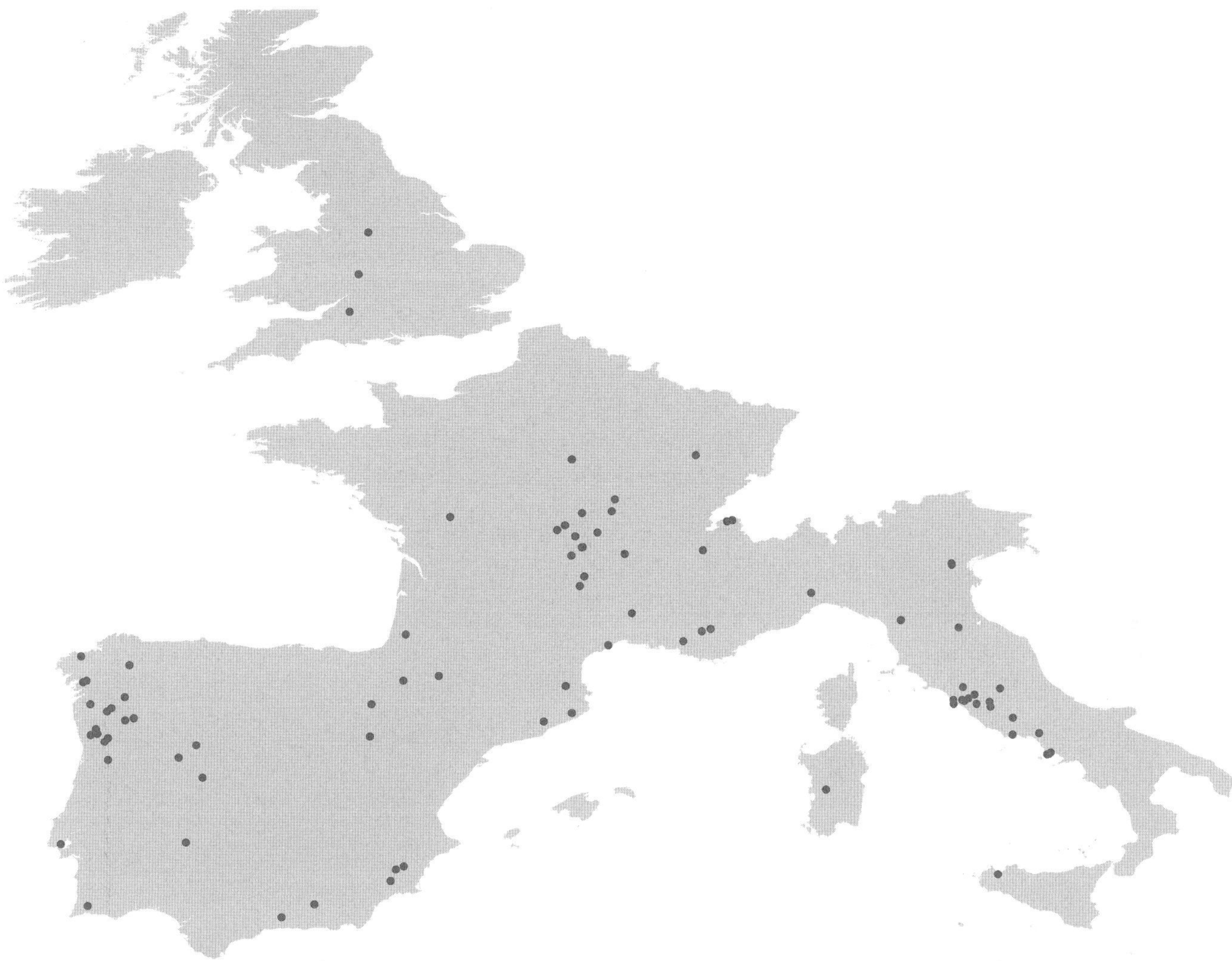

Fig. 26.2. Main Roman spas in the Western Empire analysed in this study

authors.[14] Unfortunately, there is very little archaeological evidence for this, apart from various objects relating to ancient doctors and some funerary stelae found at or near several building complexes with mineral-medicinal waters. It is not certain, however, if they can be interpreted in this sense.[15]

We propose that, at the beginning, springs were used in a natural way, keeping structures to a minimum. We have named these Type 1: 'Rural or plain type and sanctuaries'[16] (Fig. 26.4) for a spa of simple construction. Gradually and in relation to the needs of the patients and the economic, political and social interests of each settlement, we can see the evolution to more important and representative buildings: Type 2 (Fig. 26.5), with more complex constructions and emphasis on the rooms for baths and treatments, along with rooms dedicated to the water cult and healing deities of the springs.

Generally speaking, these buildings were organised around a main room with a central pool of square, circular or rectangular shape. In some cases they were complemented by other rooms with pools for different uses. These *natationes* were the natural solution for the use of the springs by pilgrims and the sick (Fig. 26.6).

In many cases, these rooms were surrounded by other smaller rooms of minor importance that were probably used for individual treatments or for having a rest during treatment[17] (Fig. 26.7). This fact argues for the possible intervention of ancient doctors in the architectural configuration of these bath buildings.

As we had already stated, we can observe an evolution in several thermal baths, especially in the case of important economic or political settlements. At a certain period in time (2nd–3rd centuries AD) we can observe how they extended their infrastructures and added different rooms, and how the

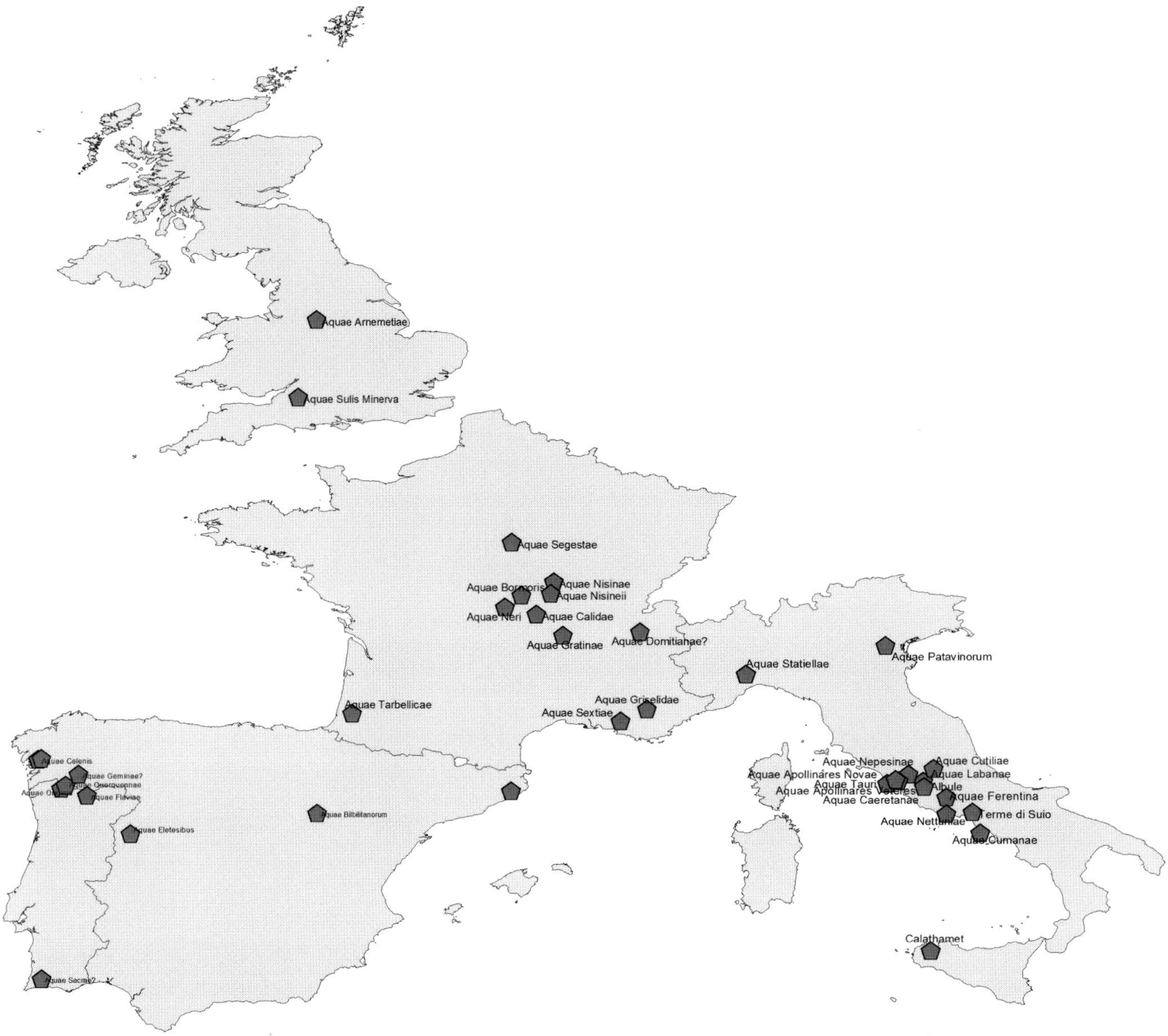

Fig. 26.3. Distribution of some '*AQUAE*' cities in the Western Empire analysed in this study

medicinal-religious uses were combined with ordinary baths in order to offer more possibilities to the visitors of these centres (Fig. 26.8).

This phenomenon was probably due to a change in the mentality and the interest of Roman people in classical bathing practices. In this way, it is suggested that, as there were more customers, the bathing areas needed to be expanded and to include new water supplies, in this case of ordinary water (e.g. Bath, England; Badenweiler, Germany, or Civitavecchia, Italy). We cannot rule out that these new parts of the spas also had a medical aim, in which the use of ordinary water and mineral water treatments was combined, as stated in the hydrotherapic regimes of classical authors.[18]

4. The role of doctors in Roman spas

Apart from the possible involvement of doctors in the designing of spas that we have postulated above, there are very few references to the presence of *medici* in thermal complexes, and the lack of any written or physical references makes it impossible to ascertain if doctors were employed in spas.

Although the richest citizens had their own personal doctors, who advised them on water treatments and other medical cures,[19] we think that usually there would have been travelling doctors or independent physicians around the spas who could prescribe treatments to the sick according to the disease of each.

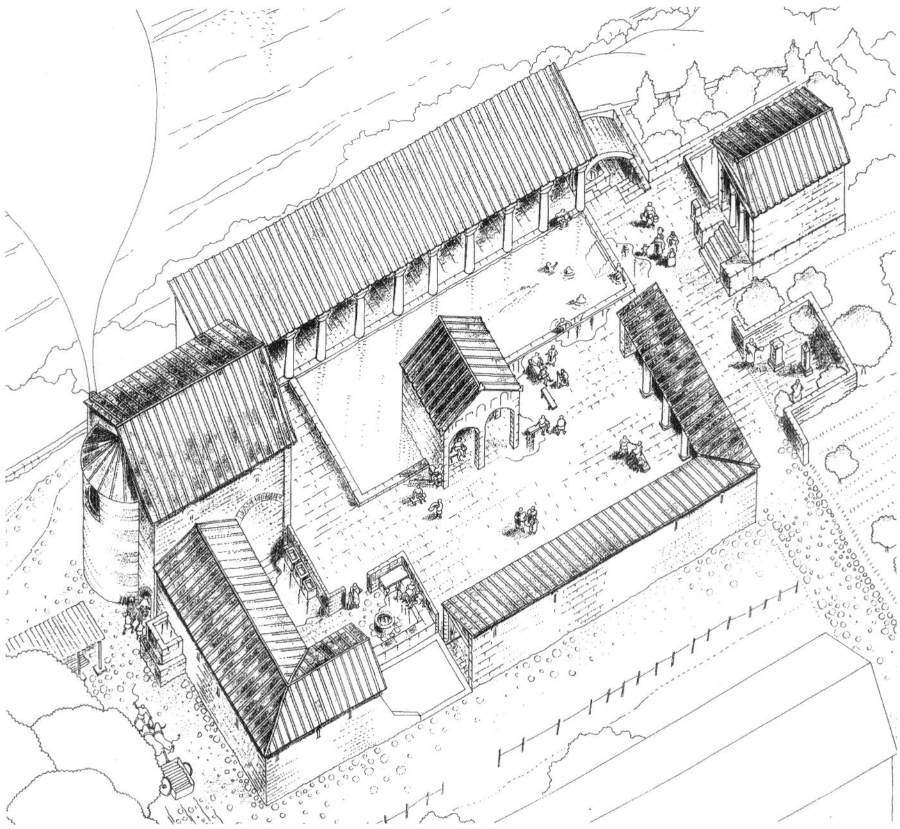

Fig. 26.4. Type 1: Design of the Roman spa and sanctuary of Bagno di Romagna, Italy (from Ortalli 2004)

We have seen that the practice of hydrotherapy, in particular with mineral-medicinal waters, is confirmed by the ancient sources. In these texts different kinds of treatments are indicated, depending on the type of waters, in order to obtain the maximum profit from these baths; and we can find in the classical authors some references to treatments almost identical to those used in modern spas today. For example, Herodotus (in Oribasius, X, III), with reference to baths with mineral waters, presents us with a kind of manual teaching doctors how to use these waters, and how they had to act in each case to obtain the best effects.

Therefore, we can confirm that, even though, at the beginning, most classical authors did not show any interest in the use of the mineral medicinal baths in the treatment of illness,[20] in later periods, mainly during the Roman Empire, the possible use of mineral waters to heal some diseases was recognised. But social mentality would have been more conservative, and the patient or pilgrim still kept the hope of divine intervention (as the votive offerings testify) as the last solution to cure their diseases.

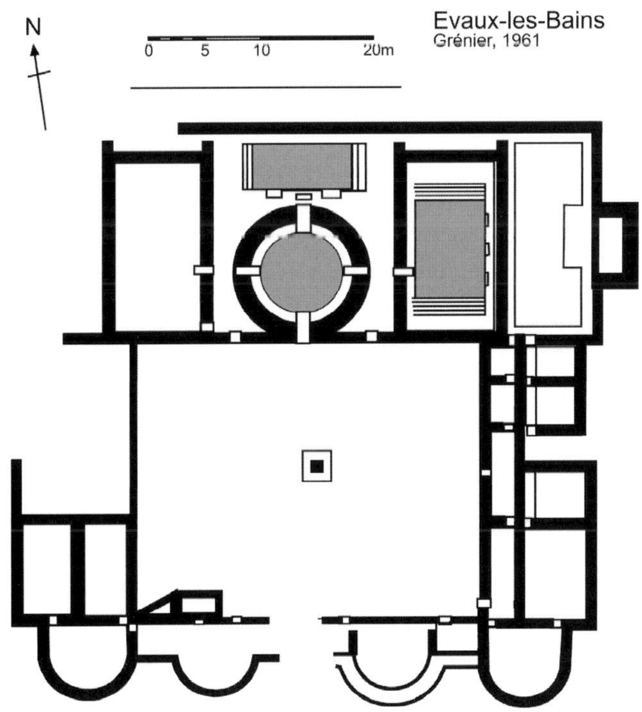

Fig. 26.5. Type 2: Évaux-les-Bains (France) (from Grènier 1960)

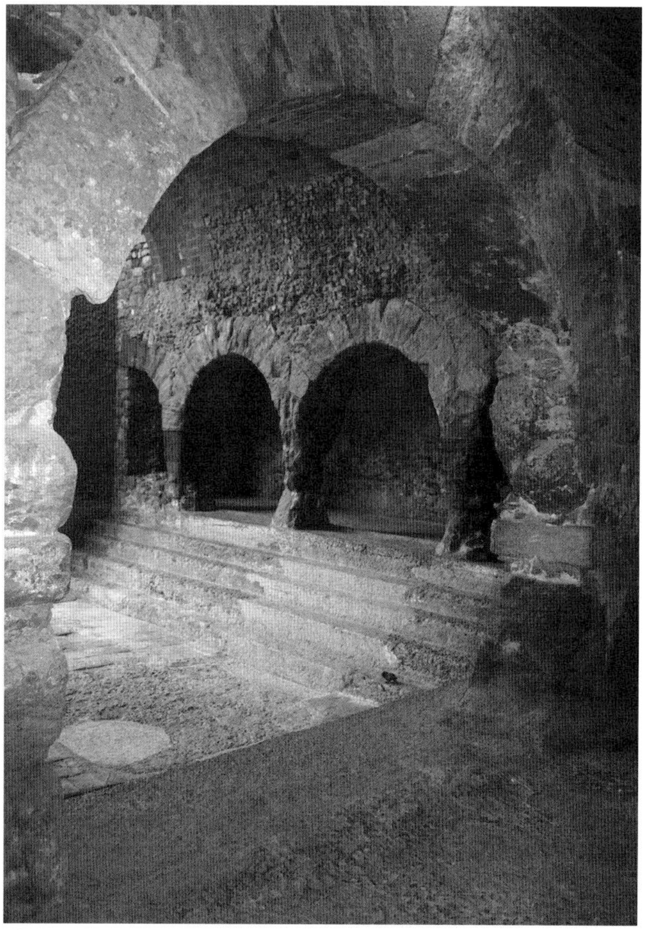

Fig. 26.6. Central swimming pool of Caldas de Montbui (Barcelona, Spain) (S. González Soutelo)

5. Some conclusions

There are very few certainties but a lot of doubts to resolve in the study of Roman healing spas. One of the issues, where there is a lot work to be done, regards the role of medicine and ancient doctors in the use of the mineral-medicinal waters. We believe that it is possible that 'scientific' medicine and doctors were involved in some way in the architectural design of these buildings, perhaps only in their theoretical conception or maybe even in a practical way. The main problem comes when we try to understand how these establishments worked internally and how the use of the waters by the patients was organised.

We still have some important issues to develop during our project. We hope that with new archaeological excavations, future discoveries and an extended revision of the classical authors we will be able to understand in a more precise way the evolution of the practice of medicine in the complex world of the Roman healing spas.

Acknowledgements

I would like to express my gratitude to Janet DeLaine for the revision of this text and for her comments.

Notes

1 This study was initially launched in the University of Santiago de Compostela, and was later continued in the Universitat Autònoma de Barcelona (UAB), thanks to a 'Juan de la Cierva' research contract from the Spanish Ministry of Culture. It has been developed in collaboration with the ICAC (Institut Català d'Arqueologia Clàssica) and the Institute of Archaeology of Oxford University.

2 For example, talking about medicine and religion, Aelius Aristides (*Hieroi Logoi*, I, 61–8: Behr 1968) described: 'From here on, the doctors stopped their criticisms, expressed extraordinary admiration for the providence of the God (Asklepios) in each particular, and said that it was some other greater disease, which he secretly cured'.

3 We must note that although, for instance, there are some examples of medical references to mineral waters as medical treatments by 'scientific' doctors, we have no reference to the health-giving use of mineral waters, for example in the *Corpus Hippocraticum*. The explanation, as Pliny the Elder mentions, could be that the classical medicine authors tried to make a clear separation between 'science' and religion (something that happened until recently): 'I wonder that Homer made no mention of hot springs, and that though he frequently speaks of a hot bath, the reason being that modern hydropathic treatment was not then a part of medicine. Sulphur waters, however, are good for the sinews, alum waters for paralysis and similar cases of collapse, waters containing bitumen and soda, such as that of Cutilia, are good for drinking and as a purge' (Pliny the Elder, *Naturalis Historia* (henceforth *NH*), XXXI, 32, trans. Jones 1975).

4 For example: Herodotus (in Oribasius, X, 5), Seneca (*Questiones Naturales*, III, I) or Vitruvius (VIII, 3, 5). Pliny the Elder mentions some mineral springs used for drinking, and he includes the opinion that people should be moderate when they drink these waters thinking that drinking a lot is healthier: 'Those make a like mistake who boast of the great quantity they can drink. I have seen some already swollen with drinking to such an extent that the rings were covered by skin, since they could not void the vast amount of water they had swallowed' (*NH,* XXXI, 32, trans. Jones 1975).

5 The main evidence is glass or pottery drinking vessels. Some examples make a more specific reference: e.g. the 'Drinker' – a Roman bronze cup representing a sick elderly woman – from Vichy (France), and some infusion cups that were found in a large quantity near a cold mineral spring (Bonnard 1908, 35 and 437; Corrocher 1985); or the bowl from Otañes (Spain), showing a scene where a young man (probably a slave) offers a glass of water from the spring to a seated elderly man (Jackson 1990, 12; Barrate 1992).

6 There were also other kinds of external uses, such as mud unction: 'The mud too of medicinal springs is used with advantage, but the application should be dried in the sun' (Pliny the Elder *NH*, XXXI, 32, trans. by Jones 1975). For

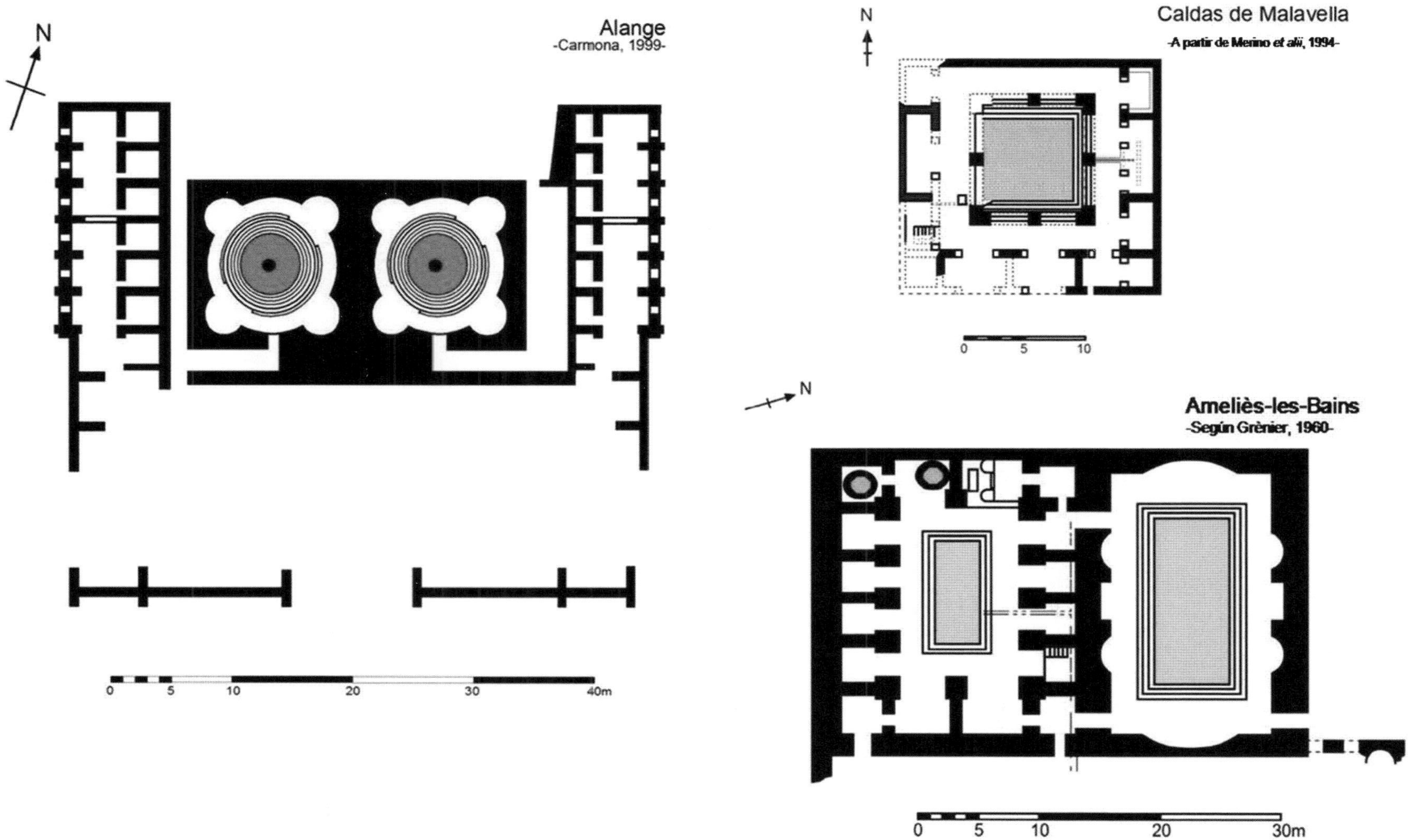

Fig. 26.7. Plans of Roman spas with characteristic rooms (Caldes de Malavella, Girona, Spain; Amèlie-les-Bains, France; Alange, Mérida, Spain) (based on Carmona Barrero 1999, Merino *et al.* 1994, and Grènier 1960, respectively)

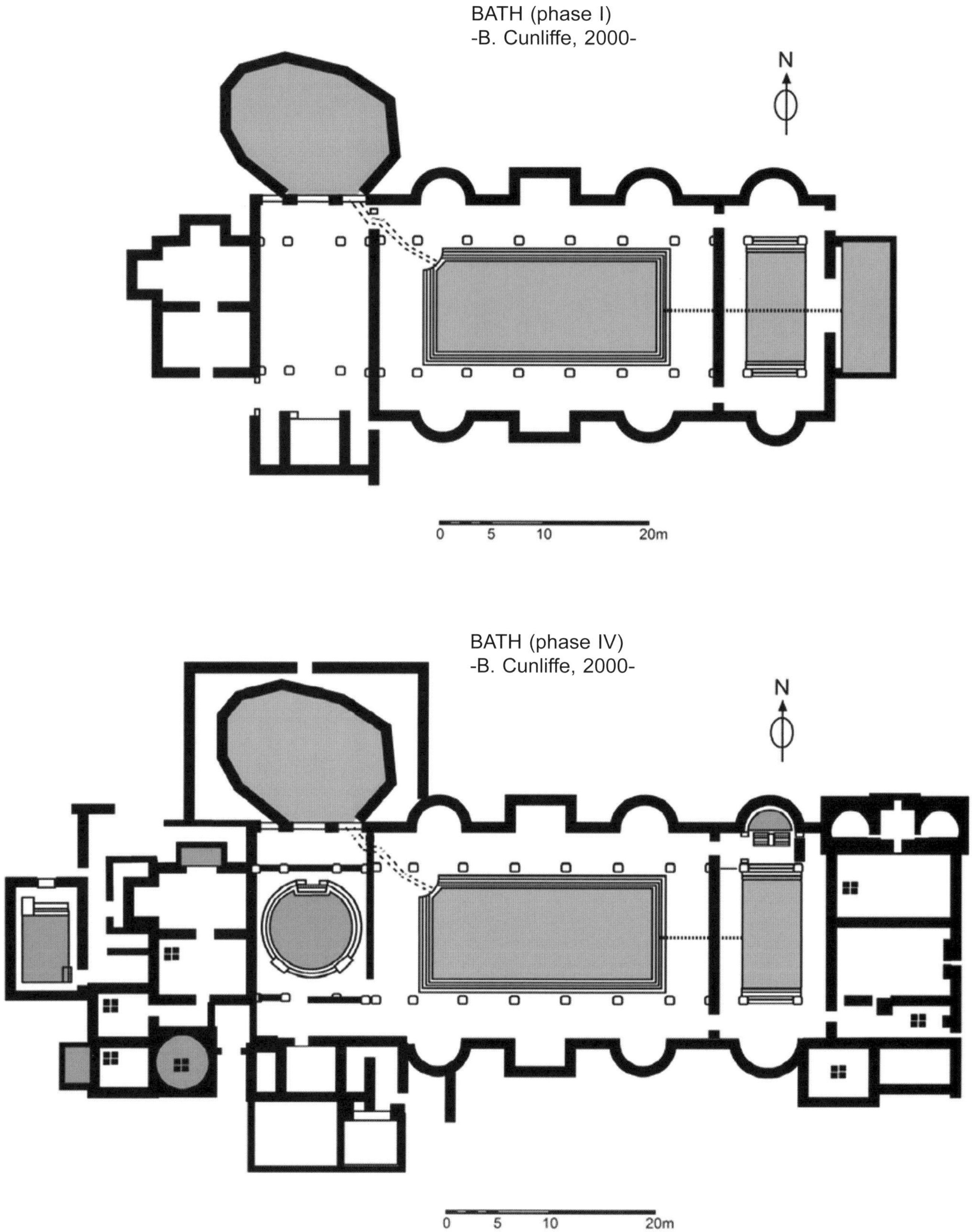

Fig. 26.8. Phases I and IV in the Roman spa at Bath (England) (from Cunliffe 2000)

example, the mud of *Aquae Mattiacae* (Wiesbaden) was very famous in antiquity (Martial, *Epigrammata* LIV, 27). The use of mineral water for a shower was also known (Antyllus, in Oribasius, X, 3, 10, trans. Bussemaker and Daremberg 1851–1876): *'Se placer sous un filet d'eau minérale est une pratique à laquelle on ne doit recourir que pour les eaux dont les propriétés sont profitables à la tête'*. There is some possible archaeological evidence for showers in a few Roman spas, in the form of pipes in the top of walls (e.g. Bourbon-Lancy, France) and in some painted images on Greek pottery (for this subject, see e.g. Bonnard 1908, 36–40; Oró Fernández 1996, 58–9; and Tölle-Kastenbein 1990).

7 As we can see, for example, in Henchir el-Hammam, with 70ºC (Laporte 2006, 299–300) or we can presume for other spas where the waters had a high temperature, like *Aquae Thibilitanae* (Hammam Meskoutine, Algeria) with 96ºC; Plombières-les-Bains (France) with 85ºC; *Aquae Flaviae* (Chaves, Portugal) with 73ºC; or Caldes de Montbui (Spain) with 70ºC.

8 'In the hills of Baiae which belong to Cumae sites are excavated for sweating-rooms. In these hot vapour rising deep down perforates the soil by the violence of its heat, and passing through it rises in these places, and so produces striking advantages in sweating-rooms' (Vitruvius, II, VI, trans. by F. Granger, 1945–1970).

9 See, e.g. Celsus (*De Medicina* II, 17) or Herodotus (in Oribasius, X, 40). Bonnard (1908, 44) suggests that there were some examples in Amélie-les-Bains and Luchon (France), while the room conserved in the Rochetas Healing Spa (Caldes de Montbui, Spain) may be considered a *laconicum* or a *concameratio sudationem* (Monleón 2002, 43–6) .

10 As we can see in classical writers' works (see also notes 4 and 5), this may explain the anatomic votive offerings found in some of these spas. These objects, which show some pathologies related to eye diseases, gout, tumours, digestive disorders, etc., represented the diseased body parts that patients wished to cure (see, for example, Vauthey and Vauthey 1985; Bourgeois and Sikora 1985, 104; Jackson 1992, 114; 2000, 160; and D'Amato 1993, 48–50). In this way, we can know which the most frequent pathologies were, and what kinds of waters were most used in each case.

11 Varro: 'So also, the hot springs (*aquae caldae*), on account of the locality and the water which gushed out there, came to be frequented for our use, since some of the springs were beneficial to one disease and others to another; and because those which they used were several in number, as at *Puteoli* and in Etruria, they called them by a plural word rather than by a singular' (*De Lingua Latina* IX, 41, 69; trans. R. G. Kent 1967).

12 Thus, we have some examples, such as: *Aquae Sulis Minerva* (Bath, England), *Aquae Calidae* (Vichy, France), *Aquae Celenae* (Caldas de Reis, Spain), *Aquae Flaviae* (Chaves, Portugal) or *Aquae Flavianae* (Henchir-el-Hammam, Algeria), etc. As Pliny the Elder said: 'Everywhere in many lands gush forth beneficent waters, here cold, there hot, there both, as among the Tarbelli, an Aquitanian tribe, and in the Pyrenees .... Water adds to the number of the gods by its various names, and founds cities, such as Puteoli in Campania, Statiellae in Liguria and Sextiae in the province of Narbonensis ...' (*NH*, XXXI, 2–3, trans. Jones 1975).

13 For example, Roman cities like Bath (England), Aachen (Germany) and Évaux-les-Bains (France).

14 E.g. Antyllus (in Oribasius, X, 3, 9), Herodotus (in Oribasius, X, 5, 6) or Celsus (*De Medicina* II, 17).

15 The evidence on *medici* being in spa areas is based on epigraphy, oculists' stamps mentioning doctors or medical instruments found near these establishments (Bonnard 1908, 48–51; Guiart 1938; Jackson 1992, 110). For example, the surgical material found in Baden, Switzerland (Jackson 1990, 9; 1992, 112), and an inscription made by a doctor in Hammam Sidi el Hadj, Algeria (Diez de Velasco 1998, 21). In our opinion, however, the presence of these objects near spas does not necessarily mean that these professionals worked in these complexes.

16 González Soutelo (2010; 2011), according to the proposal of Yegül (1992, 110–7). Examples of these sanctuaries could be that of Fortuna at Murcia, and those at Djebel Oust, Algeria and Chianciano Terme, Italy.

17 These rooms have been frequently found in spas we have studied. Some examples can be found in Amèlies-les-Bains, France and Alange or Caldes de Malavella, Spain, among others.

18 E.g. Celsus (*De Medicina* II, 17) and Herodotus (in Oribasius, X, 5).

19 As we can see, for example, in the case of Augustus and his doctor Musa (Suetonius, *Aug*, 81, 1, 94).

20 As Pliny the Elder says (*NH*, XXXI, 32). Also, as can be seen in the *Corpus Hippocraticum* (VII/XVII–XVIII) and in other classical medical authors, the quantity and importance of references to mineral waters were very scarce in relation to the total dedicated to other medical therapies.

Bibliography

Barrate, Fr. 1992: 'La coupe en argent de Castro Urdiales', 43–54 in *Les eaux thermales et les cultes des eaux en Gaule et dans les provinces voisines. Actes du colloque 28–30 septembre 1990, Aix-les-Bains*, Tours and Turin.

Behr, C. A. 1968: *Aelius Aristides and the Sacred Tales*, Amsterdam.

Bonnard, L. 1908: *Gaule Thermale. Sources et stations thermales et minérales de la Gaule à l'époque gallo-romaine*, Paris.

Bourgeois, C. and Sikora, E. 1985: 'Médicine des yeux dans le sanctuaire de l'eau de Pouillé (Loir-et-Cher)', 39–102 in Chevalier 1985.

Carmona Barrero, J. D. 1999: *AQUAE. Análisis del desarrollo histórico-arquitectónico de Alange y sus baños romanos*, Alange.

Chevallier, R. (ed.) 1985: *La médicine en Gaule: villes d'eaux, sanctuaires des eaux*, Paris.

Corrocher, J. 1985: 'Les eaux thermales de Vichy dans l'antiquité', 25–38 in A. Pelletier (éd.), *La médicine en Gaule: villes d'eaux, sanctuaires des eaux*, Paris.

Cunliffe, B. 2000: *Roman Bath Discovered*, Bath.

D'Amato, Cl. 1993: *La medicina.* (Vita e costume dei romani antichi, 15), Rome.

Diez de Velasco, F. 1985: 'Balnearios y dioses de las aguas termales en la Galicia romana', *Archivo Español de Arqueología*, No. 58, 151–2, 69–98.

Diez de Velasco, F. 1998: *Termalismo y religión. La sacralización del agua termal en la Península Ibérica y el Norte de África en el mundo antiguo* (ILU. Revista de Ciencia de las Religiones, Monografías, no. 1), Madrid.

González Soutelo, S. 2010: 'La configuración arquitectónica de los balnearios de aguas mineromedicinales en época romana: Una propuesta de estudio', *Bollettino di Archeologia On-line*, 1–9.

González Soutelo, S. 2011: *El valor del agua en el mundo antiguo. Sistemas hidráulicos y aguas mineromedicinales en el contexto de la Galicia romana.* (Galicia Histórica, Fundación Barrié), A Coruña.

Grènier, A. 1960: *Manuel d'archéologie gallo-romaine. Vol. IV: Les monuments des eaux. Villes d'eau et sanctuaires de l'eau*, Paris.

Guiart, J. 1938: *Gaule et la médicine gauloise, les villes d'eau de la Gaule romaine*, Paris.

Jackson, R. 1990: 'Water and spas in the classical world', *The Medical History of Waters and Spas*, London.

Jackson, R. 1992: 'Spas, waters and hydrotherapy in the Roman World', 107–16 in J. Delaine and D. E. Johnston (eds), *Roman Baths and Bathing. I: Bathing and Society, Vol. II: Design and Context*. Bath.

Jackson, R. 2000: *Doctors and Diseases in the Roman Empire*, London.

Laporte, J.-P. 2006: 'Henchir el-Hammam (antique *Aquae Flavianae*)', *Aouras* 3, 283–322.

Merino i Serra, J., Nolla i Brufau, J. Mª. and Santos i Retolaza, M. 1994: *Aquae Calidae: Presencia romana a la Selva*, Girona.

Monleón, A. 2002: 'Les termes romanes de Caldes de Montbui', 35–46, in *Historia termal de Caldes de Montbui*, Caldes de Montbui.

Oribasius: Bussemaker, U. C. and Daremberg, C. 1851–1876: *Oeuvres d'Oribase*, Vols 1–6, Paris.

Oró Fernández, E. 1996: 'Balneario romano: aspectos médicos, funcionales y religiosos', 23–151 in A. González Blanco *et al.* (eds), *Balneario romano y la Cueva Negra de Fortuna (Murcia): Homenaje al profesor Ph. Rahtz* (Antigüedad y Cristianismo, XIII), Murcia.

Ortalli, J. 2004: *Bagno di Romagna nell'antichità. Le terme, l'insidiamento, il territorio*, Rome.

Peréx Agorreta, Mª J. (ed.) 1997: *Actas del Congresso de Termalismo Antiguo. Ier Congreso Peninsular, Arnedillo (La Rioja, 1996)*, Madrid.

Pliny the Elder, *Natural History*, vol. 8, trans. by W. H. S. Jones, Cambridge, Mass. and London, 1975.

Tölle-Kastenbein, R. 1990: 'Duschen in archaischer Zeit', 191–202 in *Frontinus-Symposium beim Kongress „Wasser Berlin", Jahrestagung 1989 in Hannover und weitere Beiträge zur historischen Entwicklung der Technik* (Schriftenreihe der Frontinus-Gesellschaft, vol. 14), Bergisch Gladbach.

Varro, *On the Latin Language*, trans. by R. G. Kent, 2 vols, Cambridge, Mass., 1958, 1967.

Vauthey, M. and Vauthey, P. 1985: 'Les ex-voto anatomiques de la Gaule romaine. Essai sur les maladies et infirmités de nos ancêtres', 111–77 in Pelletier, A. (ed.), *La médicine en Gaule. Villes d'eaux, sanctuaires des eaux.* Paris.

Vitruvius, *De architectura*, trans. by F. Granger, 2 vols, Cambridge, Mass., 1945–1970.

Yegül, F. 1992: *Baths and Bathing in Classical Antiquity*, New York.

Part VII

Skeletal Remains

27. Health Care and Survival of a Child with Cranial Trauma at *Augusta Emerita* (Mérida, Spain)

Filipa Cortesão Silva, Juana Márquez Pérez, João Rosa and Ana Luísa Santos

Among the individuals recovered in a funerary area south of Augusta Emerita *(Mérida, Spain) was a child who was about 3 years old. According to the grave goods, this burial is dated to the second half of the 1st to the 2nd century AD. The observation of the skull revealed a severe traumatic lesion affecting the frontal and right zygomatic areas, with signs of bone remodelling, also visible on images produced by the Three-Dimensional Computed Tomography. The consequences of the lesion on the child's health and the health assistance that allowed his/her survival for some time are discussed. According to literature, the Romans had the medical knowledge, namely surgery, to deal with this type of problem.*

Introduction

Our knowledge of the history of medicine can benefit from the study of prehistoric and historic human skeletons. This type of material can reveal medical practices in addition to information about the history of diseases. Trauma is among the pathologies that can be analysed and is the key issue of this work. According to Cook and Powell (2006) the interdisciplinary study of trauma began in the last decades, with aspects such as frequency of fractures, their causes and possible treatments among the obtained data.

In paleopathological literature the diagnosis on non-adults is rare due to the difficulties of identifying these lesions in children and the lack of success in examining children for such pathology (Lewis 2007). However, in the past, as today, fractures in childhood may have been common (Roberts 2000).

Most fractures observed in children from multiple periods in the past are located on the skull, limbs, clavicles, or the ribs (e.g. Lewis 2007). Among the cranial fractures reported, Lewis (1999, in Lewis 2007) documented three cases of head injury (blunt force) in rural Wharram Percy (late medieval England). In one of these cases, the child, who was 5 years old, had no evidence of healing suggesting a subdural haematoma and subsequent death. Furthermore, there are also several bibliographic references to skull lesions observed in infants and children caught up in warfare and massacres at different places and dates (Lewis 2007). Regarding healed skull fractures, only a few cases were noticed. Rühli *et al.* (2002) studied a child cranial vault fragment found at Vilmar-Weyer, Germany, from the early medieval period, which presents a semicircular lesion with signs of bone remodelling on its edges. A Multislice Computed Tomography confirmed the diagnosis. Another example concerning healed fractures on a right parietal bone was found on a 2 year old girl from the 4th century AD in Lisieux, Normandy (Blondiaux *et al.* 2002). These authors interpreted the skull lesions as a result of child abuse.

Our research concerns a case which comes from a funerary area of the colony of *Augusta Emerita*, the capital of Lusitania. This Roman province extended over a region that today corresponds to the southern territories of Portugal and Spain. *Augusta Emerita*, now called Mérida, is a city located in the Extremadura province, in Spain. This paper aims to describe a cranial case of trauma on a Roman child, its effects on the child's health and the possible health assistance that allowed his or her survival.

Material and methods

In 2005, Grave A 33 (archaeological intervention number 5036) situated in a funerary area located in the south of

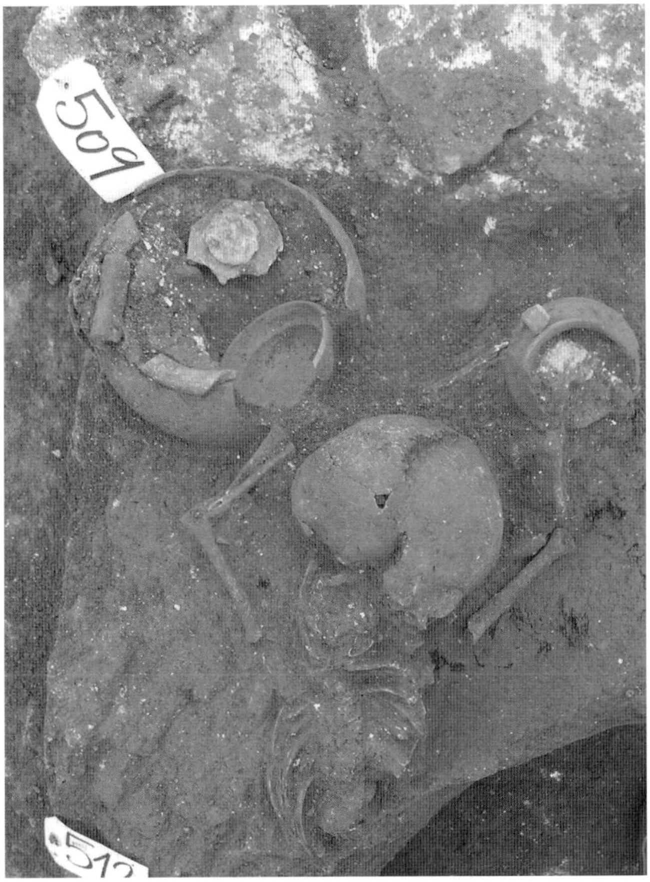

Fig. 27.1. Child burial in situ in Grave A 33 at *Augusta Emerita*, with the head facing north and the face lying on its left side. Note that the arms are raised up, one on each side of the head

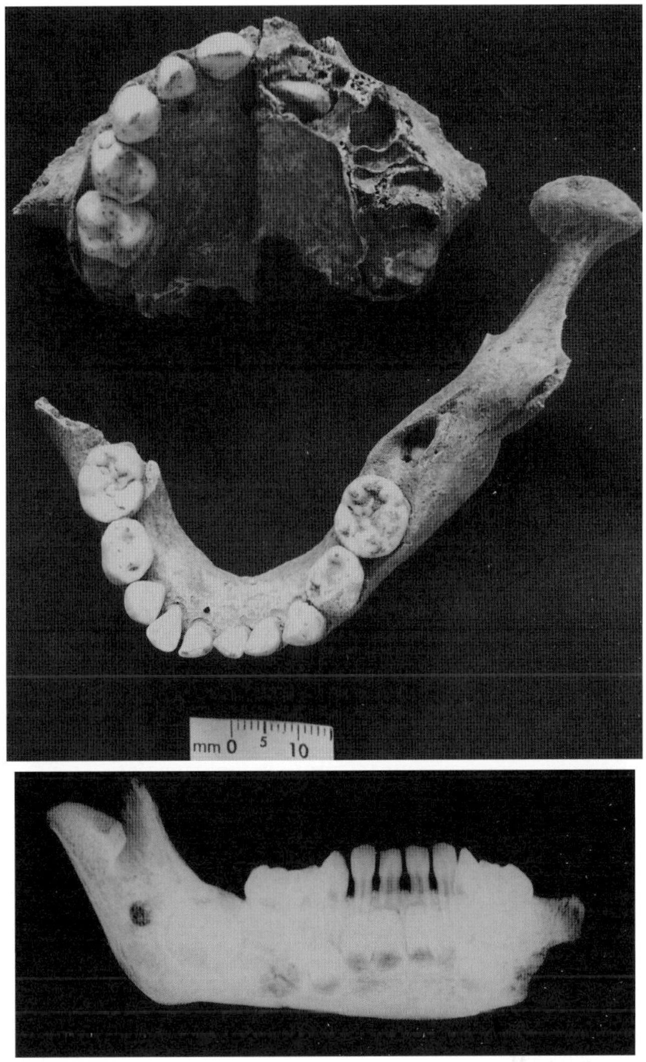

Fig. 27.2. Maxilla and mandible of the child illustrating the tooth erupted. A radiograph of the mandible where the dental development can be seen

Augusta Emerita was excavated by Juana Márquez Pérez. According to the grave goods – two ceramic vessels – this grave dates to the second half of the 1st to the 2nd century AD. Among the individuals recovered (Silva *et al.* 2008) there is a child (stratigraphic unit number 325) inhumed in supine position, with the head facing north and the face lying on the left side (Fig. 27.1). Only the skull, thorax and upper limbs were present. The arms were raised up, one on each side of the head, corresponding to an atypical burial body posture. The pelvis and the lower limbs of this individual were not preserved, probably due to the violation of the nearby burial A 34.

Later, in 2008, this individual was cleaned and studied in the laboratory. Since the skull was fragmented it was necessary to perform its reconstruction. The age at death was estimated based on Ubelaker (1989) and Scheuer and Black (2000). Measurements of the long bones were taken with a Mitutoyo digital caliper (precision 0.01 mm). The skull was radiographed (GE Healthcare, Senographe DC, reference 5131764-7-1PT) and submitted to Three-Dimensional Computed Tomography (3D-CT), using a Siemens Somatom Volume Zoom 4 VA47C.

Description of the child

According to the sequence of teeth formation and eruption (Ubelaker 1989), this individual was 3 years±12 months old (Fig. 27.2). However, long bone lengths indicated an age at death between 1½ and 3 years (Table 27.1).

The sex of this individual was not determined because, macroscopically, it is impossible to perform a reliable estimation at such a young age, or more precisely before adolescence, when the development of sexual dimorphism in the skeleton occurs (Scheuer and Black 2000).

Table 27.1. Age at death estimation based on the measurements of the long bones

Bone	*Measurement*	*Author*	*Size (mm)*	*Age at death (years)*
Right clavicle	Maximum length	Black and Scheuer 1996b*	66.5	2–3
Left humerus	Diaphyseal length	Maresh, 1970*	119.2	1.5
Right radius	Diaphyseal length	Gindhart, 1973*	91.6	1.5

* These works were cited in Scheuer and Black (2000)

The identification of a severe traumatic lesion on the frontal bone, with a length of about 4 cm, occurred during the gluing of the cranial bone pieces. The area shows irregular surfaces and signs of bone remodelling which indicate an ante mortem lesion (Fig. 27.3). Besides, an increasing thickness near the orbit and on the orbital surface of the right zygomatic bone was also noticed (Fig. 27.4). These facts were confirmed by the images obtained by 3D-CT, where different bone densities between the area affected by the lesion and the other parts of the bone can be identified (Fig. 27.5).

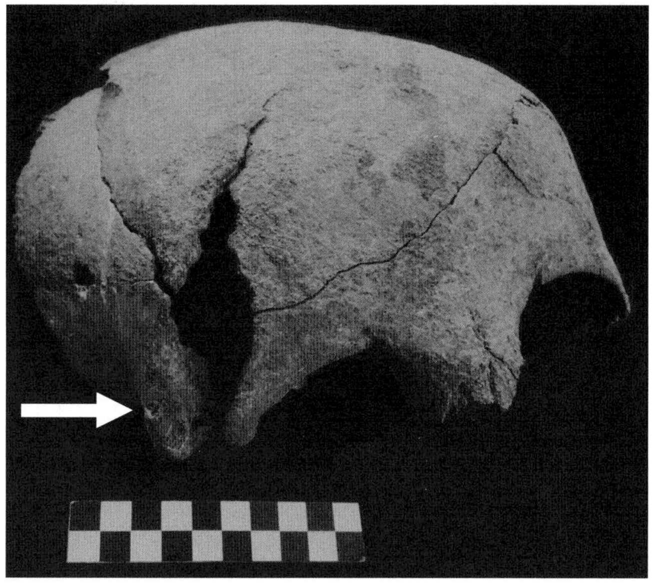

Fig. 27.3. Frontal bone in right antero-lateral view showing the fracture with bone remodelling on the edge of the lesion

Discussion

Studying trauma in bones from ancient populations gives us information about occupation, personal relationships, mortuary behaviour, accidents, subsistence and trauma treatment (Roberts 2000; Lewis 2007). Brasili *et al.* (2004) pointed out that from the type and degree of repair of the lesion it is possible to identify its etiology and possible applied treatments. Furthermore, since

> 'children were involved in many aspects of life within a community, and performed many subsistence and occupational activities, evidence for trauma in their remains helps to unravel questions such as the age of apprenticeship, child abuse, parental care, the home environment and, in case of peri-mortem cuts during autopsy, the development of paediatrics' (Lewis 2007, 169).

In *Augusta Emerita*, among the human remains recovered from Grave A 33, was an inhumed child that shows a cranial trauma. This individual dates from the 1st to the 2nd century AD, and was around 3 years old at the moment of death. The injury is located in the frontal and right zygomatic bones, and may have resulted in a primary brain lesion. Most certainly there was also a cutaneous wound. The edges of the bone lesion show signs of remodelling which, according to the medical experience of one of the authors [J. R.], suggested a survival period of between 3 weeks and 2 months. The location of the fracture, just above the orbit, and the involvement of the zygomatic area indicate that there was probably some degree of eye involvement and vision loss on the right eye. It is unlikely that vision loss occurred as a consequence of neurological damage. Despite the fact that immediate death did not occur, the trauma certainly caused some degree of unconsciousness or coma. It is also very likely that small pieces of bone, resulting from the impact, provoked the tearing of the *dura mater*, putting the brain in direct communication with the skin and opening an entrance to micro-organisms. In open or compound fractures, the exposure to microorganisms was obviously a danger in antiquity due to the risk of infection (Roberts 2000), as in this case. Thus, an infection of the wound with progression to the meninges and adjacent brain was most certainly a complication and probably another factor contributing to the child's death.

A careful observation did not identify any signs of surgery in the frontal bone. However, the Romans had the medical knowledge to treat cranial fractures as can be seen on documents from antiquity (see Jackson 2005; Kshettry *et al.* 2007). These documents contain descriptions of head surgery, including by trepanation, to treat 'direct or indirect trauma, caused by accidental injuries or battle wounds' (Jackson, 2005). There is an interesting case of a trepanation made on a hydrocephalic child who was 5–6 years old, dated from the end of the 1st century or the start of the 2nd century AD, on the site of the ancient town of *Fidenae*, near Rome

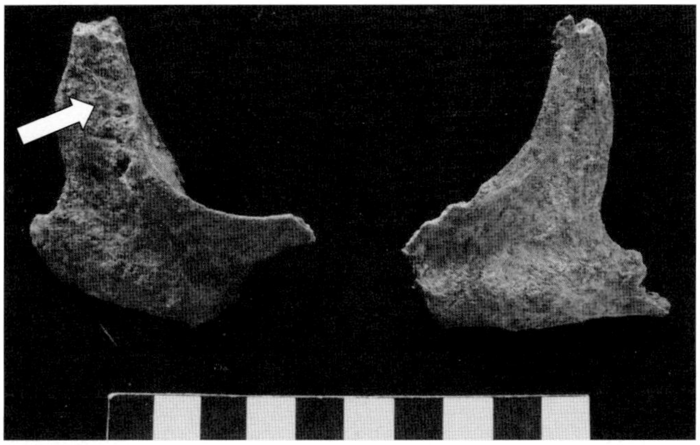

Fig. 27.4. The right zygomatic depicts an increase in the thickness near the orbit in comparison to the left one

(Mariani-Constantini *et al.* 2000). Several burials with medical instruments (e.g. Bejarano Osorio 2002; Márquez Pérez 2006) and epigraphic sources were found in *Augusta Emerita*, with the name and occupation of the person (e.g. Sanabria Escudero 1964). These finds indicate the presence of medical practitioners in the city.

Regarding the treatment of skull fractures with skin wounds, trepanation was an option but was not considered inevitable: Celsus (VIII, 4, 10–12 in Jackson 2005) proposed an initial treatment with plasters and medicated dressing. He also recognized that '[a] fractured bone unless it is treated causes severe inflammations, and is treated afterwards with greater difficulty' (*De med.* VIII, 4,7 in Jackson 2005, 112). *On Wounds in the Head*, of Hippocrates, is 'the first manuscript of antiquity dealing with cranial trauma in such detail and clarity' (Panourias *et al.* 2005, 187). In this book, he said that if the major sub-cranial blood vessels were avoided, skull operations presented less risk than surgery on many other parts of the body, but infection was a constant danger (in Jackson 2005).

The survival of the child found in *Augusta Emerita* probably depended not only on medical assistance but also on nutritional aid, since the comatose state which emerged after the accident created feeding difficulties that could lead to malnutrition and/or dehydration and cause an earlier death. These problems represented a challenge to the carer, in particular the feeding of the child, who was probably fed artificially at some point with a tube or a bottle. Unfortunately, hitherto in Mérida no such devices have been identified. However, these bottles were found in Roman child burials from Pauvadou and Saint-Lambert, exhibited in the Musée Archéologique Municipal de Frèjus (France), and recently mentioned by Trigalet (2009) in a paper about maternity and childhood. According to literaturary sources, children were breastfed until they were 3 years old and weaning was gradual (Fildes 1986 in Dupras *et al.* 2001). Meanwhile, food supplements such as boiled honey or a mixture of

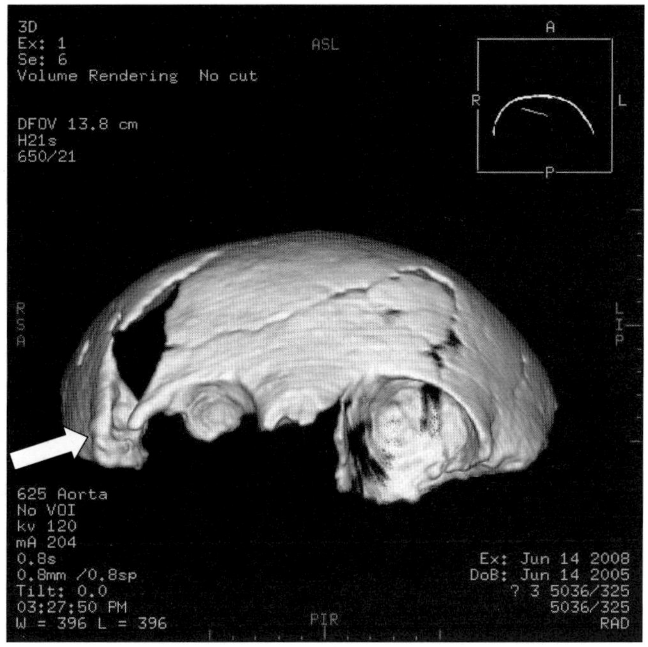

Fig. 27.5. Frontal bone observed by 3D-CT confirmed different bone densities around the area affected by the lesion

honey and goat's, cow's or sheep's milk were introduced using bottle feeding (Dupras *et al.* 2001).

Even nowadays cranial fractures are common in children in this age group (Lyons *et al.* 1999). Clinical data show that the bone affected by the lesion varies according to the age of the individual (Glencross and Stuart-Macadam 2000). Infants and young children, who are not yet able to walk, are more prone to have skull fractures (Kowal-Vern *et al.* 1992) as well as clavicular fractures (Glencross and Stuart-Macadam 2000). On the other hand, there is a prevalence of limb fractures when children become ambulatory (Cheng and Shen 1993). Today this kind of accident is more common in boys in the proportion of 1.2 to 1.5–1 (Towner and Scott 2008).

In Roman society, child mortality was high. Rawson (2003, 341) points out that in the age group of birth to 5 years old the mortality rate was probably nearly 50%. Nowadays, according to UNICEF (2009), this rate is 68‰ worldwide and 6‰ in industrialised countries. After diseases, trauma was the second cause of death (Coulon 2004). Based on Roman sources, Laes (2004) gives a picture of the kind of accidents affecting children, e.g. falls, accidents with chariots on crowded streets, sporting activities at the gymnasium or drowning in a river or swimming pool.

Conclusions

The observation of the skull of the child from *Augusta Emerita*, revealed a severe cranial trauma with signs of bone remodelling. Given the characteristics of the bone lesion and the possible consequences of the accident on the child's health, we estimate his or her survival for a period of between 3 weeks and 2 months. Survival for such a long time after such a violent head trauma could only have been possible with a relatively high level of care and assistance.

From a medical point of view the cause of death may have been multifactorial: trauma with direct brain injury was the initial mechanism followed by coma, or at least some mental status disturbance. It is impossible to know if the child was assisted by a Roman healer. However, it is known that the Romans had the medical knowledge, namely surgery, to deal with cranial trauma such as the case described here. This study also illustrates the importance of a multidisciplinary dialogue to understand the history of disease and medicine during the study of skeletons from past populations.

Acknowledgements

Our gratitude is due to the following institutions: the Consorcio de Mérida, Spain, Clínica Universitária de Imagiologia, University of Coimbra Hospital and Fundação para a Ciência e a Tecnologia, both in Portugal. We would also like to thank Dr Mary Lewis, Professor Demetrios Michaelides and to the participants of the *Medicine in the Ancient Mediterranean World* for their suggestions.

Bibliography

Bejarano Osorio, A. M. 2002: 'Nuevas aportaciones al conocimiento de la medicina y farmacéutica en la ciudad de *Augusta Emerita'*, *Mérida excavaciones arqueológicas* 2000 6, Mérida, 397–421.

Blondiaux, G., Blondiaux, J., Secousse, F., Cotten, A., Danze, P.-M. and Flipo, R.-M. 2002: 'Rickets and child abuse: the case of a two year old girl from the 4th century in Lisieux (Normandy)', *International Journal of Osteoarchaeology* 12, 209–15.

Brasili, P., Bianchi, E. and Ventrella, A. R. 2004: 'Traumatic events and life-style in Ancient Italian populations', *Collegium Anthropologicum* 28(1), 179–91.

Cheng, J. C. Y. and Shen, W. Y. 1993: 'Limb fracture pattern in different pediatric age groups: a study of 3,350 children', *Journal of Orthopaedic Trauma* 7, 15–22.

Cook, D. C. and Powell, M. C. 2006: 'The evolution of American paleopathology', 281–322 in J. E. Buikstra and L. A. Beck (eds), *Bioarchaeology: the Contextual Analysis of Human Remains*, Amsterdam.

Coulon, G. 2004: *L'enfant en Gaule Romaine*, Paris.

Dupras, T., Schwarcz, H. P. and Fairgrieve, S. I. 2001: 'Infant feeding and weaning practices in Roman Egypt', *American Journal of Physical Anthropology* 115, 204–12.

Glencross, B. and Stuart-Macadam, P. 2000: 'Childhood trauma in the archaeological record', *International Journal of Osteoarchaeology* 10, 198–209.

Jackson, R. 2005: 'Holding on to the health? Bone surgery and instrumentation in the Roman Empire', 97–119 in H. King (ed.), *Health in Antiquity*, London.

Kowal-Vern, A., Paxton, T. P., Ros, S. P., Lietz, H. Fitzgerald, M. and Gamelli, R. L. 1992: 'Fractures in the under-3-year-old age cohort', *Clinical Pediatrics* 31, 653–9.

Kshettry, V. R., Mindea, S. A. and Hunt Batjer, H. 2007: 'The management of cranial injuries in antiquity and beyond', *Neurosurgical Focus* 23(1), 1–8.

Laes, C. 2004: 'Children and accidents in Roman Antiquity', *Ancient Society* 34, 153–70.

Lewis, M. 2007: *The Bioarchaeology of Children: Perspectives from Biological and Forensic Anthropology*, Cambridge.

Lyons, R. A., Delahunty, A. M., Kraus, D., Heaven, M., McCabe, M., Allen, H. and Nash, P. 1999: 'Children's fractures: a population based study', *Injury Prevention* 5, 129–32.

Mariani-Constantini, R., Catalano, P., Gennaro, F., Tota, G. and Angeletti, L. 2000: 'New light on cranial surgery in ancient Rome', *The Lancet* 355, 305–7.

Márquez Pérez, J. 2006: *Los Columbarios: arquitectura y paisaje funerario en Augusta Emerita* (Ataecina: colección de estudios históricos de la Lusitania, 2) Mérida.

Panourias, I. G., Skiadas, P. K., Sakas, D. E. and Marketos, S. G. 2005: 'Hippocrates, a pioneer in the treatment of head injuries', *Neurosurgery* 57, 181–9.

Rawson, B. 2003: *Children and Childhood in Roman Italy*, Oxford.

Roberts, C. 2000: 'Trauma in biocultural perspective: past, present and future work in Britain', 337–56 in M. Cox and S. Mays (eds), *Human Osteology in Archaeology and Forensic Science*, London.

Rühli, F. J., Lanz, C., Ulrich-Bochsler, S. and Alt, K. W. 2002: 'State-of-the-art imaging in palaeopathology: the value of Multislice Computed Tomography in visualizing doubtful cranial lesions', *International Journal of Osteoarchaeology* 12, 372–9.

Sanabria Escudero, M. 1964: 'La medicina emeritense en las épocas romana y visigoda', *Revista de Estudios Extremeños* 20 (1), 53–84.

Scheuer, L. and Black, S. 2000: *Developmental Juvenile Osteology*, London.

Silva, F. C., Pérez, J. M., Rosa, J. and Santos, A. L. 2008: 'Cranial trauma on a child from a double Roman burial at *Augusta Emerita*, Spain', *Paleopathology Association: scientific program & abstracts. 17th European Meeting of the Paleopathology Association, 25–7 August 2008, Copenhagen, Denmark. Supplement to the Paleopathology Newsletter, 62.*

Towner, E. and Scott, I. 2008: 'Chapter 1. Child injuries in context', 1–28 in M. Peden, K. Oyegbite *et al.* (eds), *World Report on Child Injury Prevention*, Geneva.

Trigalet, V. 2009: 'Maternité et petite enfance', *Histoire antique* 41, 64–73.

Ubelaker, D. 1989: *Human Skeletal Remains: Excavation, Analysis, Interpretation*, Washington.

UNICEF 2009: http://www.unicef.org/index.php.

28. A Multidisciplinary Approach for the Study of the 11th–15th Century AD Human Skeletal Remains from *Palaion Demarheion*, Nicosia, Cyprus

Popi Chrysostomou and Yiannis Violaris

The present paper outlines the results of a research study of the human skeletal remains excavated between 2002 and 2004 at the site of Palaion Demarheion *in Nicosia, Cyprus. The study, funded by the Cyprus Research Promotion Foundation, is an innovative, interdisciplinary approach in the fields of archaeology, anthropology, genetics and medicine, aiming to gain an insight into the Byzantine and medieval society of Nicosia.*

The anthropological analyses recorded the biological profile of a minimum number of 209 individuals and evaluated the traditional methods for stature estimation against data obtained from the Byzantine and medieval skeletal material of Cyprus. A genetic study was conducted on 47 samples on a mitochondrial and Y-chromosome level, and the data were combined with the results of the palaeodemographic study in order to evaluate the presence of an incoming foreign population. In addition, 12 samples were genetically analysed in order to determine the occurrence of beta-thalassaemia. Part of this collection is currently housed at the Archaeological Research Unit of the University of Cyprus and serves as a teaching collection.

The present paper serves as an introduction to the research project and is not an exhaustive presentation of the work conducted. A more thorough presentation of the methodological tools and detailed discussions of each research topic is beyond the scope of this paper.

Introduction

The site of *Palaion Demarheion* ('Old Municipality') was accidentally discovered in June 2002 during construction works for the new Nicosia City Hall, in the old city within the Venetian walls (Fig. 28.1). Rescue excavations, undertaken by the Department of Antiquities between 2002 and 2006, under the direction of Yiannis Violaris, testify to the continuous use of the site from the Byzantine period to British rule (11th–20th century AD). The majority of finds date to the Byzantine and Frankish era, and include a plethora of movable antiquities, architectural remains of monumental public or private buildings, workshop areas (for the production of glass, jewellery and pottery), wells, a water cistern and many other unidentified architectural remains. Perhaps the most important buildings that came to light are two churches (Fig. 28.2).

The first church, conventionally named Church A′, is a complex of two small single-aisle churches. The foundations of the northern part of the church are associated with pottery dating to the 12th century AD. The southern part is associated with two architectural phases. The first phase dates to the second half of the 12th or the beginning of the 13th century. Unfortunately, most of the stratigraphy of this complex was destroyed during construction works, therefore little information is preserved about the history of these buildings. An associated cemetery was found surrounding this church; the excavated burials date from the 12th to the 13th century.

The second church, conventionally named Church B′, has two main architectural phases. The earliest construction phase dates towards the end of the 11th or early 12th century AD and was destroyed by fire in the early 13th century. The church was rebuilt during the 13th century. After the destruction of this second phase, the area of the church was used as a cemetery until the 15th century; most of the area around the church was used as a cemetery at least from the 12th century.

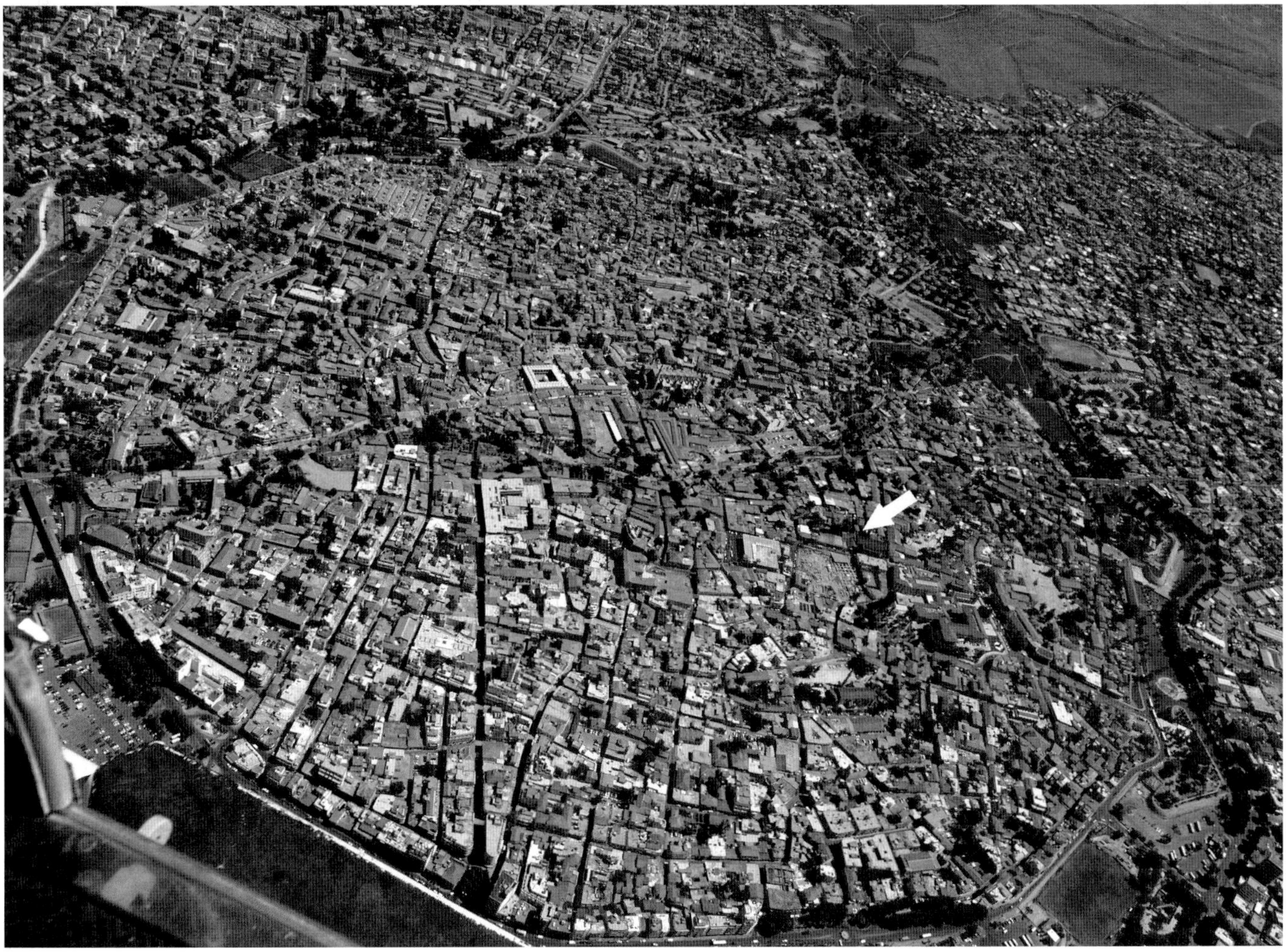

Fig. 28.1. Aerial photograph (taken in 2005) of Nicosia within the Venetian walls. the white arrow indicates the site of *Palaion Demarheion* (Department of Antiquities)

Burial customs

The archaeological evidence (tombstones, funerary artefacts, grave typology), together with the anthropological data (palaeodemography, palaeopathology) and other historical sources were evaluated in order to understand the burial customs of the society under study. Ethnographic studies also played an important role in the interpretation of the data, since many of the Byzantine and medieval funerary beliefs survive until the present time. Thus, the funerary study examined parameters of the population both from a biological and a religious context.

The excavated skeletal remains were located well within the city limits and were directly associated with the two churches. Three main types of graves were recorded: (a) cist tombs built with rectangular limestone, the inner walls covered with plaster and sealed with stone slabs (Fig. 28.3); (b) simple pits with or without a wooden coffin (Fig. 28.4); and (c) simple pits covered with stone slabs with or without a wooden coffin. There is no evidence to suggest that the grave types reflect social status. The various types most probably reflect chronological variations as well as differences in the religious customs of the different groups buried in the cemeteries.

The graves were shallow and did not typically exceed 50 cm in depth. Most synchronous burials were aligned in an orderly fashion in rows in the immediate periphery of the churches. Most of them, however, were partly or entirely superimposed on earlier burials. The disturbance of earlier burials was more frequent in the later periods and was most probably due to lack of space from the increasing cemetery population. In the 14th and 15th centuries simple rectangular headstones made of Cypriot schist marked the burials. In both churches, there was no clear pattern in grave location between male and female burials, however infant/child burials clustered in specific parts of the cemetery closer to the churches, especially near the apses.

Inhumation was the standard type of burial. Often the disturbed elements of earlier burials were carefully arranged

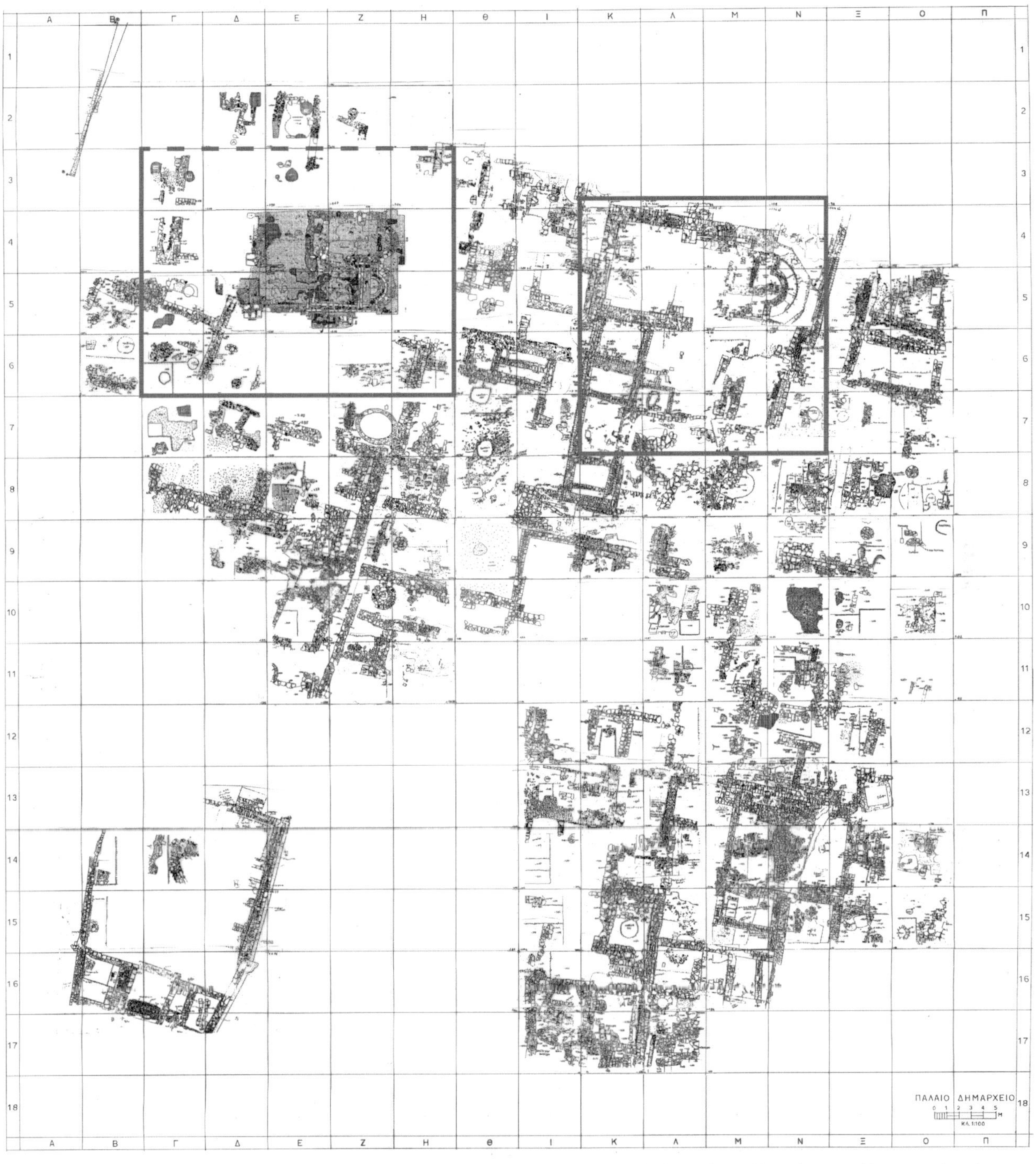

Fig. 28.2. Plan of the excavations at *Palaion Demarheion*. The rectangle on the left outlines Church A′ and its associated cemetery, whereas the rectangle on the right indicates the boundaries of the cemetery associated with Church B′ (Department of Antiquities)

around the newly inhumed body. In some cases, the disturbed bones were placed in separate small trenches. The remains that were found in anatomical position were oriented east–west and were placed in a supine position. There were variations in the position of the hands: on most occasions both hands were folded in the abdominal region, whereas the second most common position was one hand on the abdominal area and the other in the middle or on the proximal

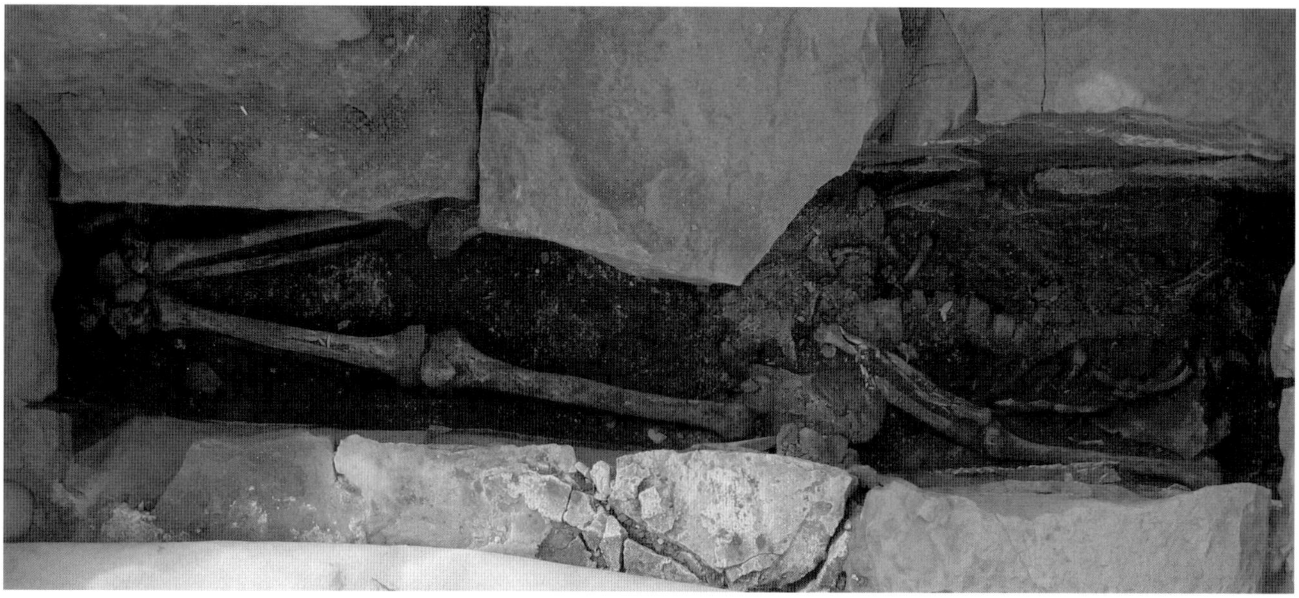

Fig. 28.3. Cist tomb associated with Church A′ (Department of Antiquities)

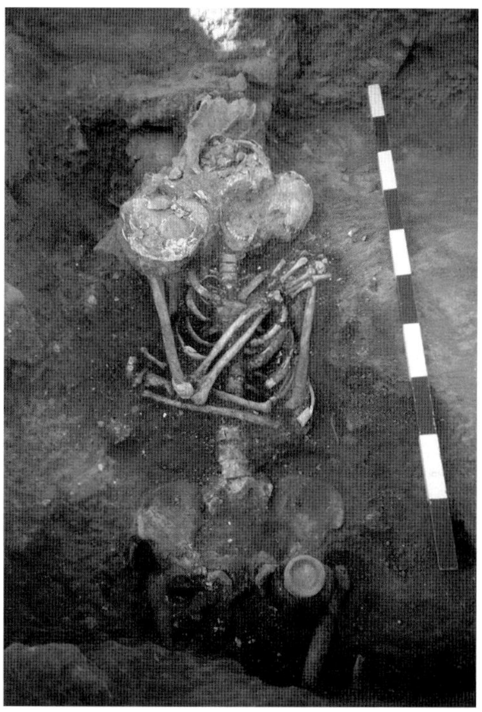

Fig. 28.4. Skeleton no. 29 recovered in situ with commingled elements around the skull. Two buckles and the base of a plate were situated in the region of the pelvis (Department of Antiquities)

end of the opposite humerus. Other variations included both hands crossed over the chest area or aligned to the sides of the skeleton. There was no pattern between hand position and gender, age or type of burial. The burials dated to the 14th and 15th century exhibited a greater diversity in hand positioning.

Headrests, simply made of earth or using one or more flat stones were often encountered under the skulls, with smaller stones situated around the calvaria. The surrounding stones were possibly used to fill the space between the coffin and the pit. The feet of the skeletons were positioned tightly side by side, due to the fact that the coffins were narrower towards the distal part of the skeleton. In many burials, iron nails defined the shape of the wooden coffins.

The skeletons were sometimes associated with rare personal belongings such as jewellery (rings, earrings, crosses) and clothing residues (buckles, buttons). In two cases coins were found within the burial fill. Eggshells, broken glass vessels and pottery sherds were frequently found in the burial fills, whereas the available evidence suggests that most of the skeletons were wrapped in shroud bands. On two occasions glazed plates were located on top of the skeletons.

Anthropological findings

The project resulted in the creation of a Byzantine/medieval human collection database. It incorporates an inventory for a minimum number of 209 individuals and records data on sex determination, age-at-death and stature estimations, congenital and acquired pathologies, dental diseases, ante-mortem and peri-mortem trauma, other metric and non-metric observations, as well as information on the archaeological context and associated findings of each skeleton. Other relevant material includes in situ drawings, excavation diaries and photographs (both during excavation and during laboratory analysis).

The anthropological study was conducted on 113 skeletons recovered in anatomical position (Figs 28.3 and 28.4) and 57 commingled cases (collective burials representing a minimum number of 96 individuals) that were excavated at the *Palaion Demarheion* during the 2002–2004 excavation seasons. Out of the skeletons recovered in situ, 55% involved 'complete' skeletons (only a few small elements missing), 6% 'almost complete' skeletons (over 70% of the elements present), 10% 'incomplete' skeletons (over 50% of the elements present) and 29% 'highly incomplete' skeletons (less than 50% of the elements present). Two thirds of the 'highly incomplete' skeletons were cases that were pending excavation at the end of the 2004 season, i.e. partly exposed but not completely excavated.

The analysis for sex determination in the adult population revealed that 10.6% did not present any conclusive data for sex assignment. Of the remaining skeletons 41.9% had female characteristics and 58.1% had male characteristics. The age-at-death distribution is described in the palaeodemography section below. The average height of females was estimated to be 160±2 cm, while for males the average height was 173±2 cm.

Besides the lesions that are described below in the "Thalassaemia" section, the most frequent pathological lesions recorded in adults, especially in females, were abnormalities associated with osteoporosis. Osteosclerotic lesions were frequently recorded in the knee and ankle regions, and periostitis was often recorded on the lower long bones. Dental disease was rare with the existence of only 5.2% incidence of caries and 8.1% of abscesses. A small number of healed fractures was also recorded.

Evaluation of stature estimations

The anthropological analyses of Cypriot collections are currently conducted based on methodologies that were developed on foreign, and oftentimes modern, populations. It is well documented that there are differences between populations (Meadows and Jantz 1995; Sarajlić and Cihlar 2007), hence the need to evaluate current practices and even create Cypriot specific sex and stature estimation equations.

Stature (height) measurements of the skeletons were taken in situ during the excavation following Kurth (1950), that is, the length from the top of the skull to the bottom of the feet (calcaneus). The maximum length of the femur was recorded both in situ in the field and under laboratory settings. Due to taphonomic constraints (fragmented skulls, disturbed elements) only a small number of skeletons was analysed during the project. A larger number of skeletal measurements were processed at a subsequent stage to include skeletons recovered in the 2005–2006 excavation seasons.

Based on the analysis, there is no significant difference between in situ femoral measurements and measurements taken in the laboratory (r=0.970, n=25). This is an important observation, since in archaeological settings where elements are extremely fragile, in situ measurements may be the only measurements available.

The in situ recorded stature of the complete skeletons was compared with the estimated stature derived by regression equations (Trotter and Gleser 1952; 1958). The latter method is based on the notion that the stature of an individual correlates with individual bone length, therefore, by using regression formulae it is possible to estimate an individual's height using the length of a skeletal element. A comparison of the two methodologies (in situ stature vs stature using regression formulae) shows that the mean values of stature derived from regression formulae overestimate female stature and underestimate male stature. In 88% of the cases the stature recorded in situ fell within the 90% prediction intervals of stature based on regression formulae.

New population-specific criteria adjusted to the Byzantine/medieval population are currently being developed.

Palaeodemographic and genetic studies

During the first systematic census of the Cypriot population in 1881, the Omeric neighbourhood, where the excavation site is located, had 335 male and 378 female inhabitants (Colonial Government 1884). No similar historic data exist for the medieval population of Nicosia, thus palaeodemographic profiles were produced during this study through life tables. Life tables present the mortality history of a hypothetical group or cohort, where through time-successive intervals the cohort loses a certain proportion of its members.

The life tables related to Church A′ and Church B′ were compared to two other European populations: a 7th century AD Italian population (Salvadei et al. 2001) and a Croatian 14th–16th century AD population (Šlaus 2000). The probability of death between the Italian and Croatian populations did not differ significantly in any age category. The same patterns were observed for the older age intervals (subadults and adults) recorded in the cemeteries of Churches A′ and B′, however the mortality rate for the infant and child cohorts were much greater in the Cypriot cemeteries. Church A′ had associated 53% infant/child mortality rate, Church B′ 33.3%, the Italian population 21.7% and the Croatian population 21.3%.

It is acknowledged that the upper layers around Church A′ were destroyed during construction works and due to the rescue nature of the excavation and the physical limitations of the site, not all areas of the plot were excavated. In particular, the northern part of the cemeteries was not excavated as it extended under a modern road. The east, west and south limits of the cemeteries were explored. It is unlikely that the high infant/child mortality can be attributed to a selective excavation methodology or to a biased anthropological sampling analysis, since it was established that there are infant burials in the unexcavated northern area, and during the 2005–2006 excavation seasons more infant than adult skeletons were excavated. Both these factors would increase further the mortality of the infant/child population.

Although selective death affecting only younger individuals could not be excluded, another hypothesis for an increased infant mortality rate, more rarely documented in the archaeological record, is the incorporation of an incoming population. This hypothesis is not only supported by the historical record, but it could also justify the high infant mortality rates of the cemeteries which are associated with the Frankish period of Cyprus. More detailed historical accounts are outlined in the Appendix of this paper.

In order to investigate the presence of a genetically diverse incoming population, forty-seven samples were analysed on a mitochondrial and Y-chromosome level. DNA was successfully extracted from thirty-two samples, fourteen of which yielded positive results in the Y-chromosome typing. Eight of the fourteen samples had good quality data and were assigned to eight different Y-haplotypes indicating heterogeneity in the male population. Sixteen samples yielded enough data to be assigned in a mitochondrial haplotype, and support the hypothesis of an incoming European population: haplotypes documented in the late 12th–early 13th century layers continue to be encountered in the 14th–15th century skeletons. The latter group, however, exhibits more diverse haplotypes which include H1, H2 and H6 that are predominantly considered as European (Stefansson *et al.* 2005)

Thalassaemia

Thalassaemia is a hereditary disease that is characterised by more than 200 mutations, the most well-known being that of beta- and alpha-thalassaemia. The frequency of this disease in the Cypriot population was extremely high until the mid-20th century (Fawdry 1946; Banton 1951) and has been documented on several archaeological collections dating as far back as the Neolithic period (Hershkovitz *et al.* 1991; Angel 1953; 1966). In the modern Cypriot population one in seven individuals is a carrier of beta-thalasseamia.

Skeletal anomalies present on a number of skeletons excavated in *Palaion Demarcheion* indicated consistency with anaemic lesions. In particular, the cranial and postcranial elements exhibited lesions that were typically reported on thalassaemic cases (cf. Lagia *et al.* 2007). A smaller number of the skeletons that presented such lesions were radiologically and molecularly studied in order to confirm or refute the hypothesis that these were associated with thalassaemia.

Twelve samples were analysed for this purpose. The polymerase chain reaction set-up was performed using primers ranging between 60–200bp, specifically designed to take into account the most common thalassaemic mutation in Cyprus (IVS 1-110 G/A). No amplifiable DNA was obtained from seven samples, and the sequence analysis performed on the five samples did not produce informative data. LightCycler Melting Curve Analysis was subsequently performed which indicated the presence of a sample with heterozygous thalassaemia. To confirm the results, ThalassoChip, a beta-thalassaemia genetic diagnostic tool which is based on arrayed primer extension (APEX) technology, was performed. The results indicated that none of the analysed samples had a G/A transition at IVSI-110.

Conclusions

The project presents an innovative interdisciplinary approach to anthropology, archaeology, history, genetics and medicine. The research conducted indicates that each discipline involved in the study of ancient human populations can contribute a wealth of information to the academic world, and an interdisciplinary study can provide a more holistic insight on past societies.

This is the first time that such a large-scale project was conducted on skeletal remains recovered on the island of Cyprus. The need of systematic studies of large skeletal collections cannot be emphasised enough. The development, via this project, of a population specific methodology for stature estimation is of immense importance and similar projects are strongly encouraged, especially for age and sex population specific methods.

One of the major outcomes of the project was the development of a Byzantine/medieval anthropological database with records of more than two hundred skeletons excavated between 2002 and 2004 at the site of *Palaion Demarheion* and the establishment of a human skeletal collection for university teaching purposes.

Another important aim of the study was to investigate the burial customs of the 11th–15th century AD population of Nicosia and compare them not only to other European populations, but also to regional historical and ethnographic records. Although the final conclusions will be drawn after the study of the excavated material in its entirety, it appears that burial customs are not so much influenced by biological factors (e.g. female vs male) or societal statuses (e.g. elite or middle class), but rather demonstrate chronological variations and differences in religious beliefs.

The preliminary results of the genetic and palaeodemographic studies indicate the presence of an incoming population, which is also supported by the historic accounts. The on-going study of the skeletal remains excavated during the 2005–2006 excavation seasons will most probably strengthen this hypothesis. Molecular studies have also indicated that skeletal elements, which exhibit lesions consistent with the disease of thalassaemia, do not have the IVSI-110 G/A transition, which is the most common thalassaemic mutation in the modern Cypriot population. Further studies are currently being conducted to identify the cause of these lesions.

The human remains recovered at *Palaion Demarheion* provide a unique source of information on the Byzantine and medieval societies of Cyprus. Future plans include the completion of the anthropological and archaeological studies of all excavated material and the thorough publication of all the data.

Acknowledgements

The project was supported by the Cyprus Research Promotion Foundation, under the National Framework Programme for Research, Technological Development and Innovation (*KOINΩ/1104/03*, 2005–2009). The participants in the project were: *Project Coordinator*: Yiannis Violaris, Department of Antiquities; *Scientific Coordinator*: Popi Chrysostomou, Department of Antiquities; *Partners*: Dr Marios Cariolou and Panagiotis Manoli, Laboratory of Forensic Sciences, Cyprus Institute of Neurology and Genetics; Dr Marina Kleanthous and George Christopoulos, Molecular Genetics Thalassaemia Department, Cyprus Institute of Neurology and Genetics; *Private Researcher*: Dr Michalis Angastiniotis; *End Users*: Dr Vassos Karageorghis, A. G. Leventis Foundation; Dr Demetrios Michaelides, Archaeological Research Unit, University of Cyprus.

Appendix
Population trends and consequences in Byzantine-medieval Cyprus

Yiannis Violaris

The following text aims to describe the population composition of Cyprus mainly during the Frankish period (1191–1489 AD). A brief introduction is given concerning the preceding Byzantine period, during which the population composition of medieval Cyprus was actually developed. Information is also given about the Venetian period which followed (1489–1570 AD). It must be noted that the burials excavated at the site of *Palaion Demarcheion* in Nicosia date from the end of the 11th or the beginning of the 12th to the 15th century, i.e. they are included in the Middle Byzantine and the Frankish periods.

When Cyprus was conquered by Richard the Lionheart during the Third Crusade (1189–1192), its ethnic composition was no different from other Byzantine territories, Asia Minor for example. The phenomenon of island insularity allowed for the persistence of a homogeneous Greek population. The ethnic composition of the Hellenistic and Roman periods was not affected to a great extent, apart from the period of the Arab raids (649–965): the main episode during this period is recorded in 688, when a large part of the local population, along with its archbishop, was relocated to the newly founded Nea Ioustinianoupolis, near Cyzicus in Asia Minor. They were sent back a few years later (Englezakis 1990; Papadopoulos 1995, 760).

During the period of Arab raids, Cyprus was culturally part of the Byzantine world and the Byzantine administration did not cease during most of the period. Despite its commercial and other contacts with neighbouring territories, as well as the movement of populations (either Christians or Arabs), the vast majority of its population consisted of Greek Christians. During these three centuries (7th–10th) its coastal areas were struck many times by raids which resulted in death, captivity and relocation of a certain percentage of the population. Cyprus finally became part of the Byzantine State again around 965. Shortly after this episode it seems that a significant change took place in the island, namely the transfer of its capital from Constantia to Nicosia (Aristeidou 2007, 299; Gounaridis 2001, 3; Nicolaou-Konnari and Schabel 2005, 14, 58, 61; Metcalf 2004, 116–20, 124).

During the Third Crusade the second most important group of the population was the Armenian which, as in other parts of the Byzantine Empire, was largely integrated in the local population. Armenian populations settled on the island in many instances, already from the early Christian period and continued to do so during the Byzantine and Frankish period. During the Frankish period the local Greek Christians still formed the majority of the population on the island: in the rural areas the Greeks were the overriding majority and the same applied in the cities, where most of the Latins lived. This applied even in Nicosia, which was the centre of the rulers of the island and of the Latin Church, as well as the place of residence of most of the Frankish nobility. In Limassol and Paphos only a handful of Frankish nobles resided and it is indicative that the Latin bishops of these cities, if they did not live abroad, they used to live in Nicosia (Coureas 2000, 33–4; Imhaus 2004, 191; Moschona 2001, 6; Nicolaou-Konnari 2006, 87–8; Papadopoulos 1995, 760–1).

The attempt to establish a crusader state by the barely 300 Knights Templar, who bought the island from Richard of England in 1191, failed after the bloody revolt of the people of Nicosia. The Templars, during their inglorious escape on the Easter Sunday of the 5th of April of 1192, slaughtered a large number of the civilians of Nicosia. The next ruler of Cyprus, Guy de Lusignan who bought the island from the Templars, did not establish a modern western state. The Frankish feudal class of the crusader states of the Middle East was transplanted into Cyprus and these nobles brought with them a middle class, which took over the state and other functions: these people were Latins but also other Christians, mainly from Syria. It should be noted, however, that despite the fact that there is information about the Latin nobility of Cyprus, there is no information at all on the rest of the Latins who arrived on the island, and this might be indicative of their very small number. Guy de Lusignan also invited nobles and knights from Western Europe as well as from the East and gave them fiefs and other incomes.

The migration trend became more intense with the gradual abolition of the crusader states of Syria and Palestine, and especially after the fall of Acre in 1291: knights, members of religious orders and monastic communities, clergy and laymen of various nationalities sought refuge in Cyprus. The island actually became the place of refuge of the Latins of the East and especially of innumerable Syrian refugees and other Christians who belonged to the eastern Christian doctrines (Nestorians, Jacobites, Copts, etc.). The latter were easily integrated into the local Greek Christian population. Syrians were encountered both in rural and urban populations in medieval Cyprus and were referred to as artisans and farmers or as small shop owners and merchants. For the first time the demographic status of the island began to change in some respects. The previous Byzantine elite, at least those who did not leave the island, changed status and dropped to the middle class, while the urban population of the Byzantine period lost its political rights. The Greek subjects were now divided into three classes: the lowest and the most numerous were the *paroikoi* or serfs, who were bound to the land, the second class were the *perperiarii* and the third one, the free men. It seems to be true that the change in the administration of the island did not affect the everyday life of the lower social classes very much, because the economic structure of the late Byzantine period remained more or less the same. Moreover, the contact of the local rural population with the new rulers was minimal, since these governed their fiefs through third parties, who were usually Greeks or Syrians. In 1237 it is mentioned that the Latin feudal lords themselves dismissed the Latins and employed Greeks for the latter purpose. It is therefore obvious that the Latin influence, at least in rural areas, was almost non-existent, and indicative is the fact that there are almost no toponyms of Frankish or Latin origin in Cyprus, while for the whole of the Frankish period only 12 chapels are recorded in rural areas (Coureas 2000, 32–4; Edbury 2007, 288, 290; Grivaud 1998, 274; Moschona 2001, 6–7; Nicolaou-Konnari 2006, 84; Nicolaou-Konnari and Schabel 2005, 3, 8–9, 39–43, 98, 103; Pardou 2001, 12–3; Richard 1995, 3, 360).

Due to the Muslim expansion and the subsequent abolition of the Crusader states, Cyprus became the centre of trade for the eastern Mediterranean: its ports were mercantile stops and places of residence and operation for many Frankish merchants and other westerners. Historical sources also mention Greek, Lombard, Bulgarian and other mercenaries, as well as numerous clerics of various rites, who ran the Latin monasteries and the churches or were engaged in all sorts of operations of occupational character. Jews were also active on the island and there were a certain number of slaves, who were mainly Muslim captives. The latter were gradually integrated with the rest of the population (Aristeidou 2007, 301; Nicolaou-Konnari and Schabel 2005, 37–8; Richard 1995, 363, 368–9).

As far as the spoken languages are concerned, apart from Greek, Syrian was widely spoken already from the Byzantine period. During the Frankish period the two languages were systematically taught and used on the island, while the Lusignans used French as the official language of the kingdom and Latin was anyway the language of European diplomacy. The French language was spread among the rest of the population, but most of them, who were peasants, used exclusively the Greek Cypriot dialect. For this reason the *Assizes*, a form of codified customary law, as well as various public documents which were addressed to the local people, were translated into the Greek Cypriot dialect. Italian was also quite widespread due to the numerous Italian merchants who settled on the island and also because many Cypriots used to study in Italy. As a result, many words and phrases of the above-mentioned languages penetrated into the local Greek dialect.

As time went by many locals entered the upper classes and some of them were also latinised. The cultural influences and intermarriages, which appear from the beginning of the Frankish period, reached a climax in the 15th century due to the Orthodox-friendly policy of the Greek queen of Cyprus, Eleni Palaiologina, wife of John II Lusignan (1460–1472). Gradually the Frankish community of the island was absorbed by the Greek way of life. The Frankish ruling class spoke in Greek and participated in the rituals of the Greek Orthodox Church. The Franks were cut off from the western world and adapted to the local historical Byzantine and Orthodox environment. This phenomenon is observed even in the royal court and among the higher social classes. Already from the middle of the 14th century the Pope complained about the large number of Latin noble and other women who attended the rituals of the Greek Orthodox churches. Even the kings attended both Latin and Orthodox churches. By the 15th century the Pope was obliged to approve intermarriages between Greeks and Latins, as well as the ritual of marriages and funerals of the Latin inhabitants of Cyprus, according to the Greek Orthodox rite. In the West it was considered that even the high ranking Latin clergy, such as Hugh the Archbishop of Nicosia, were more Orthodox Greeks rather than Latins. It is worth mentioning here that the last representatives of the Frankish dynasty of Cyprus, Jacob and Charlotte, were children of Greeks, raised according to the Greek way and Greek was indeed their native tongue. Charlotte, who was the daughter of John II and Eleni Palaiologina, was referred to as Greek and did not speak any French. She was the last legitimate heiress of the Lusignan throne but she was ousted by her stepbrother James the Bastard, son of John II and the Greek Marietta of Patras. Had James got married, as he planned, to Princess Zoe Palaiologina, daughter of the despot of the Peloponnese, and not to the Venetian Catherina Cornaro, the history of medieval Cyprus would have been vastly different. James set himself apart and despised the Francs. His death, however, as well as that of his small son shortly after, gave absolute power to the Venetian presence on the island and disrupted the progressive predominance of the Greek element (Balletto 1995, 41; Moschona 2001, 7–8; Nicolaou-Konnari 2006, 93, 97, 99; Nicolaou-Konnari and Schabel 2005, 25–6, 53–4, 64; Pardou 2001, 13).

As far as the church is concerned, it is known that the Francs imposed heavy institutional constraints on the Greek Orthodox Church. The dioceses were reduced from fourteen to four and were under the respective dioceses of the Latin Church. The Greek Orthodox Archdiocese was abolished and the property of the church was confiscated. The Greek Orthodox bishops were transferred to isolated villages and were subject to the respective Latin bishops. They acted as intermediaries between the Greek clergy and the Greek monks on one hand, and the Latin bishops on the other. In 1260 the Latin Church issued the *Bulla Cypria*, which subjected the Greek bishops to the Latins, but it recognised their broad jurisdiction on matters of family, hereditary and civic law. This was actually the epilogue of the persecution of the Orthodox by the Latin Church. In 1237 the Latin king himself was permitted by the Pope to worship at the palace's chapel and not in the Latin cathedral of Ayia Sophia. Moreover, the barons did not pay any taxes to the Latin Church, ignoring the aphorisms which were drawn against them. From the 14th century the Latin churches were empty and many Latin bishops and archbishops resided in Italy and appointed an official to deal with their economic matters and dispatch the incomes to them. In 1368 even the Latin cathedral was empty of worshippers, both on Sundays and other holidays, and Latin women of all classes attended exclusively the Orthodox churches. The nominal unification of the Churches, declared at the Ferrara-Florence Council (1439), relieved the Latins of Cyprus from any hesitation, since the two doctrines were equated and the believers could follow one or the other indiscriminately (Coureas 2000, 34–5; Edbury 2007, 293–5; Nicolaou-Konnari and Schabel 2005, 9–10, 86; Pardou 2001, 12–3).

Bearing in mind the available evidence, it would be rational to assume that the population of Cyprus during the Frankish period started to increase from the beginning of the 13th century until the big plague epidemic of 1347. At this point it reached its maximum which was not reached again until the 16th century. During the second half of the 14th century the population was reduced to a great extent due to epidemics and then it started to increase again during the first half of the 15th century. In the course of the Venetian period the population experienced a steady rise. The demographic evolution of Cyprus during the Frankish period coincides in general with the demographic trends which have been proposed for other European countries of the Mediterranean basin. One of the reasons for the increase in population during the Venetian period is the reduction of the plague epidemics and the absence of armed conflicts on the island. During the same period an influx from the rural areas to the cities can be observed. The demographic composition of the population of the island is not, however, different from the previous period. Especially the rural areas continued to be inhabited almost exclusively by the Greeks (Grivaud 1998, 277; Grivaud 2003, 49, 52; Imhaus 2004, 191–3).

Bibliography

Angel, J. L. 1953: 'Appendix II. The human remains from Khirokitia', 416–30 in P. Dikaios, *Khirokitia*, London.

Angel, J. L. 1966: 'Porotic hyperostosis, anaemias, malarias and marshes in the prehistoric eastern Mediterranean', *Science* 153, 760–3.

Aristeidou: Αριστείδου, Αικ. Χ. 2007: 'Σημαντικές πτυχές της Φραγκοκρατίας', 296–331 in A. Marangou *et al.* (eds), *Κύπρος. Από την αρχαιότητα έως σήμερα*, Athens.

Balletto, L. 1995: 'Ethnic groups, cross-social and cross-cultural contacts on fifteenth-century Cyprus', *Mediterranean Historical Review* 10 (1–2), 35–48.

Banton, A. 1951: 'A genetic study of Mediterranean anaemia in Cyprus', *Annual Journal of Human Genetics* 3, 47–64.

Colonial Government 1884: *Report on the Census of Cyprus, 1881 with Appendix* (by F. W. Barry), London.

Coureas, N. 2000: 'The Latin Elite on Cyprus: trying to keep apart', *Journal of Mediterranean Studies* 10 (1–2), 31–45.

Englezakis: Εγγλεζάκης, Π. Β. 1990: Κύπρος, Νέα Ιουστινιανούπολις, Nicosia.

Edbury, P. 2007: '1191 μ.Χ.: Κατάκτηση, συνέχεια και αλλαγή', 282–95 in A. Marangou *et al.* (eds), *Κύπρος. Από την αρχαιότητα έως σήμερα*, Athens.

Fawdry, A. L. 1946: 'Erythroblastic anaemia in childhood (Cooley's anaemia) in Cyprus', *Lancet* I, 171–7.

Gounaridis: Γουναρίδης, Π. 2001: 'Από τους Βυζαντινούς στους Σταυροφόρους', 2–4 in *Επτά Ημέρες 16.9.2001, Κύπρος Μεσαιωνική, Καθημερινή*, Athens.

Grivaud, G. 1998: 'Villages désertés à Chypre (fin XIIe–fin XIXe siécle)', *Μελέται και Υπομνήματα III*, 67–101, Nicosia.

Grivaud, G. 2003: 'Κάτοικοι και πληθυσμός', 49–54 in V.

Karageorghis, Chr. Maltezou and L. Loizou-Hadjigavriel (eds), *Κύπρος: Πετράδι στο Στέμμα της Βενετίας*, Nicosia.

Hershkovitz, I., Ring, B., Speirs, M., Galili, E., Kisley, M., Edelson, G. and Hershkovitz, A. 1991: 'Possible congenital haemolytic anemia in pre-historic coastal inhabitants of Israel', *American Journal of Physical Anthropology* 85, 7–13.

Imhaus, B. 2004: 'Quelques remarques sur la démographie Chypriote', 191–8 in B. Imhaus (ed.), *Lacrimae Cypriae. Les larmes de Chypre*, vol. 2, Nicosia.

Kurth, G. 1950: 'Über die Verwendbarkeit der Grablange vor- und fruhgeschichtlicher Reihengraberserien zur Bestimmung einer genauen Korperhohe', *Zeitschrift fur Morphologie und Anthropologie* 42, 293–306.

Lagia, A., Eliopoulos, C. and Manolis, S. 2007: 'Thalassemia: macroscopic and radiological study of a case', *International Journal of Osteoarchaeology* 17, 269–85.

Meadows, I. and Jantz, R. L. 1995: 'Allometric secular change in the long bones from the 1800's to the present', *Journal of Forensic Sciences* 40, 762–7.

Metcalf, D. M. 2004: *Byzantine Lead Seals from Cyprus*, Nicosia.

Moschona: Μοσχονά, Ν. Γ. 2001: 'Η φυσιογνωμία της Κύπρου στην περίοδο των Φράγκων', in 5–8, *Επτά Ημέρες 16.9.2001, Κύπρος Μεσαιωνική, Καθημερινή*, Athens.

Nicolaou-Konnari, A. and Schabel, C. (eds) 2005: *Cyprus: Society and Culture 1191–1374*, Boston.

Nikolaou-Konnari: Νικολάου-Κονναρή, Α. 2006: 'Η Κύπρος των Λουζινιανών και η Ευρώπη, 1192–1489', 77–111 in E. Hadjipaschali, P. Lisioti and A. Liritsas (eds), *Η Κύπρος ήταν πάντα Ευρώπη*, Nicosia.

Papadopoulos: Παπαδόπουλος, Θ. 1995: 'Δομή και λειτουργία του φεουδαρχικού πολιτεύματος', 759–84 in Θ. Παπαδόπουλος (επιμ.), *Ιστορία της Κύπρου*, τόμ. Δ', *Μεσαιωνικόν Βασίλειον, Ενετοκρατία*, Nicosia.

Pardou: Πάρδου, Α. 2001: 'Η αντίσταση της κυπριακής κοινωνίας και η αφομοίωση των κυριάρχων', in 12–3, *Επτά Ημέρες 16.9.2001, Κύπρος Μεσαιωνική, Καθημερινή*, Athens.

Richard, J. 1995: 'Η σύσταση και οι βάσεις του μεσαιωνικού βασιλείου (1192–1205)', 1–19 in Θ. Παπαδόπουλος (επιμ.), *Ιστορία της Κύπρου*, τόμ. Δ', *Μεσαιωνικόν Βασίλειον, Ενετοκρατία*, Nicosia.

Salvadei, L., Ricci, F. and Manzi, G. 2001: 'Porotic hyperostosis as a marker of health and nutritional conditions during childhood: studies at the transition between Imperial Rome and the early Middle Ages', *American Journal of Human Biology* 13, 709–17.

Sarajlić, N. and Cihlar, Z. 2007: 'Diverse stature estimation formulae applied to a Bosnian population', *Bosnian Journal of Basic Medical Sciences* 7(2), 136–9.

Šlaus, M. 2000: 'Biocultural analysis of sex differences in mortality profiles and stress levels in the late medieval population from Nova Rača, Croatia', *American Journal of Physical Anthropology* 111, 193–209.

Stefansson, H., Helgason, A., Thorleifsson, G. *et al.* 2005: 'A common inversion under selection in Europeans', *Nature Genetics* 37, 129–37.

Trotter, M. and Gleser, G. 1952: 'Estimation of stature from long bones of American Whites and Negroes', *American Journal of Physical Anthropology* 10, 463–514.

Trotter, M. and Gleser, G 1958: 'A re-evaluation of estimation of stature based on measurements of stature taken during life and of long bones after death', *American Journal of Physical Anthropology* 16, 79–123.

1st International CAPP Symposium 'New Approaches to Archaeological Human Remains in Cyprus'

29. Introduction to the Cyprus Ancient Population Project (CAPP) and the First CAPP Symposium

Kirsi O. Lorentz

The Cyprus Ancient Population Project (CAPP) was set up to promote the development of human bioarchaeological research and education in Cyprus. This paper provides a brief introduction to CAPP, as well as a brief outline of the history of the study of archaeological human remains in Cyprus, in order to provide a view of the contextual setting within which the CAPP network and CAPP symposia have been established.

While the foundations for research on archaeological human remains were laid relatively early in Cyprus (see e.g. Virchow 1884), the development of systematic, problem-oriented research on the remains of the archaeological Cypriot populations, as well as educational provisions and institutional infrastructures for physical anthropology and human bioarchaeology are still in their infancy in Cyprus (Lorentz 2011b). Basic research on archaeological human remains has a relatively long history in Cyprus: Cypriot human skeletal remains appear as part of scientific treatises as early as the 19'th century (e.g. Virchow 1884), and the early part of the 20th century sees the publication of several treatises and reports focusing exclusively on Cypriot human remains as well as some further comparative work (e.g. Buxton 1920a; 1920b; 1931; Fürst 1933; Guest 1936; Schaeffer 1935; Rix 1938; Rix and Buxton 1938). The majority of this early work has a tendency to focus exclusively on the human skull, in keeping with the research history of the discipline in general. After the Second World War physical anthropological research activity on the island resumed, and Angel, Charles, and other scholars analysed and published several Cypriot human skeletal series during the mid-20th century (Angel 1953; 1955; 1961; 1964; 1966; 1967; 1969a; 1969b; Axmacher and Hjortsjö 1959; Charles 1960; 1962; 1963; 1964; 1966; 1967; Hjortsjö 1947; Kurth 1958; Rix 1950). During the 1970s some of these already established physical anthropologists continued their research activity on Cypriot skeletal series (see e.g. Angel 1972a; 1972b; 1978; Charles 1970), and were joined by a few new researchers (Longmore 1975; Schulte-Campbell 1979; Schwartz 1974; Walker 1975). During the 1980s the number of researchers analysing Cypriot skeletal series increased further (Domurad 1985; 1986a; 1986b; 1987a; 1987b; 1988; Cadogan and Domurad 1985; Downs 1982; Fischer 1986; Fischer and Norén 1988; Galloway 1985; Moyer 1984; 1985; 1989; Musgrave and Evans 1980; Schulte-Campbell 1983; 1986; 1989; Solivères 1981), and a few of these researchers focused specifically on the human dentition (Fischer and Norén 1988; Lunt 1980; 1985; Nyqvist 1980; Taramides 1983). While palaeopathological analyses of Cypriot skeletal series can be said to have begun with Angel's focus on porotic hyperostosis (Angel 1966; 1967; 1978), and continued with notes on dental palaeopathologies in the 1980s (see e.g. Lunt 1980; 1985), it was not until the 1990s that systematic problem-oriented studies of postcranial palaeopathologies in Cyprus began to appear (Agelarakis 1997; Fox-Leonard 1997), together with reports on specific skeletal series (Agelarakis, Kanta and Stampolides 1998; Domurad 1992; Fessas 1990; Fox 1996; 1997; Herscher and Fox 1994; Le Mort 1994; 1995; Lunt 1994; 1995; Moyer 1997). While the necessary, detailed reporting on specific human skeletal series continued during the first decade of the 21st century (Crewe *et al.* 2005; Fox 2001; 2002; 2003, 2006; 2007; Harper 2002; Lorentz 2001; 2004a; 2006a; 2008e; 2009b; 2009c; Lorentz *et al.* 2011; Lunt 2006; Lunt and Watt 2003; Moyer 2004; 2005; 2006; 2007; Parks *et al.* 2000; 2001; Parras 2006a; Schulte-Campbell 2003; Tucker and Clegget 2007), the new millennium saw the publication of further problem-oriented and comparative studies on a variety of topics (Baker, Terhune and Papalexandrou 2007; Fox 2005; Harper 2010; Le Mort 2000; 2007; 2008; Lorentz 2002; 2003a; 2003b; 2006b; 2007; 2008d; 2009a; 2010a; Parras 2004; 2006b), theoretically informed human bioarchaeology (Lorentz 2004b, 2005; 2008a; 2008b; 2008c; 2010b) including *Anthropologie de Terrain* (Lorentz 2011a; forthcoming), syntheses (Harper 2008; Harper and Fox 2008), and studies employing state-of-the-art scientific methodologies and techniques such as palaeoparasitology (Harter-Lailheuge *et al.* 2005) and strontium isotope analyses for investigating residential mobility (Lorentz *et al.* in prep.).

Research activity focusing on archaeological human remains in Cyprus thus stretches back over a century, but no formal education in relevant fields in Cyprus has been or is available, nor has there ever been a scientific meeting focusing on archaeological human remains in Cyprus in particular, making such a forum long overdue. Given the increasing frequency with which archaeological human remains are found in Cyprus, both as part of research excavations, and on rescue/salvage operations, it was felt that there was a need to promote the establishment of human bioarchaeology as an academic endeavour in Cyprus, through a network of researchers engaging in human remains research on the island. Until now, unfortunately, most, if not all archaeological human remains research in Cyprus has been conducted within the framework of periodic expeditions, mostly by human bone specialists residing abroad, with no permanent positions for archaeological human remains specialists on the island of Cyprus itself.

It is in response to this situation that the Cyprus Ancient Populations Project (CAPP) was established. CAPP is a collaborative international research network for physical anthropologists, palaeopathologists and bioarchaeologists working on ancient Cypriot human remains. Its period coverage extends from the earliest prehistory to historical periods. CAPP aims to promote (1) the preparation of the *Cyprus Human Skeletal Data Base*; (2) international symposia on human skeletal remains research in Cyprus, leading to the preparation of an up-to-date synthesis on ancient Cypriot populations; (3) comparative, problem-oriented, collaborative analyses of ancient Cypriot skeletal populations based on network participants' work at various sites; and (4) training and placements for local/Cypriot students and researchers, with view to promoting excellence in physical anthropology, palaeopathology and bioarchaeology in Cyprus. Further aspects, responsive to the network participants' research vision, will be developed through network discussions. Researchers interested in participating in the CAPP research network are kindly requested to contact the network coordinator (author of this paper).

The following steps forward have already been taken in the framework of the CAPP network. The preparation of the *Cyprus Human Skeletal Data Base* (a research resource for physical anthropologists, palaeopathologists and bioarchaeologists) is under way in conjunction with the CAPP website preparation. This CAPP Symposium is the first in a series of planned *international symposia on human skeletal remains research* in Cyprus. Since the 1st CAPP symposium took place, and until the publication of this volume, research on Cypriot human remains has also been presented and discussed within several conferences and scientific meetings, including the 7ICAANE (12–16 April 2010, London) workshop on *Human Remains in the Ancient Near East: Advances, Problems and Potential*, and further, within the framework of the 1st ICASEMNE (1st International Congress on Archaeological Sciences in the Eastern Mediterranean and the Near East) congress held in Paphos, Cyprus 29 April–1 May 2010. Publications on these are in preparation. Comparative, problem oriented, collaborative analyses of ancient Cypriot skeletal populations are ongoing, and some results were already presented during the 1st CAPP symposium. Training and placements for local and Cypriot students and researchers has begun, including placements on a variety of projects, internships at the Cyprus Institute Human Bioarchaeology Laboratory, and focused training within e.g. the Souskiou-*Laona* Human Bioarchaeology Fieldschool in Cyprus.

We, as the CAPP network, feel strongly that the integration on 'ancient bones, books and biomedical sciences' – or the so-called AB3 approach as Prof. Dutour helpfully put it in the congress on Biomedical Sciences in Archaeology in Crete – is vital in furthering our understanding of the human past, and are therefore particularly pleased to present this first international CAPP Symposium as part of this Congress on the Medicine in the Ancient Mediterranean World. We thank you all in advance for your participation.

Acknowledgements

Professor Demetrios Michaelides has been vital in making it possible to realise this first international symposium on human remains from ancient Cyprus, and I would like to acknowledge here his vision and support. When I first discussed the possibility of organising a symposium on human remains in Cyprus Professor Michaelides immediately responded by inviting the CAPP network participants to organise this symposium in conjunction with this congress on the Medicine in the Ancient Mediterranean World. We are indebted to Prof. Michaelides' vision. We also hope to continue to discuss some of the issues that came up in the congress on Biomedical Sciences in Archaeology, held in Crete, especially with particular focus on Cyprus, and Cypriot human remains.

Bibliography

Agelarakis, A. 1997: 'Paleopathology and its contributions to the decipherment of the human condition in antiquity: the case of two populations from Malloura in Cyprus', *Report of the Department of Antiquities, Cyprus*, 239–50.

Agelarakis, A., Kanta, P. and Stampolides, N. 1998: 'The osseous record in the Western Necropolis of Amathous: an archaeo-anthropological investigation', 217–32 in V. Karageorghis and N. C. Stampolides (eds), *Proceedings of the International Symposium: The Eastern Mediterranean, Cyprus-Dodecanese-Crete 16th–6th c. B.C., Rethymnon, Crete*, Athens.

Angel, J. L. 1953: 'The human remains from Khirokitia', 416–30 in P. Dikaios, *Khirokitia*, London.

Angel, J. L. 1955: 'The skulls', in J. Du Plat Taylor, 'Roman tombs at Kambi Vasa', *Report of the Department of Antiquities, Cyprus* 1940–1948, 68–76.

Angel, J. L. 1961: 'Neolithic crania from Sotira', 223–9 in P. Dikaios, *Sotira*, Philadelphia.

Angel, J. L. 1964: 'Osteoporosis: thalassemia?', *American Journal of Physical Anthropology* 22, 363–73.

Angel, J. L. 1966: 'Porotic hyperostosis, anemias, malarias, and marshes in the prehistoric Eastern Mediterranean', *Science* 153, 760–3.

Angel, J. L. 1967: 'Porotic hyperostosis or osteoporosis symmetrica', 378–89 in D. Brothwell and A. T. Sandison (eds), *Diseases in Antiquity*, Springfield, IL.

Angel J. L. 1969a: 'The bases of paleodemography', *American Journal of Physical Anthropology* 30, 427–37.

Angel, J. L. 1969b: 'Paleodemography and evolution', *American Journal of Physical Anthropology* 31, 343–53.

Angel, J. L. 1972a: 'Genetic and social factors in a Cypriote village', *Human Biology* 44, 53–80.

Angel, J. L. 1972b: 'Late Bronze Age Cypriotes from Bamboula', 148–65 in J. L. Benson (ed.), *Bamboula at Kourion*, Philadelphia.

Angel, J. L. 1978: 'Porotic hyperostosis in the Eastern Mediterranean', *Medical College of Virginia Quarterly* 14, 1–16.

Axmacher, B. and Hjortsjö, C.-H. 1959: *Examen anthropologique des crânes constituent la materiel préhistorique mis à jour à la suite des fouilles effectuées par les archéologues français à Iskender, Chypre* (Lunds Universitets årsskrift, N.f., avd. 2 bd 55, nr. 2), Lund.

Baker, B. J., Terhune, C. E. and Papalexandrou, A. 2007: *Sew Long: A Seamstress Buried at Medieval Polis* (American Journal of Physical Anthropology Supplement 132: 67).

Buxton L. H. D. 1920a: 'The inhabitants of the Eastern Mediterranean', *Biometrika* 13, 92–112.

Buxton L. H. D. 1920b: 'The Anthropology of Cyprus', *Journal of the Royal Anthropological Institute of Great Britain and Ireland* 50, 183–235.

Buxton L. H. D. 1931: 'Künstlich deformierte Schädel von Cypern', *Anthropologischer Anzeiger* 7, 236–40.

Cadogan, G. and Domurad, M. R. 1985: 'Maroni V', *Report of the Department of Antiquities, Cyprus*, 77–81.

Charles, R.-P. 1960: 'Observation sur les crânes de Chrysopolitissa', in V. Karageorghis, 'Fouilles de Kition 1959', *Bulletin de Correspondance hellénique* 84, 583–8.

Charles, R.-P. 1962: *Le peuplement de Chypre dans l'Antiquité*, Paris.

Charles, R.-P. 1963: 'Note sure les restes humains d'Iskender', 245–9 in J. Deshayes, *La Nécropole de Ktima*, Paris.

Charles, R.-P. 1964: 'Étude anthropologique de sujets d'Idalion', *Report of the Department of Antiquities, Cyprus*, 85.

Charles, R.-P. 1966: 'Étude des crânes de la tombe I de Karpasha', *Report of the Department of Antiquities, Cyprus*, 41–50.

Charles, R.-P. 1967: 'Étude des restes humains de tombe 31', 148–52 in V. Karageorghis (ed.), *Excavations in the Necropolis of Salamis* I, Nicosia.

Charles R.-P. 1970: 'Étude des restes humains des tombes de Cellarka nécropole de Salamine (Chypre)', 279–92 in V. Karageorghis (ed.), *Excavations in the Necropolis of Salamis* II, Nicosia.

Crewe, L., Lorentz, K. O., Peltenburg, E. and Spanou, S. 2005: 'Treatments of the dead: investigations at Souskiou-*Laona* Chalcolithic cemetery, 2001–2004', *Report of the Department of Antiquities, Cyprus*, 41–68.

Domurad, M. R. 1985: 'The human remains', in D. Michaelides and M. Snyczer, 'A Phoenician graffito from Tomb 103/84 at Nea Paphos', *Report of the Department of Antiquities, Cyprus*, 256.

Domurad, M. R. 1986a: *The Populations of Ancient Cyprus*, PhD Dissertation, University of Cincinnati.

Domurad M. R. 1986b: 'The human remains', in E. J. Peltenburg, 'Excavations at Kissonerga-*Mosphilia* 1985', *Report of the Department of Antiquities, Cyprus*, 36.

Domurad M. R. 1987a: 'The burials', in E. J. Peltenburg, 'Excavations at Kissonerga-*Mosphilia* 1986', *Report of the Department of Antiquities, Cyprus*, 5.

Domurad M. R. 1987b: 'The skeletal remains from Aghios Giorghios 1985', in M. Yon and O. Callot, 'Nouvelles découvertes dans la nécropole ouest de Kition (Aghios Giorghios, époque classique)', *Report of the Department of Antiquities, Cyprus*, 168–9.

Domurad M. R. 1988: 'The human remains', in D. Michaelides and J. Młynarczyk, 'Tombs P.M. 2520 and P.M. 2737 from the Eastern Necropolis of Nea Paphos', *Report of the Department of Antiquities, Cyprus*, Part 2, 169–70.

Domurad, M. R. 1992: 'The population of ancient Amathus', 145–74 in V. Karageorghis, O. Picard and C. Tytgat (eds), *Études Chypriotes XIV: La nécropole D'Amathonte, tombes 113–367*, Nicosia.

Downs, D. 1982: 'The human remains', in E. Peltenburg, 'Lemba Archaeological Project, Cyprus, 1979: Preliminary Report', *Levant* 14, 51–2.

Fessas, C. 1990: 'The Ayios Theodoros, Larnaca skulls', in P. Flourentzos, 'Excavations in an Archaic necropolis at Ayios Theodoros', *Report of the Department of Antiquities, Cyprus*, 117–20.

Fischer, P. M. 1986: *Prehistoric Cypriot Skulls*, Göteborg.

Fischer, P. M. and Norén, J. 1988: 'Enamel defects in teeth from a prehistoric Cypriot population', *Ossa* 13, 87–96.

Fox, S. C. 1996: 'The human skeletal remains from Alassa-*Ayia Mavri*, Cyprus', 39–64 in P. Flourentzos (ed.), *Excavations in the Kouris River Valley II*, Nicosia.

Fox, S. C. 1997: 'The human skeletal remains from Tomb 1, Mari village, Larnaka District, Cyprus', in M. Hadjicosti, 'The family tomb of a warrior of the Cypro-Archaic I period at Mari', *Report of the Department of Antiquities, Cyprus*, 264–5.

Fox, S. C. 2001: 'The human skeletal remains from Kouklia-*Eliomylia* (KM 393, T. 125), in S. Hadjisavvas, 'An enigmatic burial at Kouklia-*Eliomylia*', *Report of the Department of Antiquities, Cyprus*, 99–102.

Fox, S. C. 2002: 'Burials in the church at Maroni *Petrera*', 38–40 in S. Manning (ed.), *The Late Roman Church at Maroni* Petrera, Oxford.

Fox, S. C. 2003: 'The human skeletal remains: a preliminary report', 274–7 in M. Rautman, *A Cypriot village of Late Antiquity: Kalavasos-*Kopetra *in the Vasilikos Valley*, (Journal of Roman Archaeology, Supplementary Series 52), Portsmouth, RI.

Fox, S. C. 2005: 'Health in Hellenistic and Roman times: the case studies of Paphos, Cyprus and Corinth, Greece', 59–82 in H. King (ed.), *Health in Antiquity*, London.

Fox, S. C. 2006: 'Human skeletal remains from the 1991 to 1998 seasons', 290–2 in D. Frankel and J. M. Webb, *Marki* Alonia. *An Early and Middle Bronze Age Settlement in Cyprus. Excavations 1995–2000* (Studies in Mediterranean Archaeology 123:2), Sävedalen.

Fox, S. C. 2007: 'The human skeletal remains from Psematismenos-*Koliokremmos/Palia*', in J. M. Webb, D. Frankel, S. W. Manning and D. A. Sewell (eds), 'Psematismenos-*Koliokremmos/Palia* Tomb PKK/94', *Report of the Department of Antiquities, Cyprus*, 131–2.

Fox-Leonard, S. C. 1997: *Comparative Health from Paleopathological Analysis of the Human Skeletal Remains Dating to the Hellenistic and Roman Periods, from Paphos, Cyprus and Corinth, Greece*, unpublished PhD dissertation, Department of Anthropology, University of Arizona.

Fürst, C. M. 1933: *Zur Kenntnis der Anthropologie der prähistorischen Bevölkerung der Insel Cypern* (Lunds Universitets årsskrift N. f., avd. 2, bd. 29, nr. 6), Lund.

Galloway, A. 1985: 'Report on the skeletal remains from the 1984 excavations, Kourion City, Grid L 9', in D. Soren and T. Davis, 'Seismic archaeology at Kourion: The 1984 campaign', *Report of the Department of Antiquities, Cyprus*, 302–6.

Guest, E. M. 1936: 'The human remains', in P. Dikaios, 'The excavations at Erimi 1933–35. Final Report', *Report of the Department of Antiquities, Cyprus*, 58–62.

Harper, N. K. 2002: 'The human remains from Pegia-*Pappara*', in E. Raptou, E. Stylianou, and E. Vassiliou, 'The Hellenistic tomb of Pegeia-*Pappara*', *Report of the Department of Antiquities, Cyprus*, 201–34.

Harper, N. K. 2008: 'Short skulls, long skulls and thalassemia: J. Lawrence Angel and the development of anthropology in Cyprus', *Near Eastern Archaeology* 71(1/2), 111–9.

Harper, N. K. 2010: 'From typology to population genetics: biodistance in Cyprus', 1–37 in S. Christodoulou and A. Satraki, *Poca 2007: Postgraduate Cypriot Archaeology Conference*, Newcastle upon Tyne.

Harper, N. and Fox, S. 2008: 'Recent research in Cypriot bioarchaeology', in *Bioarchaeology in the Near East* (e-journal) 2008(2), 1–38. Available at http://www.anthropology.uw.edu.pl/02/bne-02-01.pdf

Harter-Lailheugue, S., Le Mort, F., Vigne, J.-D., Guilane, J., Le Brun, A. and Bouchet, F. 2005: 'Premières données parasitologiques sur les populations humaines précéramiques chypriotes (VIIIe et VIIe millénaires av. J. C.)', *Paléorient* 31, 43–54.

Herscher, E. and Fox S. C. 1994: 'A Middle Bronze tomb from Western Cyprus', *Report of the Department of Antiquities, Cyprus*, 69–80.

Hjortsjö, C.-H. 1947: *To the Knowledge of the Prehistoric Craniology of Cyprus*, Lund.

Kurth, G. 1958: 'Zur Stellung den neolitischen Menschenreste von Khirokitia auf Cypern', *Homo* 104, 213–26.

Le Mort, F. 1994: 'Les sepultures', 157–95 in A. Le Brun, *Fouilles récentes à Khirokitia (Chypre) 1988–1991*, Paris.

Le Mort, F. 1995: 'Le peuplement de Chypre: Rapport des données anthropologiques', *Paléorient* 212, 111–21.

Le Mort, F. 2000: 'The Neolithic subadult skeletons from Khirokitia (Cyprus): taphonomy and mortality', *Anthropologie* 38, 63–70.

Le Mort, F. 2007: 'Artificial cranial deformation in the Aceramic Neolithic Near East: evidence from Cyprus', 151–8 in M. Faerman, L. K. Horwitz, T. Kahana and U. Zilberman (eds), *Faces from the Past: Diachronic Patterns in the Biology of Human Populations from the Eastern Mediterranean. Papers in Honor of Patricia Smith*, Oxford.

Le Mort, F. 2008: 'Infant burials in Pre-Pottery Neolithic Cyprus: evidence from Khirokitia', 23–32 in K. Bacvarov (ed.), *Babies Reborn: Infant/Child Burials in Pre- and Protohistory*, Oxford.

Longmore, B. 1975: 'The dentition of the Philia-*Drakos* Site A skulls', in M. Walker, 'Early Neolithic skeletons from Philia *Drakos*, Site A (Cyprus)', *Australian Journal of Biblical Archaeology* 2, 77–89.

Lorentz, K. O. 2001: 'The human skeletal remains from Tremithousa Tomb PM 3397', *Report of the Department of Antiquities, Cyprus*, 206–12.

Lorentz, K. O. 2002: 'Cultures of physical modifications', 203–10 in G. Muskett, A. Koltsida and M. Georgiadis (eds) *Symposium on Mediterranean Archaeology (SOMA 2002, University of Liverpool)* (British Archaeological Report International Series 1040), Oxford.

Lorentz, K. O. 2003a: *Minding the Body: The Growing Body in Cyprus from the Aceramic Neolithic to the Late Bronze Age*, unpublished PhD thesis, Department of Archaeology, University of Cambridge.

Lorentz, K. O. 2003b: 'Cultures of physical modifications: child bodies in ancient Cyprus', *Stanford Journal of Archaeology*. Available at http://archaeology.stanford.edu/journal/newdraft/2003_Journal/lorentz/index.html

Lorentz, K. O. 2004a: 'Human skeletal remains from the tomb TSR', 233–7 in S. Bezzola (ed.), *Lucerne fittili dagli scavi di Palaepaphos (Cipro)*, Mainz am Rhein.

Lorentz, K. O. 2004b: 'Age and gender in Eastern Mediterranean prehistory: depictions, burials and skeletal evidence', *Ethnographisch-archäologische Zeitschrift* 45, 297–315.

Lorentz, K. O. 2005: 'Late Bronze Age burial practices: age as a form of social difference', 41–56 in V. Karageorghis, H. Matthäus and S. Rogge (eds), *Cyprus: Religion and Society from the Late Bronze Age to the End of the Archaic Period*, Mohnesee-Wamel.

Lorentz, K. O. 2006a: 'Human skeletal remains from the 1999 and 2000 seasons', 293–7 in D. Frankel and J. Webb (eds), *Marki* Alonia. *An Early and Middle Bronze Age Settlement in Cyprus. Excavations 1995–2000*, (Studies in Mediterranean Archaeology 123:2), Sävedalen.

Lorentz, K. O. 2006b: 'Headshaping at Marki and its socio-cultural significance', 297–303 in D. Frankel and J. Webb (eds), *Marki* Alonia. *An Early and Middle Bronze Age Settlement in Cyprus. Excavations 1995–2000* (Studies in Mediterranean Archaeology 123:2), Sävedalen.

Lorentz K. O. 2007: 'Teeth as tools: health and disease at Shahr-e Sokhte' [in Farsi], 321–2 in *Proceedings of the 9th International Symposium of Iranian Archaeology, Iranian Center for Archaeological Research (ICAR)*, Tehran.

Lorentz, K. O. 2008a: 'Crafting the head: the human body as Art?', 415–32 in J. M. Córdoba, M. Molist, M. Carmen Pérez, I. Rubio and S. Martínez (eds), *Proceedings of the Fifth International Congress on the Archaeology of the Ancient Near East*, Madrid.

Lorentz, K. O. 2008b: 'From bodies to bones and back: theory and human bioarchaeology', 273–303 in H. Schutkowski (ed.), *Between Biology and Culture,* Cambridge.

Lorentz, K. O. 2008c: 'From life course to longue durée: headshaping as gendered capital?', 281–311 in D. Bolger (ed.), *Gender through Time in the Ancient Near East*, Walnut Creek.

Lorentz, K. O. 2008d: 'Activity induced patterns of dental abrasion and ante-mortem tooth loss at 3rd millennium BC Shahr-e Sokhte (Iran)', *Iran* XLVI, 319–27.

Lorentz, K. O. 2008e: 'Human skeletal remains from KA Tomb I', 216–23 in F. G. Maier (ed.), *Nordost-Tor und persische Belagerungsrampe in Alt-Paphos* (Ausgrabungen in Alt-Paphos auf Cypern 6), Berlin.

Lorentz, K. O. 2009a: 'The malleable body: headshaping in Greece and the surrounding regions', 75–98 in L. Schepartz, S. C. Fox and C. Bourbou, *New Directions in the Skeletal Biology of Greece,* Princeton.

Lorentz, K. O. 2009b: 'Human remains from the Attic sarcophagus M.P. 3509 in Paphos', Appendix in E. Raptou, 'Sarcophage attique trouvé a Paphos', *Report of the Department of Antiquities, Cyprus,* 253–60.

Lorentz, K. O. 2009c: 'Human remains in the Cyprus Museum', 265–81 in J. Webb, D. Frankel, E. Eriksson and J. B. Hennessy, *The Bronze Age Cemeteries at Karmi Palealona and Lapatsa in Cyprus. Excavations by J.R.B. Stewart* (Studies in Mediterranean Archaeology 136), Sävedalen.

Lorentz K. O. 2010a: 'Ubaid headshaping: negotiations of identity through physical appearance?', 125–48 in R. A. Carter and G. Philip (eds), *Beyond the Ubaid: Transformation and Integration in the Late Prehistoric Societies of the Middle East*, Chicago.

Lorentz, K. O. 2010b: 'Parts to a whole: Manipulations of the body in the prehistoric Eastern Mediterranean', 20–9 in K. Rebay-Salisbury, M. L. Stig Sørensen and J. Hughes (eds), *Body Parts and Wholes: Changing Relations and Meanings*, Oxford.

Lorentz, K. O. 2011a: 'Human bioarchaeology of the Cypriot Chalcolithic: analyses at Souskiou-Laona cemetery', 613–22 in A. Demetriou (ed.), *Proceedings of the IV International Cyprological Congress*, vol. I.1, Nicosia.

Lorentz, K. O. 2011b: 'Cyprus', 99–112 in N. Márquez-Grant and L. Fibiger (eds), *The Routledge Handbook of Archaeological Human Remains and Legislation: An International Guide to Laws and Practice in the Excavation and Treatment of Archaeological Human Remains*, Abington and New York.

Lorentz, K. O. forthcoming: 'Orderly disposal: human remains at Chalcolithic Souskiou-Laona, Cyprus', in P. Karsgaard (ed.), *Death and Discard: the Transformations of Places, People, Animals and Things in the Ancient Near East* (BANEA Monograph 2), Oxford.

Lorentz, K. O., Pages-Camagna, S., Coquinot, Y. and Pitzalis, D. 2011: 'Natural and material sciences applied to the analysis of the Larnaca-Liperti Tomb 128 painted sarcophagi and human remains', 45–119 in P. Flourentzos, *Two Exceptional Sarcophagi from Larnaka*, Nicosia.

Lorentz *et al.* in preparation [working title] 'Strontium isotopes in investigating residential mobility in Late Bronze Age Cyprus'.

Lunt, D. A. 1980: 'Evidence of tooth extraction in a Cypriot mandible of the Hellenistic or Early Roman Period, c. 150 B.C. to 100 A.D.', *British Dental Journal* 173, 242.

Lunt, D. A. 1985: 'Report on the human dentitions', 54–8, 150–3, 245–9 in E. J. Peltenburg *et al.*, *Lemba Archaeological Project 1. Excavations at Lemba*-Lakkous *1976–1983* (Studies in Mediterranean Archaeology 70:1), Göteborg.

Lunt, D. A. 1994: 'Report on the human dentitions from Souskiou-*Vathrykakas*, 1972', in F. G. Maier and M.-L. von Wartburg, 'Excavations at Kouklia (Palaipaphos. Seventeenth preliminary report: seasons 1991 and 1992', *Report of the Department of Antiquities, Cyprus,* 120–8.

Lunt, D. A. 1995: 'Lemba *Lakkous* and Kissonerga *Mosphilia*: evidence from the dentition in Chalcolithic Cyprus', 56–61 in S. Campbell and A. Green (eds), *Archaeology of Death in the Ancient Near East*, Oxford.

Lunt, D. A. 2006: 'The human dentition', 45–53 in E. Peltenburg (ed.), *The Chalcolithic Cemetery of Souskiou*-Vathrykakas, *Cyprus*, Nicosia.

Lunt, D. A. and Watt, M. E. 2003: 'The dentitions', 46–7 in E. Peltenburg (ed.), *The Lemba Archaeological Project, III, 1: The Colonisation and Settlement of Cyprus: Investigations at Kissonerga*-Mylouthkia, *1976–1996* (Studies in Mediterranean Archaeology 70.4), Jonsered.

Moyer, C. J. 1984: 'Report on the human skeletal remains from Amathonte, Cyprus', in P. Aupert and C. Tytgat, 'Deux tombes géométriques de la nécropole nord d'Amathonte', *Bulletin de Correspondance hellénique* 108, 649–53.

Moyer, C. J. 1985: 'The human skeletal remains', in I. A. Todd, 'A Middle Bronze Age tomb at Psematismenos-*Trelloukkas*', *Report of the Department of Antiquities, Cyprus*, 55–77.

Moyer, C. J. 1989: 'Human skeletal remains', 58–69 in A. K. South, P. Russell and P. Schuster Keswani, *Vasilikos Valley Project 3: Kalavasos*-Ayios Dhimitrios *II* (Studies in Mediterranean Archaeology 71.3), Göteborg.

Moyer, C. J. 1997: 'Human remains from Marki-*Alonia*, Cyprus', *Report of the Department of Antiquities, Cyprus*, 111–8.

Moyer, C. J. 2004: 'Human skeletal remains', 198–9 in I. A. Todd and P. Croft, *Vasilikos Valley Project 8: Excavations at Kalavasos*-Ayious (Studies in Mediterranean Archaeology 71.8), Sävedalen.

Moyer, C. J. 2005: 'Human burials', 1–17 in I. A. Todd, *Vasilikos*

Valley Project 7: Excavations at Kalavasos-Tenta *II* (Studies in Mediterranean Archaeology 71.7), Sävedalen.

Moyer, C. J. 2006: 'Human remains from LVII–1, Context 963', 286–9 in D. Frankel and J. M. Webb (eds), *Marki Alonia: An Early and Middle Bronze Age Settlement in Cyprus Excavations 1995–2000* (Studies in Mediterranean Archaeology 123:2), Sävedalen.

Moyer, C. J. 2007: 'Human skeletal remains', 262–324 in I. A. Todd, *Vasilikos Valley Project 11: Kalavasos Village Tombs 52–79* (Studies in Mediterranean Archaeology 71:11), Sävedalen.

Musgrave, J. H. and Evans, S. P. 1980: 'By strangers honor'd: a statistical study of ancient crania from Crete, Mainland Greece, Cyprus, Israel and Egypt', *Journal of Mediterranean Anthropology and Archaeology* 1, 50–107.

Nyqvist, E. 1980: 'Human teeth from Kition', *Opuscula Atheniensia* 13, 185–8.

Parks, D. A., Mavromatis, C. M. and Harper, N. K. 2000: 'Preliminary report of excavations at Kourion's Amathous Gate Cemetery, 1999', *Report of the Department of Antiquities, Cyprus,* 305–16.

Parks, D. A., Mavromatis, C. M. and Harper, N. K. 2001: 'Preliminary report of excavations at Kourion's Amathous Gate Cemetery, 2000', *Report of the Department of Antiquities, Cyprus,* 232–45.

Parras, Z. 2004: *The Biological Affinities of the Eastern Mediterranean in the Chalcolithic and Bronze Age: A Regional Dental Non-Metric Approach*, Oxford.

Parras, Z. 2006a: 'The human remains', 53–66 in E. J. Peltenburg (ed.), *The Chalcolithic Cemetery of Souskiou*-Vathyrkakas, *Cyprus*, Nicosia.

Parras, Z. 2006b: 'Looking for immigrants at Kissonerga-*Mosphilia* in the Late Chalcolithic: a dental non-metric perspective of Chalcolithic and Early Bronze Age Southwest Cyprus', 63–74 in A. P. McCarthy (ed.), *Island Dialogues. Cyprus in the Mediterranean Network* (University of Edinburgh Archaeology Occasional Paper 21), Edinburgh.

Rix, M. M. 1938: 'Description of Skeleton No. 2', in P. Dikaios, 'The excavations at Erimi 1933–35. Final report', *Report of the Department of Antiquities, Cyprus*, 80.

Rix, M. M. 1950: 'Cranial measurements', 373 in E. Stewart and J. Stewart (eds), *Vounous 1937–1938: Field Report on the Excavations Sponsored by the British School of Archaeology at Athens*, Lund.

Rix, M. M. and Buxton, L. H. 1938: 'The anthropology of prehistoric Cyprus', *Man* 38, 91–2.

Schaeffer, C. F. A. 1935: 'Crania Cypria antiqua', *L'Anthropologie* 45, 218–21.

Schulte-Campbell, C. 1979: 'Human skeletal remains', in I. A. Todd, 'Vasilikos Valley Project, 1977–1978: an interim report', *Report of the Department of Antiquities, Cyprus,* 49–50.

Schulte-Campbell, C. 1983: 'The human remains from Palaepaphos-Skales', 439–55 in V. Karageorghis, *Palaepaphos*-Skales, *An Iron Age cemetery in Cyprus*, Konstanz.

Schulte-Campbell, C. 1986: 'Human skeletal remains', 168–79 in I. A. Todd (ed.), *Vasilikos Valley Project 1: The Bronze Age Cemetery in Kalavasos Village* (Studies in Mediterranean Archaeology 71:1), Göteborg.

Schulte-Campbell, C. 1989: 'A Late Cypriot IIC tomb: Idalion Tomb 1.76. Introduction and skeletal remains', 119–35 in L. E. Stager and A. M. Walker (eds), *American Expedition to Idalion, Cyprus, 1973–1980*, Chicago.

Schulte-Campbell, C. 2003: 'The human skeletal remains', 423–38 in S. Swiny, G. Rapp and E. Herscher (eds), *Sotira Kaminoudhia: An Early Bronze Age Site in Cyprus* (Cyprus American Archaeological Research Institute Monograph Series 2), Boston.

Schwartz, J. H. 1974: 'The human remains from Kition and Hala Sultan Tekke: a cultural interpretation', 151–62 in V. Karageorghis (ed.), *Excavations at Kition I. The Tombs*, Nicosia.

Solivères, O. M. 1981: 'Étude des crânes du Cap Andreas-*Kastros*', 83–7 in A. Le Brun, *Un site néolithique précéramique en Chypre: Cap Andreas*-Kastros, Paris.

Taramides, G. 1983: 'The teeth of Neolithic Cypriots (5800–3000 B.C.), *Odontostomatoloyiki Proodos* 37, 213–8 [in Greek].

Tucker, K. and Clegget, S. 2007: 'Human remains from Tomb 789', 131–4 in D. Frankel and J. M. Webb (eds), *The Bronze Age Cemeteries at Deneia in Cyprus* (Studies in Mediterranean Archaeology 135), Sävedalen.

Virchow R. 1884: *Über alte Schädel von Assos und Cypern* (Abhandlungen der Königlichen Akademie der Wissenschaften zu Berlin, physikalischen-mathematischen Klasse 2), Berlin.

Walker, M. 1975: 'Early Neolithic skeletons from Philia-*Drakos*, Site A (Cyprus)', *Australian Journal of Biblical Archaeology* 2, 77–89.

30. My Side of the Mountain: Initial Colonisation and Biological Regionalism on Cyprus through the Neolithic and Chalcolithic

Zissis Parras

*In recent years there has been an increase in the number of sites studied from the Early Neolithic on Cyprus. This study briefly explains how dental non-metric traits from human remains are used to illustrate the dynamics of the first Cypriots and how they initially settled the island and created a longstanding and unique culture well into the Chalcolithic period. The data for this study come from four Neolithic sites (Kholetria-*Ortos*, Kissonerga-*Mylouthkia*, Kalavasos-*Tenta *and Sotira-*Teppes*) and four Chalcolithic sites (Agios Savvas, Kissonerga-*Mosphilia*, Lemba-*Lakkous *and Souskiou-*Vathyrkakas*) all located around the southern region of Cyprus. By comparing human remains from different sites throughout the Neolithic to the Chalcolithic, one of the topics discussed is how biological and cultural regionalism is reflected across time and space. In addition this discussion also introduces the idea that biological regionalism was a result of initial colonisation which may have contributed to the minor cultural differences observed throughout the island.*

Introduction

The study of archaeology and prehistory is never as simple as many of us wish it were. Ancient societies are rarely, if ever, explained in straightforward terms, with simple cause and effect scenarios. When considering the complex nature of the colonisation of prehistoric Cyprus, there are the established theories on how it may have occurred and also the idea that suggests a greater level of complexity in initial colonisation. The modern science of archaeology, in all its specialties, is beginning to examine the many levels of the complex nature of early Cypriot colonisation. Todd has suggested the early period in Cypriot colonisation perhaps included different groups from the mainland, each one exhibiting different cultural characteristics related to their points of origin (Todd 1989; 2005). To date, the discussion has tended to focus on more traditional material culture studies, and there has been limited discussion of the ancient population of Cyprus with reference to their physical remains. With a growing number of large samples of well-dated human remains from the Neolithic and Chalcolithic periods, this theory of different groups arriving from different parts of the mainland can now be examined.

Among the Early Neolithic sites on Cyprus there is evidence of cultural differences in terms of architecture, stone tool types, subsistence patterns and even the presence or absence of cattle (Croft 2003; Peltenburg *et al.* 2001; Simmons 1994; 1996; 2003; Todd 2005). These cultural differences relate to the different parts of the mainland from where they likely originated. At present no single site has yielded enough specific cultural evidence to positively pinpoint a particular location on the mainland from where these early colonists came. In general the region many archaeologists point to is the area from southern Anatolia through to the Levant where the cultural remains are the most similar with the earliest colonists on Cyprus (Guilaine and Briois 2001; Hansen 2001; Moyer 2005; Peltenburg *et al.* 2001; Stanley Price 1977; Steel 2004; Todd 1989; 2005). This idea of cultural differences between local groups has also been suggested for the Late Neolithic as well as the later Chalcolithic period (Bolger 1989; 1991; 2007; Clarke 2001). Therefore there are some indications of cultural variation within the general Neolithic culture of Cyprus, which may result in evidence for biological variation as well. Some of the earlier anthropological studies conducted on the few human remains from prehistoric Cyprus have identified biological variation between the Neolithic populations of Sotira and Khirokitia (Angel 1961; Domurad 1986).

The present study has discovered biological evidence of different groups present at sites around Neolithic Cyprus. This study also suggests that these local biological differences persisted throughout the Neolithic and into the Chalcolithic period. This evidence is based on examining dental non-metric traits on human remains from four Neolithic and four Chalcolithic sites. This bioarchaeological approach to understanding the biological constitution of ancient populations is new for Cyprus, and this is the first time it has been used on Neolithic human remains. More recently, in other parts of the Eastern Mediterranean, dental non-metric analysis has been applied to address other specific archaeological problems (Johnson and Lovell 1994; Parras 2004; Ullinger *et al.* 2005). This current research is still in the preliminary stage due to the need to gather more dental non-metric data from other Neolithic sites. Therefore the results of this study should be viewed tentatively until other data can be collected.

Materials

The data for this study come from four Neolithic sites (Kholetria-*Ortos*, Kissonerga-*Mylouthkia*, Kalavasos-*Tenta* and Sotira-*Teppes*) and four Chalcolithic sites (Agios Savvas, Kissonerga-*Mosphilia*, Lemba-*Lakkous* and Souskiou-*Vathyrkakas*) all located around the southern region of Cyprus (Fig. 30.1; Table 30.1).

Kissonerga-*Mylouthkia* (hereafter *Mylouthkia*) is a multi-period site with levels from the Aceramic Neolithic and the Early and Middle Chalcolithic periods. There is no evidence of continuous occupation from the Neolithic through to the Chalcolithic (Peltenburg *et al.* 2001; Croft 2003). The site is located approximately 10 km north of Paphos. The earlier phase of the site is a semi-sedentary farming community where the main features are two Cypro-PPNB wells (Croft 2003; Peltenburg *et al.* 2003). The Neolithic human remains were discovered mostly in Well 133, and one infant skeleton was found in Well 116. Therefore the dental non-metric data for the Neolithic period come from Well 133 and Period 1B (Late Cypro-PPNB) (Fox, Lunt and Watt 2003). There are also human remains from the Early and Middle Chalcolithic periods included in this study. All of the human skeletal remains from both time periods were identified and analysed by S. Fox; the human dentition was analysed by D. Lunt and M. Watt (Fox, Lunt and Watt 2003); both collections are located in the Paphos District Museum on Cyprus.

Kalavassos-*Tenta* (hereafter *Tenta*) is an Aceramic Neolithic site where the earliest phase (Period 5) is

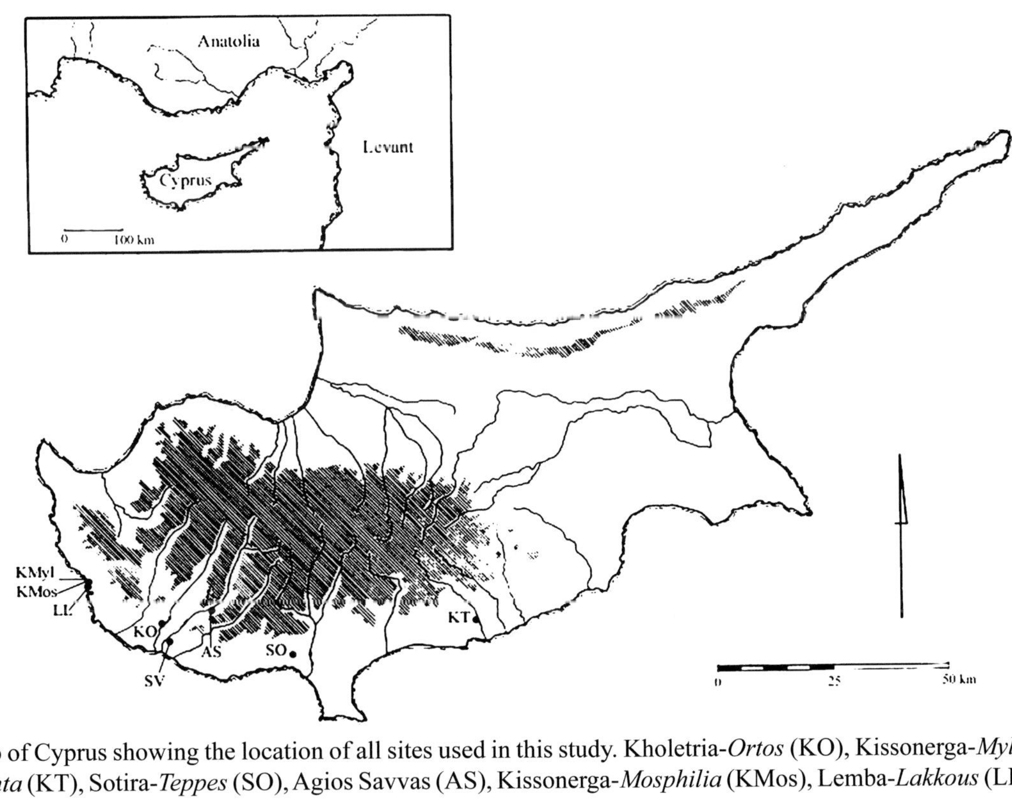

Fig. 30.1. Map of Cyprus showing the location of all sites used in this study. Kholetria-*Ortos* (KO), Kissonerga-*Mylouthkia* (KMyl), Kalavasos-*Tenta* (KT), Sotira-*Teppes* (SO), Agios Savvas (AS), Kissonerga-*Mosphilia* (KMos), Lemba-*Lakkous* (LL) and Souskiou-*Vathyrkakas* (SV)

Table 30.1. List of all sites in this study. Minimum number of Individuals (MNI) represents individuals with teeth available for dental non-metric analysis

Sites	*Abbreviation*	*Period(s)*	*MNI*	*Teeth*
Kissonerga-*Mylouthkia*	KMyl	Aceramic Neolithic & Middle to Late Chalcolithic	7	30
Kalavasos-*Tenta*	KT	Aceramic Neolithic	7	24
Kholetria-*Ortos*	KO	Aceramic Neolithic	4	10
Sotira-*Teppes*	SO	Ceramic Neolithic	8	130
Ayios Savvas	AS	Middle Chalcolithic	5	28
Souskiou-*Vathyrkakas*	SV	Middle Chalcolithic	138	943
Lemba-*Lakkous*	LL	Middle to Late Chalcolithic	42	426
Kissonerga-*Mosphilia*	KMos	Middle to Late Chalcolithic	54	508
Totals			**265**	**2,099**

contemporary with the earliest phases from Parekklisha *Shillourokambos* and *Mylouthkia* (Todd 2005). The excavation at *Tenta* began in the 1970s and over the years many people have studied the human remains from the site. C. J. Moyer studied the remains recently and compiled a comprehensive anthropological report and analysis of all the remains excavated since the 1970s (Moyer 2005). The condition of the skeletal assemblage from *Tenta* is considered poor. Even though many complete skeletons were found in anatomical position, many of the bones were encrusted with a hard crystalline deposit that obscured many of the dental traits (Moyer 2005). The human remains are located in the Larnaka District Museum on Cyprus.

Kholetria-*Ortos* (hereafter *Ortos*) is a large Aceramic Neolithic settlement located approximately 20 km east of Paphos (Simmons 1994). The site was excavated in the mid 1990s by a team from the University of Nevada led by Alan Simmons (Simmons 1994; 1996). The site is located on a prominent hill overlooking the Xeropotamos River (north of Souskiou-*Vathyrkakas*), and covers approximately 2.4 hectares. Calibrated BC dates suggest a range from 5,950 to 6,385 cal. BC (Simmons 1996, 40). The few human remains are very fragmentary and have been identified and analysed by S. Fox, then of the University of Arizona, and are located at the Kouklia Museum on Cyprus (Simmons 1994).

Sotira-*Teppes* (hereafter Sotira) is a Ceramic Neolithic site (Dikaios 1961). Porphyrios Dikaios excavated the site in the 1940s and the 1950s and the human remains were studied by J. L. Angel and R.-P. Charles (Angel 1961; Charles 1962). The human remains are in very good condition and are located in the Limasol District Museum on Cyprus.

Kissonerga-*Mosphilia* (hereafter Kissonerga) and Lemba-*Lakkous* (hereafter Lemba) are both located along the coast in the northern part of the Ktima Lowlands approximately 1–2 km apart. Occupation at Kissonerga has been identified as early as the Aceramic Neolithic up to the Early Bronze Age. The human remains are from the Middle, Late Chalcolithic and the Early Bronze periods only (Parras 2004; Peltenburg *et al.* 1998). Lemba was inhabited during the Early through Late Chalcolithic periods and the human remains are only from tombs throughout the Middle and Late periods (Peltenburg *et al.* 1985). Lemba and Kissonerga are both village sites where the people were buried intramurally between the houses.

Souskiou-*Vathyrkakas* (hereafter *Vathyrkakas*) is located approximately 20 km southeast of Lemba and situated on the edge of a plateau, approximately 100 m in elevation, bordering a deep ravine, which leads off from the river Diarrhizos, which flows from the north (Parras 2006; Peltenburg 2006). *Vathyrkakas* is the earliest recorded group of cemeteries in western Cyprus (Peltenburg *et al.* 1985). The cemeteries are dated to the Middle Chalcolithic (Peltenburg 2006). *Vathyrkakas* is unique for the Chalcolithic period on Cyprus because all known Neolithic and Chalcolithic burials have always been found beneath or very near the people's houses.

Agios Savvas is a Middle Chalcolithic settlement site located roughly 30 km east of Paphos on the Dhiarizos river (north of Souskiou-*Vathyrkakas*) (Rupp *et al.* 1999). The site was excavated under the direction of David Rupp, then of Brock University. The pottery dates the site to the early part of the Middle Chalcolithic and does not extend into the Late Chalcolithic period (Clarke and Rupp 1995; Rupp and D'Annibale 1995; Rupp *et al.* 1999). The few human remains are in poor condition and have been identified and analysed by S. Fox, then of the University of Arizona, and are currently located at the Kouklia Museum on Cyprus.

Bioarchaeological method

This study used 35 dental traits from the list prepared by

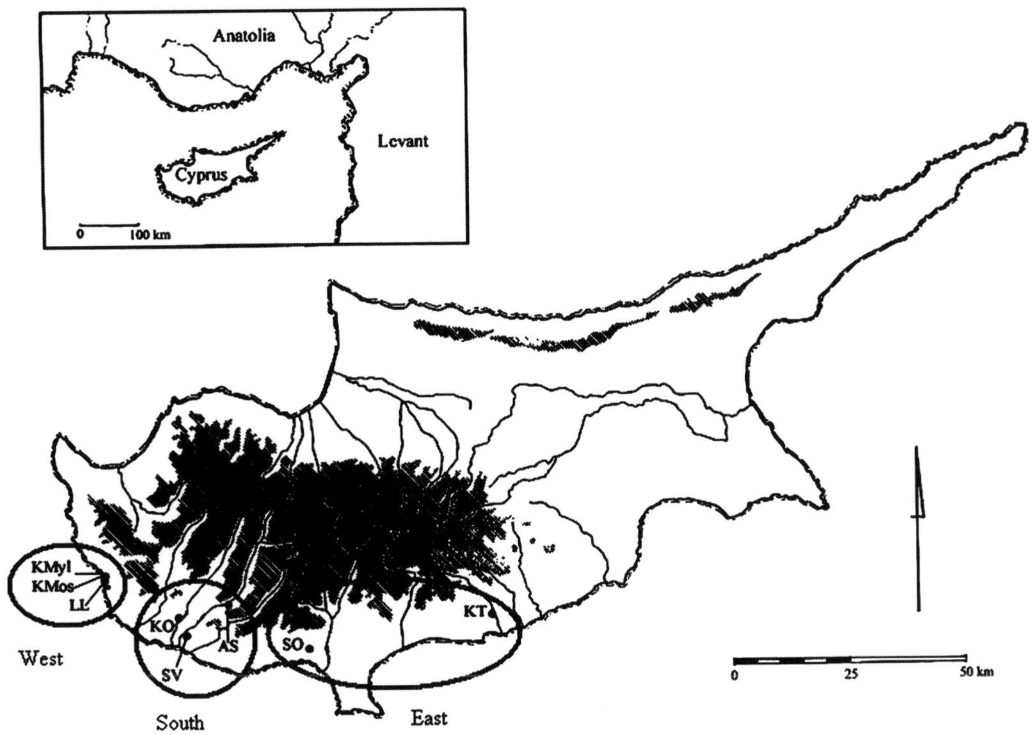

Fig. 30.2. Map of Cyprus showing location of geographic groups. Kholetria-*Ortos* (KO), Kissonerga-*Mylouthkia* (KMyl), Kalavasos-*Tenta* (KT), Sotira-*Teppes* (SO), Agios Savvas (AS), Kissonerga-*Mosphilia* (KMos), Lemba-*Lakkous* (LL) and Souskiou-*Vathyrkakas* (SV)

Arizona State University (ASU) (Turner, Nichol and Scott 1991). The ASU list and variations of it have been used in other non-metric studies (Berry 1978; Cucina *et al.* 1999; Hemphill, Lukacs and Kennedy 1991; Irish 1995; 1997; 1998; 2000; 2005; Irish and Turner 1990; Johnson and Lovell 1994; Lee and Goose 1972; Stringer, Humphrey and Compton 1997; Turner 1979; 1987; Turner and Markowitz 1990; Turner and Swindler 1978; Ullinger *et al.* 2005). Dental non-metric traits are very useful for bio-distance studies since they are durable, possess a high genetic component and require no special tools to record (Irish 2000; Scott and Turner 1997; Turner 1986; Turner, Nichol and Scott 1991).

Dental traits were recorded from the permanent dentition. Permanent teeth form in children at a very young age, and it was possible to include individuals from as young as one year old (Fig. 30.2). The inclusion of such data is advantageous for two reasons: first, a broader selection of the population was included, and second, given the high infant mortality rate in prehistoric populations, there was a high proportion of young unworn teeth to examine for traits. The fact that certain traits are not fully formed at a young age is not a concern for the analysis, any more than fully developed adult teeth that are heavily worn, thus obscuring trait identification.

In this study, traits were counted from both sides of the dentition and the side with the greatest expression was scored (Irish 2005; Turner 1985). According to Turner, this method:

> '... gives the maximal amount of information, takes into account possible asymmetry arising from developmental factors, and further benefits by the fact that such a counting procedure is consistent with developmental and genetic theory'. (Turner 1985, 263)

The data from both sexes were pooled since trait differences between males and females are not considered significant (Berry and Berry 1967; Hanihara 1992; Irish 1997; 2000; 2005; Turner, Nichol and Scott 1991). After recording the traits from the dentition, frequencies were determined for each trait for all sites in this study (Tables 30.2 and 30.3). Traditionally when larger samples are present, the frequencies are used with Smith's mean measure of divergence (MMD) distance statistic (Berry 1963; 1976; Irish 2000). This statistic assumes phenetic similarity and approximates cladistic relationship (Irish 1997; 2000). According to Irish (2000, 398), 'This multivariate technique provides a quantitative estimate of biological divergence among samples based on the degree of phenetic similarity for all traits'. It is assumed that phenetic similarity in dental morphology reflects the underlying genetic similarity

Table 30.2. Trait frequencies from all Neolithic sites (n represents all teeth and N represents teeth with traits present). For tooth abbreviation explanations see Appendix

Neolithic Samples				*KMyl*			*KO*			*KT*			*SO*	
Number of Individuals				*3*			*4*			*7*			*8*	
Traits	*Tooth*	*Range*	*N*	*%*	*n*	*N*	*%*	*n*	*N*	*%*	*n*	*N*	*%*	*n*
Shovelling	UI1	(2–7)	1	50	2	0	0	0	1	100	1	1	20	5
Labial convexity	UI1	(2–4)	0	0	2	0	0	1	0	0	1	1	20	5
Interruption groove	UI2	1	0	0	3	0	0	1	0	0	1	0	0	3
Tuberculum dentale	UI2	(2–6)	1	33	3	0	0	1	1	100	1	0	0	4
Canine distal accessory ridge	UC	(2–5)	0	0	2	0	0	1	0	0	1	0	0	3
Hypocone expression	UM2	(3–5)	0	0	0	1	100	1	0	0	0	3	100	3
Cusp 5	UM1	(2–5)	0	0	1	0	0	0	0	0	1	0	0	2
Carabelli trait	UM1	(2–7)	1	50	2	0	0	1	2	100	2	0	0	3
Enamel extension	UP1	(1–3)	0	0	3	0	0	0	0	0	1	0	0	0
Upper premolar root number	UP1	2+	0	0	2	0	0	0	0	0	0	1	100	1
Upper molar root number	UM2	3+	1	50	2	1	100	1	0	0	0	0	0	1
Peg shaped third molar	UM3	2	0	0	2	0	0	0	0	0	1	1	33	3
Odontome	LP1	1	0	0	2	0	0	0	0	0	1	0	0	2
Lower premolar lingual cusps	LP2	(2–9)	2	100	2	0	0	0	0	0	0	4	100	4
Anterior Fovea	LM1	(2–4)	0	0	0	0	0	0	0	0	2	0	0	0
Lower molar groove pattern	LM2	Y	0	0	0	0	0	2	0	0	1	0	0	5
Deflecting wrinkle	LM1	(2–3)	0	0	0	0	0	0	1	33	3	0	0	0
Distal trigonid crest	LM1	1	0	0	0	0	0	1	0	0	2	0	0	0
Cusp 5 (hypocunulid)	LM2	(1–5)	0	0	0	1	50	2	0	0	1	0	0	5
Cusp 6 (tuberculum sextum)	LM1	(1–5)	0	0	0	0	0	2	1	33	3	0	0	5
Cusp 7 (tuberculum intermidium)	UM1	(2–4)	0	0	1	0	0	1	0	0	1	0	0	0
Lower canine root number	LC	2+	0	0	1	0	0	0	0	0	0	0	0	0
Tomes' root	LP1	(3–5)	0	0	2	0	0	1	0	0	0	0	0	0

(Guatelli-Steinberg, Irish and Lukacs 2001; Irish 2000). The samples in this study are not large enough to employ the MMD equation and even grouping all of the Neolithic sites together is still too small a sample for the requirements for the MMD equation to function properly. A second reason the MMD could not be used in this study is due to the fact that for this analysis, at least three adequate samples are needed. For example, the following study compared the Neolithic with the Chalcolithic group and there was not a third group available for the MMD comparison. These are just a few of the reasons why these preliminary results are based on data that cannot be proven statistically significant at this time. Considering this last point, the following results do suggest some noteworthy patterns and it will be interesting to see if these patterns remain consistent when more data are gathered in the future.

The dichotomised breakpoints used for the analysis (Table 30.4) followed those of Turner (1987), Scott and Turner (1997) with the following modifications. The *lower* canine distal accessory trait was used instead of the *upper*, since it was present in more of the samples. In samples in which it was present in both upper and lower (LL and KMos), the lower canine trait always showed a higher expression in the lower tooth. The enamel extension trait from the upper *first premolar* has been included instead of the upper *first molar*, which has been recommended for use by Scott and Turner (1997). Again, this was done since the trait found on the *premolar* is more common in these samples from Cyprus. The selection of these two traits maximised the number of traits compared and also included the highest frequencies where possible.

Dental non-metric results grouped by time period

The first comparison examined the dental traits by time period. Individual traits from all Neolithic sites (Table 30.2) were grouped, as were traits from all Chalcolithic sites (Table 30.3). The difference in number of individuals between the two time periods should be pointed out. The much lower number of individuals from the Neolithic is a concern with dental non-metric studies, since the larger the number of individuals the more reliable the results are.

The overall results show that out of 35 dental traits, 23 are present on Cyprus from the Neolithic to the Chalcolithic,

Table 30.3. Trait frequencies from all Chalcolithic sites (n represents all teeth and N represents teeth with traits present)

Chalcolithic Samples				*SV*			*KMos*			*LL*			*AS*			*KMyl*	
Number of Individuals				*138*			*54*			*42*			*5*			*4*	
Traits	*Tooth*	*Range*	*N*	*%*	*n*	*N*	*%*	*n*	*N*	*%*	*n*	*N*	*%*	*n*	*N*	*%*	*n*
Shovelling	UI1	(2–7)	5	19.2	26	14	51.9	27	4	16.7	24	0	0	1	0	0	1
Labial convexity	UI1	(2–4)	4	16.7	24	0	0	0	0	0	5	0	0	1	0	0	1
Interruption groove	UI2	1	11	32.4	34	3	13	23	2	12.5	16	0	0	1	0	0	2
Tuberculum dentale	UI2	(2–6)	7	21.2	33	10	43.5	23	10	66.7	15	0	0	1	0	0	2
Canine distal accessory ridge	UC	(2–5)	2	4.55	44	3	17.6	17	5	50	10	1	100	1	0	0	1
Hypocone expression	UM2	(3–5)	23	92	25	8	44.4	18	9	56.3	16	1	1	1	0	0	1
Cusp 5	UM1	(2–5)	8	33.3	24	3	10.7	28	1	4.76	21	2	66	3	0	0	2
Carabelli trait	UM1	(2–7)	3	10.7	28	7	25	28	8	38.1	21	2	66	3	1	33	3
Enamel extension	UP1	(1–3)	1	3.85	26	1	4.35	23	0	0	13	0	0	1	0	0	1
Upper premolar root number	UP1	2+	9	52.9	17	1	50	2	4	100	4	0	0	0	0	0	1
Upper molar root number	UM2	3+	0	0	0	0	0	0	0	0	1	1	100	1	0	0	0
Peg shaped third molar	UM3	2	0	0	26	0	0	12	0	0	7	0	0	1	0	0	1
Odontome	LP1	1	4	10.3	39	0	0	13	0	0	13	0	0	1	0	0	0
Lower premolar lingual cusps	LP2	(2–9)	22	95.7	23	6	66.7	9	1	50	2	1	100	1	0	0	0
Anterior Fovea	LM1	(2–4)	2	4.35	46	0	0	14	0	0	16	0	0	2	1	100	1
Lower molar groove pattern	LM2	Y	13	27.7	47	0	0	16	1	10	10	0	0	1	0	0	1
Deflecting wrinkle	LM1	(2–3)	7	16.3	43	5	31.3	16	7	38.9	18	1	50	2	0	0	1
Distal trigonid crest	LM1	1	7	17.1	41	0	0	16	0	0	16	0	0	3	0	0	1
Cusp 5 (hypocunulid)	LM2	(1–5)	11	26.2	42	0	0	13	2	22.2	9	0	0	1	1	100	1
Cusp 6 (tuberculum sextum)	LM1	(1–5)	2	4.26	47	0	0	17	0	0	17	0	0	4	0	0	1
Cusp 7 (tuberculum intermidium)	UM1	(2–4)	0	0	28	0	0	27	0	0	18	0	0	3	0	0	3
Lower canine root number	LC	2+	0	0	0	1	50	2	0	0	0	0	0	1	0	0	0
Tomes' root	LP1	(3–5)	0	0	0	0	0	1	1	16.7	6	0	0	1	0	0	0

with 13 traits from the Neolithic (22 people) and 22 traits from the Chalcolithic (241 people) (Table 30.4). Two traits that show similarities between time periods are the labial convexity and tuberculum dentale traits. While four traits, the shovelling, Carabelli, upper molar root number and the deflecting wrinkle trait, are less similar between time periods. The peg shaped third molar trait is not found in the Chalcolithic period but only in the Neolithic (Sotira). The sites from the Neolithic are located in the West, South and the East, as are the Chalcolithic sites (Fig. 30.1). Even though the Neolithic group is a very small sample, it represents a wide geographic area. Looking at this group as a random sample, it could still be representative of the traits present during the Neolithic, regardless of its small sample size.

Temporal results in terms of colonisation

How these results relate to current theories on Cypriot colonisation is not yet clear since there are aspects of the earliest migration to Cyprus that are not known at this point. Unknown variables such as the duration of migration from the mainland to the various sites, and how diverse were the biological affinities (genetic make-up) of the different groups migrating to the island? These two points would affect the distribution and likely the frequency of traits in the Neolithic. Even though the Neolithic sample represents sites from only around the southern region of Cyprus, it is also limited to only four sites and clearly there is the possibility of not being representative of the entire Neolithic period. How this relates to the archaeological evidence and the difference in technology between the mainland and Cyprus cannot be addressed at this time, due to the limited focus of this study.

Dental non-metric results grouped by region

The samples were also compared by region. All of the sites come from southern Cyprus and were organised into 3 groups: a West group, a South group and an East group (Table 30.5). These groups are based on the assumption that sites in similar micro-regions will also have similar biological relatedness due to the need to find mates close by (Fig. 30.2).

A comment regarding the East group made up of Sotira

Table 30.4. Traits from Neolithic and Chalcolithic groups (n represents all teeth and N represents teeth with traits present)

Samples			*Neolithic KMyl, SOT KT, KO*			*Chalcholithic KMyl, KO LL, SV, KMos*		
Number of Individuals				*22*			*241*	
Traits	*Tooth*	*Range*	*N*	*%*	*n*	*N*	*%*	*n*
Shovelling	UI1	(2–7)	3	38	8	22	29	75
Labial convexity	UI1	(2–4)	1	11	9	4	13	31
Interruption groove	UI2	1	0	–	8	16	22	74
Tuberculum dentale	UI2	(2–6)	2	22	9	15	21	72
Canine distal accessory ridge	UC	(2–5)	0	–	7	9	12	75
Hypocone expression	UM2	(3–5)	4	100	4	40	68	59
Cusp 5	UM1	(2–5)	0	–	4	13	18	74
Carabelli trait	UM1	(2–7)	3	38	8	18	23	79
Enamel extension	UP1	(1–3)	0	–	4	2	3	62
Upper premolar root number	UP1	2+	1	33	3	14	58	24
Upper molar root number	UM2	3+	2	50	4	1	50	2
Peg shaped third molar	UM3	2	1	17	6	0	–	46
Odontome	LP1	1	0	–	5	4	6	65
Lower premolar lingual cusps	LP2	(2–9)	6	100	6	30	86	35
Anterior Fovea	LM1	(2–4)	0	–	2	3	4	74
Lower molar groove pattern	LM2	Y	0	–	8	14	20	71
Deflecting wrinkle	LM1	(2–3)	1	33	3	20	27	75
Distal trigonid crest	LM1	1	0	0	3	7	10	72
Cusp 5 (hypocunulid)	LM2	(1–5)	1	13	8	14	23	62
Cusp 6 (tuberculum sextum)	LM1	(1–5)	1	10	10	2	2	81
Cusp 7 (tuberculum intermidium)	UM1	(2–4)	0	–	3	0	–	75
Lower canine root number	LC	2+	0	–	1	1	33	3
Tomes' root	LP1	(3–5)	0	–	3	1	14	7

and *Tenta*: compared with the other groups, these two sites are not as close geographically and it could be argued this is not an appropriate grouping. Initially it was considered to include Sotira with the South group that would have left *Tenta* on its own, therefore the two sites were grouped in this way in order to maximise the data.

Out of 23 traits present from all sites, 18 are present in the West, 20 are present in the South, and 11 are present in the East (Table 30.6). First of all this suggests that all of the traits are not found only in one region, regardless of time. Specifically there are two traits only found in the West (Lower canine root number and Tomes' root), one trait only found in the South (Odontome) and one trait only found in the East (Peg shaped third molar). Two traits, Upper premolar root number and Anterior fovea, have similar frequencies between the South and the West, while two other, Labial convexity and Cusp 6, with the South and the East. This suggests that the distribution of traits and similar frequencies is spread in a geographic pattern from West to East, with the greatest number and similarities of traits occurring in the middle (South). There are also two other traits between West and East that share similar frequencies (Shovelling and the Deflecting wrinkle traits).

Ignoring the smaller sample that makes up the East group, the two larger samples (West and South) each have enough people that one would expect them to have more traits present as well. That is not the case and we can see that even in these large groups some traits are absent. It should be noted that these groups now span approximately 5000 years and roughly 100 km of distance, therefore they are not only reflecting a geographic distribution but they are also exhibiting this pattern across time. This evidence supports the idea that, not only were there different biological groups originally settling the island, but also there was not a complete movement of people throughout the island over the course of the Neolithic and Chalcolithic periods. This is referred to as biological regionalism and is irrespective of cultural similarities or differences between groups.

Table 30.5. List of sites grouped by region

West (MNI – 104)	*South (MNI – 147)*	*East (MNI – 15)*
Kissonerga-*Mylouthkia*	Kholetria-*Ortos*	Kalavasos-Tenta
Kissonerga-*Mosphilia*	Agios Savvas	Sotira-*Teppes*
Lemba-*Lakkous*	Souskiou-*Vathyrkakas*	

Table 30.6. Trait frequencies of geographic groups (n represents all teeth and N represents teeth with traits present)

Groups				*West Kmyl, LL,KMos*			*South KO, SA,SV*			*East SOT, KT*	
Number of Individuals				*104*			*147*			*15*	
Traits	*Tooth*	*Range*	*N*	*%*	*n*	*N*	*%*	*n*	*N*	*%*	*n*
Shovelling	UI1	(2–7)	19	35	54	5	19	27	2	33	6
Labial convexity	UI1	(2–4)	0	–	8	4	15	26	1	17	6
Interruption groove	UI2	1	5	11	44	11	31	36	0	–	4
Tuberculum dentale	UI2	(2–6)	9	21	43	7	20	35	1	20	5
Canine distal accessory ridge	UC	(2–5)	8	16	50	1	3	30	0	–	4
Hypocone expression	UM2	(3–5)	17	49	35	25	93	27	3	100	3
Cusp 5	UM1	(2–5)	4	8	52	10	37	27	0	–	3
Carabelli trait	UM1	(2–7)	17	31	54	5	16	32	2	40	5
Enamel extension	UP1	(1–3)	1	3	40	1	4	27	0	–	1
Upper premolar root number	UP1	2+	5	56	9	9	53	17	1	100	1
Upper molar root number	UM2	3+	1	33	3	2	100	2	0	–	1
Peg shaped third molar	UM3	2	0	–	22	0	–	27	1	25	4
Odontome	LP1	1	0	–	28	4	10	40	0	–	3
Lower premolar lingual cusps	LP2	(2–9)	9	69	13	23	96	24	4	100	4
Anterior Fovea	LM1	(2–4)	1	3	31	2	4	48	0	–	2
Lower molar groove pattern	LM2	Y	1	4	27	13	26	50	0	–	6
Deflecting wrinkle	LM1	(2–3)	12	34	35	8	18	45	1	33	3
Distal trigonid crest	LM1	1	0	–	33	7	16	45	0		2
Cusp 5 (hypocunulid)	LM2	(1–5)	3	13	23	12	27	45	0	–	6
Cusp 6 (tuberculum sextum)	LM1	(1–5)	0	–	35	2	4	53	1	13	8
Cusp 7 (tuberculum intermidium)	UM1	(2–4)	0	–	49	0	–	32	0	–	1
Lower canine root number	LC	2+	1	33	3	0	–	1	0	–	0
Tomes' root	LP1	(3–5)	1	11	9	0	–	2	0	–	0

Discussion

There is definite need for caution with these data since some of the samples are small and there are limited human remains from the Neolithic period. When trying to understand a population's gene pool, adequate numbers of human remains are essential for reliable conclusions. Considering this last point, these results show biological distinctions between the Neolithic and Chalcolithic periods as well as between the regions. Given the relatively homogenous culture represented during the later Neolithic and Chalcolithic periods, Cyprus does not show homogeneous biological affinities. How these results relate to our current understanding of the initial colonisation and development of prehistoric Cypriot culture will need to be considered.

Having no other dental non-metric studies from Neolithic or Chalcolithic Cyprus to compare with, the following discussion focuses on the theory that the effects of biological regionalism over time affects our understanding of colonisation and the development of culture in Cyprus. It should be noted that the discussion will not attempt to use the different cultural assemblages from the various sites to assist in identifying biological differences between groups. The caution stated by Bar-Yosef (2001, 130) is one that definitely applies to these data. 'At that point in the discussion we enter the treacherous field of equating archaeological finds with people'.

Considering the idea that different groups migrated from the mainland each with different biological affinities as well as cultural assemblages, is supported archaeologically from different sites around the island. This study supports the idea already put forward, and in doing so, the discussion considers other possibilities not considered by examining only the cultural remains. As Cyprus moved from the Aceramic to the Ceramic Neolithic and became more homogeneous culturally, it may not have become biologically homogeneous. This suggests that when culture and ideas are transmitted it may not be necessary for large numbers of people to move around in order for culture to be distributed. Also, any slight cultural differences between groups can be explained through the biological differences that were already present. It has been suggested that culturally homogeneous groups may still feel the need to express their own individual nature for example in different ceramic styles (Bolger 2007; Clarke 2001).

One way to consider the colonisation to Cyprus is that it may have happened in two stages: the first stage could have been made up of groups from the mainland that initially settled the island and the second stage was made up of people who later joined these initial sites. There is some evidence that after initial colonisation contact was maintained between the founding population and the specific mainland sites (Guilaine and Briois 2001; Peltenburg *et al.* 2001; Vigne *et al.* 2000). For the Neolithic site of Parekklisha-*Shillourokambos*, Vigne and colleagues suggest not a single crossing but numerous return voyages from Cyprus to the mainland would have to have occurred (Vigne *et al.* 2000). This was undoubtedly the source for the transmission of foreign artefacts (such as obsidian) and from where more settlers would have arrived. In terms of biological affinities, this would influence the concentration of existing traits, thus resulting in higher frequencies. When more Neolithic dental non-metric data are gathered from larger samples, this theory will eventually be tested.

After the colonisation period subsided the different groups (sites), each with their own cultural assemblages, could have easily exchanged ideas as well as biological affinities among the other sites on the island. Therefore identifying the cultural signature of a particular site and trying to relate it back to a specific region on the mainland may be difficult since it assumes individual groups would stay culturally static after initial colonisation. These sites would have organised themselves along specific social, political and trade networks and these relationships will also have dictated their biological intermixing (Corruccini 1972; Scott and Dahlberg 1982; Scott and Turner 1997). These early social relationships may also be the foundation for the biological regionalism which continued into the Chalcolithic period (Parras 2008).

Conclusion

The intention of this research is not to imply that biological data should be used to replace cultural data as a means to identify ancient groups or people. Instead, by including a biological profile along with cultural data we can begin to develop a more comprehensive picture of prehistoric Cyprus and perhaps begin to appreciate the complex nature of ancient people. There is a clear relationship between cultural and biological identity, and the purpose of this research is not to define this cultural and biological relationship, but merely to examine specific groups and observe how this relationship works and whether there is change over time within and between specific groups.

One of the goals of this research is to demonstrate how examining dental traits provides a clearer understanding of ancient Cyprus in a biological way, as well as to provide new insight regarding the spread of culture relative to the spread of biological affinities. Eventually more Neolithic and Chalcolithic data will be collected by the author and a more detailed picture of the complex nature of culture and biology from prehistoric Cyprus will emerge.

Acknowledgements

First I would like to thank Dr Kirsi Lorentz for allowing me the opportunity to present an earlier version of this paper at the conference, and special thanks to Michelle Gamble (Newcastle University) who actually read the paper on my behalf since I was not able to attend the conference myself. Secondly, I would like to extend my thanks to the people who allowed me to study the human remains from their respective sites. Drs David Rupp (Ayios Savvas), Ian Todd (Kalavasos-*Tenta*), Edgar Peltenburg (Kissonerga-*Mylouthkia*), Alan Simmons (Kholetria-*Ortos*), Pavlos Flourentsos (Sotira-*Teppes*) and the Department of Antiquities of Cyprus. Many thanks also to the directors and staff of the Cypriot district museums of Paphos, Kouklia, Limassol and Larnaca. Their constant, generous help was always invaluable and led to a quick and efficient study of the human remains. Thanks to Paul Croft and the Lemba Archaeological Centre, where I stayed while in the Paphos district. Paul helped me with my car rental that made my travel to the various museums much easier. I would also like to thank Nicole Wright and Paula Kyriakou for proof-reading final drafts of this manuscript; their comments were greatly appreciated. Finally a special thanks to the late Dr Danielle Parks, her constant support of my research was always positive and encouraging.

Appendix 1. Explanation of tooth abbreviations

Traits	*Tooth abbreviation*	*Tooth*
Shovelling	UI1	First Upper Incisor
Labial convexity	UI1	First Upper Incisor
Interruption groove	UI2	Second Upper Incisor
Tuberculum dentale	UI2	Second Upper Incisor
Canine distal accessory ridge	UC	Upper Canine
Hypocone expression	UM2	Second Upper Molar
Cusp 5	UM1	First Upper Molar
Carabelli trait	UM1	First Upper Molar
Enamel extension	UP1	First Upper Premolar
Upper premolar root number	UP1	First Upper Premolar
Upper molar root number	UM2	Second Upper Molar
Peg shaped third molar	UM3	Third Upper Molar
Odontome	LP1	First Lower Premolar
Lower premolar lingual cusps	LP2	Second Lower Premolar
Anterior fovea	LM1	First Lower Molar
Lower molar groove pattern	LM2	Second Lower Molar
Deflecting wrinkle	LM1	First Lower Molar
Distal trigonid crest	LM1	First Lower Molar
Cusp 5 (hypocunulid)	LM2	Second Lower Molar
Cusp 6 (tuberculum sextum)	LM1	First Lower Molar
Cusp 7 (tuberculum intermidium)	UM1	First Upper Premolar
Lower canine root number	LC	Lower Canine
Tomes' root	LP1	First Lower Premolar

Bibliography

Angel, J. L. 1961: 'Appendix 1: Neolithic crania from Sotira', 223–9 in P. Dikaios, *Sotira*, Philadelphia.

Bar-Yosef, O. 2001: 'The world around Cyprus: from the Epi-paleolithic foragers to the collapse of the PPNB civilization', 129–64 in S. Swiny (ed.), *The Earliest Prehistory of Cyprus: From Colonization to Exploitation*, Boston.

Berry, A. C. 1976: 'The anthropological value of minor variants of the dental crown', *American Journal of Physical Anthropology* 45, 257–68.

Berry, A. C. 1978: 'Anthropological and familial studies on minor variants of the dental crown', 81–98 in P. M. Butler and K. A. Joysey (eds), *Development, Function and Evolution of Teeth*, London.

Berry, A. C. and Berry, R. J. 1967: 'Epigenetic variation in the human cranium', *Journal of Anatomy* 101(2), 361–79.

Berry, R. J. 1963: 'Epigenetic polymorphism in wild populations of *Mus musculus*,' *Genetical Research* 4, 193–220.

Bolger, D. L. 1989: 'Regionalism, cultural variation and the culture-area concept in later prehistoric Cypriot studies', 142–52 in E. Peltenburg (ed.), *Early Society in Cyprus*, Edinburgh.

Bolger, D. L. 1991: 'The evolution of the Chalcolithic painted style', *Bulletin of the American Schools of Oriental Research* 282/283, 81–93.

Bolger, D. L. 2007: 'Cultural interaction in 3rd millennium B.C. Cyprus: evidence of ceramics', 163–88 in S. Antoniadou and A. Pace (eds), *Mediterranean Crossroads*, Athens.

Charles, R.-P. 1962: *Le peuplement de Chypre dans l'antiquité. Étude anthropologique* (Études Chypriotes 2), Paris.

Clarke, J. T. 2001: 'Style and society in Ceramic Neolithic Cyprus', *Levant* 33, 65–80.

Clarke, J. T. and Rupp, D. W. 1995: 'Prastio-Agios Savvas tis Karonis Monastery (Paphos District): 1993 field season Middle Chalcolithic ceramics,' *Report of the Department of Antiquities, Cyprus*, 49–60.

Corruccini, R. S. 1972: 'The biological relationships of some prehistoric and historic Pueblo populations', *American Journal of Physical Anthropology* 37, 373–88.

Croft, P. 2003: 'The animal bones', 49–58, 225–37 in Peltenburg *et al.*, *Lemba Archaeological Project III.1 The colonisaion and settlement of Cyprus: Investigations at Kissonerga-Mylouthkia 1976–1996* (Studies in Mediterranean Archaeology 70:4), Jonsered.

Cucina, A., Lucci, M., Vargiu, R. and Coppa, A. 1999: 'Dental evidence of biological affinity and environmental conditions in prehistoric Trentino (Italy) samples from the Neolithic to the Early Bronze Age', *International Journal of Osteo-archaeology* 9, 404–16.

Dikaios, P. 1961: *Sotira*, Philadelphia.

Domurad, M. R. 1986: *The Populations of Ancient Cyprus*, Unpublished Ph.D. Dissertation, University of Cincinnati.

Fox, S., Lunt, D. and Watt, M. 2003: 'Human remains', 43–7, 221–4 in Peltenburg *et al. Lemba Archaeological Project III.1 The colonisaion and settlement of Cyprus: Investigations at Kissonerga-Mylouthkia 1976–1996* (Studies in Mediterranean Archaeology 70:4), Jonsered.

Guatelli-Steinberg, D., Irish, J. D. and Lukacs, J. R. 2001: 'Canary islands-north African population affinities: measure of divergence based on dental morphology', *Homo* 52(2), 173–88.

Guilaine, J. and Briois, F. 2001: 'Parekklisha Shillourokambos: an early Neolithic site in Cyprus', 37–54 in S. Swiny (ed.), *The Earliest Prehistory of Cyprus: From Colonization to Exploitation*, Boston.

Hanihara, T. 1992: 'Dental and cranial affinities among populations of East Asia and the Pacific: the basic populations in East Asia, IV', *American Journal of Physical Anthropology* 88, 163–82.

Hansen, J. 2001: 'Aceramic Neolithic plant remains in Cyprus: clues to their origins?', 119–28 in S. Swiny (ed.), *The Earliest Prehistory of Cyprus: From Colonization to Exploitation*, Boston.

Hemphill, B. E., Lukacs, J. R. and Kennedy, K. A. R. 1991: 'Biological adaptations and affinities of Bronze Age Harappans', 137–82 in R. H. Meadow (ed.), *Harappa Excavations 1986–1990: A Multidisciplinary Approach to Third Millennium Urbanism*, Madison.

Irish, J. D. 1995: 'High frequency archaic dental traits in modern sub-Saharan African populations (abstract)', *American Journal of Physical Anthropology* Supplement 20(182), 117.

Irish, J. D. 1997: 'Characteristic high and low frequency dental traits in Sub-Saharan African populations', *American Journal of Physical Anthropology* 102(4), 455–67.

Irish, J. D. 1998: 'Ancestral dental traits in recent Sub-Saharan Africans and the origin of modern humans', *Journal of Human Evolution* 34(1), 81–98.

Irish, J. D. 2000: 'The Iberomaurusian enigma: North African progenitor or dead end?', *Journal of Human Evolution* 39, 393–410.

Irish, J. D. 2005: 'Population continuity vs. discontinuity revisited: dental affinities among late Paleolithic through Christian-era Nubians', *American Journal of Physical Anthropology* 128, 520–35.

Irish, J. D and Turner II, C. G. 1990: 'West African dental affinity of Late Pleistocene Nubians: peopling of the Eurafrican-South Asian triangle II', *Homo* 41, 42–53.

Johnson, A. L. and Lovell, N. C. 1994: 'Biological differentiation at Predynastic Naqada, Egypt: an analysis of dental morphological traits', *American Journal of Physical Anthropology* 93, 427–33.

Lee, G. T. R. and Goose, D. H. 1972: 'The inheritance of dental traits in a Chinese population in the United Kingdom', *Journal of Medical Genetics* 9, 336–9.

Moyer, C. J. 2005: 'Human burials', 1–17 in I. A. Todd (ed.), *Vasilikos Valley Project 7: Excavations at Kalavasos-Tenta Vol. II* (Studies in Mediterranean Archaeology 71:7), Sävedalen.

Parras, Z. 2004: *The Biological Affinities of the Eastern Mediterranean in the Chalcolithic and Bronze Age: A Regional Dental Non-metric Approach'* (British Archaeological Reports International Series S1305), Oxford.

Parras, Z. 2006: 'Osteological evidence', 53–66 in E. Peltenburg (ed.), *The Chalcolithic Cemetery of Souskiou*-Vathyrkakas, *Cyprus. Investigations of Four Missions from 1950 to 1997*, Nicosia.

Parras, Z. 2008: 'Looking for immigrants at Kissonerga-*Mosphilia* in the Late Chalcolithic: A dental non-metric perspective of Chalcolithic and Early Bronze Age Southwest Cyprus', 63–74 in A. McCarthy (ed.), *Island Dialogues: Proceedings of the Postgraduate Cypriot Archaeology Conference (POCA), 2006*, Edinburgh.

Peltenburg, E. J. (ed.) 2006: *The Chalcolithic Cemetery of Souskiou*-Vathyrkakas, *Cyprus. Investigations of Four Missions from 1950 to 1997*, Nicosia.

Peltenburg, E. J. *et al.* 1985: *Lemba Archaeological Project Vol. 1: Excavations at Lemba* Lakkous, *1976–1983* (Studies in Mediterranean Archaeology 70:1), Göteborg.

Peltenburg, E. J. *et al.* 1998: *Lemba Archaeological Project Volume II.1A: Excavations at Kissonerga*-Mosphilia, *1979–1992* (Studies in Mediterranean Archaeology 70:2), Jonsered.

Peltenburg, E. J., Croft, P., Jackson, A., McCartney, C and Murray, M. 2001: 'Well-established colonists: *Mylouthkia* 1 and the Cypro-Pre-Pottery Neolithic B', 61–93 in S. Swiny (ed), *The Earliest Prehistory of Cyprus: From Colonization to Exploitation*, Boston.

Peltenburg, E. J. *et al.* 2003: *Lemba Archaeological Project III.1 The colonisaion and settlement of Cyprus: Investigations at Kissonerga-Mylouthkia 1976–1996* (Studies in Mediterranean Archaeology 70:4), Jonsered.

Rupp, D. W., Fox, S. C., Herscher, E., McClellan, M. C., Clarke, J. T., D'Annibale, C., Gregory, T. E. and Critchley, J. 1999: 'Prastio: Agios Savvas tis Karonis Monastery (Paphos District, Cyprus): 1994–1995 field season and 1992–1995 artifact analysis', *Bulletin of the American Schools of Oriental Research* 316, 23–88.

Rupp, D. W. and D'Annibale, C. 1995: 'Preliminary report of the 1994 field season of the Western Cyprus Project at Prastio-Agios Savvas tis Karonis Monastery (Paphos District)', *Report of the Department of Antiquities, Cyprus*, 33–48.

Scott, G. R. and Dahlberg, A. 1982: 'Microdifferentiation in tooth crown morphology among Indians of the American southwest', 259–91 in B. Kurtén (ed.), *Teeth: Form, Function, and Evolution*, New York.

Scott, G. R. and Turner II, G. C. 1997: '*The Anthropology of Modern Human Teeth: Dental Morphology and its Variation in Recent Human Populations*, Cambridge.

Simmons, A. H. 1994: 'Early Neolithic settlement in Western Cyprus: preliminary report on the 1992–1993 test excavations at Kholetria *Ortos*', *Bulletin of the American Schools of Oriental Research* 295, 1–14.

Simmons, A. H. 1996: 'Preliminary report on multidisciplinary investigation at Neolithic Kholetria-*Ortos,* Paphos District', *Report of the Department of Antiquities, Cyprus*, 29–44.

Simmons, A. H. 2003: 'Villages without walls, cows without corals', 61–70 in J. Guilaine and A. Le Brun (eds), *Le Néolithique de Chypre. Actes du colloque international organisé par le Département des Antiquités de Chypre et l'École française d'Athènes Nicosie 17–19 Mai 2001* (Bulletin de Correspondance hellénique Supplément 43), Athens.

Stanley Price, N. P. 1977: 'Colonization and continuity in the early prehistory of Cyprus', *World Archaeology* 9(1), 27–41.

Steel, L. 2004: *Cyprus Before History. From the Earliest Settlers to the End of the Bronze Age*, London.

Stringer, C. B., Humphrey, L. T. and Compton, T. 1997: 'Cladistic analysis of dental traits in recent humans using a fossil outgroup', *Journal of Human Evolution* 32, 389–402.

Todd, I. A. 1989, 'Early prehistoric society: a view from the Vasilikos valley', 2–13 in E. Peltenburg (ed.), *Early Society in Cyprus*, Edinburgh.

Todd, I. A. (ed.) 2005: *Vasilikos Valley Project 7: Excavations at Kalavasos*-Tenta *Vol. II* (Studies in Mediterranean Archaeology 71:7), Sävedalen.

Turner II, C. G. 1979: 'Dental anthropological indications of agriculture among the Jomon people of central Japan: X. Peopling of the Pacific', *American Journal of Physical Anthropology* 51, 619–35.

Turner II, C. G. 1985: 'Expression count: A method for calculating morphological dental trait frequencies by using adjustable weighting coefficients with standard ranked scales', *American Journal of Physical Anthropology* 68, 263–7.

Turner II, C. G. 1986: 'Dentochronological separation estimates for Pacific Rim populations', *Science* 232, 1140–2.

Turner II, C. G. 1987: 'Late Pleistocene and Holocene population history of East Asia based on dental variation', *American Journal of Physical Anthropology* 73, 305–21.

Turner II, C. G., and Markowitz, M. A. 1990: 'Dental discontinuity between Late Pleistocene and recent Nubians: peopling of the Eurafrican-South Asian triangle I', *Homo* 41, 32–41.

Turner II, C. G., Nichol, C. R. and Scott, G. R. 1991: 'Scoring procedure for key morphological traits of the permanent dentition: The Arizona State University Dental Anthropology System', 13–31 in M. A. Kelly and C. S. Larsen (eds), *Advances in Dental Anthropology*, New York.

Turner II, C. G. and Swindler, D. R. 1978: 'The dentition of New Britain West Nakanai Melanesians', *American Journal of Physical Anthropology* 49, 361–72.

Ullinger, J. M., Sheridan, S. G., Hawkey, D. E., Turner II, C. G. and Cooley, R. 2005: 'Bioarchaeological analysis of cultural transition in the southern Levant using dental nonmetric traits', *American Journal of Physical Anthropology* 128, 466–76.

Vigne, J.-D., Carrère, I., Saliége, J.-F., Person, A., Bcherens, H., Guilaine, J. and Briois, J. F. 2000: 'Predomestic cattle, sheep, goat and pig during the late 9th and the 8th millennium Cal. BC on Cyprus: Preliminary results of Shillourokambos (Parekklisha, Limassol)', 83–106 in M. Mashkour, A. M. Choyke, H. Buitenhuis and F. Poplin (eds), *Archaeozoology of the Near East IV A: Proceedings of the fourth international symposium on the archaeozoology of southwestern Asia and adjacent areas,* Groningen.

31. Ante-mortem Tooth Loss in Chalcolithic Populations of Cyprus: Comparisons between Cemetery and Settlement

Kirsi O. Lorentz

*This paper aims to further the understanding of human health and disease in prehistoric Cyprus through a focus on the dental health of Chalcolithic populations. In particular, anti-mortem tooth loss was systematically assessed in the human skeletal series excavated from the Middle Chalcolithic cemetery site of Souskiou-*Laona*, where 137 tombs containing both intact and disturbed burial contexts, with several primary and secondary inhumations in each tomb, were excavated in 2001–2006. The results were compared to anti-mortem tooth loss (AMTL) within skeletal series from the contemporary Souskiou-*Vathyrkakas *cemeteries, as well as from the Chalcolithic settlement sites in Western Cyprus.*

Introduction

Our sources for understanding pre-Bronze Age Cyprus are currently largely confined to settlement sites. In contrast, information for the succeeding Early and Middle Bronze Age until now comes almost exclusively from extra-mural cemeteries. The four discrete Middle Chalcolithic cemeteries 2.5 km inland from Palaepaphos (southwest Cyprus) form an exception to this general limitation on our reconstructions. Two of these cemeteries have been extensively looted, and subsequently excavated without proper recording and recovery of human skeletal remains, while one of these cemeteries remains unexcavated. The fourth cemetery site, Souskiou-*Laona*, is the only scientifically excavated extramural Chalcolithic cemetery on the whole island of Cyprus, and the only one with detailed physical anthropological recording and analysis of the skeletal population both in the field and in the laboratory (on-going). In this paper the skeletal population from this unique site, crucial for the understanding of the Chalcolithic populations on the island, is compared with what is known of the other, incompletely recorded Chalcolithic skeletal populations. This paper uses data collected first-hand from the skeletal series in Souskiou-*Laona*, and published skeletal reports on three further Chalcolithic sites.

The aim of this paper is to investigate possible differences in palaeopathology between populations buried in the settlements, and those buried in the cemeteries. Due to the constraints imposed by poor recovery and limited publication of the settlement sites on investigating postcranial skeletal pathologies, as well as dental pathologies, ante-mortem tooth loss (see, for example Fig. 31.12) is focused on here. Questions such as 'what is the prevalence of ante-mortem tooth loss (AMTL) within Chalcolithic populations in Cyprus?' and 'are there differences or similarities in AMTL between settlement and cemetery populations during the Chalcolithic?' will be addressed.

Materials and methods

This paper compares palaeopathological data from two settlement sites (Lemba-*Lakkous*, Kissonerga-*Mosphilia*), and two cemetery sites (Souskiou-*Laona*, Souskiou-*Vathyrkakas*). The sites are located in Western Cyprus. There are no other known Chalcolithic mortuary populations of substantial size from the island.

MNI (minimum number of individuals)

Souskiou-*Vathyrkakas* has been extensively looted and rather poorly excavated during the years, and thus it has been possible to establish only an overall MNI (minimum number of individuals) for the site: MNI for subadults is *c.* 69; MNI for adults *c.* 112–31; juveniles form 34–38% of Souskiou-*Vathyrkakas* population. Total MNI for the site is thus *c.* 181– 200.

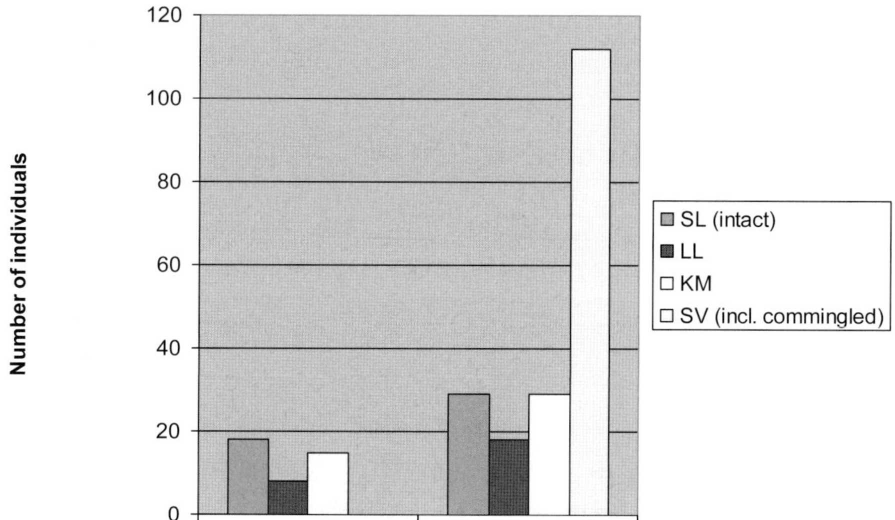

	adults/adolescents (>13 yrs) with sufficient dental data	Total adults/adolescents (>13 yrs)
SL (intact)	18	29
LL	8	18
KM	15	29
SV (incl. commingled)	0	112

Fig. 31.1. Number of adult/adolescent individuals (>13 years) with sufficient dental data for inclusion in the analysis of AMTL by tooth type in comparison with the total number of adult/adolescent individuals recovered from Souskiou-*Laona*, Lemba-*Lakkous*, Kissonerga-*Mosphilia* and Souskiou-*Vathyrkakas*

As to Lemba-*Lakkous*, Lunt writes: 'From the evidence of the dentition, there would appear to be 31 children' (Lunt 1985, 245). An additional three children have been identified from cranial fragments. Twenty-five of these died between birth and 6 years of age. Additionally, there are four adolescents between 14 and 18 years of age, and 14 adults (20 or over). This makes the total number of individuals from Lemba-*Lakkous* 52.

The site of Kissonerga-*Mosphilia* 'yielded a mortuary population of 77 individuals from interments, or 89 including identifiable internments outside facilities' (Lunt and Watt 1998, 101). There are 47 subadult individuals between birth and 12.9 years, six adolescents between 13 and 20 years of age, and 23 adults over 20 years of age (Lunt and Watt 1998, 83, table 4.8).

The analysis of the Souskiou-*Laona* population is on-going, and the final MNI estimate for the site will take into account all skeletal material found on the site, retrieved from the following find contexts: articulated intact primary inhumations, disarticulated secondary bone stacks, commingled remains from looters spoil. The cemetery has been extensively looted in the past; however, the excavated tombs on the site have yielded 29 intact individuals. Of these 29 individuals, 18 have jaw bones or jaw bone fragments accessible for analysis. It should be noted that the analysis for the Souskiou-*Laona* skeletal remains is on-going (by the author), and only the intact articulated individuals recovered from the site are included within this analysis. These 29 intact adult individuals retrieved from Souskiou-*Laona* so far, represent a significant addition to the Chalcolithic skeletal series, given that there are only 14 adults from Lemba-*Lakkous*, and 23 adults from Kissonerga-*Mosphilia*. Figure 31.1 shows the age distribution on the sites. Note the higher prevalence of subadults under the age of 13 in the settlement sites (Lemba-*Lakkous* and Kissonerga-*Mosphlia*).

A fully comprehensive palaeopathological analysis takes into account both dental and skeletal pathologies. Unfortunately, there has been a tradition of publishing only the dental remains from Chalcolithic sites (Lunt 1985; Lunt and Watt 1998). This is likely due to the perceived poor preservation on the Chalcolithic sites. However, with appropriate excavation and recovery strategies and careful analysis in the laboratory it is possible to recover data on pathologies of the postcranial skeleton also, even on the Cypriot Chalcolithic populations where the frequently poor state of preservation forms a major obstacle. Material from Souskiou-*Laona* demonstrates this potential. This is all the

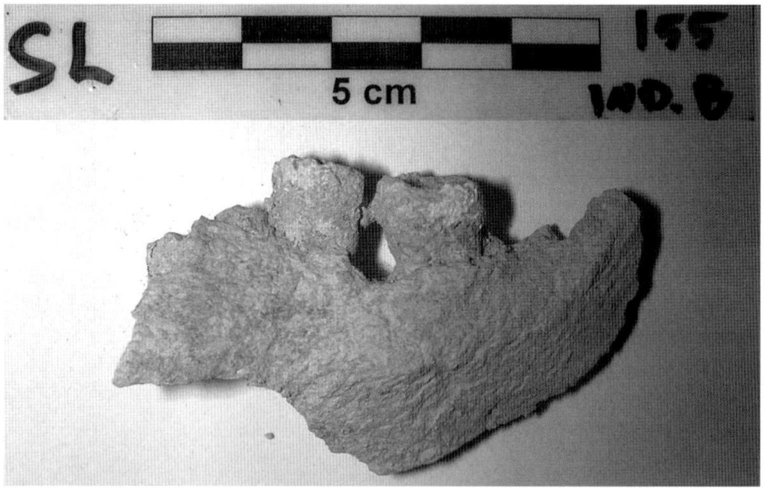

Fig. 31.2. Mandible fragment, Souskiou-*Laona* Tomb 155, Individual B. Note the poor preservation status of the enamel (photograph by K. O. Lorentz)

more important, as these poorly preserved skeletal series are all we have – they form our only window to Chalcolithic populations on the island of Cyprus.

AMTL was recorded when a tooth socket showed evidence of alveolar bone absorption (remodelling) (after Eshed, Gopher and Hershkovitz 2006; Frayer 1989; Ortner and Putschar 1985). Frequencies were calculated based on the number of teeth affected. Eshed, Gopher and Hershkovitz recently published an article (2006) where they advocate the use of simple and robust methods for recording AMTL and other dental pathologies, in order to maximise sample size while minimising inter-observer error. The more comprehensive classification schemes for alveolar bone loss, *e.g.* by Karn *et al.* (1984) and Kerr (1991) could not be used due to poor preservation of the Chalcolithic alveolae. Karn *et al.* (1984) devised a comprehensive classification scheme for vertical bone loss in the alveolae due to periodontal disease. Kerr (1991) developed a scoring scheme for the thinning of cortical bone at the crest of the approximal wall, another change in early periodontitis. Unfortunately, the poor preservation of the Chalcolithic skeletal material does not allow these types of assessment.

AMTL within the Souskiou-*Laona* skeletal series was observed first hand, while data for Lemba-*Lakkous* and Kissonerga-*Mosphilia* were tabulated from published reports, where available. It should be noted, however, that due to missing data, the larger percentages for AMTL at Lemba-*Lakkous* and Kissonerga-*Mosphilia* may not be fully reliable. For Souskiou-*Vathyrkakas* there are no data available by tooth type.

The major limitation of the current study is the inability to introduce two important factors to our analysis: sex and age. Due to the fragmentary nature of the material, the number of adults that could be accurately sexed and aged is too small for proper statistical analysis. Only qualitative data can be provided here. Both males and females suffered from AMTL. In no series did any individual younger than 16–18 years of age display AMTL, and the only adolescent displaying AMTL (at Lemba-*Lakkous*) displays extensive caries lesions, leading Lunt (1985, 152) to state that AMTL in this young individual is likely due to extensive caries rather than periodontal disease.

Preservation

Poor preservation status of the Chalcolithic human remains has been perceived as one of the main hindrances for palaeopathological studies. Very few palaeopathological analyses have been conducted, and published reports mostly concentrate on the dentition. Therefore, a brief look at the preservation status is needed here.

With a few exceptions, the bones from these Cypriot Chalcolithic sites were in poor condition. They were extremely brittle and fragile, and in many cases had disintegrated in the soil. Some elements were encased in a hard, concreted layer of soil, especially near the bottom of the rock-cut burial features. Even apparently complete elements had disintegrated within the soil into small fragments. The teeth were also in rather poor condition (Fig. 31.2). In most specimens there was evidence of post-mortem destruction of enamel, resulting in a chalky appearance of the enamel, and, in more advanced cases, a loss of surface enamel which varied in severity from a slight pitting of the surface to severe erosion in which loss was sufficient to remove minor morphological features and render measurements of the tooth inaccurate. This post-mortem erosion has destroyed the finer surface features of the teeth in some cases (Fig. 31.2). In many cases alveolae show extensive

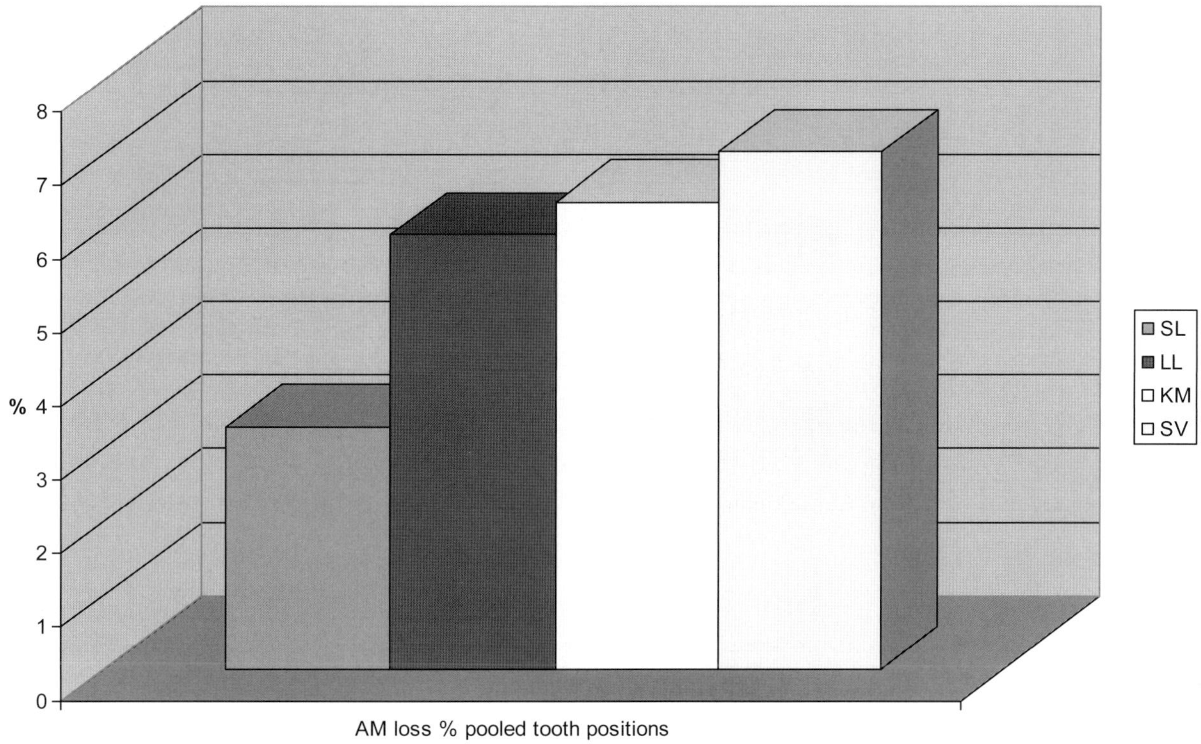

Fig. 31.3. Overall AMTL percentage by pooled tooth positions at Souskiou-*Laona*, Lemba-*Lakkous*, Kissonerga-*Mosphilia* and Souskiou-*Vathyrkakas*

post-mortem damage. In comparison with Lemba-*Lakkous* and Kissonerga-*Mosphilia*, the Souskiou-*Laona* dentitions tended to be in overall poorer state of preservation.

In Souskiou-*Vathyrkakas*, by far the most poorly preserved skeletal series, there were no intact mandibles, and '[t]here were [indeed] relatively few jaw fragments in the Souskiou-*Vathyrkakas* material: compared to a total of 1351 erupted permanent teeth, there were only 417 tooth sockets in jaw fragments, and relatively few of these had the tooth *in situ'* (Parras 2006, 50). Some alveolae have partly survived allowing some assessment of AMTL, but almost no postcranial elements remain in sufficiently good preservation status to allow analysis, having suffered taphonomic and chemical degradation, damage through excavation and ravages by rodents and insects in their current storage area.

Bone preservation is equally poor on cemetery sites as on settlement sites, if not even poorer on cemetery sites where the combined effects of looting and taphonomic processes have taken their toll. What differs between the sites, however, are the standards of recovery, curation and analysis of skeletal remains affecting the potential for comparative palaeopathological analysis. At Lemba-*Lakkous*, Kissonerga-*Mosphilia* and Souskiou-*Vathyrkakas* skeletal remains were excavated and recovered by individuals most often not trained in physical anthropology, resulting in fresh breakages, and considerable loss of bone elements and surface detail. The continuous presence of physical anthropologists on site in Souskiou-*Laona* is a significant step forward for palaeopathological research in Cyprus.

It should be noted that this paper is not advocating making detailed palaeopathological analysis and attempting detailed palaeopathological inferences on poorly preserved skeletal material where better preserved representative skeletal series are present, but given the unique nature, and particularly the great importance of these Chalcolithic populations to the understanding of Cypriot prehistory, it is important that all available remains are analysed with the highest resolution possible. This requires care both in the field and in the laboratory, as well as, at times, using the less complicated/detailed recording schemes to ensure compatibility of data.

Results: ante-mortem tooth loss (AMTL) at Souskiou-*Laona*

An overall AMTL rate for the Chalcolithic Cypriot populations ranges between 3% and *c*. 7% (Fig. 31.3). Figure 31.1 shows the number of adult/adolescent individuals recovered from each Chalcolithic site included within this study, as well as those included in the analysis of AMTL by tooth type. Only individuals over the age of 13 were included in the comparative analysis – none of the younger subadults showed any signs of AMTL. Other inclusion

Sample size by tooth type

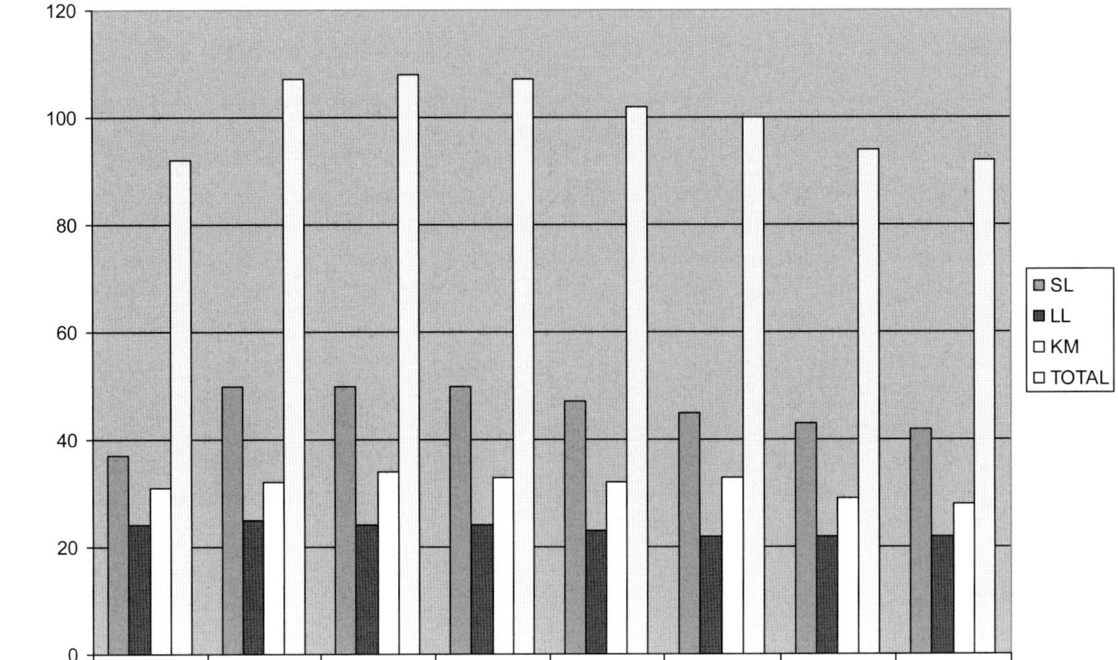

	M3	M2	M1	PM2	PM1	C	I2	I1
SL	37	50	50	50	47	45	43	42
LL	24	25	24	24	23	22	22	22
KM	31	32	34	33	32	33	29	28
TOTAL	92	107	108	107	102	100	94	92

TOOTH TYPE

Fig. 31.4. Sample size by tooth type; Souskiou-*Laona*, Lemba-*Lakkous*, Kissonerga-*Mosphilia* and Souskiou-*Vathyrkakas* populations

criteria were the presence of alveoli (all sites) and, where relevant, the sufficient detail of published data.

Due to poor excavation and recovery strategies none of the material from Souskiou-*Vathyrkakas* fills these criteria. The only data available from Souskiou-*Vathyrkakas* is by pooled tooth positions (Fig. 31.3). These kinds of data are necessarily very general and somewhat misleading given that different tooth positions are differentially affected by the various underlying causes of ante-mortem tooth loss (most commonly periodontal disease or caries). Thus, detailed data by tooth type are required.

One advantage of exploring AMTL by tooth type here is that this produces a more evenly distributed sample size (Fig. 31.4). The chart in Figure 31.5 shows AMTL by tooth type in Souskiou-*Laona*, Lemba-*Lakkous*, and Kissonerga-*Mosphilia*. AMTL concentrates exclusively on the molars and premolars. Further, highest rates of AMTL seem to occur in the first molar, a tendency that is confirmed by pooled data for the Chalcolithic (Fig. 31.6). The second most affected tooth type is the second molar.

There are differences in the areas affected between the populations: Kissonerga-*Mosphilia* shows the widest range of tooth positions affected, including both premolars and all three molars, while in Lemba-*Lakkous* AMTL has affected the molars only. In Souskiou-*Laona* AMTL is limited to the first molar and the teeth immediately adjacent to it (M2 and PM2). To explore this pattern further, AMTL was explored by jaw and tooth type.

The chart in Figure 31.7 shows how AMTL is distributed in the maxilla and mandible. It seems that in the maxilla the M1 and PM2 are most often affected, while it is the M1 and M2 that are most often affected in the mandible (these teeth are in occlusion with each other in normal dentitions). The pooled data for the Chalcolithic confirms this. Eshed, Golpher and Hershkovitz (2006, 153) found a more evenly distributed pattern in the maxilla in Natufian and Neolithic populations of the Levant.

This pattern is also visible when the cemetery population is compared with the settlement populations (Fig. 31.8). This chart also shows that while in the cemetery population AMTL is limited to two teeth on each side, in the settlement populations a full range of premolars and molars are affected.

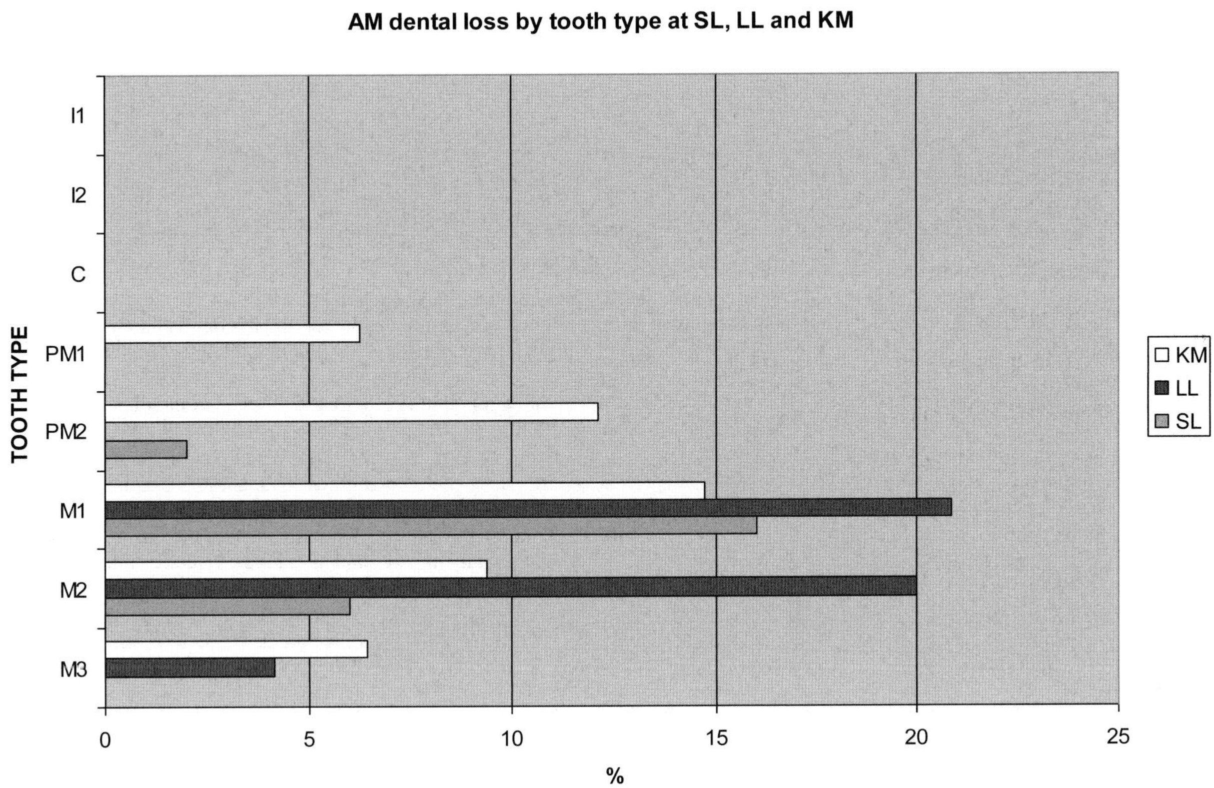

Fig. 31.5. AMTL by tooth type at Souskiou-*Laona*, Lemba-*Lakkous* and Kissonerga-*Mosphilia*

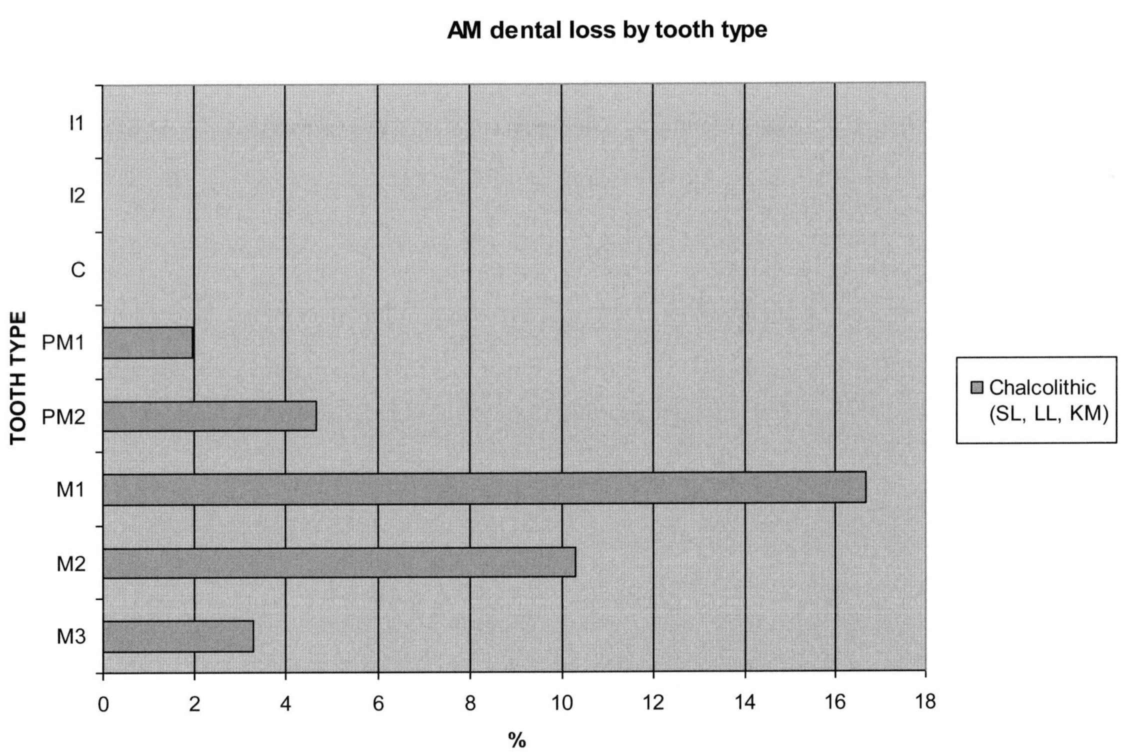

Fig. 31.6. Pooled data for AMTL by tooth type in Chalcolithic Cypriot populations (pooled data includes data from Souskiou-*Laona*, Lemba-*Lakkous* and Kissonerga-*Mosphilia*)

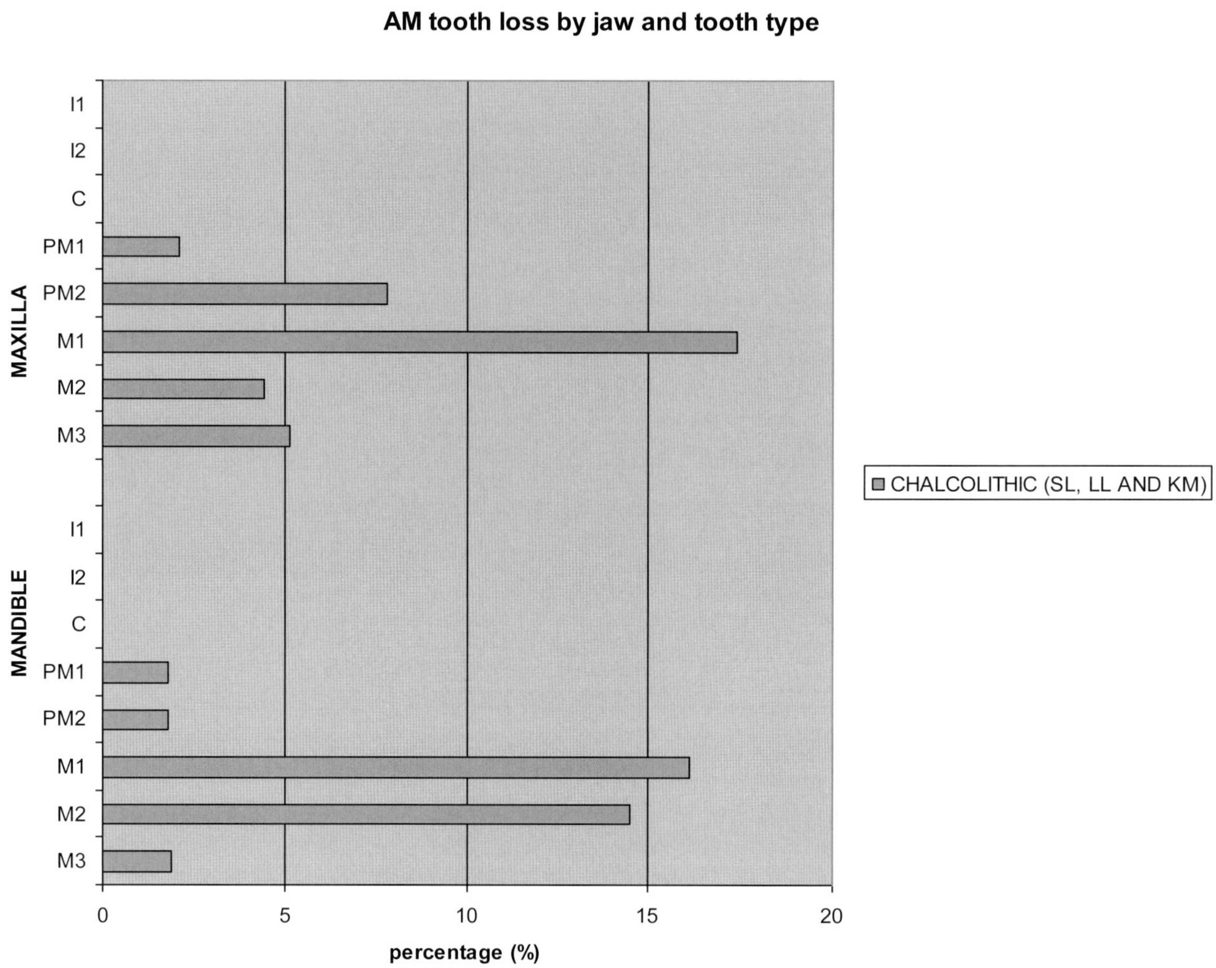

Fig. 31.7. Pooled data for AMTL by jaw and tooth type in Chalcolithic Cypriot populations (pooled data includes data from Souskiou-*Laona*, Lemba-*Lakkous* and Kissonerga-*Mosphilia*)

AMTL due to periodontal disease is usually symmetrical (Hillson 2005, 304–7, 311–3). In order to investigate the patterning as to side, data by jaw, side and tooth type were produced (Fig. 31.9). There are no significant differences in the Souskiou-*Laona* data. Pooled data for the Chalcolithic confirm this (Fig. 31.10).

Discussion: common causes of ante-mortem tooth loss

Periodontal disease and caries are two major factors associated with tooth loss in archaeological populations (Clarke and Hirsch 1991; Hillson 1986; Backett and Lovell 1994; Cook 1984; Lukacs 1992). Quantifying rates of caries and periodontal changes would thus be needed in order to be able to investigate possible causes of AMTL in the Cypriot Chalcolithic. However, no systematic data on periodontal changes by tooth type from Lemba-*Lakkous*, Kissonerga-*Mosphilia* or Souskiou-*Vathyrkakas* have been published. Pooled data on caries occurrence is available, but poor preservation status of some of the crowns may affect the results. The relatively low rates of caries in all series may preclude caries as a major cause of AMTL in the Chalcolithic.

Comparative material in sufficient detail on AMTL in contemporary skeletal series is hard to come by. Thus only general remarks on skeletal series from surrounding regions are made here. Eshed, Gopher and Hershkovitz (2006, 150) found relatively low AMTL rates for the Natufian and Neolithic populations in the southern Levant (mandible: Natufian 3.7%, Neolithic 4.5%; maxilla: Natufian 2%, Neolithic 0.6%) in connection with low rates of periodontal disease and caries. They attribute this to the scarcity of sticky foodstuffs in the diet of these hunter-gatherer and early agricultural populations. They found that the Natufians lost significantly more anterior teeth (incisors and canine) than did the Neolithic populations, while AMTL in the lower

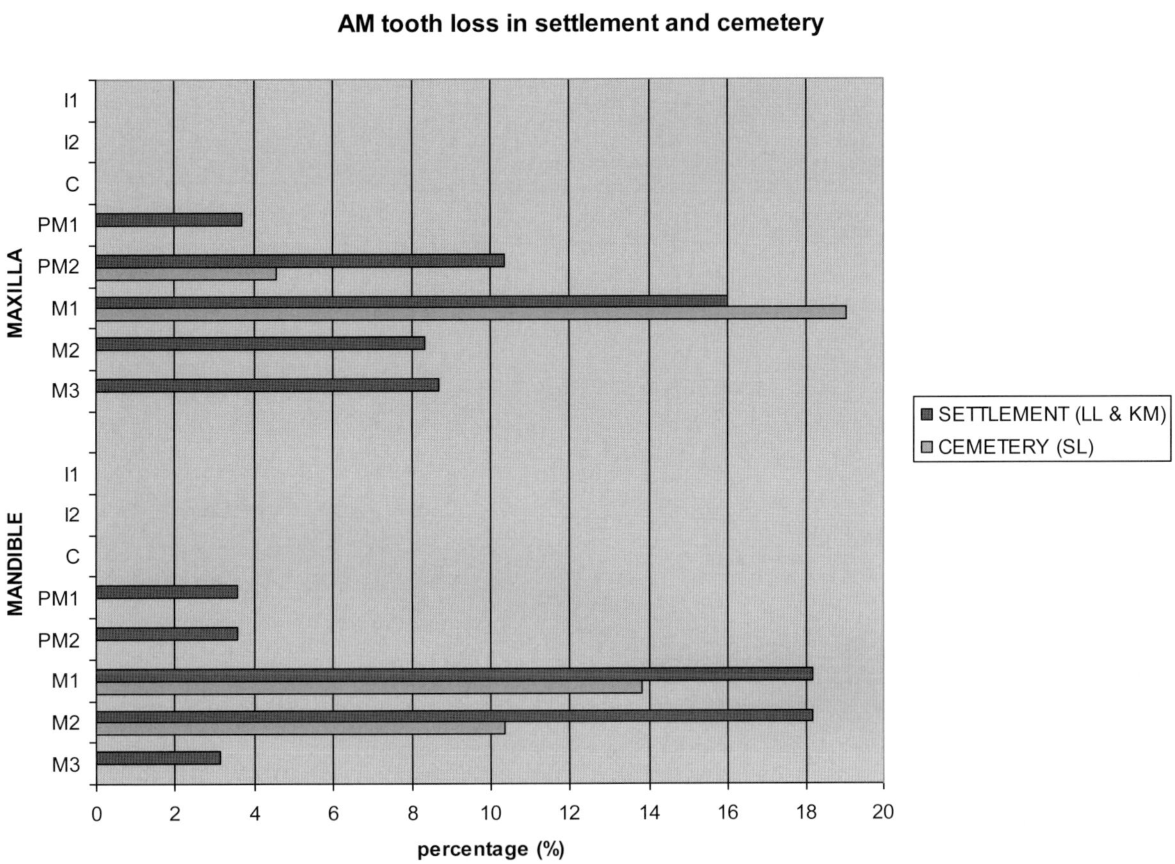

Fig. 31.8. AMTL by jaw and tooth type in cemetery (Souskiou-*Laona*) and settlement (Lemba-*Lakkous,* Kissonerga-*Mosphilia*) populations

molars were more common in the Neolithic population, being especially so in the first molar, where the rate for the Neolithic was double compared to that of the Natufian (14.1% vs. 6.1% respectively). As no anterior teeth were affected by AMTL in the Chalcolithic series, and the AMTL clearly concentrates on the M1 area, it may be said that AMTL pattern in Chalcolithic Cyprus is more similar to the Neolithic rather than the Natufian pattern. This is consistent with the suspected similarities in nutrition and food related practices.

As to modern populations in the Eastern Mediterranean region, Sayegh *et al.* (2004, 125–6) found that the reasons for tooth loss in disadvantaged Jordanians with limited access to dental care *(N=2200;* study over four years; 3069 teeth lost) included, in the order of magnitude, caries (46.9%), periodontal disease (18%), combination of caries and periodontal disease (8%), preprosthetic reasons (19.4%), orthodontic reasons (4%), eruption problems (2.8%), and trauma (0.7%).

As to periodontal changes in the Chalcolithic populations, periodontal pockets, shallow sockets and visible reduction of alveolar height were observed in some specimens in all the series, though poor preservation status precludes detailed statistical analysis. The general pattern of AMTL at these Chalcolithic series is, however, consistent with AMTL pattern due to periodontal disease as detailed by Hillson 1996.

Shahr-i Sokhta

When the AMTL rates and locations within the Cypriot Chalcolithic series are compared for example with the roughly contemporary, 3rd millennium BC material from Shahr-i Sokhta, Iran (Lorentz 2007; 2008), the differences in AMTL patterns and dental wear are poignant. The overall AMTL rate within a sample of the extensive Shahr-i Sokhta skeletal series is very high: 15% of all tooth positions (N=974) are affected.[1] Further, the AMTL rate for incisors (9% for central incisors and 8% for lateral incisors) and canines (5%) within the Shahr-i Sokhta sample is very high. It is notable that within the Cypriot Chalcolithic series there is no involvement of these anterior teeth in terms of AMTL. While AMTL due to periodontal disease is usually symmetrical (Hillson 2005, 304–7, 311–3, and most often initially affects molars and premolars, AMTL in individual dentitions at Shahr-i Sokhta is often asymmetrical, and in

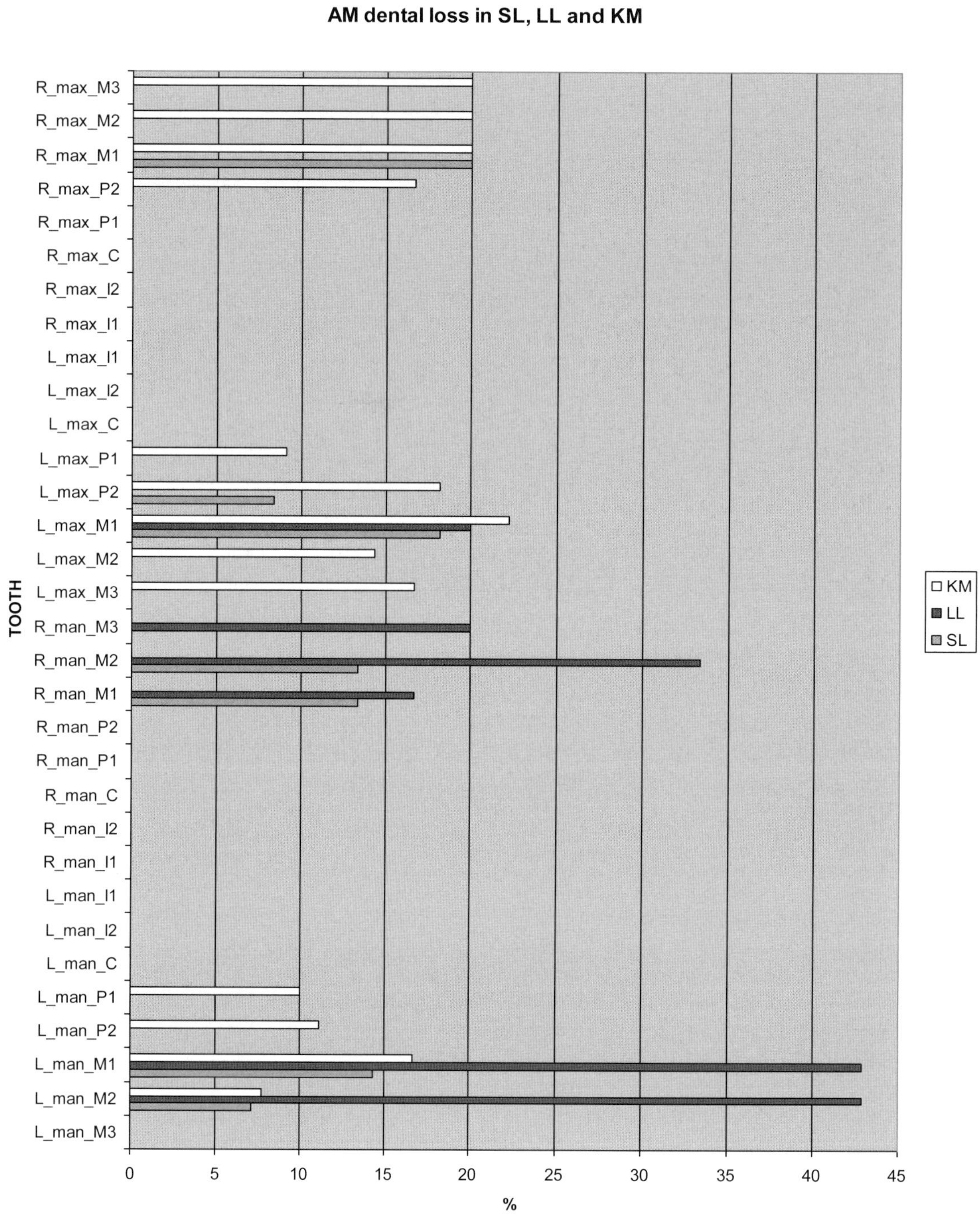

Fig. 31.9. AMTL by jaw, side and tooth type in Souskiou-*Laona*, Lemba-*Lakkous* and Kissonerga-*Mosphilia*

some cases involves only the incisors and canines. Caries does not seem to be a major cause of AMTL at Shahr-i Sokhta (Lorentz 2007, 324–5; 2008, 324–5). The general pattern of AMTL at this Shahr-i Sokhta sample cannot thus be fully explained by reference to periodontal disease or caries. Several dentitions within the Shahr-i Sokhta sample show dental abrasion that is diffuse and irregular in direction, severity and distribution (Lorentz 2007, 324–5; 2008, 322). The pattern of AMTL and dental wear within the Shahr-i Sokhta skeletal series points to the use of teeth in non-masticatory activities, or as 'a third hand'.

The two skeletal series (Shahr-i Sokhta and Souskiou-

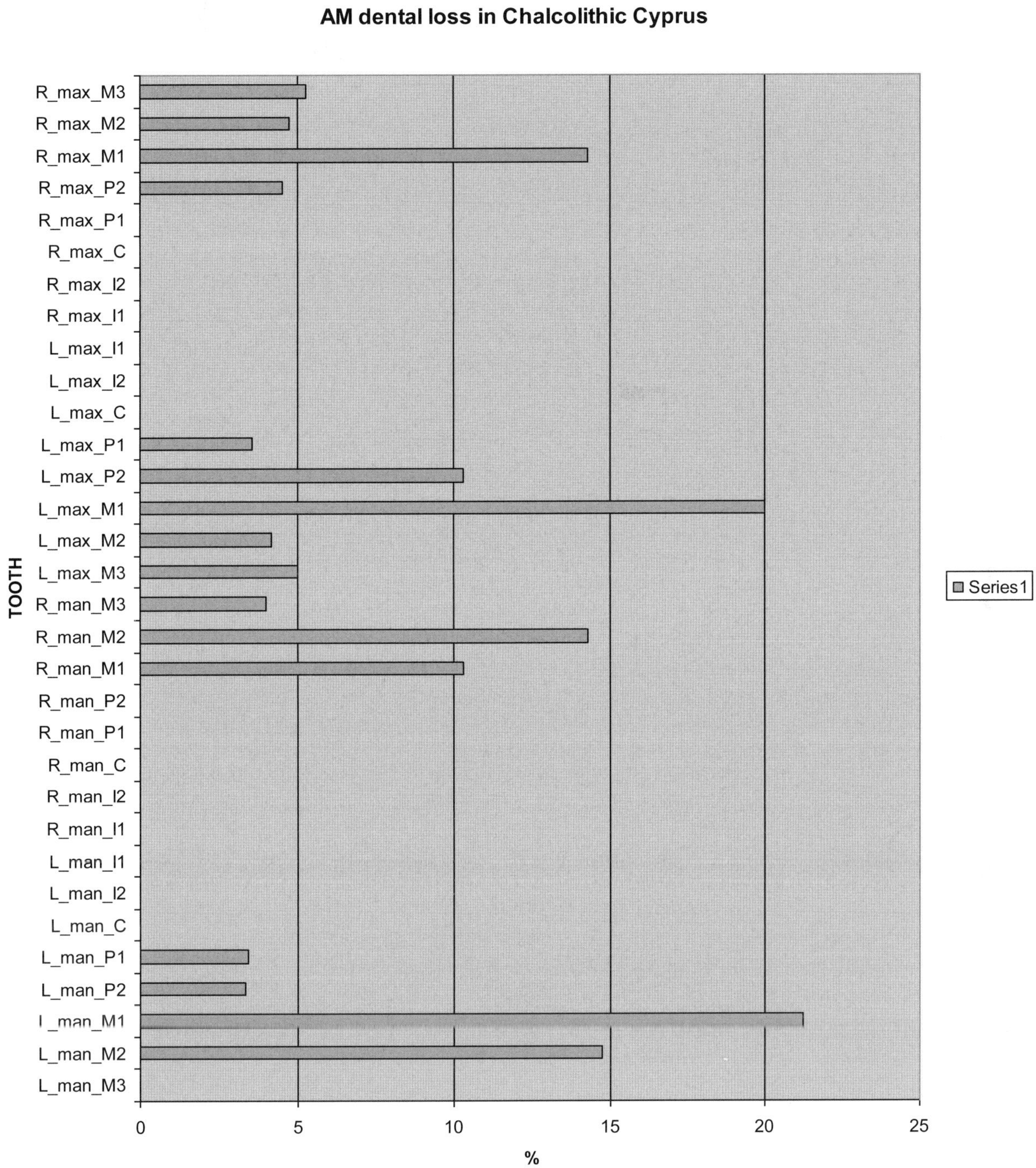

Fig. 31.10. Pooled data for AMTL by jaw, side and tooth type in Chalcolithic Cyprus (pooled data includes data from Souskiou-*Laona*, Lemba-*Lakkous* and Kissonerga-*Mosphilia*)

Laona) thus show very different patterns of AMTL (Fig. 31.11a–b) and dental wear, pointing to differential diagnosis as to the aetiology of these particular patterns. The patterning of AMTL and dental wear within the Chalcolithic Cypriot series is consistent with periodontal disease and normal masticatory use of dentition, respectively, while the patterning of AMTL and dental wear within the Iranian Shahr-i Sokhta series is consistent with the use of teeth as tools – something that is supported by rich contextual evidence for large-scale craft activities on the site, ranging from basketry to bead manufacture.[2]

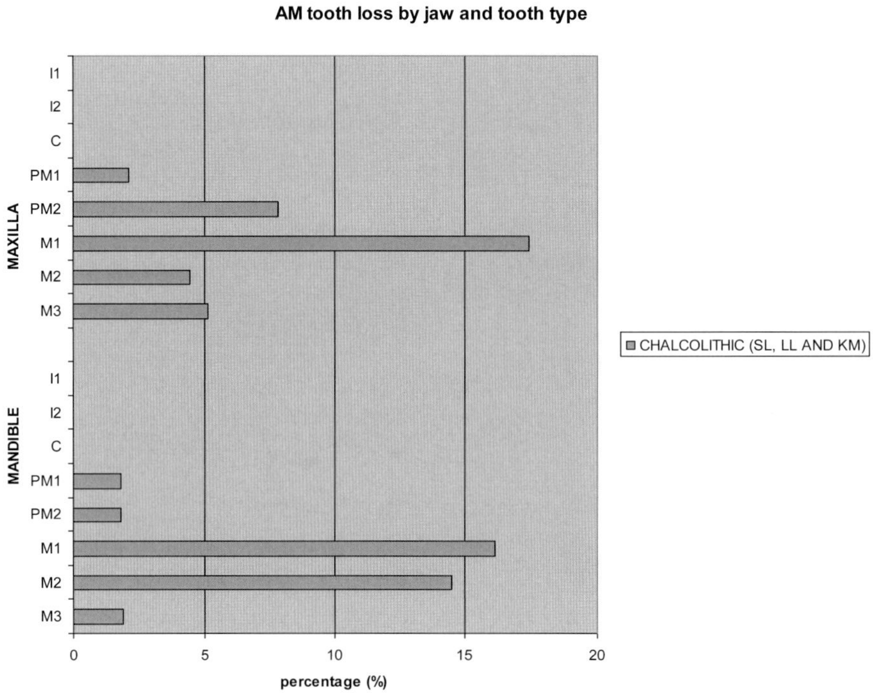

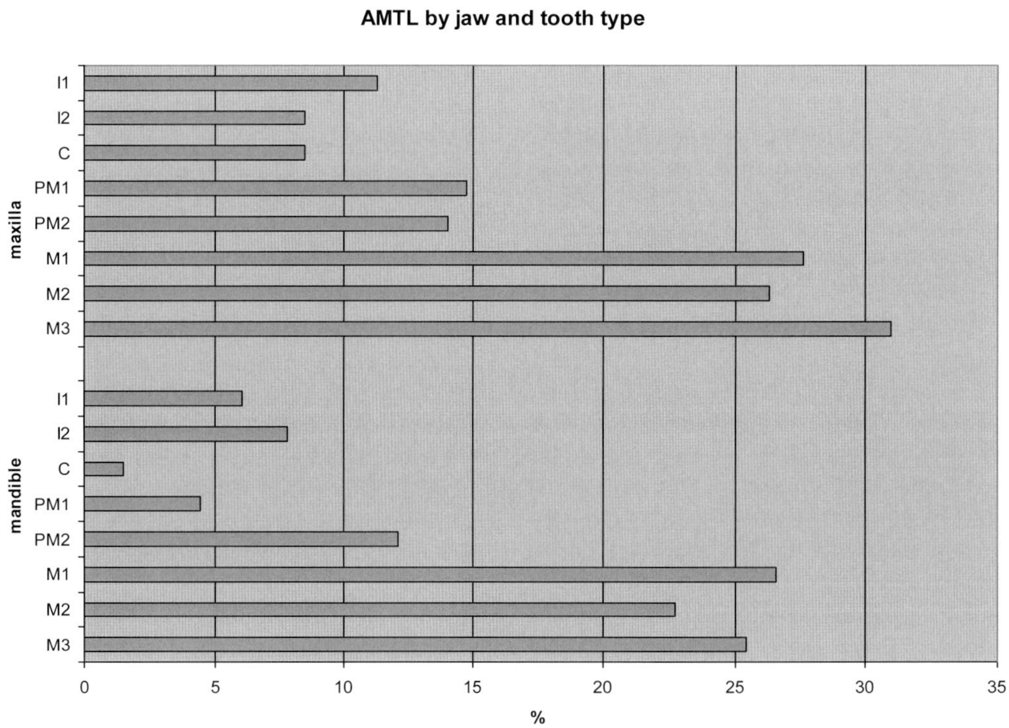

Fig. 31.11. AMTL by jaw and tooth-type in (a) Chalcolithic Cyprus; at (b) Shahr-i Sokhta

Conclusion

The overall AMTL rate in pooled tooth positions in Cypriot Chalcolithic (all four sites) is 5.6%.[3] Symmetrical bilateral ante-mortem tooth loss occurs in both the cemetery and settlement populations, although in cemetery populations the area affected is more limited (the first molar and adjacent teeth; Fig. 31.12). While in the cemetery population AMTL is limited to two teeth on each side, in the settlement populations a full range of premolars and molars are affected. This may indicate differences in the extent of

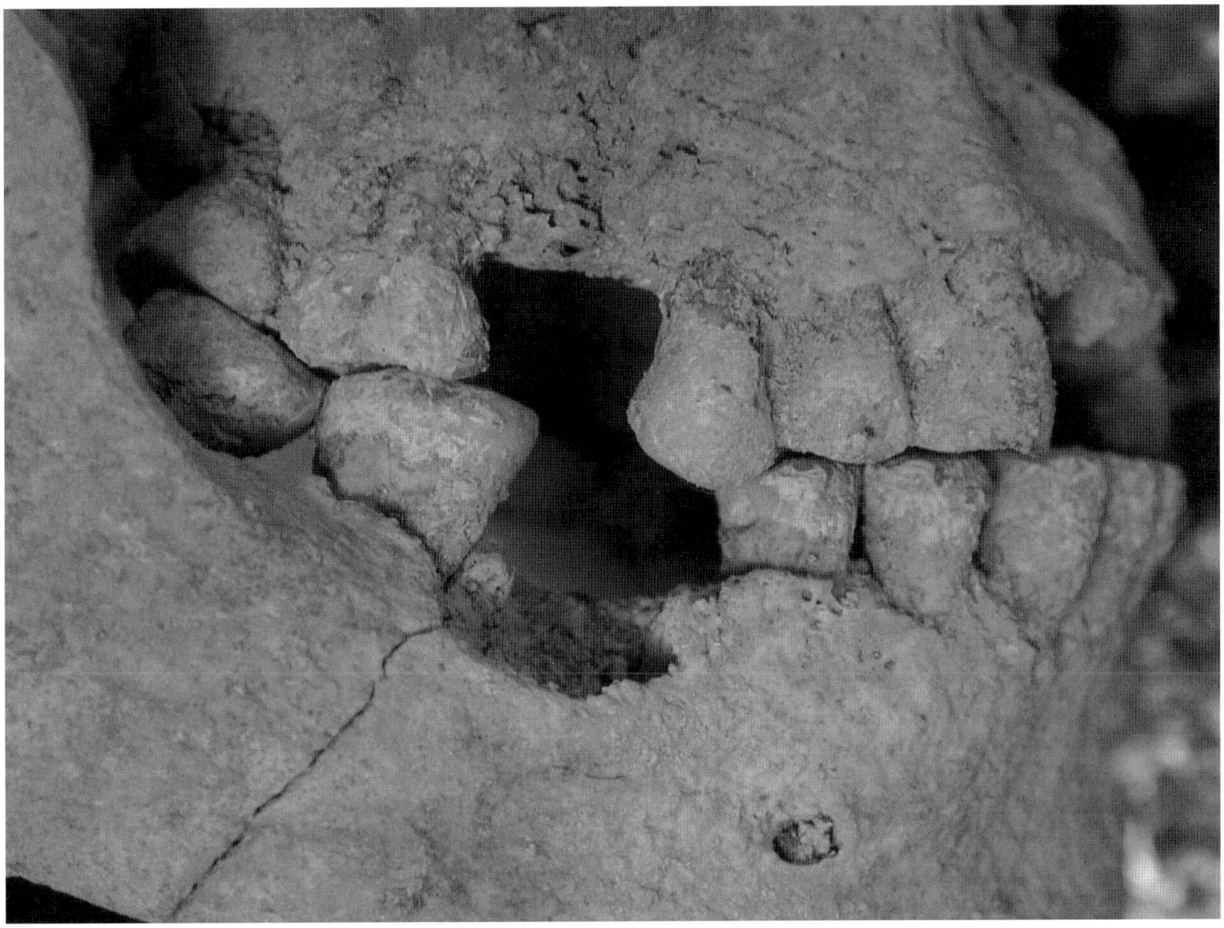

Fig. 31.12. Souskiou-*Laona* Tomb 200, Individual D. Note the AMTL, and alveolar remodeling at different stages in the maxilla and the mandible (photograph by Lorentz)

periodontal disease, or differences in age profiles of the populations. Unfortunately, the sample sizes and lack of published detail preclude a detailed analysis by age or sex here.

Postcranial pathologies at Souskiou-*Laona* include fractures both in upper and lower extremities. The skeletal population of Souskiou-*Laona* is so far the only skeletal population from Chalcolithic Cyprus that has been recovered fully, and thus the only one that allows analyses according to current palaeopathological standards. Souskiou-*Laona* thus holds an important position both in terms of the light it throws on pre-Bronze Age populations in Cyprus, and in terms of illustrating the potential for palaeopathological analyses on skeletal series where preservation is less than ideal, but recovery is systematic and complete.

There is still a large amount of very basic recording to be carried out on ante-mortem tooth loss in archaeological material, and the major challenge is to standardise recording, also in poorly preserved remains, using systems with sufficient detail as to tooth type and position, so that broader comparisons on ante-mortem tooth loss can be made.

In summary, until now, investigation of the Chalcolithic populations of Cyprus has been somewhat limited: for example only dental analyses have been published from Kissonerga-*Mosphilia* and Lemba-*Lakkous*, but the skeletal remains from these sites remain unpublished (work is ongoing on these). Until recently, Chalcolithic Cypriot human remains, as well as in many cases Cypriot prehistoric human remains in general, were only used to arrive at estimates of sex and age. This paper has, however, shown that investigation of palaeopathologies is possible – to an extent – even in the poorly preserved human skeletal series of Cypriot prehistory. Such investigations are our only chance of gaining glimpses of the health status of prehistoric populations, and as such should always be undertaken to the fullest extent possible.

Notes

1 Much lower rates of AMTL have been found in the Natufian and Neolithic populations of the Levant (3.7% and 4.5% respectively) (Eshed, Gopher and Hershkovitz 2006, 150). Further, the AMTL rate for incisors (9% for central incisors

and 8% for lateral incisors) and canines (5%) within the Shahr-i Sokhta sample is very high when compared, for lack of closer parallels, with the Neolithic populations of the Levant, which have 0–1% AMTL of anterior teeth (Eshed, Gopher and Hershkovitz 2006, 150), and the Chalcolithic populations of Cyprus with 0% AMTL, showing no involvement of incisors or canines in either maxilla or mandible.

2 Shahr-i Sokhta is a vast urban site, while the Chalcolithic Cypriot skeletal series included within this study relate to village-based, small-scale populations.

3 If Souskiou-*Vathyrkakas* is discounted from analysis it is 4.9%.

Bibliography

Backett, S. and Lovell, N. C. 1994: 'Dental disease evidence for agricultural intensification in the Nubian C-Group', *International Journal of Osteoarchaeology* 1994(4), 223–40.

Clarke, N. G. and Hirsch, R. S. 1991: 'Physiological, pulpal, and periodontal factors influencing alveolar bone', 241–66 in M A. Kelley and C. S. Larsen (eds), *Advances in Dental Anthropology,* New York.

Cook, D. C. 1984: 'Subsistence and health in the Lower Illinois Valley: osteological evidence', 235–69 in M. N. Cohen and G. J. Armelagos (eds), *Palaeopathology at the Origins of Agriculture,* New York.

Eshed, V., Gopher, A. and Hershkovitz, I. 2006: 'Tooth wear and dental pathology at the advent of agriculture: new evidence from the Levant', *American Journal of Physical Anthropology* 130, 145–59.

Frayer, D. W. 1989: 'Oral pathologies in the European Upper Palaeolithic and Mesolithic', 255–62 in I. Hershkovitz (ed.), *People and Culture in Change. Proceedings of the Second Symposium on Upper Paleolithic, Mesolithic and Neolithic Populations of Europe and the Mediterranean Basin* (British Archaeological Report International Series 508), Oxford.

Hillson, S. 2005: *Teeth* (Cambridge Manuals in Archaeology), 2nd edition, Cambridge.

Hillson, S. 1996: *Dental Anthropology*, Cambridge.

Karn, K. W., Shockett, H. P., Moffitt, W. C. and Gray, J. L. 1984 'Topographic classification of deformities of the alveolar process', *Journal of Periodontology* 55, 336–40.

Kerr, N. W. 1991 'Prevalence and natural history of periodontal disease in Scotland – the medieval period (900–1600 AD)', *Journal of Periodontal Research* 26, 346–54.

Lorentz, K. O. 2007: 'Teeth as tools: health and disease at Shahr-e Sokhta' [in Farsi], 321–32 in *Proceedings of the 9th International Symposium of Iranian Archaeology*, ICAR, Iranian Center For Archaeological Research, Tehran.

Lorentz, K. O. 2008: 'Activity induced patterns of dental abrasion and ante-mortem tooth loss at 3rd millennium BC Shahr-i Sokhta (Iran): Preliminary results', *Iran* XLVI, 319–27, 333–4.

Lukacs, J. R. 1992: 'Dental paleopathology and agricultural intensification in south Asia: new evidence from Bronze Age Harappa', *American Journal of Physical Anthropology* 87, 133–50.

Lunt, D. A. 1985: 'Report on the human dentitions', 54–8, 150–3, 245–9 in E. J. Peltenburg *et al.*, *Lemba Archaeological Project 1. Excavations at Lemba*-Lakkous *1976–1983* (Studies in Mediterranean Archaeology 70:1), Göteborg.

Lunt, D. A. and Watt, M. E. 1998: 'The human dentitions', 73–82 in E. Peltenburg (ed.), *Lemba Archaeological Project Vol. II.1A: Excavations at Kissonerga*-Mosphilia *1979–1992* (Studies in Mediterranean Archaeology 70:2), Jonsered.

Lunt, D. A. and Watt, M. E. 2006: 'The human dentition', 45–53 in E. Peltenburg (ed.), *The Chalcolithic Cemetery of Souskiou-Vathrykakas, Cyprus*, Nicosia.

Ortner, D. and Putschar, W. G. J. 1985: *Identification of Pathological Conditions in Human Skeletal Remains,* 2nd edition, Washington DC.

Parras, Z. 2006: 'The human remains', 53–66 in E. Peltenburg (ed.), *The Chalcolithic Cemetery of Souskiou-Vathrykakas, Cyprus*, Nicosia.

Sayegh, A., Hilow, H. and Bedi, R. 2004: 'Pattern of tooth loss in recipients of free dental treatment at the University Hospital of Amman, Jordan', *Journal of Oral Rehabilitation* 31(2), 124–30.

32. A Preliminary Look at the Health Status of Chalcolithic Populations: Inferences from Linear Enamel Hypoplasias

Michelle Gamble and Kirsi O. Lorentz

*This paper aims to contribute to the understanding of the health status of Chalcolithic populations in Cyprus, through presenting the results of macroscopic analyses of linear enamel hypoplasias (LEH) on the permanent canine teeth within the skeletal series deriving from Souskiou-*Laona *cemetery with comparison to samples from the Chalcolithic settlement sites of Lemba-*Lakkous *and Kissonerga-*Mosphilia. *A maximum of 24.4% of individuals (based on the maxillary right permanent canine tooth) displayed LEH. There was no statistically significant difference between males and females or amongst age at death groups. These results seem to indicate that the Chalcolithic population did not suffer a high occurrence of physiological stress in childhood during the period of canine crown formation. Whether this truly reflects a healthy population will require further palaeopathological study.*

> 'For I would have you know, Sancho, that a mouth without teeth is like a mill without a millstone, and that a tooth is much more worthy of esteem than a diamond'
>
> *Don Quixote* (Cervantes 1605, 146).

Introduction

'The study of disease in earlier societies stands firmly in the purview of the discipline of the history of medicine' (Waldron 2007, 1). Every individual in a society is affected by health and disease, and gaining insight into the diseases and stresses suffered by individuals in the past will provide a clearer image of their life experiences. Palaeopathology is the study of physical suffering in the past. In prehistoric populations, where there are limited textual and pictorial resources, the best source for examining disease is the remains of the people themselves.

Discussions of human remains have been included in archaeological site reports for Cyprus since the early 1930s (e.g. Angel 1953; 1961; Charles 1963; Gjerstad 1934a; 1934b; Guest 1936). These reports tend to focus solely on the crania recovered, and problem oriented analysis is all but absent. Current studies of human remains are taking a more problem oriented focus, and recent works provide invaluable information in regards to past populations' health status, burial and other cultural practices, biological affinity and lifestyle (see e.g. Baker, Terhune and Papalexandrou 2007; Fox 2005; Harper 2010; Harter-Lailheugue *et al.* 2005; Le Mort 2000; 2007; 2008; Lorentz 2006; 2008a; 2008b; 2008c; 2009; 2010; Parras 2004; 2006; for further references see Harper and Fox 2008 and Lorentz 2011b). As of now, there is no comprehensive palaeopathological study of the Chalcolithic populations in Cyprus.

The Souskiou-*Laona* cemetery represents the first Chalcolithic cemetery excavation in Cyprus which was completed with consistent and modern anthropological techniques allowing for comprehensive recording. It is the earliest completely excavated cemetery in Cyprus. Therefore, the human remains from this excavation have the potential to provide a vast and varied amount of information about the Chalcolithic population on Cyprus. This paper aims to contribute to the understanding of the general health status in the southwest of Cyprus during the Chalcolithic period (3900–2400 BC – for previous work, see Lorentz, this volume). This will be achieved through the presentation of the results of macroscopic analyses of linear enamel hypoplasias (hereafter LEH) on the permanent canine teeth. In particular, this paper focuses on the occurrence of LEH within the skeletal series deriving from the Souskiou-*Laona* cemetery and comparisons with two contemporary skeletal series from the settlement sites of Lemba-*Lakkous* and Kissonerga-*Mosphilia*.

At the time of publication, the only study specifically focusing on LEH in Cyprus which could be located is Fischer and Norén's examination of enamel defects from Late Bronze Age and Cypro-Geometric Iron Age sites (1989). This study examines macroscopically visible dental defects in a histological analysis with polarised light and microradiography. Fischer and Norén were interested in providing an age of occurrence for the dental defects within the various populations. They observed that the onset of the defects was primarily estimated at between two and five years of age (Fischer and Norén 1989, 96). They compared their findings to modern populations and found that 'the morphological appearance of enamel aberrations' were very similar to those in the past (*ibid.*, 90). They do not at this point extrapolate to gain further insight into the life experiences of the population. The only comprehensive palaeopathological study from Cyprus at this time is for the Hellenistic and Roman periods by Fox-Leonard (1997). In her study, she observed that 9.1% of the population she examined at Paphos exhibited LEH (1997, 429).

In general, dental enamel hypoplasia is a deficiency in the amount or thickness of dental enamel, resulting from a disruption in the secretory/matrix formation phase of amelogensis (enamel formation) (Goodman and Armelagos 1985, 479; Sarnat and Schour 1941; Skinner and Goodman 1992, 155). It represents an area of decreased enamel thickness, appearing as a linear horizontal groove in the surface of a tooth. Within physical anthropological studies LEH is viewed as an indicator of general health status, as it has a non-specific aetiology, representing a period of physiological stress during enamel formation (Aufderheide and Rodriguez-Martin 1998, 405; Boldsen 2007, 132; Cutress and Suckling 1982; Fitzgerald *et al.* 2006, 179; Goodman and Armelagos 1988; Roberts and Manchester 2005, 75). It can be observed with the naked eye and is best viewed on the buccal or labial side of the tooth (Goodman and Rose 1990, 280–1; Skinner and Goodman 1992, 157). Instrumental methods of analysis have been developed by a number of researchers (Dirks *et al.* 2002; Hillson 1996; Reid and Dean 2006) and will be undertaken in the future.

Materials and methods

The Souskiou-*Laona* cemetery is located in the southwest of Cyprus on a ridge in the Dhiarizos River Valley, approximately 300 m northwest of a contemporaneous settlement site just outside modern Kouklia (Crewe *et al.* 2005, 44). A total of 137 burial facilities, dating to *c.* 3000 BC have been excavated, containing individuals in both articulated and commingled contexts and various states of preservation (Crewe *et al.* 2005). Preliminary papers on the contextual evidence and some preliminary results of the skeletal analysis from the site have been published recently

Table 32.1. Total number of canine teeth examined (Max = maxillary, Man = mandibular, L = left and R = right)

Tooth location	*Cemetery*	*Settlement Series*			*Total Canines*
		Mosphilia	*Lemba*	*Total*	
Max L	33	3	13	16	*49*
Man L	37	0	11	11	*48*
Max R	30	2	13	15	*45*
Man R	37	0	9	9	*46*
Totals	*137*	5	46	*51*	*188*

(Crewe *et al.* 2005; Lorentz 2011a, forthcoming a; Gamble and Lorentz forthcoming). Full results of skeletal analyses will be published in due course (Lorentz forthcoming b).

The LEH data from Souskiou-*Laona* were compared to LEH data collected for the skeletal series from the settlement sites of Lemba-*Lakkous* and Kissonerga-*Mosphilia*, both of which are located in the Paphos district in the southwest of Cyprus. The sites were excavated over the course of three decades by the Lemba Archaeological Research Project, under the direction of Edgar Peltenburg (Peltenburg *et al.* 1985; 1998). These settlement sites provide a good sample for comparison, not only for their geographical proximity to Souskiou-*Laona*, but also because of Parras' findings that the individuals from Souskiou-*Vathyrkakas* and the two settlement sites are biologically closely related (Parras 2004, 61). Because of the small sample size from Kissonerga-*Mosphilia* and the similarities in burial programme, these individuals were grouped with the Lemba-*Lakkous* material to create the 'combined settlement' series, whilst, Souskiou-*Laona* is referred to as the 'cemetery' series (Table 32.1). The demographic profile of the settlement series contained a high proportion of individuals with deciduous dentition which were not involved in this study.

The dentitions of both Kissonerga-*Mosphilia* and Lemba-*Lakkous* have been previously examined by D. A. Lunt (1985; Baxevani *et al.* 1998) whose results differed from those in this study. She examined 150 burial contexts from both sites (56 at Lemba-*Lakkous* and 94 at Kissonerga-*Mosphilia*). Only four contexts were observed as displaying the defect (one from Lemba-*Lakkous* and three from Kissonerga-*Mosphilia*). Therefore, according to Lunt's publication, only 2.7% of the settlement series display LEH (from Lunt 1985 and Baxevani *et al.* 1998). As presented below, there is a significant difference in the results of the current study.

The dentitions of 67 individuals from Souskiou-*Laona*, 45 individuals from Lemba-*Lakkous* and nine individuals from Kissonerga-*Mosphilia* were examined for this study. Of these, an overall total of 58 individuals had at least one canine tooth. Demographic data were collected by individual. Some of the individuals did not have canine teeth, due to recovery and/or preservation. The results presented within this paper are based strictly on the data derived from the canine dentition (Table 32.1).

In order to create a manageable sample size given the time constraints of the study and because of prior studies indicating the increased frequency of LEH on particular teeth (Goodman and Armelagos 1985), the permanent canine tooth was selected to represent the occurrence of LEH within the populations. The enamel of all four canine teeth in the dental arc forms within a relatively limited period (1.4/1.5–5.2/6.2 years for the lower canine and 1.7–4.8/5.3 years for the upper canine) (Reid and Dean 2006, 343; Schwartz 1995, 192 modified from Ten Cate 1989) which makes understanding the timeframe of the defect occurrence easier and facilitates comparative observations.

Due to the context of the skeletal material (commingled and articulated individuals) it was necessary to record the canine teeth based on tooth quadrants. This means that it was recorded whether the tooth was mandibular or maxillary and whether it comes from the left or right side of the mouth. This eliminated the possibility of double or multiple counting, reflecting a more accurate prevalence regarding individuals among the population. It must be remembered that as this study focused only on the permanent canine teeth, it does not deal with the deciduous dentition.

Preservation is an issue for skeletal analyses in Cyprus. Therefore, due to the pitted and chalky surface condition of some of the teeth observed during a pilot study, it was decided not to assess levels of hypoplastic pitting as it was difficult to distinguish between pitting caused by environmental processes and potential pitting caused by physiological stress. The poor surface preservation is a result of taphonomic conditions at the cemetery, which have caused the enamel to flake off and may eventually lead to the destruction of the entire crown.

In order to assess the presence or absence of LEH, robust methods of examination were used. Two phases of examination of the canine teeth were undertaken: (1) an initial macroscopic or visual assessment, followed by (2) a microscopic inspection, using a basic optical microscope. The tooth surface was examined and described using a list of descriptive features which were created specifically for this study (for further description and discussion of tooth preservation level and the methods developed for dealing with poorly preserved material see Gamble and Lorentz forthcoming). The level of crown completeness and tooth completeness were also assessed. This allowed for a quantitative analysis of preservation which presents a more accurate representation of the prevalence of LEH (Gamble and Lorentz forthcoming).

Standard methods of age and sex estimation were employed where the preservation and contextual association of the material permitted. Sex estimates were most often based on cranial and mandibular features as the pelvic bones did not survive. Adult aging was based on tooth wear (Buikstra and Ubelaker 1994; Miles 1963; Moorrees, Fanning and Hunt 1963; White and Folkens 2005, 298–391). It should be noted that the reference populations on which these estimation methods are based are not Cypriot and that there may be some variation between populations (see Baxevani *et al.* 1998, 102; Walker, Dean and Shapiro 1991). However, as there are no age and sex estimation methods specific to Cypriot populations, the methods employed are the best ones currently available. For quantitative analyses, the median of the estimated age range was utilised to allow for grouping of data within an age at death table based on Buikstra and Ubelaker (1994). A basic descriptive statistical analysis was conducted to investigate the occurrence of LEH within and between age and sex groups and burial locations.

Results

Just under 21% (n=39) of the 188 canine teeth examined exhibited LEH. Overall, of the 137 canine teeth from the cemetery series, 19% (n=26) displayed one or more LEH, while 25.5% (n=13) of the 51 canines from the combined settlement series exhibited the defect. These general numbers do not refer to individuals but to the canine teeth grouped as a whole. As discussed above, in order to gain an idea about the maximum number of individuals displaying the defect, the canine teeth were recorded by quadrant within the dental arc.

The maxillary right canines from the settlement display the highest percentage (25.8%) of LEH from that site and also the highest percentage overall of the canines from both series. The mandibular left canines from the combined settlement series display the highest percentage (27.3%) of LEH, as well as the highest percentage for a tooth quadrant group for both series' (Table 32.2). The maximum discrepancy between quadrant groups is 12.1%.

Overall (including both the combined settlement series and the cemetery series), sex estimation was possible for 28 individuals (11 males and 17 females). All 11 males of the sample come from the cemetery as neither of the two males examined from the combined settlement series had canine teeth. Ten of the females are from the cemetery series

Table 32.2. Percentage of canines with LEH by burial location and quadrant within the dental arcs

Tooth location	*Cemetery*	*Settlement*	*Totals*
Max L	15.2 (n=5/33)	25.0 (n=4/16)	18.4
Man L	21.6 (n=8/37)	27.3 (n=3/11)	22.9
Max R	25.8 (n=7/30)	26.7 (n=4/15)	24.4
Man R	16.2 (n=6/37)	22.2 (n=2/9)	17.4
Totals	18.97	25.5	20.7

Table 32.3. Percentage of canines with LEH in tooth quadrants by sex

Tooth location	*Male*	*Female*	*Indeterminate sex*
Max L	16.7	23.5	15.4
Man L	22.0	23.5	22.7
Max R	33.3	40.0	12.5
Man R	18.2	25.0	13.0

and seven are from the combined settlement series. A minimum number of six females (out of 17) and two males (out of 11) displayed LEH. The canine teeth which displayed the highest prevalence of LEH amongst both males and females was the maxillary right (Table 32.3). Females in general displayed slightly higher levels of frequency of the defect, though this did not prove to be statistically significant (Gamble 2007).

It was possible to estimate the age at death for 36 individuals overall within both series (combined settlement and cemetery). An additional 16 individuals for whom an exact age could not be assigned are called 'general', reflecting an individual with permanent dentition for whom a specific age cannot be estimated. While those of indeterminate age represent individuals for whom it was impossible to establish even a general idea of age (Table 32.4).

Of these individuals with an estimated age at death, the majority fell within the 'young adult' category (aged 21–35 years at death [n=19]) (based on Buikstra and Ubelaker 1994). This group also displays the highest prevalence of LEH on a tooth quadrant basis (53.8% of canines with LEH are from this age group). The highest prevalence of LEH within this group was on the maxillary right canine (Table 32.5). Interestingly, on an individual basis, by establishing a minimum number of individuals based on the canine teeth in each quadrant, there are more adolescents with LEH. Adolescents only comprise 13.9% of the individuals for whom age could be estimated. When examined on a tooth quadrant basis, there was no statistically significant difference in prevalence between the age groups (at a 10% probability [p=0.076]).

Discussion

'Interpretations of defects in ancient hard tissues are inferences rather than precise diagnoses. They are probability statements based on the best available scientific evidence' (Skinner and Goodman 1992, 160; for description and discussion of the osteological paradox and its impact on osteological analyses see Wood *et al.* 1992 and Wright and Yoder 2003). The relatively low occurrence of LEH in both the cemetery and the settlement series is consistent with the hypothesis that they experienced rather low levels of physiological stress in childhood. When compared to other LEH studies of prehistoric groups, which range from 52% to 98% prevalence, the Chalcolithic population on Cyprus had a much lower prevalence of LEH at 21% (Table 32.6). These results more closely resemble the low prevalence observed in the later Hellenistic and Roman periods on Cyprus (Fox-Leonard 1997, 429).

Goodman found that the relationship between LEH and life expectancy is inversely correlated (Goodman 1991). This means that as the frequency of LEH increased, the life expectancy decreased. He theorises three possible reasons for this: first, an inherent increased susceptibility to stress may cause an increased frequency of hypoplasias; second, an individual who was exposed to stress may suffer a loss of ability to respond to other stresses; and third, it may result

Table 32.4. Percentage of individuals with LEH by age at death group

Indeterminate (n=3)	*Infant* (0–3y) (n=1)	*Child* (4–12y) (n=6)	*Adolescent* (13–20y) (n=5)	*Young Adult* (21–35y) (n=19)	*Adult* (36–50y) (n=5)	*General* (n=16)
33.3 (n=1/3)	0.0 (n=0/1)	16.7 (n=1/6)	40.0 (n=2/5)	36.8 (n=7/19)	20.0 (n=1/5)	31.3 (n=5/16)

Table 32.5. Percentage of permanent canines with LEH in tooth quadrants by age at death (reflected as a % of all canines with LEH [n=39])

Tooth location	*Indeterminate*	*Infant (0–3y)*	*Child (4–12y)*	*Adolescent (13–20y)*	*Young Adult (21–35y)*	*Adult (36–50y)*	*General*
Max L	0.0	0.0	2.6	2.6	12.8	0.0	5.1
Man L	0.0	0.0	0.0	0.0	12.8	2.6	12.8
Max R	0.0	0.0	0.0	5.1	17.9	2.6	2.6
Man R	2.6	0.0	2.6	2.6	10.3	0.0	2.6
Total	2.6	0.0	5.1	10.3	53.8	5.1	23.1

Table 32.6. A brief selection of previous LEH studies for comparison

Site	*LEH Prevalence*	*Period*	*Canines examined?*	*Reference*
Souskiou-*Laona* Cemetery, Cyprus	19%	Middle Chalcolithic *c.* 3000 BC	Yes	
Kissonerga-*Mosphilia* and Lemba-*Lakkous*, Cyprus	25.5%	Middle to Late Chalcolithic 3500–2300 BC	Yes	
Dickson Mound, Illinois	66%	950–1300	Yes (not exclusively)	Goodman *et al.* (1980)
Trentino, Italy	85.7–92.9%	Copper Age	Yes (% relates to canine teeth)	Cucina (2002)
Fort Center, Florida	98%	200–600/800 AD	Yes (% relates to canine teeth)	Cucina and Işcan (1997)
Pasión River sites, Guatemala	59%	600 BC–600 AD	Yes (% relates to canine teeth)	Wright (1997)
Ajios Jakovos, Enkomi and Lapithos, Cyprus	52% (estimate)	1575 BC–850 BC	Unknown, teeth examined not recorded	Fischer and Norén (1989)

from increased exposure to stressors due to behaviour or culture (*ibid.*, 283). Thus, it must be kept in mind that the effect of a stressor on an individual is due not only to the characteristics of the stressor, but also to the individual's biological response to the stress (*ibid.*, 286). These studies also indicate that there is a certain cultural buffering involved in stress and that there are those who are able to avoid stress due to differential social status which can have an impact on longevity (*ibid.*, 284).

The correlation between age at death and the prevalence of LEH is not clearly defined within the Chalcolithic Cypriot populations. Overall, the greatest number of individuals have an age at death between 20 35 years, however it is within the adolescent age group (ages 13–20 years) that a higher percentage of individuals displayed the dental defect (40.0%). Goodman's discussion is a reminder that while there is an inverse correlation between longevity and high frequency of LEH in many previous cases, there are other cultural and biological considerations which must be understood in order to address the variability in expression amongst age groups (Goodman 1991, 283, 286). Further research is needed to examine the role of the possible connection between childhood physiological stresses and adult age at death within the Chalcolithic populations of Cyprus (including an examination of the deciduous dentition for LEH). The differences in occurrence between sex groups did not prove to be statistically significant which implies that both males and females experienced a similar susceptibility to the defect and/or a similar exposure to physiological stressors. There is a maximum of 12.1% difference amongst all the quadrants within both series (15.2–27.3% maxillary left from the cemetery and mandibular left from the combined settlement series respectively). This variation, based on tooth location, is most likely due to recovery and preservation. There is continued discussion on which teeth display the highest prevalence of dental defects and what might account for variation amongst teeth (e.g. see Goodman and Armelagos 1985; King, Humphrey and Hillson 2005, 552; Saunders and Keenleyside 1999).

As LEH is generally linked to metabolic distress, nutrition, disease, lifestyle and labour can all be involved in the occurrence of a lesion. A number of scholars have made interpretative suggestions as to the economy and lifestyle during the middle Chalcolithic period in southwest Cyprus (e.g. Croft 1991; Murray 1998; Peltenburg 1991a; 1991b; Peltenburg *et al.* 1991; 1998; Steel 2004). In general, they were an agro-pastoralist society, increasingly focusing on agriculture and animal husbandry at this stage. According to faunal and archaeobotanical studies, diet was rather diverse, and with variability and low population concentrations, it should have been possible to acquire the nutrients required for a relatively healthy subsistence (Croft 1991; Murray 1998). During this period, domestic structures were more permanent and it seems that there was more of a focus on the family unit (Peltenburg 1991a; Peltenburg *et al.* 1998). It is described by Peltenburg as a 'flourishing' period with specialised buildings and complex ritual (Peltenburg 1991a, 26). There is increased social differentiation, based on an increase of luxury items in the middle Chalcolithic which is elaborated in the late Chalcolithic (*ibid.*, 28–30). Until further, more concrete patterns of health status can be discerned from within the population, it is difficult to infer which aspects of life may be affecting the prevalence of LEH.

Recent publications (Peltenburg *et al.* 2001; Peltenburg and Wasse 2004) have emphasised the close links between the earlier Neolithic populations of Cyprus and the Near East. Therefore, a very brief survey of palaeopathological research, specifically looking at LEH studies, from the continent would be beneficial to compare to the Cypriot material. At the time of publication, there were no studies located which specifically focused on LEH prevalence in prehistoric periods in this part of the world. There are, however, studies by: Zias (1989; 1991), Goldstein, Arensburg and Nathan (1976) and Hershkovitz *et al.* (1991; 1992) published on disease and palaeopathology in Israel, and Eshed *et al.* (2006; 2010) have studied dental disease and palaeopathology in the Levant at the Nautufian–Neolithic transition. A new online journal, edited by Soltysiak, called *Bioarchaeology of the Near East*, has contributed to the dissemination of studies of human remains in the Near East from the prehistoric periods (2007; 2008). This publication includes human remains reports from current excavations. More importantly, it indicates that there is an increasing number of problem oriented human remains studies from this part of the world and will most likely in the future provide more comparative specialist studies in palaeopathology. These palaeopathological and bioarchaeological studies have the potential to significantly expand our understanding of the complex socio-cultural transformations during prehistory within this region.

Conclusions

The overall low prevalence (a maximum of 24.4% of individuals and a minimum of 17.4% of individuals based on the maxillary right and the mandibular right respectively) of LEH determined by this preliminary study is consistent with the hypothesis that the Cypriot Chalcolithic populations included within this analysis were relatively healthy during the period of the permanent canine enamel formation (1.4/1.5–5.2/6.2 years for the lower canine and 1.7–4.8/5.3 years for the upper canine) (Reid and Dean 2006, 343; Schwartz 1995, 192 modified from Ten Cate 1989, 275–98). Contextual archaeological evidence shows that the Chalcolithic period ushered in significant changes in domestic space, subsistence economy and gender relations. Yet, the social inequality that these changes supposedly brought about, according to Steel (2004, 93), Bolger (2003, 78, 80–1) and Peltenburg (1991b, 107, 117), are at this point not evidenced in the general health status of the population, as viewed through this pilot study focusing on LEH. This could imply that the mortuary populations of both sites came from living groups which shared a similar frequency of stresses in life, regardless of possible social structure.

There is no statistically significant difference in the results between males and females, though females display a slightly higher rate of LEH than males. Therefore males and females likely experienced similar incidences of physiological stress during the period of permanent canine formation. 48.2% of the individuals for whom an age at death could be assessed were between the ages of 21–35 years. This relatively young age at death is consistent with the expected pre-industrial population mortality (Boldsen 2007). However it must be noted that of these 19 individuals only a maximum of seven individuals (36.8%) displayed LEH. This would seem to indicate that the occurrence of LEH does not seem to have a direct correlation to an early age at death within this population. However, since this study does not include deciduous dentition the interpretation and inferences made in regards to the relationship between LEH and age at death are limited (for further discussion about the relationship between LEH occurrence and age at death see Boldsen 2007; Goodman 1991; Goodman and Armelagos 1988; Skinner and Goodman 1992, 160; King, Humphrey and Hillson 2005).

It is hoped that the palaeopathological research on the rest of the skeletal material from Souskiou-*Laona*, Kissonerga-*Mosphilia* and Lemba-*Lakkous*, which is currently being conducted, will be able to elucidate further the health status of the Chalcolithic populations. The incidences of LEH, as observed within these samples, seem to indicate that either: 1) the Chalcolithic Cypriot population did not face a lot of physiological stress in childhood and/or 2) they were not particularly susceptible to this particular defect. As Goodman and Armelagos (1988) and Skinner and Goodman (1992) have discussed, LEH can be indicative of the general health status of a population. The results of this preliminary study on LEH are, therefore, consistent with the hypothesis that the Chalcolithic Cypriot populations included within this analysis were relatively healthy during childhood. A better understanding of the health and disease processes within the population will aid in providing a clearer representation of the life experiences of the Chalcolithic peoples in Cyprus.

Acknowledgements

The authors would like to thank Professor Edgar Peltenburg for his permission to examine the skeletal material from all three sites as well as the staff of the Paphos District Museum for their help in accessing the dental remains from Lemba-*Lakkous* and Kissonerga-*Mosphilia*. Warm thanks are also extended to Professor Demetrios Michaelides for his efforts in organising the Medicine in the Ancient Mediterranean Conference, Nicosia, as well as, providing the opportunity to present this paper in the conference proceedings.

Bibliography

Angel, J. L. 1953: 'Appendix II: The human remains from Khirokitia,' 416–30 in P. Dikaios, *Khirokitia*, London.

Angel, J. L. 1961: 'Appendix 1: Neolithic crania from Sotira', 223–9 in P. Dikaios, *Sotira*, Philadelphia.

Aufderheide, A. C. and Rodríguez-Martin, C. 1998: *The Cambridge Encyclopedia of Human Paleopathology*, Cambridge.

Baker B. J., Terhune, C. E. and Papalexandrou, A. 2007: 'Sew long: a seamstress buried at Medieval Polis', *American Journal of Physical Anthropology Supplement* 132, 67.

Baxevani, E., Lunt, D. A., Peltenburg, E. and Watt, M. E. 1998: 'Chapter 16: Mortuary evidence', 87–120 in E. Peltenburg, D. Bolger, P. Croft, E. Goring, B. Irving, D. A. Lunt, S. W. Manning, M. A. Murray, C. McCartney, J. S. Ridout-Sharpe, G. Thomas, M. E. Watt and C. Elliott-Xenophontos, *Lemba Archaeological Project, Cyprus,* Vol. II.1B (Part 1): *Excavations at Kissonerga-Mosphilia, 1979–1992*, Edinburgh.

Boldsen, J. L. 2007: 'Early childhood stress and adult age mortality – a study of dental enamel hypoplasia in the Medieval Danish village of Tirup', *American Journal of Physical Anthropology* 132, 59–66.

Bolger, D. L. 2003: *Gender in Ancient Cyprus*, Walnut Creek.

Buikstra, J. E. and Ubelaker, D. H. 1994: *Standards for Data Collection from Human Remains*, Fayetteville.

Cervantes, M. de 1605: *Don Quixote*, translation by J. Rutherford (2000), London.

Charles, R.-P. 1963: *Le peuplement de Chypre dans l'antiquité: Étude anthropologique* (Études Chypriotes 2), Paris.

Crewe, L., Lorentz, K., Peltenburg, E. and Spanou, S. 2005: 'Treatments of the dead: a preliminary report of investigations at Souskiou-*Laona* Chalcolithic cemetery, 2001–2004', *Report of the Department of Antiquities, Cyprus*, 41–67.

Croft, P. W. 1991: 'Man and beast in Chalcolithic Cyprus', *Bulletin of the American Schools of Oriental Research* 282/3, 63–79.

Cucina, A. 2002: 'Brief communication: diachronic investigation of linear enamel hypoplasia in prehistoric skeletal samples from Trentino, Italy', *American Journal of Physical Anthropology* 119, 283–7.

Cucina, A. and Işcan, M. Y. 1997: 'Assessment of enamel hypoplasia in a high status burial site', *American Journal of Human Biology* 9, 213–22.

Cutress, P. and Suckling, D. 1982: 'The assessment of non carious defects of the enamel', *International Dental Journal* 32, 109–20.

Dirks, W., Reid, D. J., Jolly, C. J., Phillips-Conroy, J. E. and Brett, F. L. 2002: 'Out of the mouths of baboons: stress, life history, and dental development in the Awash National Park Hybrid Zone, Ethiopia', *American Journal of Physical Anthropology* 118, 239–52.

Eshed, V., Gopher, A. and Hershkovitz, I. 2006: 'Tooth wear and dental pathology at the advent of agriculture: new evidence from the Levant', *American Journal of Physical Anthropology*, 130, 145–59.

Eshed, V., Gopher, A., Pinhasi, R. and Hershkovitz, I. 2010: 'Paleopathology and the origin of agriculture in the Levant', *American Journal of Physical Anthropology*, 143, 121–33.

Fischer, P. M. and Norén, J. G. 1989: 'Enamel defects in teeth from a prehistoric Cypriot population', *Ossa* 13, 87–96.

Fitzgerald, C., Saunders, S., Bondioli, L. and Macchiarelli, R. 2006: 'Health of infants in an Imperial Roman skeletal sample: perspective from dental microstructure', *American Journal of Physical Anthropology* 130, 179–89.

Fox, S. C. 2005: 'Health in Hellenistic and Roman times: the case studies of Paphos, Cyprus and Corinth, Greece', 59–82 in H. King (ed.), *Health in Antiquity*, London.

Fox-Leonard, S. C. 1997: *Comparing Health from Paleopathological Analysis of the Human Skeletal Remains Dating to the Hellenistic and Roman Periods, from Paphos, Cyprus and Corinth, Greece,* Unpublished Ph.D. Dissertation, University of Arizona.

Gamble, M. 2007: *A preliminary investigation into the general health status of the Chalcolithic population in Cyprus: using dental defects as a reflection of non-specific incidences of stress in childhood*, Unpublished M.A. Dissertation, Newcastle University.

Gamble, M. and Lorentz, K. O. forthcoming: 'Assessing growth disruptions and preservation levels: preliminary results on linear enamel hypoplasias at the Souskiou-*Laona* Chalcolithic cemetery, Cyprus', in A. Jacobs and K. Nys (eds), *Proceedings of the 8th Postgraduate Cypriot Archaeology Conference, Brussels, Belgium*, Göteborg.

Gjerstad, E. 1934a: 'Lapithos', 13–276 in E. Gjerstad, J. Lindros, E. Sjöqvist and A. Westholm, *The Swedish Cyprus Expedition: Finds and Results of the Excavations in Cyprus, 1927–1931* Vol. 1, Stockholm.

Gjerstad, E. 1934b: 'Enkomi', 467–575 in E. Gjerstad, J. Lindros, E. Sjöqvist and A. Westholm, *The Swedish Cyprus Expedition: Finds and Results of the Excavations in Cyprus, 1927–1931* Vol. 1, Stockholm.

Goldstein, M. S., Arensburg, B. and Nathan, H. 1976: 'Pathology of Bedouin skeletal remains from two sites in Israel', *American Journal of Physical Anthropology* 45(3), 621–40.

Goodman, A. H. 1991: 'Stress, adaptation, and enamel developmental defects', 280–7 in D. J. Ortner and A. C. Aufderheide (eds), *Human Paleopathology: Current Syntheses and Future Options*, Washington, DC.

Goodman, A. H., Armelagos, G. J. and Rose, J. C. 1980: 'Enamel hypoplasias as indicators of stress in three prehistoric populations for Illinois', *Human Biology* 52, 515–28.

Goodman, A. H. and Armelagos, G. J. 1985: 'Factors affecting the distribution of enamel hypoplasia within the human permanent dentition', *American Journal of Physical Anthropology* 68, 479–93.

Goodman, A. and Armelagos, G. J. 1988: 'Childhood stress and decreased longevity in a prehistoric population', *American Anthropologist* 90(4), 936–44.

Goodman, A. H. and Rose, J. C. 1990: 'Dental enamel hypoplasias as indicators of nutritional status', 279–94 in M. A. Kelley and C. S. Larsen (eds), *Advances in Dental Anthropology*, New York.

Guest, E. M. 1936: 'The human remains,' in P. Dikaios, 'The excavations at Erimi, 1933–1935 final report', *Report of the Department of Antiquities, Cyprus*, 58–62.

Harper, N. K. 2010: 'From Typology to Population Genetics: Biodistance in Cyprus', 1–37 in S. Christodoulou and A. Satraki, *POCA 2007. Postgraduate Cypriot Archaeology Conference, Nicosia*, Newcastle upon Tyne.

Harper, N. K. and Fox, S. C. 2008: 'Recent research in Cypriot bioarchaeology', *Bioarchaeology of the Near East* 2, 1–38.

Harter-Lailheugue, S., Le Mort, F., Vigne, J.-D., Guilane, J., Le Bruno, A. and Bouchet, F. 2005: 'Premières données parasitologiques sur les populations humaines précéramiques chypriotes (VIIIe et VIIe millénaires av. J. C.)', *Paléorient* 31, 43–54.

Hershkovitz, I., Ring, B., Speirs, M., Galili, E., Kislev, M., Edelson,

G. and Hershkovitz, A. 1991: 'Possible congenital hemolytic anemia in prehistoric coastal inhabitants of Israel', *American Journal of Physical Anthropology* 85, 7–13.

Hershkovitz, I., Speirs, M., Katznelson, A. and Arensburg, B. 1992: 'Unusual pathological condition in the lower extremities of a skeleton from ancient Israel', *American Journal of Physical Anthropology* 88, 23–6.

Hillson, S. 1996: *Dental Anthropology*, Cambridge.

King, T., Humphrey, L. T. and Hillson, S. 2005: 'Linear enamel hypoplasias as indicators of systemic physiological stress: evidence from two known age-at-death and sex populations from postmedieval London', *American Journal of Physical Anthropology* 128, 547–59.

Le Mort, F. 2000: 'The Neolithic subadult skeletons from Khirokitia (Cyprus): taphonomy and mortality', *Anthropologie* 38, 63–70.

Le Mort, F. 2007: 'Artificial cranial deformation in the Aceramic Neolithic Near East: evidence from Cyprus', 151–8 in M. Faerman, L. K. Horwitz, T. Kahana and U. Zilberman (eds), *Faces from the Past: Diachronic Patterns in the Biology of Human Populations from the Eastern Mediterranean. Papers in Honor of Patricia Smith*, Oxford.

Le Mort, F. 2008: 'Infant burials in Pre-Pottery Neolithic Cyprus: evidence from Khirokitia', 23–32 in K. Bacvarov (ed.), *Babies Reborn: Infant/Child Burials in Pre- and Protohistory*, Oxford.

Lorentz, K. O. 2006: 'Headshaping at Marki and its socio-cultural significance', 297–303 in D. Frankel and J. Webb (eds), *Marki Alonia. An Early and Middle Bronze Age Settlement in Cyprus. Excavations 1995–2000*, Sävedalen.

Lorentz, K. O. 2008a: 'Crafting the head: the human body as art?', 415–32 in J. M. Córdoba, M. Molist, M. Carmen Pérez, I. Rubio and S. Martínez (eds), *Proceedings of the Fifth International Congress on the Archaeology of the Ancient Near East, Madrid, April 3–8, 2006*, Madrid.

Lorentz, K. O. 2008b: 'From bodies to bones and back: theory and human bioarchaeology', 273–303 in H. Schutkowski (ed.), *Between Biology and Culture*, Cambridge.

Lorentz, K. O. 2008c: 'From life course to longue durée: headshaping as gendered capital?', 281–311 in D. Bolger (ed.), *Gender through Time in the Ancient Near East*, Walnut Creek.

Lorentz, K. O. 2009: 'The malleable body: headshaping in Greece and the surrounding regions', 75–98 in L. Schepartz, S. C. Fox and C. Bourbou (eds), *New Directions in the Skeletal Biology of Greece*, Princeton.

Lorentz, K. O. 2010: 'Parts to a whole: manipulations of the body in prehistoric Eastern Mediterranean', 20–29 in K. Rebay-Salisbury, M. L. Stig Sørensen and J. Hughes (eds), *Body Parts and Bodies Whole: Changing Relations and Meanings*, Oxford.

Lorentz, K. O. 2011a: 'Human bioarchaeology of the Cypriot Chalcolithic: Analyses at Souskiou-*Laona* cemetery', 613–21 in A. Demetriou (ed.), *Proceedings of the IV. International Cyprological Congress, Lefkosia 29 April–3 May 2008*, Lefkosia.

Lorentz, K. O. 2011b: 'Cyprus', in N. Márquez-Grant and L. Fibiger (eds), *Physical Anthropology and Legislation: European Perspectives and Beyond.*

Lorentz, K. O. forthcoming a: 'Orderly disposal: human remains at Chalcolithic Souskiou-Laona, Cyprus', in P. Karsgaard (ed.), *Death and Discard: The Transformations of Places, People, Animals and Things in the Ancient Near East, BANEA Monograph* 2, Oxford.

Lorentz, K. O. forthcoming b: 'The Human Remains from Souskiou-*Laona (OpC)* Cemetery'. [Working title].

Lunt, D. A. 1985: 'Report on the human dentitions', 54–8, 150–3 in E. Peltenburg *et al.*, *Lemba Archaeological Project, Cyprus,* Vol. I: *Excavations at Lemba-Lakkous, 1976–1983*, Göteborg.

Miles, A. E. W. 1963: 'Dentition in the estimation of age', *Journal of Dental Research* 42, 255–63.

Moorrees, C. F. A., Fanning, E. A. and Hunt, Jr., E. E. 1963: 'Age variation of formation stages for ten permanent teeth', *Journal of Dental Research* 42, 1490–502.

Murray, M. A. 1998: 'Chapter 11: Archaeobotanical report', 215–23 in E. Peltenburg *et al.*, *Lemba Archaeological Project, Cyprus,* Vol. II.1B (Part 1*): Excavations at Kissonerga-Mosphilia, 1979–1992,* Edinburgh.

Parras, Z. 2004: *The Biological Affinities of the Eastern Mediterranean in the Chalcolithic and Bronze Age: A Regional Dental Non-Metric Approach* (British Archaeological Report International Series 1305), Oxford.

Parras, Z. 2006: 'Looking for immigrants at Kissonerga-Mosphilia in the Late Chalcolithic: a dental non-metric perspective of Chalcolithic and Early Bronze Age southwest Cyprus', 63–74 in A. P. McCarthy (ed.), *Island Dialogues. Cyprus in the Mediterranean Network*, Edinburgh.

Peltenburg, E. 1991a: 'Kissonerga-Mosphilia: a major Chalcolithic site in Cyprus', *Bulletin of the American Schools of Oriental Research* 282/3, 17–35.

Peltenburg, E. 1991b: 'Local exchange in prehistoric Cyprus: an initial assessment of picrolite', *Bulletin of the American Schools of Oriental Research* 282/3, 107–25.

Peltenburg, E., Baird, D., Betts, A., Colledge, S., Croft, P., Elliott, C., Lawrence, T., Lunt, D. A., Niklasson, K., Renault-Miskovsky, J., Ridout Sharpe, J. S., Slater, E., Stewart, J. D. and Xenophontos, C. 1985: *Lemba Archaeological Project, Cyprus,* Vol. I: *Excavations at Lemba-Lakkous, 1976–1983*, Göteborg.

Peltenburg, E., Betts, A., Bolger, D., Croft, P., Elliott, C., Goring, E., Murray, M. A., Ridout-Sharpe, J. S. and Thomas, G. 1991: *Lemba Archaeological Project, Cyprus* II.2: *A Ceremonial Area at Kissonerga*, Göteborg.

Peltenburg, E., Bolger, D., Croft, P., Goring, E., Irving, B., Lunt, D. A, Manning, S. W., Murray, M. A., McCartney, C., Ridout-Sharpe, J. S., Thomas, G., Watt, M. E. and Elliott-Xenophontos, C. 1998: *Lemba Archaeological Project, Cyprus,* Vol. II.1B (Part 1): *Excavations at Kissonerga-Mosphilia, 1979–1992*, Edinburgh.

Peltenburg, E., Colledge, S., Croft, P., Jackson, A., McCartney, C. and Murray, M. A. 2001: 'Neolithic dispersals from the Levantine corridor: a Mediterranean perspective', *Levant* 35, 35–64.

Peltenburg, E. and Wasse, A. (eds) 2004: *Neolithic Revolution: New Perspectives on Southwest Asia in Light of Recent Discoveries on Cyprus*, Oxford.

Reid, D. J. and Dean, M. C. 2006: 'Variation in modern human enamel formation times', *Journal of Human Evolution* 50(3), 329–46.

Roberts, C. A. and Manchester, K. 2005: *The Archaeology of Disease*, 3rd edition, Stroud.

Sarnat, B. G. and Schour, I. 1941: 'Enamel hypoplasia (chronologic enamel aplasia) in relation to systemic disease: a chronologic, morphologic and etiologic classification', *The Journal of the American Dental Association* 28, 1989–2000.

Saunders, S. R. and Keenleyside, A. 1999: 'Enamel hypoplasia in a Canadian historic sample', *American Journal of Human Biology* 11, 513–24.

Schwartz, J. H. 1995: *Skeleton Keys: An Introduction to Human Skeletal Morphology, Development, and Analysis*, Oxford.

Skinner, M. and Goodman, A. H. 1992: 'Anthropological uses of developmental defects of enamel', 153–74 in S. Saunders and M. Katzenberg (eds), *Skeletal Biology of Past Peoples: Research Methods*, New York.

Soltysiak, A. (ed.) 2007: *Bioarchaeology of the Near East*, Available from <http://www.anthropology.uw.edu.pl/> [Accessed on 28–11-09].

Soltysiak, A. (ed.) 2008: *Bioarchaeology of the Near East*, Available from <http://www.anthropology.uw.edu.pl/> [Accessed on 28-11-09].

Steel, L. 2004: *Cyprus Before History: From the Earliest Settlers to the End of the Bronze Age*, London.

Ten Cate, A. R. 1989: 'Physiological tooth movement: eruption and shedding', 275–98 in A. R. Ten Cate (ed.), *Oral Histology: Development, Structure, and Function*, St. Louis.

Waldron, T. 2007: *Palaeoepidemiology: The Measure of Disease in the Human Past*, (University College London Institute of Archaeology Publications), London.

Walker, P. L., Dean, G. and Shapiro, P. 1991: 'Estimating age from tooth wear in archaeological populations', 169–78 in M. A. Kelley and C. S. Larsen (eds), *Advances in Dental Anthropology*, New York.

White, T. D. and Folkens, P. A. 2005: *The Human Bone Manual*, London, San Diego and Burlington.

Wood, J. W., Milner, G. R., Harpending, H. C., Weiss, K. M., Cohen, M. N., Eisenberg, L. E., Hutchinson, D. L., Jankauskas, R., Esnys, G., Katzenberg, M. A., Lukacs, J. R., McGrath, J. W., Roth, E. A., Ubelaker, D. H. and Wilkinson, R. G. 1992: 'The osteological paradox: problems in inferring prehistoric health from skeletal samples', *Current Anthropology* 33, 343–70.

Wright, L. 1997: 'Intertooth patterns of hypoplasia expression: implications for childhood health in the Classic Maya collapse', *American Journal of Physical Anthropology* 102, 233–47.

Wright, L. E. and Yoder, C. J. 2003: 'Recent progress in bioarchaeology: approaches to the osteological paradox', *Journal of Archaeological Research* 11(1), 43–70.

Zias, J. 1989: 'Lust and leprosy: confusion or correlation?', *Bulletin of the American Schools of Oriental Research* 275, 27–31.

Zias, J. 1991: 'Current archaeological research in Israel: death and disease in ancient Israel', *Biblical Archaeologist* 54(3), 147–59.

33. A Preliminary Analysis of Trauma Patterns in Early Christian Cyprus

Sherry C. Fox, Ioanna Moutafi, Eleanna Prevedorou and Despina Pilides

*Human skeletal remains from four Early Christian ecclesiastical sites in Cyprus have been analysed in an effort to discern the common burial customs, the demographic profiles (sex and age) of individuals from the site, along with pathological data such as the common diseases, and in particular, evidence for trauma from individuals dating to this time period on the island. There are few skeletal studies on Cypriot material from the Early Christian period. The largest site under study, the Hill of Agios Georgios (St George's Hill), is an inland site, located on a rise adjacent to the Pediaios River outside the Venetian walled city of the capital, Nicosia. Four churches and their associated cemeteries dating from around the 7th century AD to the post-medieval period have been excavated at the Hill of Agios Georgios where today a chapel dedicated to St George the Healer is situated. To date, approximately 28 of the total 216 individuals from the site have been recovered from Early Christian contexts. The other, smaller church/basilica sites of Kalavasos-*Kopetra *(n=21), Alassa-*Ayia Mavri *(n=26), and Maroni-*Petrera *(n=6), are located near the south coast. Patterns have emerged between the smaller, coastal sites when compared to the larger, inland site of the Hill of Agios Georgios. The pattern is particularly evident when examining evidence for trauma such as fracture types and locations. Reasons for the different patterns in this preliminary study will be discussed.*

Introduction

Trauma patterns can lend insight into the way of life in the past. The purpose of this study is to present the patterns of trauma exhibited among the human skeletal remains that date from the late 4th to the mid-7th centuries AD, from a period known synonymously as the Late Roman, Early Christian or Early Byzantine in Cyprus, referred to hereafter as the Early Christian period. One question is to test whether life was riskier in rural or urban Byzantine Cyprus through the analysis of a specific type of trauma, bone fractures. Another question is to determine whether there are sex differences in the prevalence of fractures. And do the location and prevalence of fractures change over time during Byzantine times on the island?

The samples from this study are derived from four Early Christian basilica sites: the urban and inland site of the Hill of Agios Georgios (St George's Hill) is compared with the combined samples from the rural sites of Kalavasos-*Kopetra*, Alassa-*Ayia Mavri* and Maroni-*Petrera*, all located near the south coast of the island, on rises, and adjacent to rivers. Results from a later, 10th–12th century AD phase from the site of the Hill of Agios Georgios are presented here to test the continuity of these trends.

The Hill of Agios Georgios is located east of the Pediaios River in the capital city of Nicosia, and the site has held religious significance throughout its history. This holds true today as a chapel dedicated to St George the Healer is situated in the central apse of one of the architectural phases at the site.

Under the direction of Dr Despina Pilides, excavations on the Hill of Agios Georgios began in 1996 by the Department of Antiquities, Cyprus, prior to construction of the new House of Representatives building designated for the site. It was the former site of the old PA.SY.D.Y. (Pancyprian Public Employees Trade Union) building, and the area is commonly referred to by that name. Dr Pilides spent 16 field seasons excavating this modern city block that additionally contained, among other things, a meteorological station and prefabricated barracks housing the offices of the Ministry of Communications and Works that were vacated in 1999 (Pilides 2003; Pilides and Destrooper-Georgiades 2008; Pilides and Olivier 2008). During one year at the site alone, Dr Pilides and her team spent 11 months in the field. They have unearthed remains dating to the Archaic, Classical, and Hellenistic periods, in addition to the four superimposed churches and associated cemeteries that dated from the Early, Middle and Late Byzantine periods and through the medieval period (Hadjisavvas 1999, 621–4; Flourentzos 2004–2005, 1678–9; 2006, 873–919).

Unfortunately, the preservation of the human remains from all four sites is only generally fair. This is common on the island as Angel (1945, 289) has previously reported for similar environments in Greece. A climate fluctuating between hot, dry summers and cool, wet winters may be in part responsible for the lack of good bone preservation along with the basic pH from the chalky, alkaline soils that predominate in Cyprus. A notable exception would include the human remains recovered from the cistern at Kalavasos-*Kopetra*. The cistern provided a more constant micro-environment allowing the bones better preservation (Fox 2003) despite the similar alkaline pH of the soil from within as compared with soil from tombs at the site.

The authors recently published an article on the burial customs of Early Christian Cyprus (Fox *et al.* 2012). The archaeological information particular to these sites, including the preferred basilica or church location, grave type, the culturally prescribed body orientation and body positioning for the period, the average number of individuals per tomb, along with biological information gleaned from the skeleton, including individual sex, age at death, reconstructed living stature, and health data will be presented. Until the last two decades, the Early Christian period in Cyprus was not well understood from a bioarchaeological perspective as the human skeletal remains had not previously received much attention (cf. Fox 1996; 2002; 2003). It should be noted that although the south coast sites have been published (Rautman 2003; Flourentzos 1996; Manning 2002), the results presented from the Hill of Agios Georgios are preliminary and include only the individuals from Early Christian contexts of the more than 216 burials excavated at the site.

Materials and methods

The individuals were sexed and aged following established methodologies. For demographic purposes, the age categories used in this study are from the *Standards for Data Collection from Human Skeletal Remain* (Buikstra and Ubelaker 1994). Adults not displaying more precise aging criteria were included in the 'Middle Adult' age category for all sites. 'Juveniles' are only reported here for demographic purposes and will not be included in this study as they show no evidence of trauma.

Of the minimally 28 individuals retrieved from Early Christian burials at the Hill of Agios Georgios, a total of four juveniles and 24 adults were recovered. The combined south coast samples yielded a different demographic pattern with predominantly younger ages, with a total of 54 individuals including 33 juveniles and 21 adults. This difference could be due to variations in burial practices between the rural, south coast sites and the urban, inland site. As for the later period from the Hill of Agios Georgios, out of the 19 individuals recovered, there are four juveniles and 15 adults.

Among the 24 adults from the Hill of Agios Georgios, sex was determined for 13 individuals, including seven males and six females. Of the 21 adults from the south coast, there are 14 males and seven females. One of the sites from the south coast, Kalavasos-*Kopetra* may have been a monastic complex, and, as such, it is not surprising to find more remains of males than females. From the 15 adults from the later phase at the Hill of Agios Georgios, seven are males, five are females and three are of indeterminate sex.

Results

The main focus of this research is on pathology. Of the 21 adults recovered from the south coast, nine demonstrate some pathological lesion, and four of the 21 (19%) show evidence of single or multiple traumata (Table 33.1). Only one individual, a young adult female, demonstrates both trauma and an additional pathology.

With regard to the Early Christian period at the Hill of Agios Georgios, of the 24 adults recovered, 16 demonstrate some pathological lesion (prevalence of 67%), a much larger percentage when compared to the south coast (43%). Eight of the 24 adults (33%) display evidence of trauma. In contrast to the situation on the south coast, all but one individual demonstrate both trauma and some other pathology. Unlike the south coast, where only fractures are observed, a variety of traumata is exhibited at the Hill of Agios Georgios. The number of fractures, however, is comparable between the two samples. From the later phase at the Hill of Agios Georgios, eight out of the 15 adults (53%) demonstrate pathological lesions, four of whom (27%) exhibit trauma. Three out of the four (75%) display both evidence of trauma and an additional pathology.

A picture of fractures is presented from both the south coast and the Hill of Agios Georgios beginning with the south coast. Something catastrophic must have taken place at Kalavasos-*Kopetra* for nine individuals to have been deposited within a cistern. One individual of indeterminate sex exhibits a pseudarthrosis of the right clavicle (Fig. 33.1). This fracture exhibits non-union which is not uncommon in the clavicle due to the mobility of the shoulder joint. A

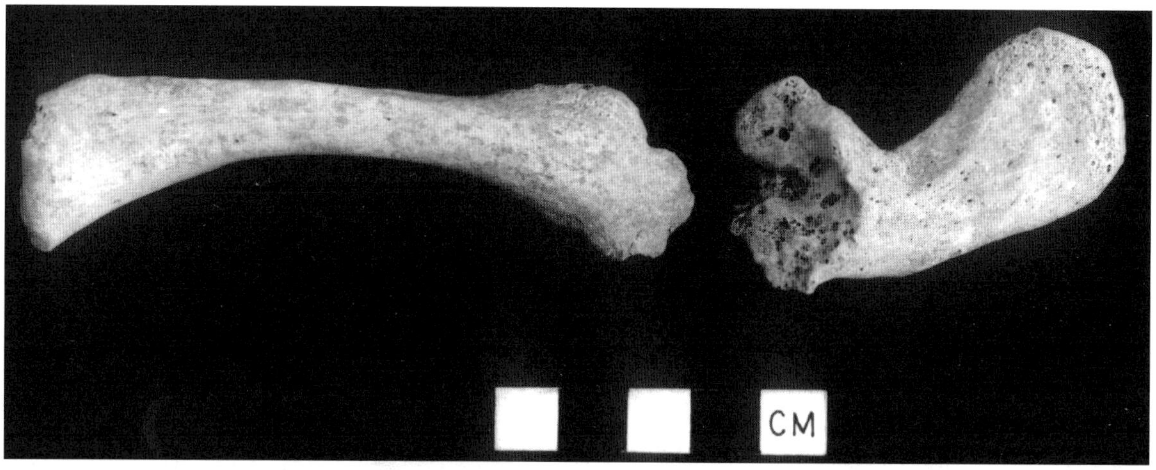

Fig. 33.1. Pseudarthrosis of a right clavicle from an individual from Kalavasos-*Kopetra*

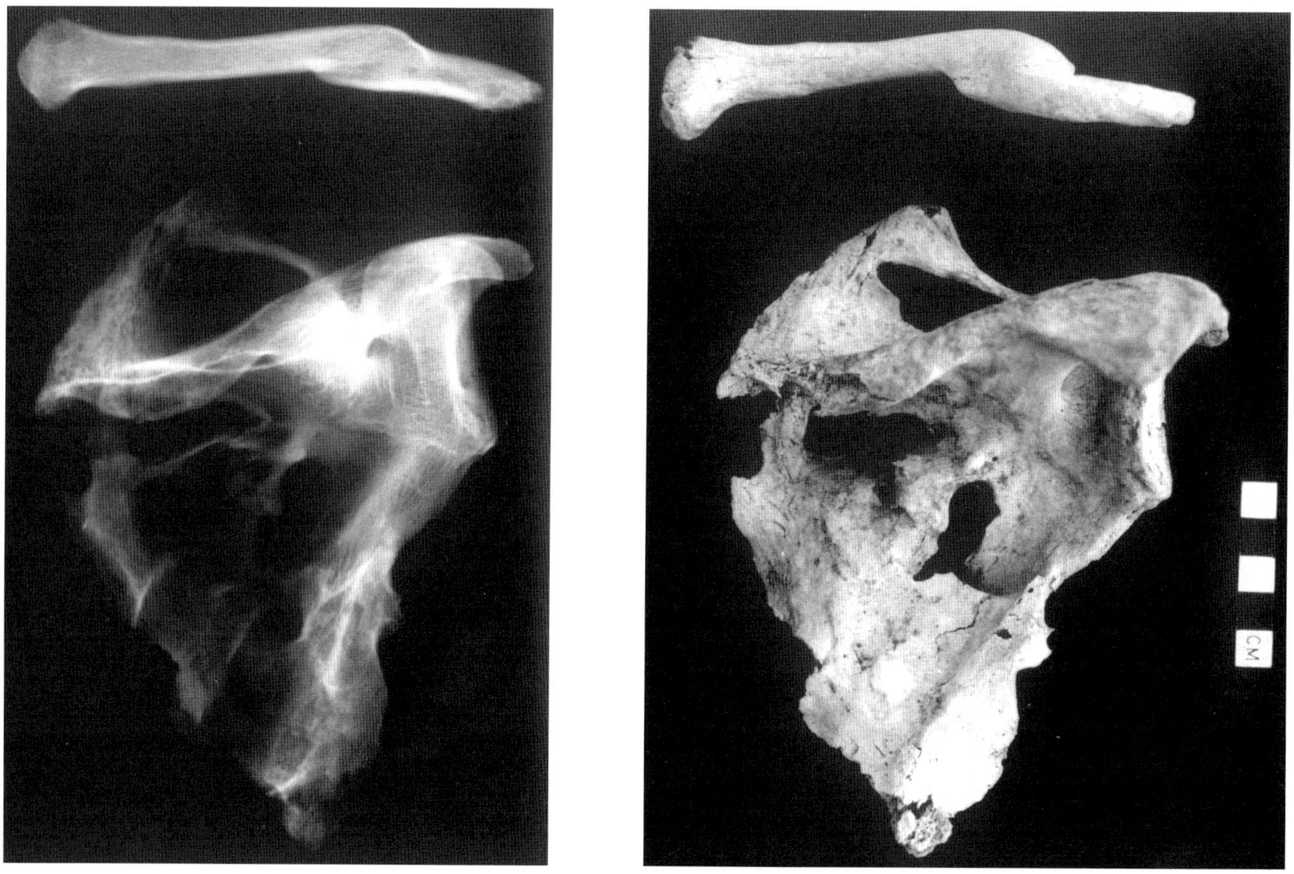

Fig. 33.2. Healed fractures of both the right clavicle and scapula from an adult male from Kalavasos-*Kopetra*

possible related trauma includes traumatic arthritis of two cervical vertebrae from the same individual, likely caused by a fall. Two middle-aged adult males were recovered from a tomb within a nearby church. The more superficial of the two displays both healed fractures of the right clavicle and scapula (Fig. 33.2) as well as two ankylosed thoracic vertebrae (Fig. 33.3). The clavicle displays an oblique, type 2 fracture, medial to the conoid tubercle. Scapular fractures are relatively uncommon and occur most often in people 40–60 years of age, according to Galloway (1999, 117). Severe injuries to this bone are indicative of major trauma. In addition to the complete transverse neck fracture that is

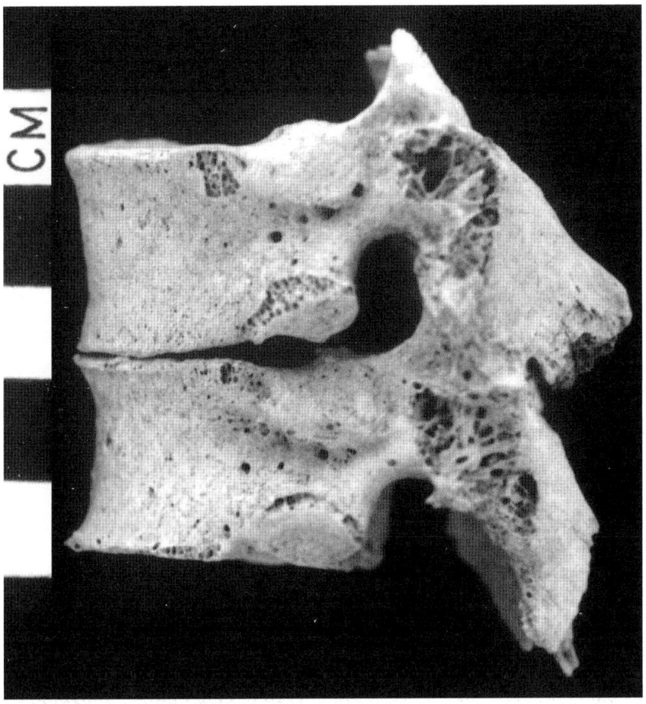

Fig. 33.3. Ankylosed thoracic vertebrae from an individual from Kalavasos-*Kopetra*

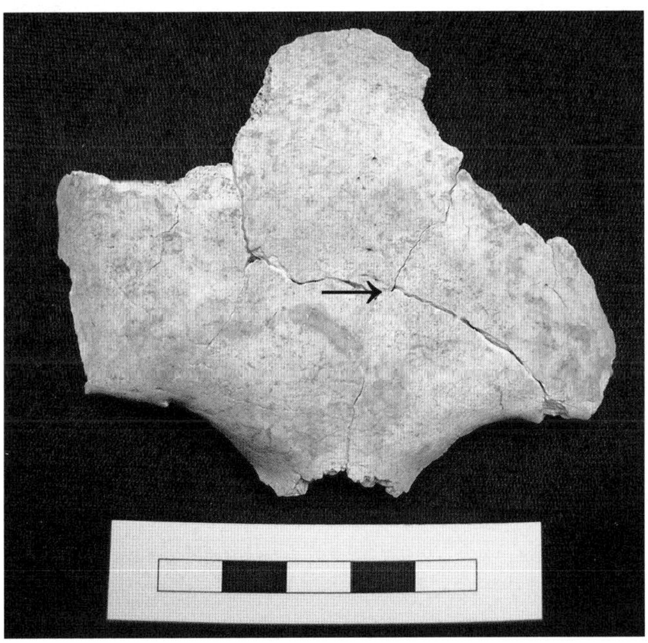
Fig. 33.4. Depressed cranial fracture of the frontal of an adult female from the Hill of Agios Georgios

healed and displaced, there is also an incomplete transverse glenoid fracture along with osteochondylar disease of the glenoid fossa. According to Galloway (*ibid.*), association

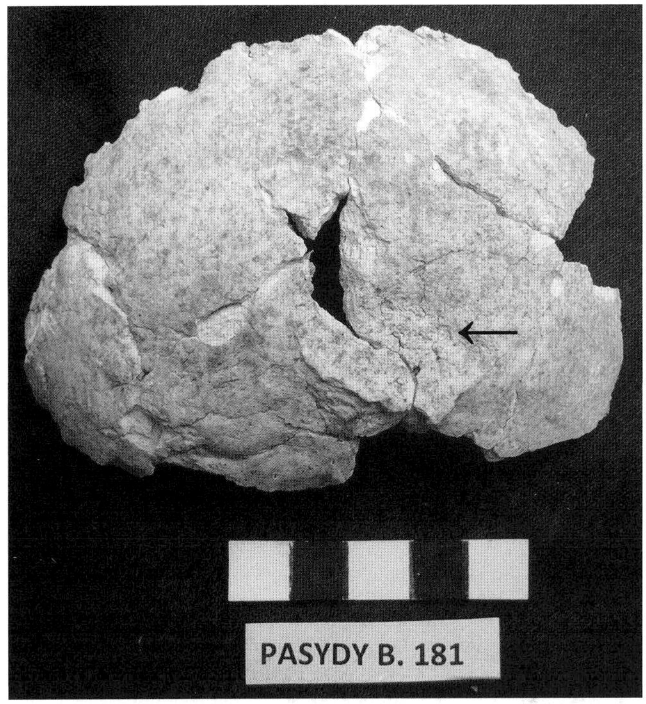

Fig. 33.5. Depressed cranial fracture of the occipital of an old adult male from the Hill of Agios Georgios

of clavicle fractures with scapular fractures occurs in 19–39% of modern cases. The left humerus from a young adult female demonstrates what appears to be a Hahn-Steinthal capitellar fracture that has not united. Capitellar fractures account for only 0.5–1% of all elbow fractures and 6% of all distal humerus fractures, and are not found among children under 10 years of age and are more common in females (*ibid.*, 120). According to Galloway, in 20% of capitellar fractures, radial head fractures are also found. Unfortunately, the radial head was not recovered from this individual, nor was the olecranon process of the ulna. Hahn-Steinthal fractures result from sheer forces from a fall onto an outstretched hand or a fall directly onto the elbow. Other fractures from the south coast include a distal fracture of the right radius of a young adult female as well as the healed fracture of the base of the right first metatarsal from another young adult female.

A different pattern of fractures emerges from the inland site of the Hill of Agios Georgios. Two depressed cranial fractures are identified at the Hill of Agios Georgios from the Early Christian period. One of these is observed in the frontal of a middle-aged female (Fig. 33.4). There is no sinus involvement upon endocranial inspection and it is well-healed. The second depressed cranial fracture appears to be a well-healed occipital fracture near the external occipital protuberance of an old adult male (Fig. 33.5). It is unfortunate that there is so much post-mortem damage to this bone. Other traumata will be described below.

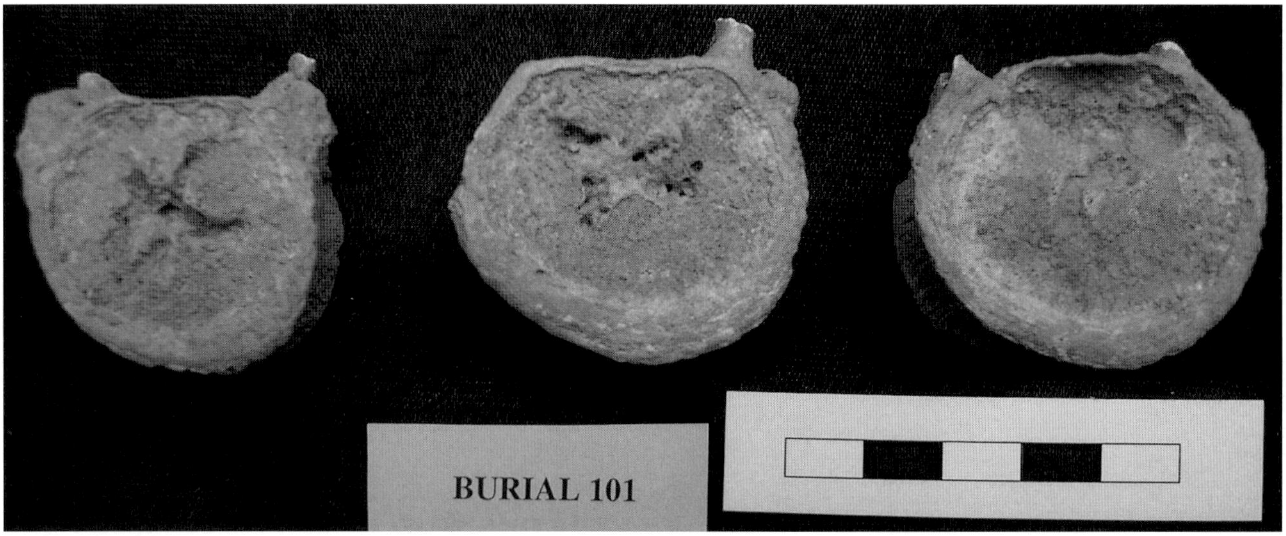

Fig. 33.6. Schmorl's nodes of a thoracic vertebra from an adult male from B 128 at the Hill of Agios Georgios

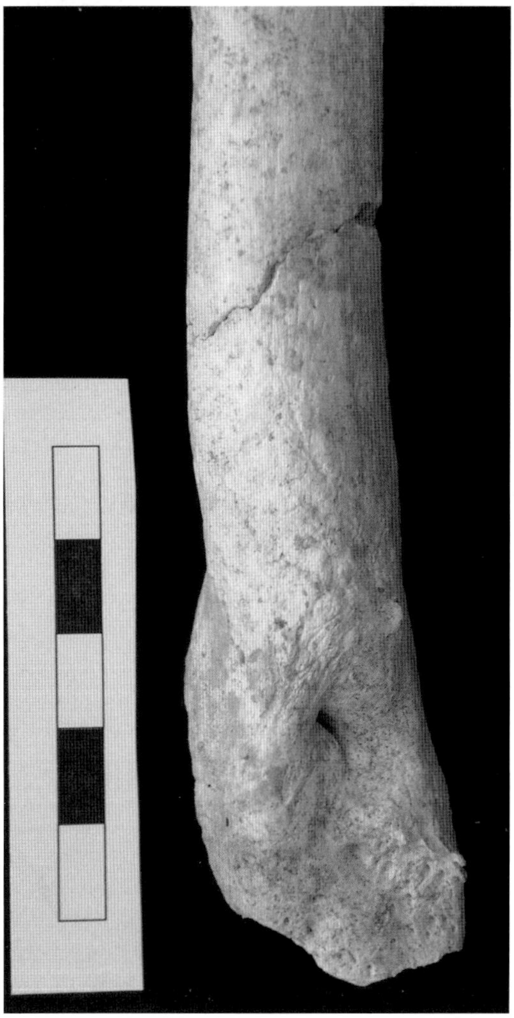
Fig. 33.7. Healed fracture and osteomyelitic infection of a humerus from an old adult male from the Hill of Agios Georgios

Schmorl's nodes are depressed fractures of the endplates of vertebral bodies caused by the evulsion of the nucleus pulposis of the intervertebral discs into the bodies. Their etiology is unknown but they could be related to traumatic episodes. Schmorl's nodes are present in three individuals from the site and from both the Early Christian and later phase such as is depicted in the thoracic vertebra from this old adult male from B 128 (Fig. 33.6) which may be associated with a single traumatic event. This case may be related to trauma of the femoral head as well. There is an angulated healed fracture of the distal right humerus from an old adult male dating to the Early Christian period, with subsequent malalignment and osteomyelitic infection with a cloaca (Fig. 33.7). It appears that the right radius from this individual demonstrates disuse atrophy as the radial neck is quite wasted when compared to a normal bone on the right (Fig. 33.8). A distal fragment of the right ulna was recovered, and, it too, appears to have atrophied. These atrophied bones of the forearm are likely related to nerve damage to the lower arm from the associated pathology of the humerus. The indeterminately sexed adult at the Early Christian Hill of Agios Georgios, demonstrates displacement and ankylosis of coccygeal elements as depicted (Fig. 33.9) in this dorsal view, likely related to a fall in a seated position. Four individuals from the Hill of Agios Georgios demonstrate traumata to bones of the hand or wrist, including one from an Early Christian context and three from the later phase. A fracture of the right fifth metacarpal of an adult of unknown sex from an Early Christian context is among the pathological lesions of the hand (Fig. 33.10). It appears to be a very well-healed fracture with callus formation at the medial aspect of the shaft. This is not the typical boxer's fracture of the fifth metacarpal, but Galloway (1999, 156) states, 'Direct blows may be blocked by the hands producing

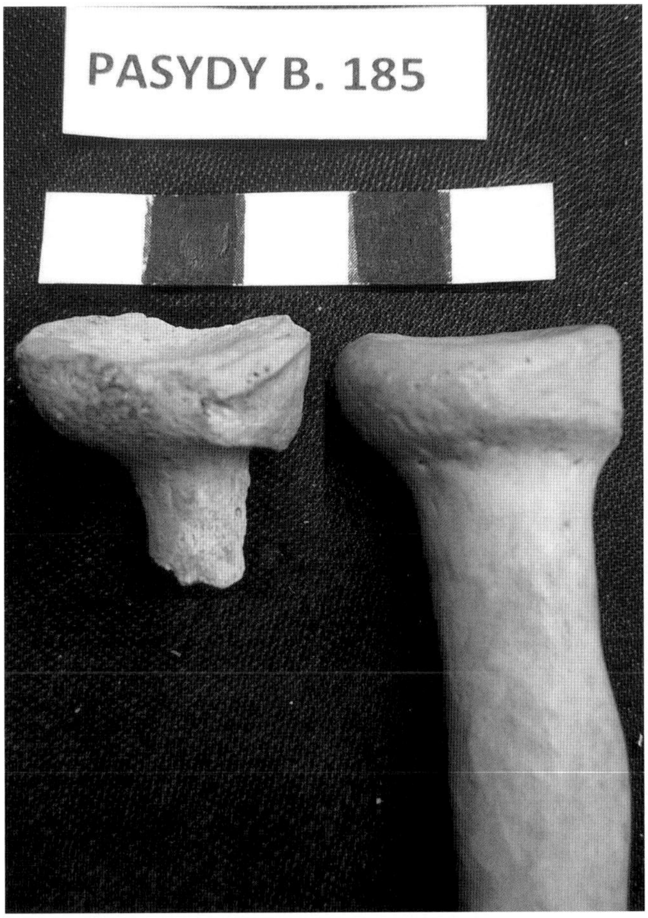

Fig. 33.8. Wasted right radius due to previous nerve damage from the same old adult male as Fig. 33.7 from the Hill of Agios Georgios

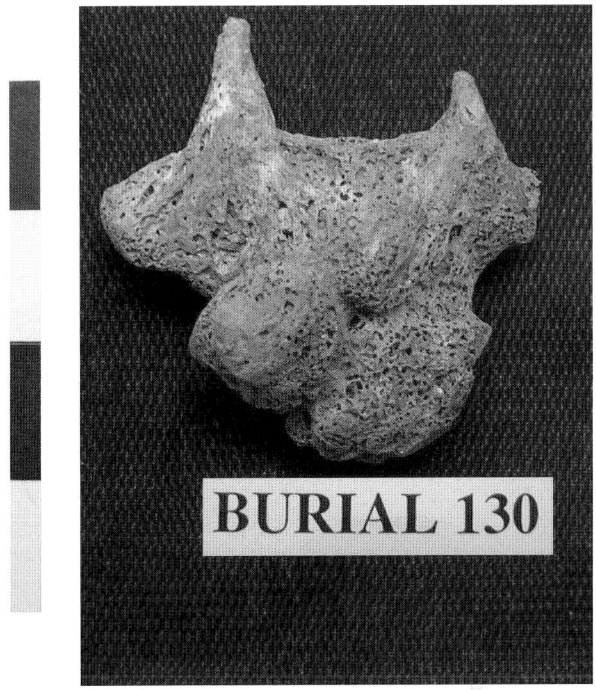

Fig. 33.9. Displacement and ankylosis of the coccygeal elements from an adult from the Hill of Agios Georgios

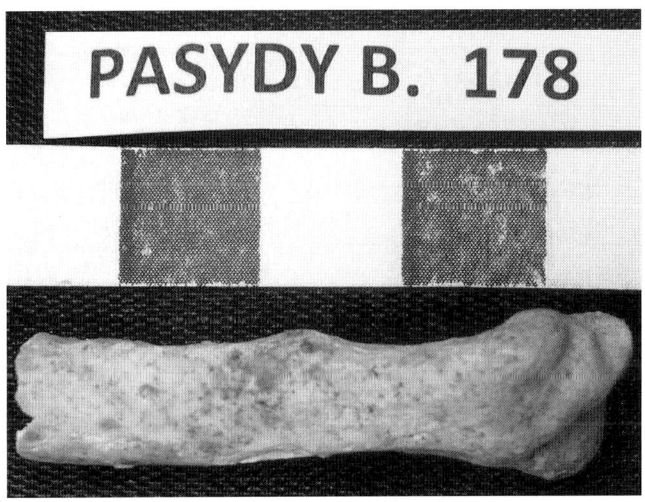

Fig. 33.10. Healed fracture of a right fifth metacarpal from an adult from the Hill of Agios Georgios

fractures of the metacarpals'. These are defensive injuries.

Parry fractures of the ulnae, forearm defensive wounds from warding off blows, are observed among two individuals from the Hill of Agios Georgios, one in an adult female and one from a middle-aged adult male, both from the later phase. The X-ray of the male demonstrates a textbook parry fracture showing both the point of impact and callus formation. A rib fracture is also included among the fractures of the people from the later phase at the Hill of Agios Georgios (Fig. 33.11). The left humerus of an old adult male demonstrates a couple of traumatic lesions, with evidence of osteochondylar disease of the capitulum, perhaps from a traumatic event that could be linked with the fracture to the left fifth metacarpal (Fig. 33.12). According to Ortner (2003, 155), 'If fracture occurs in or near the physis, the trauma may result in premature fusion of the growth plate and result in abnormal length of the affected bone. The severity of the abnormal length will depend on the age of the individual at the time of the injury'. Figure 33.12 shows the normal right fifth metacarpal for comparison. There are relatively very few traumata observed among lower body bones. A femur from an old adult of indeterminate sex demonstrates what appears to be an injury to the anterior proximal aspect of the long bone probably an example of myositis ossificans of the origin of vastus intermedius (Fig. 33.13). Other differential diagnoses should be included, such as a sharp implement wound. Lastly, an amputation of the first proximal hand phalanx from a medieval phase at the Hill of Agios

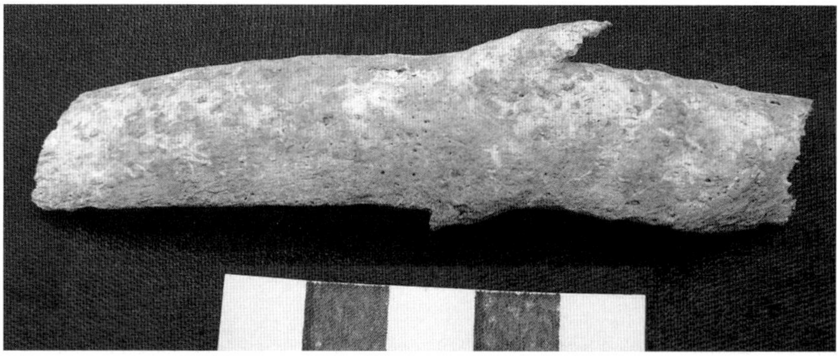

Fig. 33.11. Rib fracture from an adult from the Hill of Agios Georgios (later phase)

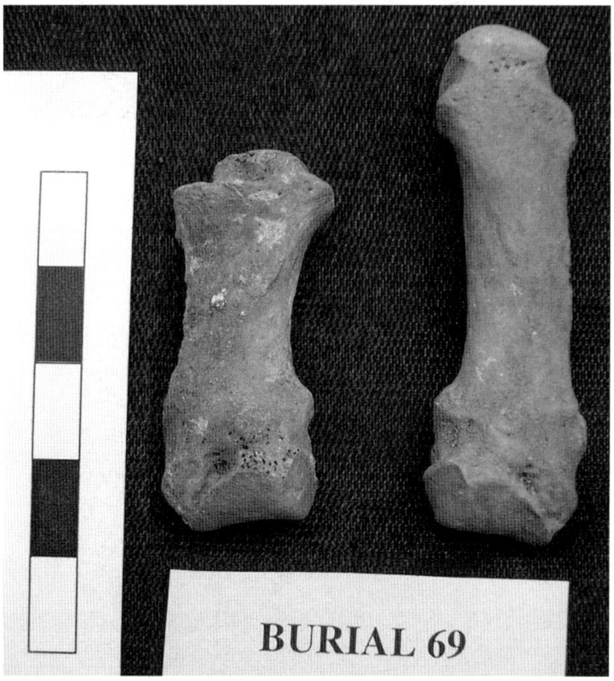

Fig. 33.12. Left fifth metacarpal with an old healed fracture at the physis compared with the normal right fifth metacarpal from the same individual from the Hill of Agios Georgios

Georgios encourages study of the later material from the site (Fig. 33.14).

Discussion and conclusions

In conclusion, some trends could be observed when comparing the rural south coast sites with the inland site of the Hill of Agios Georgios. There is a much greater prevalence of pathology at the Hill of Agios Georgios, including trauma. This can, in part, be explained by the demographic differences between the two samples, with the older individuals at the Hill of Agios Georgios having the opportunity to acquire more traumata. The second difference is that males at the Hill of Agios Georgios have a greater propensity for traumatic lesions. This difference cannot be explained on the basis of the demographic profile. In fact, the south coast has more males than the Hill of Agios Georgios. Although, very small subsamples, the mode for trauma is that young adult females exhibit more traumatic injuries on the south coast while old adult males tend to display them at the Hill of Agios Georgios. Three of the four sexed individuals expressing trauma in Early Christian deposits at the Hill of Agios Georgios are male. These results are similar to findings of Bourbou (2004, 57) at Early Byzantine Eleutherna with all five fractures found among males at the site. Additionally, Angel (1974) found that males exhibited twice the number of fractures as females from his large sample derived mostly from Greek archaeological sites. With regard to the location of injuries, there is a predominance of upper body trauma. It should be noted that cranial fractures and hand injuries are completely absent from the south coast. Again, cranial injuries are seen among the remains from the Early Christian phase, and hand injuries among both Early Christian and later phases at the Hill of Agios Georgios. Further differences in the types of fracture and or injuries are observed. Two parry fractures are identified among ulnae of individuals from the Hill of Agios Georgios, from the 10th–12th century phase. On the south coast, conversely, the only fracture to a forearm bone is a distal radial fracture as a result of a fall. The most commonly fractured bone is the right clavicle among individuals from the south coast and hand injuries are the most prevalent trauma among individuals from the inland site. With regard to the severity of the trauma, the impression is that the severity is greater among individuals from the south coast. Severe trauma is exhibited inland, but all of the traumata demonstrated at the coast are in the form of fractures and three of the four are severe, including one

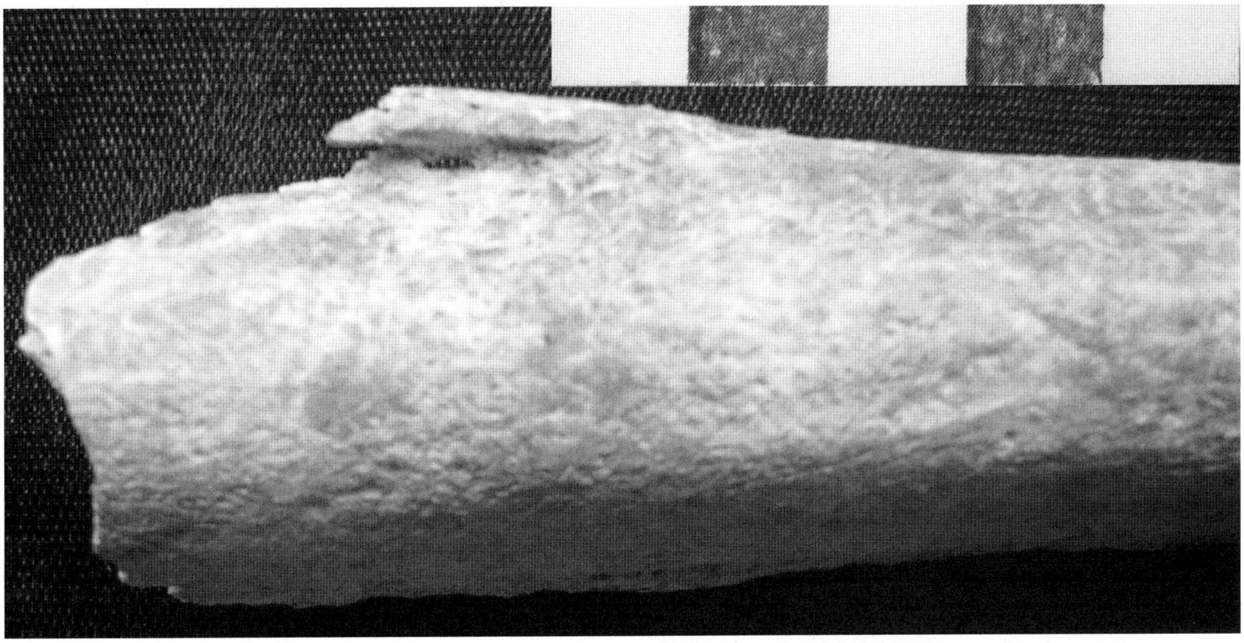

Fig. 33.13. Possible myositis ossificans of a femur from the Hill of Agios Georgios

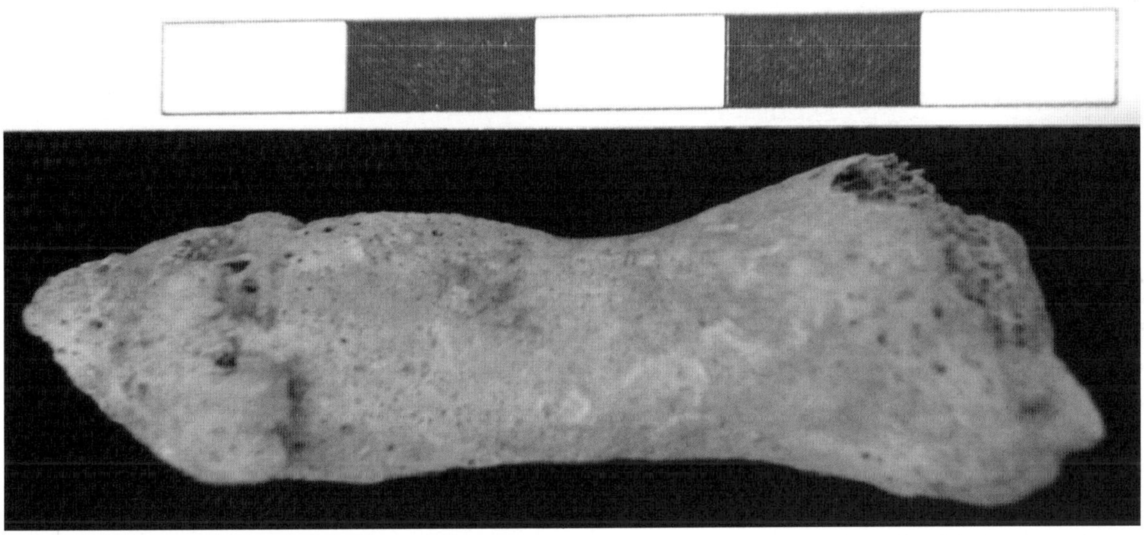

Fig. 33.14. Amputation of a proximal hand phalanx from a medieval phase at the Hill of Agios Georgios

individual with three fractures in two bones, and another individual with fractures in two bones. Not one individual from the Hill of Agios Georgios possesses more than a single fracture. Again, falls appear to have been responsible for these fractures among the individuals from the south coast. Falls are responsible for many of the injuries observed among individuals from the Hill of Agios Georgios as well. However, the trauma observed at the Hill of Agios Georgios expresses greater variability. The sample size is far too small at this point to make sweeping generalisations and, as such, simple trends are stated. Furthermore, the 'strong circumstantial evidence of malevolent intent' that Walker (2001, 567) suggests is necessary to indicate violent injury in bioarchaeology is lacking. In contrast to the south coast sample, the trend for depressed cranial fractures, and hand trauma exists at the Hill of Agios Georgios in the Early Christian period, and parry fractures and hand trauma are demonstrated to have occurred in the later phase. Additionally, males exhibited far more traumata than females at the Hill of Agios Georgios.

It is obvious that additional factors explaining these patterns could be at play, including cultural, behavioural, or occupational differences. Future excavations at the Hill of Agios Georgios and study of the later material may help shed light on the way of life at the inland and urban centre when compared to the coastal and rural south coast sites.

Acknowlegements

The authors thank Prof. Demetrios Michaelides for the organisation of the conference from which these proceedings emanated and his unfailing patience. The Department of Antiquities of Cyprus is warmly acknowledged for supporting Dr Despina Pilides' excavations on which part of these results were founded and for allowing the human skeletal material to be temporarily transferred to the Wiener Laboratory at the American School of Classical Studies at Athens for analyses. The Global History of Human Health Project for Europe, funded by the National Science Foundation, helped support one of the authors, Ms Ioanna Moutafi. Dr Malcolm Wiener, the Wiener Laboratory and the American School of Classical Studies at Athens are appreciated for their support of Dr Sherry C. Fox. The Department of Antiquities of Cyprus is also greatly acknowledged, along with Profs Marcus Rautman and Sturt Manning, and Dr Pavlos Flourentzos for their permission for Dr Sherry C. Fox to study the human skeletal remains from their sites: Kalavasos-*Kopetra*, Maroni-*Petrera* and Alassa-*Ayia Mavri*, respectively.

Bibliography

Angel, J. L. 1945: 'Skeletal material from Attica', *Hesperia* 14, 279–363.

Angel, J. L. 1974: 'Patterns of fractures from Neolithic to modern times', *Anthropologiai Közlemények* 18, 9–18.

Bourbou, C. 2004: *The People of Early Byzantine Eleutherna and Messene (6th–7th centuries A.D.): A Bioarchaeological Approach,* Athens.

Buikstra, J. E. and Ubelaker, D. H. 1994: *Standards for Data Collection from Human Skeletal Remains* (Arkansas Archeological Survey Research Series 44), Fayetteville.

Flourentzos, P. 1996: *Excavations in the Kouris River Valley II. The Basilica of Alassa*, Nicosia.

Flourentzos, P. 2004–2005: 'Chronique de fouilles et découvertes archéologiques à Chypre en 2003,' *Bulletin de Correspondence héllenique* 130, 1635–708.

Flourentzos, P. 2006: 'Chronique de fouilles et découvertes archéologiques à Chypre en 2005,' *Bulletin de Correspondence héllenique* 130, 873–919.

Fox, S. C. 1996: 'The human skeletal remains from Alassa-*Ayia Mavri*, Cyprus', Appendix (39–64) in P. Flourentzos, *Excavations in the Kouris River Valley II. The Basilica of Alassa*, Nicosia.

Fox, S. C. 2002: 'Burials in the church at Maroni *Petrera*', 38–40 in S. Manning, *The Late Roman Church at Maroni* Petrera, Oxford and Oakville.

Fox, S. C. 2003: 'The human skeletal remains: a preliminary report,' Appendix 5 in M. Rautman, *A Cypriot village of Late Antiquity: Kalavasos*-Kopetra *in the Vasilikos Valley*, (Journal of Roman Archaeology, Supplementary Series 52), Portsmouth, RI.

Fox, S. C., Moutafi, I., Prevedorou, E. and Pilides, D. 2012: 'The burial customs of Early Christian Cyprus: A bioarchaeological approach' 60–79 in M. Perry (ed.), *Bioarchaeology and Behavior: The People of the Ancient Near East*, Gainsville.

Galloway, A. (ed.) 1999: *Broken Bones,* Springfield.

Hadjisavvas, S. 1999, 'Chronique de fouilles et découvertes archéologiques à Chypre en 1998', *Bulletin de Correspondence héllenique* 123, 599–633.

Manning, S. 2002: *The Late Roman Church at Maroni* Petrera, Oxford.

Ortner, D. 2003: *Identification of Pathological Conditions in Human Skeletal Remains*, Amsterdam.

Pilides, D. 2003, 'Excavations at the Hill of Agios Georgios (PA. SY.D.Y.), Nicosia, 2002 Season. Preliminary Report' (with an Appendix by Andrea Berlin and Jeffery Pilacinski) in *Report of the Department of Antiquities Cyprus*, 181–237.

Pilides, D. and Olivier, J. P. 2008: 'A Black Glazed Cup from the Hill of Agios Georgios, Lefkosia, belonging to a 'wanax'', *Report of the Department of Antiquities Cyprus*, 337–52.

Pilides, D. and Destrooper-Georgiades, A. 2008: 'A hoard of silver coins from the plot on the corner of Nikokreontos and Hadjopoullou Streets, (east extension of the settlement of the Hill of Agios Georgios, Lefkosia)', *Report of the Department of Antiquities Cyprus*, 308–35.

Rautman, M. 2003: *A Cypriot Village of Late Antiquity: Kalavasos-*Kopetra *in the Vasilikos Valley*, (Journal of Roman Archaeology Supplementary Series 52), Portsmouth, RI.

Walker, P. L. 2001: 'A bioarchaeological perspective on the history of violence,' *Annual Review of Anthropology* 30, 573–96.

Part VIII

Asklepios and Incubation

34. The Development of the Practice of Incubation in the Ancient World

Juliette Harrisson

There has been much debate concerning how to define incubation, and where to look for its origins. This paper defines incubation 'as a practice in which a person performs a ritual act and then sleeps in a sacred place, with the deliberate intention of receiving a divine dream', and argues that 'incubation' in its strictest sense did not exist before the development of the practice in healing shrines in ancient Greece. The various examples of 'incubation' that have been identified elsewhere represent stages in the development of ideas concerning dreams that would eventually lead to the development of incubation proper.

Much has been written about the practice of incubation in the ancient world, but research on this subject has been complicated by opposing definitions of what does or does not constitute incubation. This paper argues that 'incubation' in its strictest sense did not exist before the well-known development of the practice in healing shrines in ancient Greece. The various examples of 'incubation' that have been identified in Egypt and the Ancient Near East represent certain stages in the development of ideas concerning dreams and oneiromancy that would eventually lead to the development of incubation proper.

The first and foremost problem in discussing ancient incubation is defining the practice, as a number of possible definitions are available. The *Oxford English Dictionary* offers several definitions, mostly related to biology; the one that concerns this paper is the fourth given meaning of the word, which is 'the practice of sleeping in a temple or sacred place for oracular purposes'. The dictionary supports this definition with a quotation from Tylor's 1871 work, *Primitive Culture*, which describes incubation at the temple of Asclepius.

The roots of the English word 'incubation' are found in Latin. The *Oxford Latin Dictionary* gives, as part (b) of the second meaning of the verb *incubo*, 'to sleep (in a temple in the hope of having inspired dreams, or of divine healing)'. Margalit has noted that the term comes from a translation of the Greek *ἐγκοιμίζω*, 'to lull to sleep (in a place)' (Margalit 1989, 263). The *Oxford Classical Dictionary* (focusing, of course, on Greece and Rome) defines incubation as 'ritual sleep in a sanctuary … in order to obtain a dream, mostly for healing' (Graf 1996, 753). Benjamin Kilborne, in his article for Mircea Eliade's *Encyclopedia of Religion*, connects incubation even more strongly with healing, referring to it as a 'Mediterranean' practice and defining it as 'sleeping in a sacred place in order to dream a cure to ailments … and to seek guidance … and knowledge of the future from a divine being'. He cross-links the practice specifically with the cult of Asclepius and speaks of it with reference only to Greece and Rome (Kilborne 1987, 485–86). Sally Butler, introducing her discussion of Mesopotamian incubation, refers to the practice at Greek and Roman sanctuaries as the 'archetype' of the technique (Butler 1998, 217). Although much of the evidence for Greco-Roman incubation does relate to healing, to include such a connection in the very definition of the word seems to be going too far; we do have examples of incubation that are not directly related to health, notably from the oracle of Trophonius (see Pausanias, 9.39.4–9.40.2, though it should be noted that, according to Pausanias, the statue of Trophonius was modelled after Asclepius; 9.39.4).

Definitions of 'incubation' among Egyptologists and scholars of the Ancient Near East show some variation. Oppenheim refers to an incubation dream as a dream experienced while sleeping in a sanctuary or a sacred place 'whether the dream is sought or not' (Oppenheim 1956, 190). Robert Gnuse defines 'dream incubation' as 'an activity in which an individual goes to a shrine or a sacred site and engages in some ritual activity … in order to obtain a revelation from the deity' (Gnuse 1993, 356). However, he complicates his definition by suggesting a 'typology' for 'dreams at holy places' which includes 'intentional dream incubation' alongside 'incidental unintentional dream incubation' and 'accidental unintentional dream incubation' (*ibid.*, 365). The suggestion that some instances of incubation are 'unintentional' seems to contradict his own definition of incubation as a ritual activity which is performed '*in order to*' receive a dream (my italics). Ann Jeffers, on the other hand, sidesteps this problem by simply defining incubation as 'a dream revelation which the person attains at a holy place', despite having earlier suggested that even the holy place is not necessarily vital (Jeffers 1996, 135, 137). C. L. Seow does not provide a specific definition of incubation, but does seem to suggest that it requires 'intentionality' (Seow 1984, 146, 147). K. Patton emphasises that 'intentional preparation and orientation were mandatory in ancient dream incubation', but within the page contradicts her own assertion by claiming that 'unintentional incubations are occasionally known in antiquity' (Patton 2004, 202–3).

The chief reason for the discrepancy among Near Eastern scholars is that a strong inclination has developed for identifying certain dream reports, some from the Old Testament, others from other sources, usually royal, as examples of 'incubation'. One of the earliest proponents of this theory was E. Ehrlich, whose chapter on incubation in his book on dreams in the Old Testament identified a number of Old Testament dream reports as examples of incubation (Ehrlich 1953, 13–57). In the case of Ugaritic literature, Margalit has suggested that this idea can be traced back to Obermann's 1946 study, which was quickly endorsed by a number of scholars (Margalit 1989, 260–1). Obermann's chief object of study was one of the few texts that do appear to represent an early form of incubation ritual, an Ugaritic poem (see below). During the course of his study, he suggests that a number of other texts may represent incubatory rituals; however, on closer examination, the evidence for this is slim.

Obermann provides some examples which he argues represent examples of incubation, but where the actual incubation ritual is not described. For example, he suggests that Job 33.15 provides a 'reference' to incubation (Obermann 1946, 10). The main problem with this suggestion is that a rather circular argument ensues; on the one hand, it is possible that incubation was understood to have taken place without needing to be described; on the other hand, why should we read something into a text that is not there? Job 33.15 states that God speaks 'in dreams and in night-visions/ when slumber has settled on humanity/ and people are asleep in bed'.[1] There is no reference to any kind of ritual, no suggestion that the communication was deliberately sought by the sleeper, and these people are specifically described as being in bed, not at a sanctuary of any kind. Obermann suggests that, if we had found a text describing incubation rites for practical purposes, we would have been able to discover more about the ritual (Obermann 1946, 9). Such speculation is, however, ultimately fruitless, as we have no such texts. Whether they existed but have been lost, or whether they never existed at all, is extremely difficult to tell, but neither possibility can arbitrarily be ruled out.

Another example will illustrate the main problems with this line of argument. Jeffers, following Obermann, claims that the dream of Keret (Keilalphabetische Texte aus Ugarit (KTU) 1.14 I:26ff), which comes to him after he has fallen asleep, weeping, on his bed, can be viewed as an example of incubation. She argues that incubation need not take place at a sanctuary and that Keret's weeping is linked to ritual weeping at times of crisis, and therefore represents a ritual action performed in order to bring on a dream (Jeffers 1996, 135).[2] This assessment, however, is not entirely convincing. It might be reasonable to suggest that incubation does not need to take place at a sanctuary, though examples of obviously incubatory practice at other sites are rare. But Jeffers' suggestion that Keret's weeping is related to ritual weeping in times of crisis and therefore 'may be part of an incubation ritual' is unsubstantiated; at no point does the text suggest that the act of weeping was deliberate, or related to ritual in any way. Falling asleep on one's bed crying is not a ritual act, nor does it suggest the desire to produce a divine dream. It is much more reasonable to read the actions of the god as motivated by sympathy for Keret, rather than brought about by ritual action.

Some have attempted to offer an explanation for the lack of description of incubation ritual in these examples. In the case of the Old Testament, Gnuse and Patton (among others) have argued that, because, in Jewish (and later Christian) theology, it is not appropriate to force God to do the bidding of a human being, and because incubation seems to represent such a manipulation of God by performing a ritual designed to make Him send the person a dream, accounts of incubation in the Old Testament have been 'suppressed' and described in vague terms, in order to hide their incubatory origin (Gnuse 1993, 367–8; Patton 2004, 218). However, this is not necessarily the case. Firstly, incubation ritual is not necessarily entirely incompatible with Jewish theology, as it represents a request for God/a god to send a dream, i.e. a prayer; (the) God is not forced or obliged to comply, and there is some evidence of later Judeo-Christian incubation.[3] Secondly, the paucity of evidence for incubation in the Ancient Near East (see below) suggests that incubation, in its classical form, was not commonly practised until later periods. There is relatively little evidence for incubation outside the Bible, so why should we read some unclear examples within it as examples of incubation? Finally, one must ask the question – if followers of these religions believed one should not order the gods to send a dream to them, and were careful to avoid referring to such a practice in their written texts, why would they go on to practise such a ritual?

Several scholars have noted these problems, and Margalit, Lindblom, and Kenik have all expressed reservations about applying the label 'incubation' to so many dream reports (see Margalit 1989, 265). Kenik, referring to Solomon's dream at Gibeon, which has been identified as incubatory, suggests that this example is neither incubatory nor historical, but a narrative device employed by the writer of Deuteronomy to establish Solomon's kingship (Kenik 1983, 182). Lindblom has investigated several examples of dreams in the Old Testament, often identified as incubation dreams, and noted that there is no mention in these cases of the dreamer having deliberately slept in a holy place for the purpose of having a divine dream; the dream came 'while they were by chance sleeping in a holy place' (Lindblom 1961, 103–5). Margalit identifies incubation as a purely Classical and Christian practice (including Classical Greece and Rome and on into Christianity) (Margalit 1989, 263).

How then, should we define incubation? The traditional assessment regarding Greece and Rome seems a little narrow – although the great majority of examples of Greco-Roman incubation are from medicinal shrines, the practice is not exclusive to medicine and healing. On the other hand, some of the definitions relating to the Ancient Near East seem excessively broad. First of all, the aspect of deliberation is vital. Incubation must refer to a deliberate ritual act, performed with the intention of experiencing a divine dream. Oppenheim has suggested that divine dreams experienced while sleeping in a sanctuary, whether sought or not, form a 'prototype' of sorts for later oneiromantic practices (Oppenheim 1956, 190). This seems very likely, but these experiences cannot be defined as ritual 'incubation' if the sleeper is not actively seeking a divine message or dream; they are stages in the development of incubatory practice, but do not yet represent full incubation. The nature of the ritual act may vary, but it must be deliberate – weeping does not qualify. There can be no 'unintentional' incubation, for it is by nature an intentional act. The relative importance of the sanctuary is more difficult. Simply entering a sanctuary, without any intention of sleeping and receiving a divine dream, is not incubation – so the argument that both of Jacob's dreams constitute incubation, including the first, where he is unaware that he is in a sacred place, is unconvincing (see for example Gnuse 1993, 363–5; Jeffers 1996, 137–8).

Margalit has suggested that, since the term 'incubation' comes from the Greek for 'to lull to sleep (in a place)' (see above), sleeping in a sacred place should be understood as essential to the practice of incubation (Margalit 1989, 263). Although one might have some reservations about considering this to be the most important aspect of incubation, as Margalit suggests – the deliberate act being, perhaps, even more important – it seems clear from the available evidence that incubation, as normally practised, involved sleeping in a sacred place. And so we arrive at a working definition for 'incubation' as *a practice in which a person performs a ritual act and then sleeps in a sacred place, with the deliberate intention of receiving a divine dream*. The dream must be deliberately sought through ritual action, or what we are looking at is not incubation.

There are, then, three elements to the incubatory ritual; sleeping in a sacred place, performing a specific ritual before sleep, and praying specifically for a dream from the god. All of these elements appear separately in various sources from Egypt and the Ancient Near East, and this has led some scholars to identify occurrences of these elements as indications of the practice of incubation. However, it is only when these three elements come together that we can call the ritual 'incubation'. The existence of these elements separately from each other in earlier sources suggests that these ideas and practices, having developed separately across the ancient world, eventually came together in the practice of incubation.

Sleeping in a sacred place is a motif that occurs several times in different sources. It has sometimes been confused with another motif, in which a person sleeps in an ordinary place, but while sleeping there, receives a divine dream, and afterwards the place becomes sacred because of this experience. An experience like this is obviously conceptually related to incubation, but does not represent incubation itself. The most commonly cited example is that of Jacob in Genesis 28, when he lies down to sleep in a 'certain place', with his head on a stone, and has a dream in which Yahweh speaks to him (Genesis 28.10–22). There is nothing in the text to suggest that Jacob knew that the site was sacred. When Jacob wakes from his dream, he declares that Yahweh must be in that place; he has discovered that the place is sacred because of the dream, rather than lying down to sleep there because it is sacred (he also performs no preparatory ritual). The idea that God (or a god) might speak to someone in a dream if they slept in a holy place is therefore clearly present in the text, but this idea stands alone; there is no corresponding ritual in order deliberately to provoke a divine dream.

Yahweh's call to Samuel has sometimes been interpreted as incubation because Samuel was sleeping in the sanctuary, but this is the only aspect of incubation present in this example. The author notes that, at the time, Yahweh spoke rarely and visions were uncommon. He then describes how Samuel was lying in Yahweh's sanctuary and heard Yahweh calling his name, though three times he mistook the voice for his father, who eventually realised what was happening, and told Samuel to tell Yahweh that he was listening (1 Samuel 3). This may be a dream, as Samuel is lying down, though the text seems to suggest that Samuel is on the edge of sleep and hears Yahweh calling. Again, Samuel's reception of the divine call while sleeping in a holy place suggests conceptualisations of sleeping and dreaming that would eventually develop into the practice of incubation. However, since Samuel does not ask for this divine message, and does not realise there is anything special about it until the fourth time, this clearly does not represent developed incubatory practice.

Turning to non-Hebrew sources, in the *Annals* of Assurbanipal, a 'seer' receives a message dream from Ishtar with a message for Assurbanipal, which occurs while Assurbanipal, who has been threatened by a rival, is praying, presumably in the temple (he says he approached her presence). While Assurbanipal prays for help, and indeed receives comforting words from the goddess himself, apparently while awake, the goddess sends a dream to a 'seer' with specific instructions concerning what Assurbanipal should do (Smith 1871, 123–6). The dream is unsolicited – Assurbanipal prays for help, but not specifically for a dream, and it comes to someone else anyway – but related to Assurbanipal's prayer, as the dream is essentially the answer to his prayer. Again, we see evidence of the idea that being physically present in the temple might encourage the god to send a divine dream, but this is not connected to any specific ritual.

A fragment from an Anatolian historical epic includes a dream attributed to a man called Kurigalzu, possibly while sleeping in Esgalia; however, the text is very unclear (Butler 1998, 235). It does appear that Kurigalzu slept in the temple, but whether he did so with the deliberate intention of soliciting a divine dream is impossible to tell, as the text has been too badly broken; it may be that this is another example of the stories of divine dreams experienced in temples that would eventually lead to the development of incubation (see Finkel 1983, 78).

There is a reference in one of the Mari letters (A.2437) to a woman who 'had a vision in the temple' (translated by Durand as '*a eu une vision dans le temple*…') (Durand 1988, 478). Unlike most of the other letters, this letter does not refer to a 'dream' ('*rêve*' in Durand's translation) but to a 'vision'; it is, therefore, unclear whether this was a dream or a waking vision. There is also no reference to the woman having deliberately slept in the temple in order to receive a dream or performing any kind of ritual to receive a dream.[4]

In Egypt, from the period of the New Kingdom, there is evidence that people sometimes slept in the temple precinct, presumably in order to try to get closer to the god (see Sauneron 1959, 40). A New Kingdom inscription devoted to Hathor refers to sleeping in the temple precinct, but makes no reference to a preliminary sacrifice, or to the expectation of receiving a divine dream (nor to any interesting dreams experienced by the subject). As K. Szpakowska has noted, the emphasis seems to be on spending a lot of time in the temple, even sleeping there (Szpakowska 2003, 146).

Ritual action followed by the reception of a divine dream is also a frequent motif, but in most cases, there is no causal link between the action and the dream; the person does not specifically pray for a dream, nor does he sleep in a sacred place. Additionally, most of these examples refer, not to just any person, but to kings, leaders and prophets.

Examples include the *Weidner Chronicle* (from a Neo-Babylonian temple library), which contains a sequence in which a god is sacrificed to and petitioned and later appears in a dream, though Butler has observed that the sacrifice and prayers are a standard form of petitioning the gods, and do not necessarily indicate that a dream is sought specifically. Butler also notes that this document is written as a glorification of Babylon and Marduk, and may not represent actual practice (Butler 1998, 234–5). Oppenheim suggested that the dream of Nabonidas which is part of his consultation of various beings is 'one of the few unequivocally described incubation-dreams in cuneiform literature'; however, as Butler has pointed out, although there is a reference to lying down at night, the vision is not specifically described as a dream, nor does it contain a precise message (Oppenheim 1956, 205; Butler 1998, 233–4).

In the Old Testament, Jacob sacrifices at Beersheba, and that night, God speaks to him in a vision (Genesis 46.1–5). Solomon's dream at Gibeon is recorded twice. 1: Kings 3.4–15 describes how Solomon offered 'a thousand' burnt offerings at Gibeon, and then Yahweh appeared to him in a dream during the night. 2: Chronicles 1.6–12 describes Solomon presenting an offering to Yahweh at Gibeon, and that night God appears to him and they have a conversation. It is these dreams in particular that lend themselves to the theory that incubatory practice was being carried out, but suppressed in writing. However, there is no reason to assume such a suppression. Solomon is a king and Jacob is a king-like character; these dreams fit better into the category of royal message dreams, which are well attested in the Ancient Near East (see Harrisson 2013, 89–90). Although sacrifice is described, there is no reference to the dreamer sleeping in a sacred place (although, since Jacob is travelling, it may be assumed that he slept where he was). The sacrifices are not directly linked to the dream by intentionality. Although there is a clear link, in that Yahweh was pleased by the sacrifice, therefore He appeared to the dreamer in a dream, there is no suggestion that the sacrifice was carried out in order to provoke a dream from the divine. Again, it is possible that incubatory practices developed from the ideas present here, that if one sacrifices to God, he may respond by sending a divine dream, but the ritual practice of incubation is not yet developed.

There is sometimes, then, a link between royal ritual action and dream reports. In some cases, it may have been politically prudent for a new king to claim to have had a divine dream to cement his claim to kingship. In this case, the king would deliberately perform a ritual act, then, the following day, proclaim that God/a god sent him a dream, confirming his suitability for kingship. In most cases, the relationship between the ritual action and the dream is not one of 'the action is performed therefore the dream is sent', but rather one of 'God/a god is pleased by the action that has been performed, therefore He chooses to send a dream'. The difference is subtle, but extremely important. Gnuse's argument that the action followed the first pattern, but the text reported it as following the second, seems spurious. Firstly, this argument is based entirely on supposition, and not based on the only substantial evidence available, the text. Secondly, it is the text that indicates how the dream was viewed by the people. What actually took place in the king's mind is a matter of speculation; if he was politically savvy, the likelihood is that his dreams were unremarkable, or if he was deeply religious, then he may have experienced a message dream, because his unconscious mind expected to. What matters, however, is that the dream was reported as a spontaneous action of a God who was pleased – whether or not the spontaneous action was expected, it could not be commanded.

The final element of incubatory ritual, the act of praying to the god, asking for a divine dream, also appears in some Near Eastern and Egyptian evidence. From Egypt, some of the *Letters to the Dead* feature a living person asking for a sign from a dead person to be shown them in a dream. However, there is no suggestion in these letters that the living person has removed to a sacred place in order to bring on a dream, or that they have performed any kind of ritual beforehand (see Szpakowska 2003, 144). It should also be noted that, in these cases, the living dreamer is petitioning a dead friend or relative, not directly petitioning a god or divine being. Although incubation often took place at the shrine of a hero, it is normally an extraordinary or heroic figure who is petitioned, not a close relative. Sometimes, a person would pray to a god or gods, asking them to send good dreams, such as the invocation to Isis in P. Chester Beatty III r. 10.10–19 (*ibid.*, 197). Oracular amuletic decrees from the Third Intermediate Period include, among other promises for health and happiness, promises from the gods that the wearer's dreams will be good (*ibid.*, 181–3).

Dream rituals are well-attested in the Ancient Near East. Butler's collection of *Rituals to Obtain a Purussû*, a relatively late source, includes various incantations performed in order 'to see an oracular decision', some of which also refer to dreams; Butler has suggested that the phrase 'to see an oracular decision' may also be translated as 'to see a dream' (Butler 1998, 222, 349–77). Similarly, the *Atrahasis* epic contains a reference to a sacrifice performed asking the god to send a dream, followed by sleeping near a river (*ibid.*, 228–31).

There are some examples of similar or related practices from the Ancient Near East which appear to fit the definition of incubation; a person makes an offering to a god, sleeps in a sacred place, and prays for a divine dream. For example, Tablet 4 of the *Epic of Gilgamesh* features Gilgamesh performing a ritual and asking the Mountain for a dream, and sleeping in a specially built hut near a mountain (which could be interpreted as a sacred space); this literary example may reflect real practice (Butler 1998, 224–7). In the clearest example, Gudea, having received an unsolicited dream from Ningirsu, crosses a river and prays, first to Ningirsu, then to Gatumdu. He offers bread and water to Gatumdu, then sets up a bed next to her statue and sleeps there, having prayed to Gatumdu for a sign and observed that he will tell his dream to his mother, an interpreter of dreams (Edzard 1997, 69–70). Gudea is patron of a temple, and the dreams relate to the building of the temple. These isolated examples relate to leaders and rulers, and so are related more closely to the tendency for leaders to legitimate their actions through divine dreams (see Harrisson 2013, 89–90) than to incubation.

Patton includes Pharaoh's famous dreams under the heading of incubation, under the loose note that 'rulers are frequent incubators of dreams' (Patton 2004, 213). Certainly there is a connection between ruling and significant dreams, but Pharaoh's dreams are omens in the form of dreams, which are closely related to royal message dreams, not incubation. Pharaoh is plagued by unwanted dreams. There is no ritual, no intentionality and no sleeping in a sacred place, so there is no incubation. Gnuse suggests that Psalms 3–5, 11, 17, 27, 57, 63 and 101 may represent 'vague allusions' to incubation (Gnuse 1993, 366). However, none of these contain a definite reference to a dream, and some do not even refer to sleeping; certainly none of them constitute allusions to incubation, however vague.

It has been seen that the ideas and practices that would eventually coalesce to form the ritual practice of incubation were present from a very early period, throughout the ancient world. However, aside from a few isolated examples from rulers and leaders, the regular ritual practice of incubation does not appear until we reach Archaic and Classical Greece; from this period onwards, evidence for incubation becomes plentiful and is particularly, though not exclusively, associated with healing and with the god Asclepius, to whom more incubation shrines are dedicated than to any other god or goddess (see Harrisson 2013, 200–1). The practice seems to date from at least the Archaic period, but the paradigmatic example of 'incubation' is the practice as carried out at the Temple of Asclepius at Epidauros in the Classical period.[5]

From Greece, incubation spread and became increasingly popular. It took off particularly in Hellenistic Egypt, where it was often connected with the god Serapis. Ray has suggested that the appearance of incubation and related practices (such as invocations to the gods to send a dream outside of a temple) in later Egyptian texts represents 'a clear change in Egyptian thought' (Ray 1976, 130). He connects this with an increasing concern with one's own fate and a desire to control it through magic or other means.

However, there is a simpler explanation; the dramatic increase in incubation and related practices was the result of invasion from Greece, where this practice reached its fullest developed form. Most of the evidence relating to incubation in Egypt is Ptolemaic or later. Egyptian ideas about dreams had prepared the ground for the practice of incubation; for example, Szpakowska has suggested that dreams were playing an increasingly important role in religious practice in the New Kingdom, while in literature, Alan Lloyd has noted that dreams become more and more important in Egyptian stories as time goes on (Szpakowska 2003, 147, 151; Lloyd 2006, 88). However, it was in the Hellenistic period, under Greek influence, that incubation took root and became popular. As more and more of the ancient world became part of the Roman Empire, the practice continued to be popular, especially in famous shrines such as that at Pergamum (see Harrisson 2013, 200–10).

It seems likely that there is a link between the various reports sometimes referred to as 'incubation' in Egypt and the Ancient Near East, and the development of the practice of incubation in Greece in the Classical period. The three separate ideas that come together in incubatory practice – that sleeping in a sacred place might encourage a god to communicate, that performing a ritual act or sacrifice might encourage the god to communicate, and that one could ask a god specifically to communicate through the medium of a dream – were all clearly present. However, it was only in Greece that these ideas coalesced into a ritual that could be repeated regularly by any suppliant, no matter what their social status was. The practice of incubation, *a practice in which a person performs a ritual act and then sleeps in a sacred place, with the deliberate intention of receiving a divine dream*, was not fully developed until the Classical period in Greece. Once developed, it spread; there is plenty of evidence of incubation in Hellenistic, Greek-ruled Egypt and the practice continued throughout the Roman period.

Notes

1 All Biblical quotations and translations are from *The New Jerusalem Bible*, Reader's Edition, Wansbrough 1990.

2 See also Obermann 1946, 10, who first suggested that this represented incubation.

3 For examples in the ancient world, see Talbot 2002, 153–4. For a comparatively more recent example from an eyewitness, see Harrison 1908, 313–4.

4 On the dreams in the Mari letters, see further Sasson 1983.

5 See further the collections of epigraphic evidence from Epidauros published by the Edlesteins (Edelstein and Edelstein 1998) and LiDonnici (LiDonnici 1995). On other incubation sites, see for example Behr 1968, 27; Edelstein and Edelstein 1998, 242–55; Petropoulou 1981. For further details on the precise rituals accompanying incubation, see Lupu 2003, 324; Burkert 1985, 267–8; Graf 2008.

Bibliography

Behr, C. A. 1968: *Aelius Aristides and the Sacred Tales*, Amsterdam.

Burkert, W. 1985: *Greek religion* (originally published in 1977 in German, and translated into English by John Raffan), Cambridge, MA.

Butler, S. 1998: *Mesopotamian Conceptions of Dreams and Dream Rituals*, Münster.

Durand, J.-M. 1988: *Archives épistolaires de Mari I/1*, Paris.

Edelstein, E. J. and Edelstein, L. 1998: *Asclepius: Collection and Interpretation of the Testimonies*, Baltimore and London.

Ehrlich, E. L. 1953: *Der Traum im Alten Testament* (Zeitschrift für die Alttestament, Wissenschaft Beihefte 73), Berlin.

Edzard, D. O. 1997, *The Royal Inscriptions from Mesopotamia, Early Periods. Gudea and his Dynasty*, Toronto.

Finkel, I. L. 1983: 'The dream of Kurigalzu and the tablet of sins', *Anatolian Studies* 33, 75–80.

Gnuse, R. 1993: 'The Temple Experience of Jaddus in the *Antiquities* of Josephus: a report of Jewish dream incubation', *The Jewish Quarterly Review*, N.S. 83(3/4), 349–68.

Graf, F. 1996: 'Incubation', 753–54 in S. Hornblower and A. Spawforth (eds), *The Oxford Classical Dictionary*, Oxford.

Graf, F. 2008: 'Incubation', in H. Cancik and H. Schneider (eds), *Brill's New Pauly*, Brill Online, url:http://www.brillonline.nl/subscriber/entry?entry=bnp_e524700 accessed 31/10/08.

Harrison, M. C. 1908: 'A survival of incubation?', *Folklore* 19(3), 313–15.

Harrisson, J. G. 2013: *Dreams and Dreaming in the Roman Empire: Cultural Memory and Imagination*, London and New York.

Jeffers, A. 1996: *Magic and Divination in Ancient Palestine and Syria*, Leiden, New York and Cologne.

Kenik, H. 1983: *Design for Kingship: The Deuteronomistic Narrative Technique in 1 Kings 3: 4–15*, Chico, CA.

Kilborne, B. 1987: 'Dreams', 482–92 in M. Eliade (ed.-in-chief), *The Encyclopedia of Religion*, Vol. 4, New York and London.

LiDonnici, L. R. 1995: *The Epidaurian Miracle Inscriptions: Text, Translation and Commentary*, Atlanta.

Lindblom, J. 1961: 'Theophanies in Holy Places in Hebrew religion', *Hebrew College Union Annual* 32, 91–106.

Lloyd, A. B. 2006: '*Heka*, dreams and prophecy in ancient Egyptian stories', 71–94 in K. Szpakowska (ed.), *Through a Glass Darkly: Magic, Dreams and Prophecy in Ancient Egypt*, Swansea.

Lupu, E. 2003: 'Sacrifice at the Amphiareion and a fragmentary sacred law from Oropos', *Hesperia* 72, 321–40.

Margalit, B. 1989: *The Ugaritic Poem of AQHT*, Berlin and New York.

Obermann, J. 1946: 'How Daniel was blessed with a son: an incubation scene in Ugaritic', *Journal of the American Oriental Society* Supplement 6, Baltimore, 1–30.

Oppenheim, A. L. 1956: 'The interpretation of dreams in the Ancient Near East. With a translation of an Assyrian dream-book', *Transactions of the American Philosophical Society*, N.S.46(3), 179–373.

Oxford Latin Dictionary, Oxford 1968.

Patton, K. 2004: '"A Great and Strange Correction": intentionality, locality, and epiphany in the category of dream incubation', *History of Religions* 43, 194–223.

Petropoulou, A. 1981: 'The Eparche Document and the early oracle at Oropus', *Greek, Roman and Byzantine Studies* 22, 39–63.

Ray, J. D. (trans.) 1976: *The Archive of Hor*, London.

Sasson, J. M. 1983: 'Mari dreams', *Journal of the American Oriental Society* 103, 283–93.

Sauneron, S. 1959: 'Les Songes et leur Interprétation dans l'Égypte Ancienne', 19–61 in A.-M. Esnoul, P. Garelli, Y. Hervouet, M. Leibovici, S. Sauneron and J. Yoyotte, *Les Songes et leur Interprétation*, Sources Orientales II, Paris.

Seow, C. L. 1984: 'The Syro-Palestinian context of Solomon's dream', *The Harvard Theological Review* 77, 141–52.

Smith, G. (trans.) 1871: *History of Assurbanipal, translated from the Cuneiform Inscriptions*, London.

Szpakowska, K. 2003: *Behind Closed Eyes: Dreams and Nightmares in Ancient Egypt*, Swansea.

Talbot, A.-M. 2002: 'Pilgrimage to healing shrines: the evidence of miracle accounts', *Dumbarton Oaks Papers* 56, 153–73.

Tylor, E. B. 1871: *Primitive Culture: Researches into the Development of Mythology, Philosophy, Religion, Language, Art and Custom*, London.

35. The Authority of Physicians as Dream Interpreters in the Pergamene Asclepieion

Ido Israelowich

The cult of Asclepius attracted the sick from all parts of Asia Minor and beyond. In the Asclepieion sick worshippers spent a night of incubation where Asclepius would send his worshippers dreams with medical prescriptions, if he deemed them worthy of cure. Despite the clear jurisdiction of the priests over the cultic activities which were performed at the temple, there is substantive evidence for regular consultations of the convalescents with physicians. This article, therefore, considers what authority physicians had in the Pergamene Asclepieion and whether they offered an alternative to the skills of the priests or worked in collaboration with them.

Introduction

The popularity of the cult of Asclepius in general and that of the Pergamene Asclepieion in particular attracted the sick from all parts of Asia Minor and beyond.[1] In the temple the sick worshippers of the god of medicine spent a night of incubation in a purposefully designated sleeping hall, the *abaton*.[2] It was believed that whilst there Asclepius would send his worshippers dreams with medical prescriptions, if he deemed them worthy of cure (Iamblichus, *de Mysteriis* 3.3; Philostratus, *Vita Apollonii* 4.11; Cicero, *De Divinatione* 2.59, 123; Aristides, *Oration* 48.31–5 K).[3] The practice of interpreting these god-sent dreams was often entrusted to the hands of the temple wardens. However, despite the clear jurisdiction of the priests over the entire cultic activities which were performed at the Asclepieion, and although incubation for the purpose of inducing the god to send dreams was a religious habit,[4] there is substantive evidence for regular consultations of the convalescents with physicians concerning the right interpretation of these dreams.[5] The most detailed picture of life in the Pergamene Asclepieion during the high Empire is found in the pages of Aelius Aristides' *Sacred Tales*. Through studying the experiences of Aristides, and then setting them in the context of his contemporaries, this article will, therefore, examine the question of what authority physicians had in the Pergamene Asclepieion. It will also consider whether the physicians offered an alternative to the skills of the priests or whether they worked in collaboration with them when it came to interpreting the dreams Asclepius sent to his worshippers.

The experience of Aelius Aristides

Aelius Arisitides' account of life in the Pergamene Asclepieion offers us the most comprehensive description of the experiences of being a sick worshipper at the temple. In order to uncover the power relations that existed between priests and physicians in the Pergamene Asclepieion it is, therefore, necessary to consider first what the work of Aristides reveals about the subject. According to Aristides, physicians played a seminal role in the temple. They helped worshippers to interpret the dreams Asclepius sent them and often provided medical supervision for the execution of the god's commands.[6] Durinog Aristides' own stay in the temple he often consulted physicians regarding the contents of his dreams. On one occasion one of the two current temple wardens, Philadelphos, had a dream vision 'which I too had' (ἥπερ κἀμοί) (Aristides, *Oration* 48.30 K). Philadelphos and Aristides both dreamt of a large congregation of worshippers in the Sacred Theatre, all wearing white garments and that Aristides was also present and that he delivered a hymn to the god (Aristides, *Oration* 48.30–3 K). Having woken up, Aristides summoned a physician by the name of Theodotos (καλῶ τὸν ἰατρὸν Θεόδοτον), and as soon as the physician arrived Aristides told him of the content of his dream (διηγοῦμαι τὰ ὀνείρατα) (Aristides, *Oration* 48.34 K). Theodotos soon realised the divine nature of this dream but did not know how to interpret it (ὁ δ' ἐθαύμαζε μὲν ὡς εἶχε δαιμονίως, ἠπόρει δὲ ὅ τι χρήσοιτο). Being at a loss, Theodotos and Aristides decided to summon the other temple warden, Asclepiacos (Aristides, *Oration* 48.34–35 K). Aristides resided at Asclepiacos' home during his period in the Pergamene Asclepieion and often discussed his dreams with him (Aristides, *Oration* 48.35 K). As soon as Asclepiacos arrived he told Aristides and Theodotos that his colleague Philadelphos just informed him that he had an identical dream. When Philadelphos was summoned by them he narrated his dream. Since the dreams agreed (ὡς δὲ συνέβαινεν τὰ ὀνείρατα) Aristides drank the curative which the dream recommended. A positive result soon followed (Aristides, *Oration* 48. 35 K).

There were other instances in the *Sacred Tales* where this practice of physicians employing the prescriptions found in dreams can also be seen. On another occasion during Aristides' period in the Pergamene Asclepieion, Asclepius commanded Aristides to spend time on songs and lyric verse, and to relax and maintain a chorus of boys. The same physician Theodotos, who was in attendance and remembered Aristides' dreams, subsequently used to order the boys to sing some of his lyric verse as a proven treatment for his ills. Aristides could report that while the boys were singing he experienced comfort (Aristides, *Oration* 50.38 K). And Theodotos had found yet another dream to be relevant to Aristides' health during his stay at the Asclepieion. It was a dream of a certain Macedonian, whom the *Sacred Tales* describe as 'one of his fellow-pilgrims' (ἑνὶ τῶν συμφοιτητῶν). Theodotos thought that this dream pertained directly to Aristides. The Macedonian dreamt that he sang a paean of Aristides in which there was the invocation 'hail Paean, Heracles Asclepius (Ἰὴ Παιὰν Ἥρακλες Ἀσκληπιέ') (Aristides, *Oration* 50.42 K). Aristides then offered the paean in common to both gods.

Moreover, this habit of employing dreams in the pursuit of cure was not limited to Theodotos. A physician of far greater significance consulted Aristides during his 'incubation which I was performing in the temple of the Saviours'. It was the Pergamene physician Satyrus, who was also Galen's teacher and a possible source for the latter diagnosis of Aelius Aristides.[7] Satyrus visited Aristides on his sickbed in Pergamon (Aristides, *Oration* 49.8–10 K). The distinguished physician disapproved of Aristides' regimen of purging large quantities of blood and prescribed him a simple plaster for his abdomen. Aristides claimed he did not have the authority to quit the bloodletting, which was Asclepius' command, but he did use the plaster (Aristides, *Oration* 49.8–10 K). From Aristides' point of view, following the regimen of Satyrus was not incompatible with abiding by Asclepius' prescriptions.

The collaboration between priests and physicians within the Asclepieion is well attested in Aristides' experiences. By choosing to convalesce in the temple of the god of medicine, Aristides demonstrated his confidence in the healing power of Asclepius. In his frequent consultations with the temple wardens regarding the contents of his dreams and the appropriate manner for understanding Asclepius' commands, which were implicit within them, Aristides expressed his trust in the fashion in which the cult was conducted. Furthermore, Aristides described Asclepiacos as a temple warden and as a physician interchangeably.[8] It appears that these categories (or disciplines), *at least to him*, did not seem mutually exclusive. Such an inclusive approach was not unique to Aristides, however, and all physicians, excluding Methodists, acknowledged the possibility of divine healing.[9] In addition to Asclepiacos who functioned as both a priest and physician there was an aged physician who aspired to replace Alexander of Abonuteichos as a priest of his shrine, and even Galen himself was a devotee of Asclepius (Lucian, *Alexander* 60).[10] The ancient physicians themselves were aware of the abilities of other kinds of healers. Scribonius Largus, for example, in the introduction to his *Compositions*, noted that some experienced healers were excluded from the medical profession, while others who were not, were deemed either incompetent or negligent. Conversely, the therapeutic measures Asclepius prescribed his sick devotees bore great resemblance to those prescribed by lay physicians (Nutton 1985, 46–7).

The wider context

A study of the authority of physicians as dream interpreters in the Pergamene Asclepieion cannot accept the testimony of Aristides in general and that of the *Sacred Tales* in particular without due criticism.[11] Aristides was not a physician. Nor was he writing a history of the Pergamene Asclepieion or a treatise about the medical procedures which were practised there. In addition, Aristides left no general work that discloses his comprehension of the nature of dreams and their role in medical practice or in divination. All remarks regarding his understanding of the nature of the health-care and the habitat of the Pergamene Asclepieion were made by Aristides in passing. Before reaching any conclusions about the authority of physicians within the temple, and their relationship with priests, it is, therefore, necessary to see Aristides' experience within the context of his contemporaries.

The Asclepieion in Pergamon can be dated further back than the Greek city of Pergamon itself, where it remained and flourished well into late antiquity (Habicht 1969, 1 with n. 3). In Roman times, particularly from the time of Domitian until the reign of Caracalla, the Pergamene Asclepieion outshone all other Asclepieia in the Graeco-Roman world and, more specifically, it gained a reputation as a sanatorium (Habicht 1969, 6–8). Marcus Aurelius himself identified the Pergamene Asclepieion as the most famous cure institution in the Roman world (Fronto, *Ad Caesarem* 3.10 (ed. Hude) 43). According to Lucian, the Pergamene Asclepieion was a rival to Zeus in popularity and appeal (Lucian, *Icaromenippus* 24).[12] Indeed, all evidence shows that patients came from all over Asia Minor to convalesce at the temple (Philostratus, *Vita Apollonii* 4.34).[13]

A social history of the city of Pergamon approves the existence of a large number of physicians who dwelled, studied, and practised in the city. The Asclepieion itself was known to attract physicians, alongside sophists, philosophers and poets. The great sophist Polemo came to Pergamon as a patient and spent a night of incubation at the temple.[14] A century later, Hermocrates was also reported to have followed the prescription of Asclepius of Pergamon (Philostratus, *Vitae Sophistarum* 2.25.5). Euarestos of Crete, a philosopher who came from Egypt, arrived in the Pergamene Asclepieion to learn about the god and his deeds (Aristides, *Oration* 50.23 K). Galen, Satyrus and Quintus are a mere fraction of the physicians who lived and practised in the city. Galen, who resided in the city for a while, seemed to have accepted the therapeutic value of the prescriptions in Asclepius' dreams. In this respect Galen was only following a long and well-established medical tradition which finds its origin in the Hippocratic Corpus, and goes through the likes of Herophilus and Rufus of Ephesus. Galen reports, for example, of a wealthy Thracian who came to Pergamum following a god-sent dream. The dream included a prescription of drinking a drug (φάρμακον) made out of vipers and instructed the patient to anoint his body. According to Galen the patient followed Asclepius' instructions and the disease was soon cured (Galen, *Subfiguratio empirica*, Cp. 10 (ed. Deichgräber) 78). Furthermore, from Galen's language it appears that physicians supported temple medicine. Galen's approval of temple medicine and of the therapeutic attributes of Asclepius' dreams again comes to the fore in a passage from his *De Sanitate tuenda*, when Galen discusses the proven ability of physicians to help the mentally ill (Galen, *De Sanitate tuenda*, 1.8.19–21 (ed. Koch) 20). 'No slight witness to that', says Galen, 'is our [i.e. physicians] ancestral god Asclepius'.[15] Galen then lists various prescriptions Asclepius gave to his sick worshippers, which the reader is to understand Galen himself was in the habit of prescribing. The overall tone of this passage is one of synergy and indicates the shared professional language and traits between physicians and Asclepius.

A fragment of another contemporary of Aristides, the sophistic declaimer Aelianus, describes how a blind person, who was instructed by Asclepius to anoint his diseased eyes with boar's fat and vinegar, actually turned to an unnamed physician for an explanation of this remedy's rationale. The physician explained that one part of the treatment contracted the tumour through its acidity and the other anointed the eyes and nourished them:

> (ὀφθαλμὼ γάρ τις ἐνόσει. εἶτα ἐπιστὰς ὅδε λέγει ὄξει λύσαντα κάρπου πιμελὴν κᾆτα ὑπαλείψασθαι. ὃ δὲ κοινοῦται τῷ συνήθει ἰατρῷ. ὃ δὲ επειρᾶτο τὰς αἰτίας λέγειν· τὸ μὲν γὰρ συστέλλειν τὸ οἴδημα τῇ δριμύτητι, τὸ δὲ ἐπιλιπαίνειν καὶ ἡσυχῇ ὑποτρέφειν ὁ εἴρων ἔλεγε) (Aelianus, *Fragment* 100).

Epictetus describes Asclepius' skills using philosophical vocabulary, which suggests he acknowledged the existence of scientific method behind it: ... ὡς ὁ Ἀσκληπιὸς εὐθὺς ὑποδεῖξαι δύνασαι, πῶς θεραπεύοντες αὖθις ἔσονται (Epictetus 4.8.28–9). Therefore, physicians and priests, not just in Pergamon but all over the Graeco-Roman world, did not use mutually exclusive professional language, nor did they avoid cross references. In fact, there is a 'striking collaboration between priest and doctor, and a remarkable lack of polemic between the two' (Nutton 1985, 46). This lack of dichotomy is particularly attested when reviewing the approaches of priests and physicians towards dreams and their comprehension of the relevance of dream to medical care.

In the Graeco-Roman world it was common in the dream experience to see the dream figure as existing objectively in space, and independent of the dreamer (Dodds 1951, 104). The Greeks never spoke of *having* a dream but of *seeing* a dream (*ibid.*, 105). Furthermore, the possibility of interaction directly with a deity in a variety of ways, and that such communication could be established via dreams, was a truism throughout classical antiquity.[16] Inscriptions and literary reports testify that the appearance of a deity in a dream bearing a command was common to the dream experience in the Graeco-Roman world (*Syll.*^{3} 663; 985; Plato, *Leges* 909e–910a; Dodds 1951, 108).[17] This almost unanimous comprehension that certain dreams are mantic explains the wide use of dreams and the stimulation of dreams as part of medical treatment,[18] frequently by incubation. Incubation, as a religiously motivated ritual aiming to secure god's cure, was extensively practised in the sanctuaries of Asclepius,[19] and in other healing sanctuaries such as that of Amphiaraus at Oropus or the oracular shrines like the Daunian ones of Calchas (Strabo 6.3.9) and Podalirius (Lycophoron *Alexandra* 1050). Sarapis and Isis also cured through dreams and incubation was practised in their temples as well. Votive offerings in the form of eyes made out of silver and gold suggest that eye treatment was offered there (Cox Miller 1994, 110). The Epidaurian *iamata*, stelai displayed in the sleeping hall (*abaton*), which included details from previous miraculous cures, provide an excellent testimony to the cures Asclepius provided, as well as to the widespread appeal of the cult.[20]

All these various approaches to the understanding of the dream-mechanism made dreams highly relevant to the practice of medicine. The Hippocratic author of the treatise *On Regimen* 4 considered dreams as an inherent part of his subject matter. As for their nature, this author held that certain dreams are godly and foretell the future of cities and individuals (Hippocrates, *On Regimen* 87). The meaning of these dreams was only accessible with the help of those who possessed the art of the interpretation of dreams. However, the dreamer was advised to consult a physician, not a dream interpreter, when the dreams concerned his physical symptoms (Hippocrates, *On Regimen* 87). The Hellenistic physician, Herophilus of Alexandria, was also interested in the nature of dreams and, like his Hippocratic predecessors, he used dreams in his medical practice. Herophilus introduced a tripartite division of dreams, which included a category of god-sent dreams and another category of dreams which result from bodily activity (Ps. Plutarch, *Placita Philosophorum* 5.1.2 (trans. von Staden) 226a–b; Ps. Galen, *Historia philosopha* 106 (trans. von Staden) 226c; Galen 6.833 K; Von Staden 1989, 306–10). It is only the latter category which interested him as a physician.

These Hippocratic views (and, indeed, Hippocratic medicine) were still pertinent during the high Roman Empire. Rufus of Ephesus, for example, a physician of the Flavian age, is another example of a physician who used dreams to form a diagnosis (Abu Ali 1992). Rufus (*Medical Questions* 5) thought that dreams are symptomatic of malfunctioning humours. Galen himself accepted that certain dreams are mantic and should be taken as messages from the gods. In fact, Galen could tell of a god-sent dream of his father, Nikon, which first encouraged him to study medicine (Galen, *De methodo medendi* 10.609 K; *De ordine librorum propriorum* 19.59 K).[21] Galen also recorded that Asclepius sent him a dream concerning his own health and advising a course of action. He then followed Asclepius' prescription and his life was saved (Galen, *In Hippocratis De humoribus* 16.221–223 K). In addition, Galen's work also provides evidence to the popularity of the temple of Asclepius and for the widespread belief in the curative contents of his dreams (Galen, *Subfiguratio empirica*, Cp. 10, (ed. Deichgräber) 78; Galen, *De Sanitate tuenda*, 1.8.19–21). The use of dreams in medical practice seemed to have been credible and important enough to Galen for compiling a whole treatise on medical diagnosis using dreams (Galen, *De dignotione ex insomnis libellis* 6.832–5 K).[22] He argued that dreams are indicative of the dreamer's constitution and that they reflect various aspects of the bodily humours (Galen, *De dignotione ex insomnis libellis* 6.832 K).

Conclusions

What, then, was the authority of physicians as dream interpreters in the Pergamene Asclepieion? Having reviewed the evidence, it is clear that physicians were practising in the city of Pergamum and within its Asclepieion. In tune with most Graeco-Roman physicians, they seemed to have acknowledged the relevance of dreams in medical care, both as symptomatic of somatic movements, and as carriers of divine prescriptions. They did not challenge the premise of the cult of Asclepius, namely that the god of medicine sends his sick worshippers dreams which include remedies and regimens, which are vital for their recuperation. More importantly, neither the evidence of the *Sacred Tales* nor that of the physicians themselves suggests that there was any distinction between the understanding of the nature of dreams by the physicians and in temple medicine. This study of the authority of physicians as dream interpreters in the Pergamene Asclepieion has, therefore, indicated that priests and physicians shared a mutual professional language when it came to dreams and their place in medical care. Physicians were authoritative as dream interpreters but only insomuch as practitioners of temple medicine,[23] and their skills tended to complete rather than challenge those of the temple wardens. While they were certainly not irrelevant, physicians offered no alternative to temple medicine, either conceptually or in practice, and no distinction between temple medicine and scientific medicine appears to have been in operation at this time.

Notes

1 For the epigraphical evidence Habicht 1969 is essential. See also Hoffmann 1998, 47.

2 Testimonies are collected in Edelstein and Edelstein 1945, T 414–442.

3 A collection of such miraculous cures from the Asclepieion in Epidaurus has been edited by LiDonnici (1995).

4 Compare with Fränkel 1895 II, no. 251; *Inscriptiones Graecae* II^2 no. 1163; Aristides *Oration* 48. 29 K. The English translations of Aelius Aristides are from Behr 1981–1986.

5 For the jurisdiction of the priests in the Asclepieion see Fränkel 1895, II, no. 251 23–6; Sokolovski 1955. One has to bear in mind that the *iatroi* and *medici* were but one group of health-care providers. They had to compete with herb-cutters, druggists, midwives, gymnastic trainers, diviners, exorcists, and priests of both private and public temples (Lloyd 1979, 38–9; Nutton 1985, 40). It is also noteworthy that throughout classical antiquity there was no institutional system of licensing physicians, and that it was left to the lay person to decide who is a physician (*Codex Theodosianus* XIII.3.10; Cohn-Haft 1956, 17; Nutton 1981, 16–20; 1985, 27).

6 See Aristides, *Oration* 48.20 K: 'when the divine manifestation was announced (i.e. the prescriptions Asclepius sent Aristides via dreams) friends escorted us with various doctors, some of them acquaintances ... there was a certain Heracleion, a doctor, a companion of ours ...'

7 Galen remarked that Aristides had a weak body and a strong soul and thought Aristides was consumptive. This diagnosis is preserved only in the Arabic translation of Galen's

Commentary on Plato's Timaeus (Schröder 1934, 33). There is no proof, however, that the famous Pergamene physician had inspected Aristides in person, or even that the two men had met. Bowersock assumed such an encounter was highly plausible. His argument is circumstantial, assuming that two men of such magnitude who dwelled in Pergamon at the same time could not have failed to make each other's acquaintance (Bowersock 1969, 61). Behr doubts it, suggesting that Galen's knowledge of Aristides' condition could have easily reached him from one of his teachers, probably Satyrus of Smyrna who personally inspected Aristides (Behr 1968, 162–3; Aristides, *Oration* 49.8 K). This Satyrus was a Greek physician who worked in the second century AD and was a student of Quintus (Galen 2.217 K) and a teacher of Galen when in Pergamon (Galen 2.224; 19.58 K). His work rested on Quintus' interpretation of the Hippocratic Corpus with a particular interest in anatomy and pharmacology (Nutton 1996).

8 Asclepiacus as a doctor: Aristides, *Oration* 49.25 K (Ἀσκληπιακὸν τὸν ἰατρόν); as a priest: Aristides, *Oration* 49.22 K (ὁ νεωκόρος <ὁ> Ἀσκληπιακός). Nutton claimed that Asclepiacos was primarily a physician, who also acted as one of the dream interpreters in the Pergamene Asclepieion (Nutton 1985, 47).

9 Compare with Edelstein 1937, 201–46; Kudlien 1968, 1–20; Nutton 1985, 23–53.

10 On Galen's religious beliefs see Kudlien 1981, *passim* and Frede 2003, *passim*.

11 On this difficulty see Müller 1987, 212. He argues: 'Wie aus seinen Aufzeichnungen wieder und wieder aufscheint, nimmt die Umwelt voll interessierter Aufmerksamkeit an seinen religiösen und medizinischen Erfahrungen Anteil. Und auch wenn das Verhalten seiner Mitpatienten in Pergamon vielleicht nicht in allem völlig identisch ist, so verläuft es doch in den gleichen Bahnen'.

12 The other contestants over Zeus' popularity were Apollo of Delphi, Artemis of Ephesus, the Thracian Bendis, and the Egyptian Anubis.

13 There is extensive evidence of votive offerings by foreigners to the god in Pergamon (Fränkel 1895 II, nos 74–8, 88, 127, 131). There are also dedications in the Asclepieion to the 'Pergamene Asclepieion' (Hepding 1933, 98).

14 Polemo's critical response to the dream Asclepius had sent him (*sic*) should not undermine the fact that when sick, Polemo chose to convalesce in the Pergamene Asclepieion, of all places (Philostratus, *Vitae Sophistarum* 1.25.4).

15 All passages from Galen's *De Sanitate tuenda* come from the translation of Edelstein and Edelstein 1998.

16 Renberg (2003) collected 1300 inscriptions (623 in Greek and 677 in Latin) which cite a direct divine communication as the motivation for a dedication or some other undertaking. See also Hanson 1980 and Weber 2000, 30.

17 Van Straten (1976) collected no less than 225 votive inscriptions, encouraged by an epiphany of a deity in a dream or a daydream.

18 Compare with Pelling 1997, 97, and Cox Miller 1994, 106–23.

19 Testimonies are collected in Edelstein and Edelstein (1945, T 414–442).

20 These inscriptions were re-edited by LiDonnici (1995). See also Furley and Bremer (2001, 209). Dillon (1994) discusses the nature of these *iamata*.

21 For Galen's life see Hankinson 2008.

22 Oberhelman 1983 is probably right arguing that the piece included in Kühn's edition is only a fraction of a bigger work.

23 Müller (1987, 226) points out that Asclepius and his earthly colleagues prescribed similar things, such as cleansing, vomiting and blood-letting.

Bibliography

Abu Ali, A. 1992: *The Medical Writings of Rufus of Ephesus*, Ph.D thesis, University of London.

Behr, C. 1968: *Aelius Aristides and the Sacred Tales*, Amsterdam.

Behr, C. 1981–1986: *P. Aelius Aristides: The Complete Works i–ii*, trans., Leiden.

Bowersock, G. 1969: *Greek Sophists in the Roman Empire*, Oxford.

Cohn-Haft, L. 1956: *The Public Physicians of Ancient Greece*, Northampton, MA.

Cox Miller, P. 1994: *Dreams in Late Antiquity: Studies in the Imagination of a Culture*, Princeton.

Dillon, M. P. J. 1994: 'The didactic nature of the Epidaurian iamata', *Zeitschrift für Papyrologie und Epigraphik* 101, 239–60.

Dodds, E. R. 1951: *The Greeks and the Irrational*, Berkeley, Los Angeles, London.

Edelstein E. and Edelstein, L. 1945: *Asclepius*, Vols I–II, Baltimore.

Edelstein, L. 1937: 'Greek medicine in its relation to religion and magic', *Bulletin of the Institute of the History of Medicine* 5, 201–46.

Fränkel, M. (ed.) 1895: *Die Inschriften von Pergamon* (Altertümer von Pergamon, Band 8/2), Berlin.

Frede, M. 2003: 'Galen's theology', 73–126 in J. Barnes and J. Jouanna (eds), *Galien et la Philosophie*, Geneva.

Furley, M. D. and Bremer, J. M. 2001: *Greek Hymns*, Vols I–II, Tübingen.

Habicht, C. 1969: *Die Inschriften des Asklepieions* (Altertümer von Pergamon. 8/3), Berlin.

Hankinson, R. J. 2008: 'The man and his work', 1–34 in R. J. Hankinson (ed.), *The Cambridge Companion to Galen*, Cambridge.

Hanson, J. S. 1980: 'Dreams and vision in the Graeco-Roman world and early Christianity', *Aufstieg und Niedergang der Römischen Welt* II 23, 1395–427.

Hepding, H. 1933: 'Ῥουφίνιον ἄλσος', *Philologus* 42, 90–103.

Hoffmann, A. 1998: 'The Roman remodeling of the Asclepieion', 41–59 in H. Koester (ed.), *Pergamon, Citadel of the Gods*, Harrisburg, PA.

Kudlien, F. 1968: 'Der Arzt des Körpes und der Arzt der Seele', *Clio Medica* 3, 1–20.

Kudlien, F. 1981: 'Galen's religious belief', 117–30 in V. Nutton (ed.), *Galen: Problems and Prospects*, London.

LiDonnici, L. R. 1995: *The Epidaurian Miracle Inscriptions*, Atlanta.

Lloyd, G. E. R. 1979: *Magic, Reason, and Experience*, Cambridge.

Müller, H. 1987: 'Ein Heilungsbericht aus dem Asklepieion von Pergamon', *Chiron* 17, 193–233.

Nutton, V. 1981: 'Continuity or rediscovery? The city physician in classical antiquity and medieval Italy', 9–46 in A. W. Russell (ed.), *The Town and State Physician in Europe from the Middle Ages to the Enlightenment*, Wolfenbüttel.

Nutton, V. 1985: 'Murders and miracles: lay attitudes towards medicine in classical antiquity', 23–53 in R. Porter (ed.), *Patients and Practitioners*, Cambridge.

Nutton, V. 1996: 'Satyrus', *Brill New Pauly* 13: 40, Leiden.

Oberhelman, S. M. 1983: '*Galen,* on diagnosis from dreams', *Journal of the History of Medicine and Allied Sciences* 38, 36–47.

Pelling, C. 1997: 'Tragical dreamer: some dreams in the Roman historians', *Greece and Rome* 44, 197–213.

Renberg, G. 2003: *Commanded by the Gods: An Epigraphical Study of Dreams and Visions in Greek and Roman Religious Life,* Ph.D dissertation, Duke University, Durham, NC.

Schröder, H. O. (ed.) 1934: *Galeni in Platonis Timaeum commentarii fragmenta* (Corpus Medicorum Graecorum Suppl. 1), Leipzig and Berlin.

Sokolowski, F. 1955: *Lois Sacrées de l'Asie Mineure*, Paris.

Van Straten, F. T. 1976: 'Daikrates' dream. A votive relief from Kos, and some other kat'onar dedications', *Bulletin Antieke Beschaving* 6, 1–38.

Von Staden, H. (ed.) 1989: *Herophilus*, Cambridge.

Weber, G. 2000: *Kaiser, Träume und Visionen in Prinzipat und Spätantike*, Stuttgart.

36. Asclepius the Divine Healer, Asclepius the Divine Physician: Epiphanies as Diagnostic and Therapeutic Tools

Georgia Petridou

The phenomenon of the ascendancy of the cult of Asclepius in the civic religion of the Greek polis is closely paralleled with the rise of the Hippocratic tradition. Asclepius manifested himself in the dreams of those in need both as a physician performing advanced surgical procedures and as a healing god who miraculously and effortlessly eliminated the pain and the cause of the disease. This paper focuses on divine epiphanies in the context of disease and healing, as well as on the usage of these divine epiphanies as diagnostic and therapeutic tools in the medicinal thought and practice of classical antiquity in general and in the cult of Asclepius in particular.

νοῦσοι δ' ἀνθρώποισιν ἐφ' ἡμέρῃ, αἳ δ' ἐπὶ νυκτὶ
αὐτόματοι φοιτῶσι κακὰ θνητοῖσι φέρουσαι
σιγῇ, ἐπεὶ φωνὴν ἐξείλετο μητίετα Ζεύς.
οὕτως οὔ τί πη ἔστι Διὸς νόον ἐξαλέασθαι.

'Out of their own accord diseases come upon men constantly
Some by the day and some by the night, bringing evil to mortals
silently; for sagacious Zeus deprived them of their voice.
Thus, there is no way to escape Zeus' design'.

Hesiod, *Works and Days* 102–5[1]

Recognising divine origins in various diseases has been a cross-cultural *topos* (Edelstein 1968, 219–24). The passage from Hesiod's *Works and Days* quoted above is indicative of this tendency in Archaic Greek thought and culture. Even though diseases are described here as having the power to inflict themselves spontaneously on the tribes of mortal men, we should not forget that initially they came out of the jar of Pandora, the first mortal woman, the gods' deadly gift to humanity. Compare the passages from Hesiod, *Works and Days* 238–45 and *Odyssey* 9.411–40, where similar ideas are found (Lloyd 2003, 15). Even in our modern western society, where the majority of the population has adopted a scientific causation of illness, research has shown that under the pressure of life-threatening or chronic disease, most of us are ready to reconsider, if only partly, a non-scientific explanation of our illness (Young 1971; Kirmayer 2006, 583–92). Yet, this is far from expecting a divine manifestation to reveal to the patient the cause and possibly the right treatment for an illness, as was often the case in the Graeco-Roman world. Visitations from healing deities in the course of a dream or waking reality (henceforth referred to as divine epiphanies) are attested by literary and epigraphic, as well as archaeological and numismatic sources from the late Archaic to the Hellenistic eras and beyond.[2] The present paper focuses on divine epiphanies in the context of disease and healing, as well as on the usage of these divine epiphanies as diagnostic and therapeutic tools in the medicinal thought and practice of classical antiquity in general and in the cult of Asclepius in particular.

Along with the fear of death, disease seems to be one of the most significant crises an individual has to face. More importantly, it seems to be unavoidable in the sense that everyone or almost everyone eventually confronts disease at some point in the course of their life. Since epiphanies take place in the context of critical situations such as war, siege, famine, drought etc. (Petridou in press, chapter 2), it comes as no surprise that they also take place in the context of both physical and psychological illnesses. One must not forget, however, that disease is not necessarily confined to the private realm. It is also of concern to the community, to the extent that the physical and psychological health of the individual is a prerequisite for a healthy and thriving community and the perpetuation of its socio-political structures and cultural values.

Generally speaking, gods are perceived to be both the ones who grant the individual and the community a healthy being, and the ones who deprive them of it (Parker 1983,

234–56; Lloyd 2003, 12–3; Willi 2008, 159). Potentially every Greek deity was able to affect negatively or positively matters of human health (Nutton 2004, 108). There is, however, a group of deities that were traditionally associated with both curative and preventive medicine, such as Apollo (with the cultic titles Paion and Epikourios) and his son Asclepius, Heracles, Athena Hygeia, and, imported from the East, Serapis and Isis, and Zeus Hypsistos, a major healing deity of later antiquity. In addition, great popularity is attested for the cult of *Heros Iatros* (ἥρως ἰατρός, the hero physician). This figure was known under different names in different places: Amphilochos in Athens, Aristomachos in Marathon, and Oresinios in Eleusis; while in Rhamnous he was known as Aristomachos and later on as Amphiaraos (Parker 1996, 176–7; Nutton 2004, 107–8). In Oropos the cult of the hero doctor Amphiaraos became the leading healing cult, which soon acquired panhellenic status and attracted visitors from all over the Greek-speaking world.

Asclepius' early career and the introduction of his cult in Athens

However, the majority of our evidence comes from Asclepius' cult. As a result, my discussion will focus primarily on Asclepius' epiphanies.[3] Asclepius started his medical career as a local hero from Epidaurus or Trikka *c.* 500 BC (Aston 2004 with more bibliography). But soon his cult acquired a panhellenic stature and spread throughout the whole Greek-speaking world. Of the several famous places where his *epidemiai* (i.e. his periodic manifestations) took place, we can single out his healing sanctuaries at Cos, Trikka, Lebena, Epidaurus, Piraeus, Pergamon, Aegae, and Pellene. But the decisive boost to Asclepius' career as a divine physician was given by his introduction to Athens.

Telemachos of Acharnai, either an Athenian (Garland 1992, 119) who imported the god or an Epidaurian (Parker 1996, 176–7) who exported his native deity, commemorated Asclepius' arrival on a double-sided relief.[4] In the first couple of lines of the fragmentary text we read with Parker (1996, 177):

> 'coming up from Zea (?) during the Great Mysteries he lodged (?) [in the Eleusinion] and summoning a snake (?) from home brought it here on [a wagon] [a reference to Telemachos in a uncertain case follows immediately as part of the same sentence]. At the same time came Health (?). And so this whole shrine was founded in the archonship of Astyphilos'.

The god was introduced to the city in the form of a snake on a chariot.[5] The exact date of Asclepius' arrival is known to us thanks to Telemachos' monument: 18th of Boedromion of 420/19 BC. The god arrived in Athens almost immediately after the signing of the Peace of Nikias (421 BC), the peace-treaty that allowed Athens to re-establish its diplomatic discourse with Epidaurus (Garland 1992, 118). According to our sources, he arrived first in the harbour of Zea in Piraeus (see the first couple of lines from the Telemachos relief quoted above) and that information ties up with the fact that it was Piraeus that was afflicted by the plague of 430 BC.[6] The plague continued to torture the Athenians up to *circa* 426. Mikalson (1984, 220) takes this plausible connection between the two historical events (namely the plague and the introduction of Asclepius' cult in Athens) one step further: the Athenian attack against Epidaurus during the Peloponnesian war aimed at an appropriation of the healing qualities of the god. His suggestion seems to me rather appealing in view of the failing of the pre-Asclepius healing deities to defend the city against the plague (cf. also Nutton 2004, 104). Sophocles was said to have provided *xenia* to Asclepius in his own house, before the god acquired his own dwelling, and for this reason received the cultic title *Dexion* (*Etymologicum Magnum* 256, 6 s.v. Δεξίων). The heroic status that Sophocles acquired post mortem as recorded by his biographers is confirmed by the two inscriptions (*Inscriptiones Graecae* II/III^2 1252= *Syll.*^{3} 1069 and *Inscriptiones Graecae* II/III^2 1253) that record celebrations and offerings to *Dexion* on behalf of the city.[7]

Asclepius' mystic epiphanies.

On his coming into Athens, Asclepius received a warm and friendly welcome from the priesthood of Demeter and Kore, the '"saviours" of older type', as Parker (1996, 179) calls them.[8] A relief from the Athenian Asclepieion (*IG* II^2 4359 = *LIMC s.v. Asklepios*, 886, no. 313) shows the god in the company of the two goddesses approached by a number of worshippers. An official day was established to celebrate the god's arrival, that was later said to have coincided with his initiation into the Eleusinian Mysteries ([Aristotle] *Athenian Constitution* 56.4; Pausanias 2.26.8. For a 2nd century AD version of the same aetiological myth, see Philostratus, *Life of Apollonius* 4.18)[9], while the newcomer god found temporary shelter in the Eleusinion (*IG* IV^2, 4960a). The very festival that commemorated the god's first arrival in the city became part of the Great Mysteries. Asclepius' other festival, the *Asclepieia* (celebrated in Elaphebolion), was part of another prestigious festival of old, that of the Great Dionysia. Both festivals in honour of Asclepius are found to be part of the poliadic aspect of old, reverent and popular mystery cults. Could this cautious arrangement of the festive calendar point to a closer relation of the very essence of these cults and subsequently to the way that the divine epiphanies take place within their cultic context? No definite answer can be given to this question.

There are, however, further structural parallels between the cult of Asclepius and that of Demeter and Kore in Eleusis that may point to some similarities on the level of content. Compare here: a) that both cults include mystic rites (*teletai*) that were confined to those initiated, b) a sacred potion called *kykeon* is mentioned in connection to both cults, c) fasting from certain types of food and sacrificing piglets are mentioned in connection with both cults, d) both cults included in their priestly personnel a *hierophantes*, a *dadouchos* and a *mystagogos*, e) both cults are concerned with the well-being of their initiate, f) and finally night-festivals (παννυχίς) were held in both cultic contexts, if we are to believe Aelius Aristides and what he says in *Orationes* 23.16, Keil (see below).

Moreover, there are a number of narratives from the imperial era where practising incubation in the Asclepieion of Pergamon (more on which in Israelowich in this volume) is described in explicit mystic imagery. Compare for instance two of the most indicative cases as reported by the ever so persistent incubant Aelius Aristides:

a) 'and neither belonging to a chorus nor sailing together nor having the same teacher is as great a thing as the boon and profit of being a fellow pilgrim to the temple of Asclepius and being initiated to the first of the holy rites by the fairest and most perfect torchbearer and leader of the mysteries, to whom every rule of necessity yields'.

   καὶ οὔτε χοροῦ σύλλογος πρᾶγμα τοσοῦτον οὔτε πλοῦ κοινωνία οὔτε διδασκάλων τῶν αὐτῶν τυχεῖν, ὅσον χρῆμα καὶ κέρδος εἰς Ἀσκληπιοῦ τε συμφοιτῆσαι καὶ τελεσθῆναι τὰ πρῶτα τῶν ἱερῶν ὑπὸ τῷ καλλίστῳ καὶ τελεωτάτῳ δᾳδούχῳ καὶ μυσταγωγῷ καὶ ᾧ πᾶς ἀνάγκης εἴκει θεσμός (*Orationes* 23.16, Keil, trans. C. A. Behr).[10]

b) 'it [*sic.* the remedy] was revealed in the clearest way possible (ἐνεργέστατα), just as countless other things also made the presence of the god manifest (ἐναργῆ τὴν παρουσίαν εἶχε τοῦ θεοῦ). For I seemed almost to touch him and to perceive that he himself was coming, and to be halfway between sleep and walking (μέσως ἔχειν ὕπνου καὶ ἐγρηγόρσεως and want to get the power of vision and to be anxious lest he depart beforehand, and to have turned my ears to listen, sometimes as in a dream, sometimes as in a waking vision (τὰ μὲν ὡς ὄναρ, τὰ δὲ ὡς ὕπαρ), and my hair was standing on end and tears of joy (καὶ τρίχες ὀρθαὶ καὶ δάκρυα σὺν χαρᾷ), and the weight of knowledge was no burden–what man could even set these things into words? But if he is one of the initiates, then he knows and understands (τις τῶν τετελεσμένων ἐστίν, σύνοιδέν τε καὶ γνωρίζει)' (*Orationes* 48.31–33 Keil, trans. C. A. Behr).

Now, one may hastily dismiss these passages as the pompous and extravagant utterances of a neurotic megalomaniac of literary tastes. However, Asclepius was strongly connected with the goddesses of Eleusis in a plethora of ancient literary and iconographical sources (of diverse chronological and generic background): in Aristophanes' *Plutus* (640), for instance, the god is called 'great light for the mortals' (μέγα βροτοῖσι φέγγος Ἀσκληπιόν), a syntactical structure that is often used to describe Demeter and Kore (compare for instance here the Homeric Hymn to Demeter 278 and Plutarch, *Themistocles* 15.2). Moreover, one of the Hippocratic treatises (*Epistulae* 2 (T 467)) draws a parallel between Asclepius and his remedies, and Triptolemos and the seeds of Demeter. We also have the testimony of a late inscription from *c.* 160 AD, where it is reported that when Marcus Julius Apellas practiced incubation in the temple of the god in Aegina, he offered common sacrifices to Asclepius, Epione and the Eleusinian goddesses (*IG* IV^{2,} 1. 126 (T 432): κοινῇ θῦσαι Ἀσκληπιῷ, Ἠπιόνῃ, Ἐλευσεινίας, . . .). More importantly, in an Orphic hymn (67.5–9), Asclepius is invoked (note the performative *elthe*) as both the giver of health and the giver of a good end of life. It is possible that Socrates asked a cock to be sacrificed to the god with this in mind (more on this in Edelstein (T 527–31); contra Most 1993, 96–111). Finally, Asclepius' affinities with the kingdom of the underworld and its goddesses are underscored in Xenophon's *Cynegeticus* (1.6), where we learn that the god was revered not only as the healer of the sick, but also as the one who revived the dead:

> . . . Ἀσκλήπιος δὲ μειζόνων ἔτυχεν, ἀνιστάναι μὲν τεθνεῶντας, νοσοῦντας δὲ ἰᾶσθαι· διὰ δὲ ταῦτα θεὸς ὢν παρ' ἀνθρώποις ἀείμνηστον κλέος ἔχει

Nevertheless the strongest indication of a close correlation between the type of mystic epiphanies in a mystery cult context and those related to the cult of Asclepius comes from the similar prohibitions which appear to have regulated the process of ritual viewing in both cases. Compare for instance the story of Aeschines (*IG* IV^2, 1, nos 121–2 A11), who climbed up a tree and tried to peer over the wall into the abaton in the temple of Asclepius in Epidaurus. Just like many other transgressors who dared to see what is not meant to be seen, he was punished for his curiosity and lost his eyesight. The benevolent god, however, restored his vision after appearing to him in the course of a dream-vision Aeschines had while he slept at the sanctuary. (More on this in Petridou 2013).

Farnell (1921, 244) thought that the relationship between Asclepius and the cult of Eleusis should not be taken further than that of a new deity being admitted by a well-established cult and thus being incorporated into the city religion. Nevertheless, the passages briefly mentioned above surely point to a more profound relation of analogy between the mystery cult of Eleusis and that of the divine newcomer.

Other myths of introduction and Asclepius' zoomorphic epiphanies

In Sikyon, almost a decade after the first arrival of the god in Zea, a certain Nicagora lead Asclepius' sacred snake on a cart drawn by mules to the god's sanctuary (Pausanias 2.10.3). Another sacred snake is involved in the story of Thersandros of Halieis, which formed the aetiological myth for the introduction of Asclepius' cult in the city of Halieis (*IG* IV^2, 1, nos 121–2, B25). Thersandros, like Sostrata from Pherae, left the god's temple in Epidaurus without achieving his initial goal, namely to acquire a vision of the god to cure his consumption (*IG* IV^2, 1, nos 121–2, B33). Nevertheless, he was completely unaware of the fact that one of the sacred snakes coiled itself around the axle of the wheels of his wagon and followed Thersandros back home. On their arrival, the snake miraculously cured Thersandros and consequently became the manifest sign of the god's interest in expanding his cult in the city of Halieis. The Halieis having consulted the Delphic oracle built a temenos to Asclepius and got to keep the sacred snake for future use!

Are we to interpret these sacred snakes as symbols of the god's presence or as his zoomorphic epiphanies? In any case, these sacred snakes functioned as a kind of zoomorphic cult-dispatcher in the other Greek cities and beyond (Garland 1992, 122). Asclepius' cult survived most gracefully the advent of Christianity: the features we have from our sources are quite impressive: by the 2nd century AD circa 320 Asclepieia are spread all over the Greco-Roman world. As late as the 3rd century AD, Asclepius entered Rome in his zoomorphic guise. A sacred snake was dispatched in a boat from Epidaurus and was received triumphantly in the capital of the Roman Empire, in an attempt to trounce the plague that had broken out the same year (Livy, *Periochae* 11; Valerius Maximus 1.8.2; Ovid, *Metamorphoses* 15.626–744). As Aston (2004, 22) very aptly puts it:

> 'The myths of arrival were a means of dealing with Asclepius' unusually 'place specific' quality: in the context of a very rapid growth in the range and popularity of his cult, they allowed more sites to have a share of his (originally exclusive) presence, after that presence had been claimed with some finality, it seems, by Epidaurus'.

Alternatively, the god, if not transported from a renowned cult centre, may manifest his presence by being born in a specific place. A god's birth epiphany (*γέννησις*) was valued even more highly than his simple visitation (*παρουσία*) (Diodorus Siculus 3.66.2). A parodied version of the ritual of the reception of Asclepius into a human community can be found in a passage from Lucian's *Alexander the Oracle-Monger* (13–14), where Alexander of Abonouteichus, the pseudo-seer, stages a birth-epiphany of Asclepius, to ratify the introduction of his pseudo-oracular/healing cult. The god manifested his godhead as an infant reptile hidden within an empty goose egg, which Alexander had cunningly buried under the foundations of a newly planned temple. But first his arrival was publicly advertised by the pseudo-prophet himself who had run through the agora naked and ecstatic heralding the god's imminent epiphany and singing hymns to appease the coming god and to secure his benevolence. The audience's response to all this was typical of those perceiving a divine manifestation: initially they were struck with awe, amazement, and even confusion, but when they finally beheld the infant reptile emerging from the cracked egg, they were overjoyed and broke into loud cheering and they all prostrated themselves in front of the snake-like god:

> καὶ οἱ παρόντες εἶδον κινούμενον καὶ περὶ τοῖς δακτύλοις εἰλούμενον, ἀνέκραγον εὐθὺς καὶ ἠσπάζοντο τὸν θεὸν καὶ τὴν πόλιν ἐμακάριζον καὶ χανδὸν ἕκαστος ἐνεπίμλατο τῶν εὐχῶν, θησαυροὺς καὶ πλούτους καὶ ὑγιείας καὶ τὰ ἄλλα ἀγαθὰ αἰτῶν παρ᾽ αὐτοῦ (Lucian, *Alexander* 14).
>
> 'Those present could see it [*sic.* the infant reptile] stirring and winding about Alexander's fingers; they raised a shout, hailed the God, blessed the city, and every mouth was full of prayers – for treasure and wealth and health and all the other good things which the god might give'.

The citizens of Abonouteichos, then, had no reservations in regarding the baby snake as the theriomorphic re-incarnation of Asclepius. Now, we cannot be sure whether the Athenians, the Sikyonians, the people of Limera, or the people of Halieis, regarded the Epidaurian snake-dispatches as symbols of the god's presence (hence as *pars pro toto* epiphanies), as fragments of Asclepius' divine essence, or as his actual zoomorphic manifestation. There are arguments to support either: Pausanias' wording (in 2.10.3), for instance, points to a zoomorphic epiphany (*δράκοντι εἰκασμένον*). Compare also Aurelius Victor's *De Viris Illustribus* 22.1 and Valerius Maximus I.8.2 etc. In an interesting passage from Marinus' *Life of Proclus* (30), the manifestation of the sacred snake is explicitly characterised as an *epiphaneia*.

However, there are a large number of these sacred snakes along with other sacred animals (e.g. dogs and horses) that populate the temples of Asclepius.[11] Are they all to be conceived of as zoomorphic manifestations of the god? In all probability, such a dilemma would not have occurred to the visiting worshippers and pilgrims at the time. Whether we regard them today as symbols of the god or his actual zoomorphic manifestations, these snakes were, for their contemporary audience, signifiers of the god's presence. Compare here the text from the 17th cure from the Epidaurian Iamata (*IG* IV^2 1, nos 121–22, A17):

> (XVII) ἀνὴρ δάκτυλον ἰάθη ὑπὸ ὄφιος· οὗτος τὸν τοῦ ποδὸς δάκτυλον ὑ/πὸ τοῦ ἀγρίου ἕλκεος δεινῶς διακείμενος μεθάμερα ὑπὸ τῶν θε/ραπόντων ἐξενειχθεὶς ἐπὶ ἑδράματός τινος καθῖζε· ὕπνου δέ νιν λαβόντος ἐν τούτωι δράκων ἐκ τοῦ ἀβάτου ἐξελθὼν τὸν δάκτυλον / ἰάσατο τᾶι γλώσσαι καὶ τοῦτο ποιήσας εἰς τὸ ἄβατον ἀνεχώρησε/πάλιν. ἐξεγερθεὶς δὲ ὡς ἦς ὑγιής, ἔφα ὄψιν ἰδεῖν,

δοκεῖν νεανίσ/κον εὐπρεπῆ τὰμ μορφὰν ἐπὶ τὸν δάκτυλον ἐπιπῆν φάρμακον.

'A man's toe was healed by a snake. He was in a terrible condition from a malignant ulceration on his toe. During the day he was carried out of the Abaton by the servants and was sitting on a seat. He fell asleep, and then a snake came out of the Abaton and healed the toe with his tongue; and when it had done this it went back into the Abaton again. When the man woke up, he was well and he said he had seen a vision: it seemed to him that a good-looking young man had sprinkled a drug over his toe' (trans. LiDonnici 1995).

What we have here is a variation of what has been termed by Hanson (1980, 1414) as a 'double dream-vision report': 'this is a narrative in which two characters each have a dream or vision. What is seen and/or heard in each of these dreams or visions can be identical, similar, or quite different. But the paired dreams will in some way be connected such that they produce what may be called a 'circumstance of mutuality' between the two dreamers'. The patient himself perceived the god as a good-looking youth who treated his ulcerous toe with a drug of some sort, while the bystanders (or rather the omniscient third-person narrator) saw a snake coming out of the *abaton* and licking the man's toe. None of these versions of the same dream-vision is more significant or more 'real' than the other. The images of Asclepius the physician and that of the god's sacred snake are more than complementary; they are two sides of the same coin. Herzog (1931, 14, no. 17) has paralleled this narrative with a celebrated votive relief from Oropos, which on the far right depicts the healing hero Amphiaraos tending Archinos' (the name of the dedicant) shoulder, while in the left a snake licks the affected part as the same dedicant sleeps (van Straten 1976, 36, fig. 10).

Towards a typology of an Asclepeian epiphany

This intimate relationship between the anthropomorphic and the zoomorphic healing deity, or perhaps between the divine physician and his reptile familiar, is also evident in a narrative from Aristophanes' *Wealth* (633–747), where Carion relates to his wife the treatment the god Plutus received from Asclepius at the temple of the god in Piraeus. What Carion witnesses is a synergy of the healing power of the divine doctor and those of his sacred snakes:

'Wife: And the god himself still hadn't come?
Carion: Not yet, but he did right after. Then I did something really funny. As he was approaching, I had an attack of wind and let out an enormous fart.
Wife: He must have been put to flight!
Carion: No, but his attendants! Iaso blushed like anything, and Panacea held her nose and turned away. My farts aren't exactly incense and myrrh.
Wife: And Asclepius himself?
Carion: He never even noticed it.
Wife: What an earthy god!
Carion: Oh, I wouldn't say earthy; remember he tastes shit for living.
Wife: Really!!
Carion: Well, I was rather frightened after that and covered myself up, while the god went round looking very carefully at all the patients. Then a boy placed by his side a stone pestle and mortar and medicine box.
Wife: A stone one?
Carion: Not the medicine box, silly.
Wife: But, you lying scoundrel, how did you see all this? You'd covered yourself up!
Carion: I saw it through my cloak; that had no shortage of holes! Well, first of all he treated Neocleides. He prepared a plaster to rub on his eyes: three heads of Tenian garlic, then he pounded in some fig juice and sea onions, and finally soaked the lot with vinegar from Sphettus. Then he turned up Neocleides' eyelids and rubbed the mixture into them, so as to give the maximum pain. He yelled and screamed, jumped up and run off. Asclepius laughed and said, 'That's got you good and plastered; no more moving the precious question in the Assembly for you now!'
Wife: What a wise and public-spirited god!
Carion: Then he came to Wealth and sat at his side. He felt his head and wiped his eyelids with a clean linen cloth, while Panacea spread a red cloth all over his head and face. Then the god gave a clucking sound and at once two enormous snakes came out of the inner shrine.
Wife: Gods save us!
Carion: They went under the red cloth and licked all round his eyelids, at least I think they did; and mistress, before you could drink down ten cups of wine, Wealth was on his feet, and he could see. I clapped my hands for joy, and woke up master. At once the god disappeared, snakes and all, into the inner shrine' (trans. Sommerstein 2003).

Aristophanes' *Wealth* along with Aelius Aristides' *Sacred Tales* (47–52) and Plautus' *Curculio* (I, 1.61–62; II, 1.216–2, 273) contain perhaps some of the most extensive literary accounts of Asclepius' epiphanies as means to diagnose and treat a disease.[12] The most informative epigraphic records, however, are from Epidaurus, Athens, Rome, Pergamon and Lebena (Nutton 2004, 109). In Epidaurus, in particular, we find lengthy accounts of the diagnostic and healing process followed there, which often consisted in lengthy descriptions of the god's divine epiphanies. These are the so-called Epidaurian Iamata. As LiDonnici (1995, 40) rightly argues, it is naïve though to treat the Epidaurian Iamata as the creations of pious patients. They are mainly the product of the Epidaurian priesthood's careful collection, arrangement and adaptation of a large variety of source material, which ranges from individual narrative and pictorial votives to oral tradition attached to temple features and state-sponsored inscriptions. The same holds true of the inscriptions from Athens, Rome and Lebena.

None of these literary or epigraphic sources provides us

with an exhaustive description of a 'paradigmatic healing process', in the sense that they all include elements that must have been particular to the time and the place the healing took place. Nevertheless, they all more or less describe a phenomenon called incubation (κατάκλισις), which could be briefly described as follows: the patient sleeps in a temple or other sacred precinct in order either to be healed by the healing deity of the sanctuary on the spot, or to obtain a remedy for subsequent healing (Harrisson in this volume). Both the healing and the remedy for subsequent healing are administered in a dream-vision (ὄνειρος, ὄναρ, ἐνύπνιον, ὅραμα, φάσμα, φάντασμα, φαντασία, ὅρασις, κ.τ.λ.).[13]

Consequently, it is worth attempting to give a rough outline of the whole process: first of all, it was the patient himself that had to sleep in the temple; alternatively we get reports of relatives or close friends, who practised incubation on behalf of the afflicted. See for instance the case of Arata from Lacedaimon, who suffered from dropsy (*IG* IV^2, 1, nos 121–22, B21). It was Arata's mother who slept in the temple of the god and dreamt of the god chopping off her daughter's head and successfully treating the disease. When she came back to Lacedaimon, she found out that Arata had had the same dream:

> (XXI) Ἀ̣ράτα [Λά]καινα ὕδρωπ[α. ὑπ]ὲρ ταύτας ἁ μάτηρ ἐνεκάθευδεν ἐλ Λακεδαίμο/νι ἔσσα[ς] καὶ ἐνύπνιον [ὁ]ρῆι· ἐδόκει τᾶς θυγατρός οὑ τὸν θεὸν ἀποταμόν/τα τὰν κ[ε]φαλὰν τὸ σῶμα κραμάσαι κάτω τὸν τράχαλον ἔχον· ὡς δ' ἐξερρύα συ/χνὸν ὑγρ[ό]ν, καταλύσαντα τὸ σῶμα τὰν κεφαλὰν πάλιν ἐπιθέμεν ἐπὶ τὸν αὐ/χένα· ἰδο[ῦ]σ̣α δὲ τὸ ἐνύπνιον τοῦτο ἀγχωρήσασα εἰς Λακεδαίμονα κατα/λαμβάνε̣[ι τ]ὰν θυγατέρα ὑγιαίνουσαν καὶ τὸ αὐτὸ ἐνύπνιον ὡρακυῖαν.

> 'Arata of Lacadaemon, dropsy. For her sake, her mother slept here, while she remained in Lacedaemon, and she saw a dream. It seemed to her the god cut off the head of her daughter and hung the body neck downwards. After much fluid had run out, he untied the body and put the head back on the neck. Having seen this dream she returned to Lacedaemon and found on her arrival that her daughter was well and that she had seen the same dream' (trans. LiDonnici 1995).

Whoever came in quest of a divine manifestation had to bathe and perform sacrifices to Asclepius and other deities that were thought of as facilitating the dream visions, such as Hermes, the bringer of dreams (more on this topic in Parker 1996, 182). There is no decisive evidence about abstinence from certain kinds of food and drink, as rightly maintained by Edelstein and Edelstein (1998, 148–9). When the night came, they would have to enter the temple or the special halls where incubation was practised (ἐνκοιμετήριον). There they would sleep and wait for a healing epiphany.

The lights of the temple must have been burning in the places where the patients were gathered, but they would all have been extinguished before the god manifested himself. Compare here the analogous sequence of events in Carion's account of Plautus being healed by Asclepius (Aristophanes, *Wealth* 649–71). Darkness, strongly associated with sleep and dreaming, facilitated the god's divine manifestation. It is important that the god received his clientele on a daily basis, unlike the other gods whose temples were open only on certain sacred calendar days. Asclepius would potentially reveal his godhead to anyone who would go to so much trouble as to sleep in his temple having performed the preparatory bathing and sacrifices (Edelstein and Edelstein 1998, 150). Or almost everyone …

Complaints on Asklepios' misdemeanours

In a passage from Philostratus' *Life of Apollonius* (1.9) we read about an Assyrian young man who made scornful remarks about not having received any healing visions, despite the fact that he came to the temple of the god and practiced incubation. At the same time, though, he did not make an effort to cut down on his luxurious and extravagant way of living. That was exactly why Asclepius did not pay a visit to the youth's dreams (ἠμελεῖτο δὴ ὑπὸ τοῦ Ἀσκληπιοῦ διὰ ταῦτα, καὶ οὐδὲ ὄναρ αυτῷ ἐφοῖτα). The god overheard his criticism and revealed himself to the youth (ἐπιμεμφομένῳ δὲ ταῦτα ἐπιστὰς ὁ θεός). It is not clear whether in waking reality or in his dreams – the formulaic *epistas* points towards to the latter – advising him to befriend Apollonius and consult him on the matter. Apollonius reproached the young man for uttering blasphemous words and explained that the god reveals himself to those who crave healing (τοῖς γὰρ βουλομένοις δίδωσι), not to those who undermine their own health. Asclepius, the divine healer seems to manifest himself only to those who make an effort to actively improve their life-style and to follow the prescribed regimen.

Nevertheless, the most frequent kind of criticism Asclepius was faced with was related to the god's 'multilocality' and his absence at the moment of need from one specific sanctuary due to his obligation to visit other patients in a different healing location. Indicative are, for instance, the complaints expressed by Themistius, the 4th century AD philosopher in the 27th of his Private Orations entitled 'On the Need to Give Thought' (*Orationes* 27.333d with Penella 1999, 164–73). Themistius reacted against the idea of Asclepius not being present in the local temple and the patient having to travel to the most prestigious Asclepieia of Epidaurus and Tricca to consult him. Similarly, in one of the Epidaurian Iamata (*IG* IV^2, 1, B23), we learn about a certain Aristagora who having suffered from tapeworm failed to encounter Asclepius in her sleep in his sanctuary in Troizen, because the god 'was out of town' (οὐκ ἐπιδαμοῦντος) attending his clientele at his temple in Epidaurus (ἀλλ' ἐν Ἐπιδαύρωι ἐόντος). Nevertheless, Asclepius' sons (τοὺς υἱοὺς τοῦ θεοῦ) proceeded with chopping off Aristagora's head and would have failed to put it back, if the god hadn't come back from Epidaurus to Troizen (ὁ θεὸς ἵκων ἐξ Ἐπιδαύρου). When the god returned from Epidaurus he reattached the head, cut open her belly, removed the tapeworm and stitched her up. This reference to the sons of Asclepius may well be to the secular doctors, collectively known as the *Asclepiadae*, who were associated with the temple (on which see Parker 1996, 177). If this is so, one may also argue that the passage neatly subordinates the prescriptive voice of secular medicine of the 4th century to the authority of the divine healer (more on the dynamic relationship between secular and temple medicine from the 4th century BC up to the imperial era below).

Similar delinquencies were not unknown even in Epidaurus, as we can conclude from Aelian's account (*Nature of Animals* 9.33) of a woman, who while suffering from tapeworm as well, came to the temple of the god to receive treatment. Just as in Aristagora's case in Troizen, the god happened to be absent (οὐκ παρῆν ὁ θεός). In her dream, the over-confident helpers of the god decapitated her and one of them pulled out the tapeworm. He could not, however, reattach her head and the woman died. Once the god returned to Epidaurus, he put the woman's head back in its place and raised her from the dead!

Media of transmission for healing epiphanies: dreams or waking reality?

The incubant would normally see the god in his sleep or in an interstitial state between sleep and waking. Incubation was, indeed, the predominant technique of acquiring healing epiphanies. Asclepius is strongly associated with dreams and dreaming. As stated above, Asclepius revealed himself primarily in dreams during the night. However, there are a few reports of dream visions of Asclepius which took place during daytime, such as those reported by Libanius in his *Autobiography* (143): 'Out of the three dream-visions I had of the god, two took place at noontide' (τρισὶ δὲ ἐνυπνίοις ὁ θεός, ὧν τὼ δύο μεθημερινώ). Philostratos informs us of yet another sophist named Antiochos, who was said to have spent many nights in the temple of the god not only on account of the divine prescriptive dreams, but also for the sake of 'all the intercourse there is between those who were awake and converse with one another, for in his case the god used to converse with him while awake' (*Vitae Sophistarum* 568). Epiphanic revelations in the course of a dream prescribing the appropriate remedy and course of action are at the heart of temple medicine practised in the name of the god, and even epitomised the medical art *per se* according to Iamblichus (*On the Mysteries* 3.3):

> οὕτως ἐν Ἀσκληπιοῦ μὲν ταὰ νοσήματα τοῖς θείοις ὀνείροις παύεται· διὰ τὴν τάξιν τῶν νύκτωρ ἐπιφανειῶν ἡ ἰατρικὴ τέχνη συνέστη ἀπὸ τῶν ἱερῶν ὀνειράτων.
>
> 'Thus, in the temples of Asclepius diseases come to an end by means of divine dreams; and, because of the order of the nocturnal epiphanies, the medical art consists of sacred dream-visions'.

To be sure, dreams used as diagnostic tools were not unique in the cult of Asclepius. On the contrary, dream diagnosis was known to and practised by the author of the Hippocratic *Regimen* (cf especially Book IV), Galen or pseudo-Galen (if we are to judge from his work *On Diagnosis from Dreams*) and Rufus, the Ephesian physician and contemporary of Galen (compare, for instance, the emphasis given on diagnostic dreams and their interpretation in his *Medical Questions*), as rightly argued by Andrew Holowchack (2001, 382–99). What is unique in Asclepius' cult is that dreams become not simply the diagnostic, but also the therapeutic, means of treating an illness.

Occasionally it is not clear at all to the perceiver whether the god appears in a dream or a waking vision. In these cases the god is described as appearing halfway between sleep and walking (μέσως ἔχειν ὕπνου καὶ ἐγρηγόρσεως), as, for instance, in the case of Aelius Aristides who was seeking remedy for his condition at the Asclepieion of Pergamon (*Sacred Tales* 48.32 quoted above). In another strange account of an Asclepius epiphany, reported this time by Pausanias (10.38.13), the god appears originally in something that feels like a dream but turns out to be something much more complicated and eerie. The story goes that Asclepius appeared to the poetess Anyte and ordered her to deliver his written message to Phalysius of Naupactus, who was blind. Initially, Anyte thought that the god revealed his will in a dream, but later on and judging from the sealed tablet she found in her hands, she concluded that the god had appeared in waking reality: τουτο ἐφάνη τῇ γυναικὶ ὄψις ὀνείρατος, ὕπαρ μέντοι ἦν αὐτίκα. καὶ εὗρέ τε ἐν ταῖς χερσὶ ταῖς αὐτῆς σεσημασμένην δέλτον. Phalysius took the divine letter in his hands and as soon as he opened the shield, he regained his vision. The story became the aetiological myth behind the introduction of the god's cult in Naupactus. Anyte's vision belongs to what Dodds (1951, 102–3) calls 'rapport dreams'. Rapport dreams are those exceptional cases of dream visions in which the deity leaves the dreamer with an unquestionable token of his/ her visitation, such as the written tablet in our narrative.

Additionally, we come across some reports of Asclepius manifesting himself in waking reality, but, admittedly, these cases occur only very rarely. In the passage from Aristophanes' *Wealth* (633–747) discussed above, for instance, Karion is not asleep when the god approaches him and blind Plutus. Another instance of the god appearing in waking reality is that of Sostrata from Pherae, who, having experienced a false pregnancy, slept in the Epidaurian Asclepieion without, however, any fruitful results (*IG* IV^2, 1, nos 121–2, B25, with Herzog 1931, 18):

vac. (XXV) Σωστράτα Φεραί[α παρ]/εκύησε. α[ὕ]τα ἐμ παντὶ ἐοῦσα φοράδạν εἰς τὸ ἱαρὸν ἀφικομένα ἐνε[κά]/θευδε. ὡς δὲ οὐθὲν ἐνύπνιον ἐναργ[ὲ]ς ἑώρη, πάλιν οἴκαδε ἀπεκομίζ̣[ε]/το. μετὰ δὲ τοῦτο συμβολῆσαί τις περὶ Κόρνους αὐτᾶι καὶ τοῖς ἑ[πομέ]νοις ἔδοξε τὰν ὄψιν εὐπρεπὴς ἀνήρ, ὃς πυθόμενος παρ' αὐτῶν τ[ὰς δυσπρα]/ξίας τὰς αὐτῶν ἐκελήσατο θέμεν τὰν κ̣λίναν, ἐφ' ἇς τὰν Σωστρ[άταν ἔφε]/ρον. ἔπειτα τὰγ κοιλίαν αὐτᾶς ἀνσχίσας ἐξαιρεῖ πλῆθος ζ[ωϋφίων πάμ]/πολυ, [δύ]ε ποδανιπτῆρας· συνράψας δὲ τὰ[ν γ]αστέρα καὶ ποήσας ὑ[γιῆ] / τὰν γ̣υναῖκα τάν τε παρουσίαν τὰν αὐτο[ῦ π]αρενεφάνιξε ὁ Ἀσκλαπιὸς καὶ ἴατρα ἐκέλ̣ετο ἀπ[ο]πέμπειν εἰς Ἐπί[δα]υρ[ον. *vac.*]

'Sostrata of Pherai, false pregnancy. This woman, borne entirely on a litter, arrived at the sanctuary and slept there. But since she saw no clear dream she was carried homeward again. Later, around Kornoi, she and her attendants met up with someone, in appearance a handsome man, who, when he heard from them their bad luck, told them to set down the couch on which Sostrata was borne. Then he cut open her belly and took out lots and lots of creatures – two footbasins full. When he had sewn up her stomach and made the woman well, Asclepius revealed his presence to her and ordered her to send offerings to Epidaurus' (trans. LiDonnici 1995).

On their way home, the woman and her attendants met a handsome man, who having learnt all about her misfortunes, cut the belly of the afflicted lady wide open and set her free from the various creatures that she was carrying within. When he had sewn up her stomach and made the woman well, Asclepius revealed his identity (τάν τε παρουσίαν τὰν αὐτο[ῦ π]αρενεφάνιξε ὁ Ἀσκλαπιός) and ordered her to send his medical fee (*iatra*) to Epidaurus. Asclepius reveals his identity only after the whole operation was brought successfully to completion and in a sense his epiphany coincides with the healing of the woman. Does that qualify us to claim that in this particular case, the healing is objectified as the god's divine manifestation? It is most significant that the corporeal manifestation of the god is presented as a belated result of the woman's practising incubation in the temple earlier.

Apparently, this story along with other similar ones (originally having sprung from a votive relief?) must have been carefully and craftily reworked by the priestly personnel, in their attempt to advertise the possibility that *prima facie* unsuccessful *katakliseis* may prove to be fruitful later on. What we read in the hymn to Asclepius as found on an inscription from the Asclepieion in Pergamon is also relevant here: '…. Saviour … summoned during night and day, you came to me when I was troubled in my heart by painful illness' (Edelstein and Edelstein T 596). Consequently, the Edelsteins (1998, 150, n. 22) are not entirely right, when they claim that Asclepius manifested his godhead only in night-time dreams in a healing context. To be fair they do mention Sostrata's example, but Carion's account in Aristophanes' *Wealth* is dismissed as poetic license. Dreams have undoubtedly been the medium of healing epiphanies par excellence, but waking reality as a most rare medium of Asclepius' epiphanies should not be excluded. Whether in dreams or in waking reality, it is significant that Asclepius' manifestations to the afflicted are taken to be the tangible proof of the god's power and divinity.

Asclepius the divine doctor

To pull the threads together, if we put Asclepius' zoomorphic epiphanies, so popular with his introduction myths, to one side, in the majority of our literary and epigraphic sources (as well as in Asclepius' most popular artistic representations), the god manifested himself in the form of a bearded man of mature age. His standard iconographical identity was that of a paternal figure resembling Zeus in everything apart from his staff with the coiled snake, or snakes which appear to accompany him. There are, of course, a small number of testimonies where Asclepius manifested himself in the likeness of a handsome young man (τὰν ὄψιν εὐπρεπὴς ἀνήρ), as in his epiphany to Sostrata (B25, discussed above). Similarly the man of Epidaurian cure A17 who had his sore toe healed by a snake, claimed, when he woke, that he dreamt of a youth with a beautiful appearance (νεανίσκον εὐπρεπῆ τὰμ μορφάν) putting some drug on his toe. In Sostrata's case, in particular, the handsome man is explicitly identified as the god Asclepius himself.

There are, in fact, a whole range of narratives from the Epidaurian Iamata which lay emphasis on the beauty and the youth of the dream figure that the patient encounters, and which seem to hint at having sex with the god for healing purposes (*IG* IV^2, I, nos 121–2, A14, B11, B19). In one of these, a man who had a stone in his penis dreamt of having sex with a beautiful boy (perhaps an anthropomorphic manifestation of the god). He had an orgasm in his sleep and ejected the stone. In another, a woman called Andromache dreamt that a beautiful boy uncovered her, and that the god touched her with his hand. 'As a result a son was born to Andromache by Arybbas'. LiDonnici (1989, 109, n. 28) rightly maintains that the stress on the baby's paternity aims at eliminating any possibility that Asklepios was the father. In a third narrative, a childless woman slept at the temple of the god and dreamt that 'a snake (in all likelihood a zoomorphic manifestation of the god) lay on her belly and as a result five children were born to her'. In all three cases, the sexual contact with these otherworldly beings takes place in the course of a dream (Petridou in press, chapter five).

Alternatively, the god manifested himself in the form of his statue. This was the case, for instance, with Domninus, who, having woken up, spoke to the statue of the god and even had a brief argument with it concerning the prescribed course of action (Suidas, s.v. Δομνῖνος). Aelius Aristides is also reported to have conversed with the god in the form of his cult statue (*Sacred Tales* 50. 50–1). On Asclepius manifesting his godhead in the course of dreams in general, see also Artemidorus, *Interpretation of Dreams* 2.37.

The god in his anthropomorphic and statuary manifestations was seen laughing (Aristophanes, *Plutus* 723) and even joking with his patients (*IG* IV^2, 1, nos 121–2, A8). The exception that verifies the rule is Asclepius' frightening manifestation to the author of the Hippocratic *Epistulae* (15, 9), where the god did not appear as a benign and calm paternal figure, but appeared in a lively posture and rather fearsome in the company of enormous snakes (compare here Aristophanes, *Plutus* 733–734). More importantly, in the majority of our sources, the god was seen cutting his patients' veins, heads, stomachs etc.; he was seen applying remedies on their skin and limbs, or simply consulting them on the appropriate course of action. In other words, Asclepius often acquired the form of a physician and even his cures, though thought of as miraculous, followed the pattern of rational and empirical medicine (Edelstein and Edelstein 1998, 345). In fact, many students of the history of Ancient Medicine would agree that the god's close cooperation with the developing art of medicine was one of the most significant reasons for the popularity of Asclepius' cult:

> 'Divine healer though he was, Asclepius had the wisdom never to resist the developing secular 'art' of medicine. On the contrary, he appropriated it: not its substance perhaps but its symbols, its aura, its prestige. We already find various medicinal instruments listed in an early inventory of the Asclepieum in the Piraeus, and represented behind the god on Telemachus' monument; and the public physicians of Athens actually sacrificed twice annually in the hero's shrine. The truest explanation for the rise of Asclepius may be that he was, as it were, in partnership with Hippocrates' (Parker 1996, 184).[14]

On the other hand, to think of Asclepius' cult exclusively in terms of medical techniques, treatments, and procedures which more or less find parallels with contemporary medicinal thought and practice would be to miss the point entirely. Asclepius' healing epiphanies carry the unmistakable hallmarks of a divine revelation and often, as seen above, the signs of a mystic experience. No matter how hard it is to think beyond the perceptual filters of an age in which the human physician and his attendants are the epicentre of the healing process, one must try not to forget that Asclepius was both a divine healer and a divine physician, both a god and a doctor.

Acknowledgements

I am indebted to John Wilkins for his useful comments and suggestions on an early draft of this paper, and to Paul Scade for improving the language of the paper significantly. I would also like to thank Demetrios Michaelides for all his pertinent remarks and corrections. Part of the research for this chapter was conducted within the 'Medicine of the Mind – Philosophy of the Body' research programme, which is led by Prof. Philip van der Eijk, and funded by the Alexander von Humboldt-Stiftung.

Notes

1 Translations, unless otherwise stated, are by the author.

2 The Edelsteins (1998) provide an informative discussion of the relevant literary and epigraphic material. Hart (2000), on the other hand, provides a review of the relevant archaeological and numismatic evidence. On a general overview on health and disease in the ancient world see King's introduction (1–11) in King (2005).

3 On the origins of Asclepius' cult and his associations with Egyptian and other Near Eastern healing deities, see Willi 2008, 160–1.

4 The monument (a T-shaped structure made of Pentelic marble) has been reconstructed from 14 fragments, which belong in collections of the National and the Epigraphical Museums in Athens, the British Museum in London, the Museo Civico in Padova, and the Museo Maffeiano in Verona. Some of these fragments appear to be copies of the original monument. Elpida Mitropoulou (1975) has assembled a catalogue of most of the fragments, including detailed measurements and photographs. An illustration of the monument as reconstructed by Luigi Beschi appears as figure 4.2 in Wickkiser (2008, 69). See also Wickkiser 2008, 67–8 for the inscription's text. On the Telemachos monument see also van Straten (1993, 259): 'The two sides of this *amphiglyphon* show the interior and the exterior of the newly founded sanctuary, and on one side there is also an indication of the Asklepieion in Piraeus, whence Asklepios had come to Athens. Telemachos himself, however, is in no way different from any other worshipper on any other votive relief of the same period. In the inscription on the pillar supporting this relief, though it is extremely succinct and matter-of-fact, we may perhaps detect a certain amount of self-confidence and pride. Telemachos declares, and he emphatically repeats it in another inscription, that he was the first to found the sanctuary of Asklepios and Hygieia and the sons and daughters of Asklepios.

5 The inscription on the Telemachos' Monument (*IG* II2 4960a), which tells us of Asclepius' advent in Athens is fragmentary. In lines 12–15 of Beschi's reconstruction (1967–1968), we read that Telemachus summoned a snake from home and brought it in a chariot to Athens. The reading ΔΡΑ]ΚΟΝΤΑ, though, is not certain. It is Körte's conjecture (*AM* 21, 1896, 316), and it has been contested by Clinton (1994, 20), who prefers to read ΔΙΑ]ΚΟΝΟΝ (with Beschi). Körte supports his suggestion with the numerous examples of zoomorphic cult-dispatchers discussed below (cf. Sikyon, Limera, Halieis, Rome). Clinton's grounds for questioning Körte's reading are not entirely convincing: he claims that a snake from Epidaurus would have had a more prominent position in the text and the name of the city would have been given extra emphasis. See also most recently Aston (2004, 21), who thinks that Clinton *et al.*'s reading of ΔΙΑ]ΚΟΝΟΝ 'is not unassailable'. This second reading ['attendant'], though, is of use to Clinton who favours the idea of Asclepius' being introduced in the

city in the form of a wooden statue of substantial size. The attendant mentioned above would have been the one appointed to take care of the god's image. The two variants, nevertheless, the statue and the snake, i.e. the anthropomorphic effigies and the zoomorphic cult-dispatcher are not contradictory (On the different forms of divine epiphany see Petridou in press, chapter six). They can in fact be complimentary and could have been combined in introducing Asclepius' authority in such a major city as Athens, perhaps to contest his major divine rivals in the realm of healing, e.g. Athena Hygeia.

6 The incubation scene in Aristophanes' *Wealth* 656–8 takes place by the sea, namely in the Asclepieion of Piraeus.

7 Connolly (1998, 20) argues that it is unlikely that the poet received heroic honours before the 330s and dismisses the story of Asklepios' *xenia* as 'Hellenistic fabrication'. As for the inscriptions, he thinks that they honour a separate local hero.

8 Although initially there may have been some dispute over the site of the god's sanctuary (Parker 1996, 177–81 with bibliography).

9 For the significance of the adoption of Asclepius by the Eleusinian priesthood, see Garland (1992, 124) and Parker (1996, 180) among others.

10 For a full list of similarities see Garland (1992, 124); on mystic epiphanies see Petridou in press and 2013. The intentional ambiguity of the mysteric imagery and terminology used by Aristeides is a topic I deal with in my current research project which is entitled 'Medicine and Mysticism in Aelius Aristeides' *Hieroi Logoi*'. On this passage see also Petsalis-Diomidis (2010, 12–4).

11 All the references are from Herzog (1931): dogs: nos 20 and 26; horses of Asclepius' chariot in no. 38; snake: no. 33; snake and god: nos 37, 42.

12 Plautus' testimony is very important because he follows a Greek original of the 3rd century. On Asclepius and temple medicine in Aelius Aristides, see Horstmanshoff 2004, 325–41.

13 More on the terminology of the dream-vision in Hanson 1980, 1407–79. On incubation see Herzog 1931; Kerenyi 1959; van Straten 1976; Hanson 1980; LiDonnici 1995; Edelstein and Edelstein 1998; Hart 2000; Holowchak 2001; Lloyd 2003 and Nutton 2003, among several others. The 'grammar' of incubation is well demonstrated in votive reliefs depicting scenes of incubation. These reliefs come from all the Asklepieia. More on this issue in van Straten 1981, 63-146.

14 On the cooperation of secular and religious healing and their practitioners see also Holowchack 2001, 386 and Nutton 2004, 110–4.

Bibliography

Aston, E. 2004: 'Asclepius and the legacy of Thessaly', *Classical Quarterly* 54(1), 18–32.

Behr, C. A. 1968: *Aristides and the Sacred Tales*, Amsterdam.

Behr, C. A. 1981: *P. Aelius Aristides: The Complete Works II*, Leiden.

Beschi, L. 1967–1968: 'Il Monumento di Telemachos, fondatore dell'Asklepieion ateniese', *Annuario della Scuola Archeologica di Atene e delle Missioni Italiane in Oriente* 45–6, n.s. 29–30, 381–436.

Clinton, K. 1994: 'The Epidauria and the arrival of Asclepius in Athens', 17–34 in R. Hägg (ed.), *Ancient Greek Cult Practice from the Epigraphical Evidence. Proceedings of the Second International Seminar on Ancient Greek Cult, Swedish Institute at Athens, 22–24 November 1991*, Stockholm.

Connolly, A. 1998: 'Was Sophocles heroised as Dexion?', *Journal of Hellenic Studies* 118, 1–21.

Dodds, E. R. 1951: *The Greeks and the Irrational*, Berkeley, Los Angeles and London.

Edelstein, L. 1968: 'Greek medicine in its relation to religion and magic', 205–46 in O. Temkin and C. L. Temkin (eds), *Ancient Medicine*, Baltimore and London.

Edelstein, E. J. L. and Edelstein, L. 1998: *Asklepius: A Collection and Interpretation of the Testimonies*, 2nd ed., Baltimore.

Farnell, L. R. 1921: *Greek Hero Cults and Ideas of Immortality*, Oxford.

Garland, R. 1992: *Introducing New Gods. The politics of Athenian religion*, Ithaca.

Hanson, J. S. 1980: 'Dreams and visions in the Graeco-Roman world and early Christianity', *Aufstieg und Niedergang der römische Welt* 23(2), 1395–427.

Hart, G. D. 2000: *Asclepius, the God of Medicine,* London.

Herzog, R. 1931: *Die Wunderheilungen von Epidauros* (Philologus Supplement 22.3), Leipzig.

Holowchak, A. M. 2001: 'Interpreting dreams for corrective regiment: diagnostic dreams in Greco-Roman medicine', *Journal of Medicine and Allied Sciences* 56(4), 382–99.

Horstmanshoff, H. F. 2004: 'Asclepius and temple medicine in Aelius Aristides' Sacred Tales', *Studies in Ancient Medicine* 27, 325–41.

Kerenyi, C. 1959: *Asklepios. Archetypal Image of the Physician's Existence,* trans. R. Mannheim, Princeton.

King, H. (ed.) 2005: *Health in Antiquity*, London and New York.

Kirmayer, L. J. 2006: 'Toward a medicine of the imagination', *New Literary History* 37, 583–605.

Körte, A. 1896: 'Die Ausgrabungen am Westabhange der Akropolis. IV. Das Heiligtum des Amysos', *Athenische Mitteilungen* 21, 287–332.

LiDonnici, L. R. 1995: *The Epidaurian Miracle Inscriptions. Text, Translation and Commentary*, Atlanta.

Lloyd, G. E. R. 2003: *In the Grip of Disease. Studies in the Greek Imagination,* Oxford.

Mikalson, J. 1984: 'Religion and the plague in Athens', 217–25 in K. J. Rigsby (ed.), *Studies Presented to Sterling Dow on his Eightieth Birthday*, Durham, NC.

Mitropoulou, E. 1975: *A new Interpretation of the Telemachos Monument*, Athens.

Most, G. W. 1993: 'A cock for Asclepius', *The Classical Quarterly* 43(1), 96–111.

Nutton, V. 2004: *Ancient Medicine*, London and New York.

Parker, R. 1983: *Miasma*, Oxford.

Parker, R. 1996: *Athenian Religion. A History*, Oxford.

Penella, R. K. 1999: *The Private Orations of Themistius*, Berkeley.

Petsalis-Diomidis, A. 2010: *Truly Beyond Wonders: The Cult of Asclepius and Aelius Aristides' Hieroi Logoi*, Oxford.

Petridou, G. 2013: '*Blessed is he, who has seen ...* The power of ritual viewing and ritual framing in Eleusis', in S. Blundell, D.

Cairns and N. Rabinowitz (eds), *Vision and Power* (Helios 40) (forthcoming).

Petridou, G. in press: *Divine Epiphany in Greek Literature and Culture*, Oxford.

Sommerstein, A. H. 2003: *Aristophanes, The Birds and Other Plays*, London.

van Straten, F. T. 1976: 'Daikrates´s dream. A votive relief from Kos and some other *kat' onar* dedications', *Bulletin Antieke Beschaving* 51, 1–38.

van Straten, F. T. 1981: 'Gifts for the Gods', 65–151 in H. S. Versnel (ed.), *Faith, Hope and Worship. Aspects of Religious Mentality in the Ancient world*, Leiden.

van Straten, F. T. 1993: 'Images of Gods and men in a changing society: self-identity in Hellenistic religion', 248–65 in A. W. Bulloch, E. S. Gruen, A. A. Long, and A. Stewart (eds), *Images and Ideologies: Self-definition in the Hellenistic World*, Berkeley.

Wickkiser, B. L. 2008: *Asklepios, Medicine, and the Politics of Healing in Fifth-century Greece: Between Craft and Cult*, Baltimore.

Willi, A. 2008: 'νόσος and ὁσίη etymological and sociocultural observations on the concepts of disease and divine (dis)favour in Ancient Greece', *Journal of Hellenic Studies* 128, 153–71.

Young, R. M. 1971: 'Scientific medicine and the social order', available from: http://human-nature.com/rmyyoung/paper/paper 87.doc [Accessed 15 August 2008].

37. Ὁ Ξενὼν τοῦ Ἁγίου Δημητρίου: Εἰκονογραφικὰ Ζητήματα

Χαραλάμπος Μπακιρτζῆς

At the end of the 6th century, there was a functioning xenon *or hospital in the basilica of Saint Demetrios in Thessaloniki. The course of treatment for the patients was based on Hippocratic medicine, together with miraculous interventions by Saint Demetrios. The treatment process was similar to that which had been implemented at the Serapeion in Thessaloniki. The iconography of the mosaics in the basilica of Saint Demetrios is linked to the function of the hospital. The mosaics are from patients restored to health and are dedicated in gratitude to Saint Demetrios, the Mother of God and other saints venerated there. In one of these there is a depiction of an angel offering Saint Demetrios a doctor's staff. The children represented are an element of the treatment process of the* xenon, *which specialised in paediatric and obstetric cases. The positioning of the mosaics indicates the 'stations' made by pilgrims and patients when going round the basilica. The mosaics of the basilica of Saint Demetrios constitute an artistic ensemble from Early Christian times which continues the tradition, inherited from the Asclepieia and Serapeia of Antiquity, of dedicating icons by way of thanks.*

Συνδυάζοντας πληροφορίες διάσπαρτες στὰ *Θαύματα τοῦ Ἁγίου Δημητρίου* κατέληξα στὸ συμπέρασμα ὅτι στὴ βασιλικὴ τοῦ Ἁγίου Δημητρίου στὴ Θεσσαλονίκη (Εἰκ. 37.1) λειτουργοῦσε στὰ τέλη τοῦ 6^{ου} αι. *ξενὼν* (νοσοκομεῖον) (*Ἁγίου Δημητρίου Θαύματα*, 368–71. Bakirtzis 2010, 398–405). Ἡ θεραπεία τῶν ἀσθενῶν στὸν ξενώνα τοῦ Ἁγίου Δημητρίου γινόταν ὄχι μόνον μὲ τὴ βοήθεια τῆς ἱπποκρατικῆς ἰατρικῆς ποὺ ἐξασκοῦσαν ἰατροί, ὅπως στὸν περίφημο ξενώνα τοῦ Σαμψὼν στὴν Κωνσταντινούπολη, ἀλλὰ καὶ μὲ τὶς θαυματουργίες τοῦ ἁγίου Δημητρίου, ὅπως συνέβαινε καὶ σὲ ἐκκλησίες ἄλλων θεραπευτῶν ἁγίων, π.χ. τοῦ ἁγίου Ἰσιδώρου στὴ Χίο ἢ τῶν ἁγίων Κύρου καὶ Ἰωάννου στὴν ἐκκλησία τῶν Εὐαγγελιστῶν ἀνατολικὰ τῆς Ἀλεξάνδρειας (Miller 1998). Ἡ θεραπευτικὴ ὡστόσο παρέμβαση τοῦ ἁγίου Δημητρίου δὲν συνίστατο σὲ φάρμακα ἢ ἰατρικὲς συμβουλές, ὅπως ὑπεδείκνυαν ἄλλοι ἅγιοι ἰατροί, π.χ. ὁ ἅγιος Ἀρτέμιος στὴν ἐκκλησία τοῦ Ἁγίου Ἰωάννη Εὐαγγελιστὴ στὴν Κωνσταντινούπολη ἢ οἱ ἅγιοι Κοσμᾶς καὶ Δαμιανὸς στὴν ἐκκλησία τους στὸ Κοσμίδιον Κωνσταντινουπόλεως, ἀλλὰ γιάτρευε ἀποκλειστικὰ μέσω τῆς σιωπηλῆς θαυματουργίας ἐμφανιζόμενος σὲ ὅραμα κατὰ τὴ διάρκεια *ἐγκοιμήσεως (incubatio)* τῶν ἀσθενῶν: *τὴν χεῖρα ἐπιτιθέντα καὶ τὸν σταυρὸν κατασημαίνειν πειρώμενον* (Lemerle 1979, 80.23–4). Ἀπὸ τὶς διηγήσεις τῶν *Θαυμάτων* δὲν προκύπτει ἀνταγωνισμὸς θαυματουργικῆς καὶ ἱπποκρατικῆς, θείας καὶ ἀνθρωπίνης ἰατρικῆς στὴ λειτουργία τοῦ ξενώνα τοῦ Ἁγίου Δημητρίου, ποὺ ἦταν σύνηθες φαινόμενο στὰ ἰατρικὰ χρονικὰ τῶν πρώτων χριστιανικῶν αἰώνων (Miller 1998, 69–71). Ἀντιθέτως λειτουργοῦσαν συμπληρωματικά. Παραβάλλοντας τὴ θεραπευτικὴ διαδικασία τοῦ ἁγίου Δημητρίου μὲ αὐτὴ ἁγίων ἰατρῶν τῆς Κωνσταντινουπόλεως διαπιστώνει κανεὶς ὅτι βρίσκεται πιὸ κοντὰ στὶς θαυματουργικὲς ἰάσεις ποὺ ἐφαρμόζονταν στὸ περίφημο Σαραπεῖον τῆς Θεσσαλονίκης, ὅπως τὶς γνωρίζουμε ἀπὸ τὶς ἐπιγραφὲς ποὺ βρέθηκαν (Koester 2007, 38–54 καὶ Τζαναβάρη 2003, 237–52), παρὰ στὶς μεθόδους τοῦ Ἀσκληπιοῦ, ὁ ὁποῖος συνεδύαζε τὴ χειρουργική, τὴ φαρμακολογία, τὴ φυσιοθεραπεία καὶ τὴ θαυματουργικὴ ἰατρικὴ διὰ τῆς ἀγγίξεως τῶν ἀσθενῶν (Dauphin 1999, 237–52).

Ἡ βασιλικὴ τοῦ Ἁγίου Δημητρίου στὴ Θεσσαλονίκη εἶναι περίφημη γιὰ τὰ προεικονομαχικὰ ψηφιδωτά της. Ἐρωτήματα γιὰ τὴ χρονολόγησή τους καὶ τὴν εἰκονογραφία τους δὲν ἔχουν τύχει ἀκόμη κοινὰ ἀποδεκτῆς ἀπαντήσεως. Ἡ ἑρμηνεία μάλιστα τοῦ εἰκονογραφικοῦ προγράμματος παραμένει ἀνοιχτὸ θέμα ἐπειδὴ δὲν συσχετίζεται μὲ τὰ

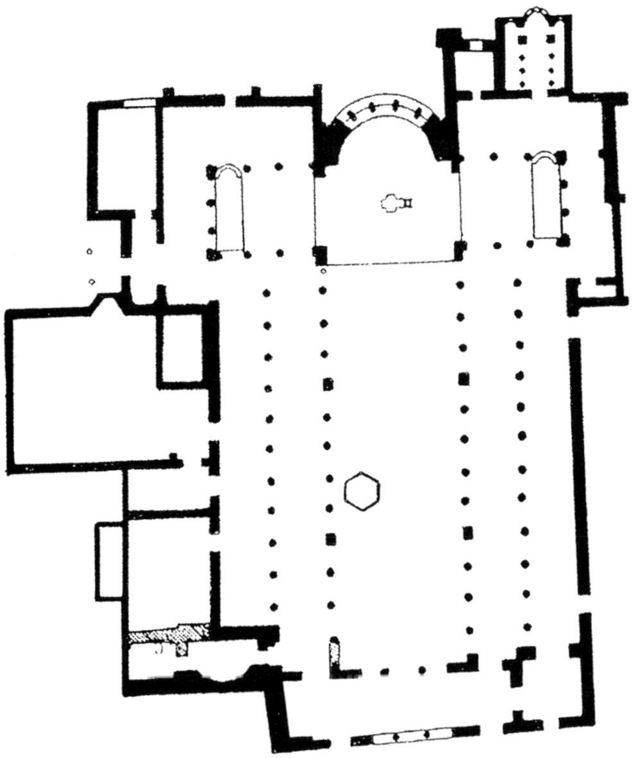

Εἰκ. 37.1. Κάτοψη βασιλικῆς Ἁγίου Δημητρίου (σχέδιο Χ. Μπακιρτζῆ)

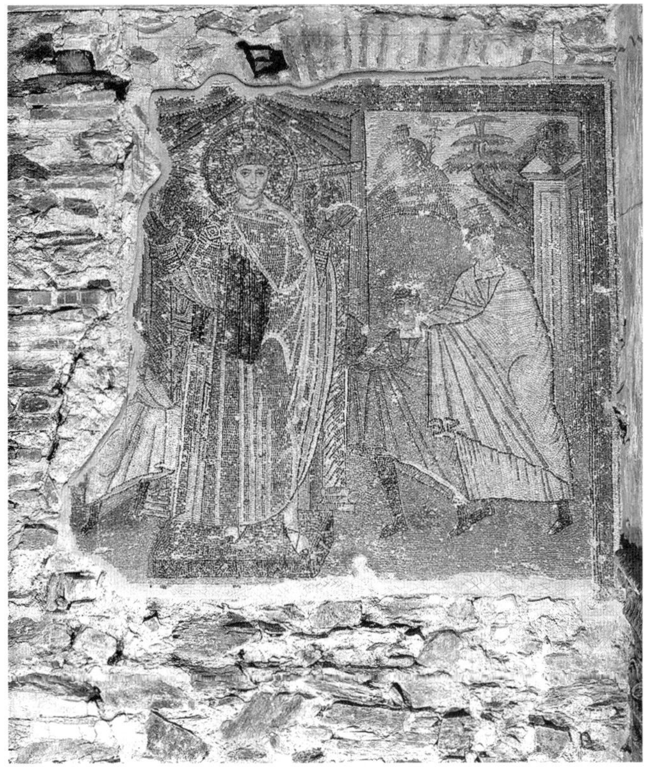

Εἰκ. 37.2. Ψηφιδωτὸ μὲ παράσταση ἁγίου Δημητρίου μὲ παιδιά (9η Ἐφορεία Βυζαντινῶν Ἀρχαιοτήτων)

εἰκονογραφικὰ προγράμματα ἄλλων παλαιοχριστιανικῶν ἐκκλησιῶν τῆς Ρώμης ἢ τῆς Ραβέννας ἢ τοῦ Parenzo κ.ἄ. Στὸ κείμενο ποὺ ἀκολουθεῖ θὰ παρουσιάσω τὴ χωροταξία τῶν ψηφιδωτῶν μέσα στὴ βασιλικὴ καὶ τὴν ἄποψή μου γιὰ τὴν ἑρμηνεία τῆς εἰκονογραφίας τους.

Τὰ ψηφιδωτά χωρίζονται σὲ δύο εὐκρινεῖς ὁμάδες, ὅπως εἶναι γενικὰ ἀποδεκτό: πρὶν καὶ μετὰ τὴν καταστροφὴ καὶ ἀναστήλωση τοῦ ναοῦ *c.* 620, ἤτοι ψηφιδωτὰ παλαιότερα τοῦ 7ου αἰώνα καὶ ψηφιδωτὰ ἀπὸ τοῦ 7ου αἰώνα καὶ ἑξῆς (Ξυγγόπουλος 1969· Μπακιρτζῆς 2012, 143). Στὴν πρώτη ὁμάδα ἀνήκουν δύο ψηφιδωτὰ στὸ δυτικὸ τοῖχο τῆς βασιλικῆς, καὶ τὰ ψηφιδωτὰ τῆς βόρειας μικρῆς κιονοστοιχίας, ποὺ εἶναι γνωστὰ μόνον ἀπὸ παλαιὲς φωτογραφίες καὶ ὑδατογραφίες.[1] Τὰ ψηφιδωτὰ τῆς δεύτερης ὁμάδας βρίσκονται στὸ ἀνατολικὸ τμῆμα τῆς βασιλικῆς, στοὺς δύο πεσσοὺς ἑκατέρωθεν τοῦ ἱεροῦ βήματος, καὶ σὲ ἄλλα σημεῖα τοῦ ναοῦ.

Α. Ψηφιδωτὰ παλαιότερα τοῦ 7ου αἰώνα

1. Τὸ πρῶτο ψηφιδωτὸ βρίσκεται πάνω ἀπὸ τὴν εἴσοδο τοῦ νάρθηκα πρὸς τὸ πρῶτο νότιο κλίτος καὶ πρὸς τὴν πλευρὰ τοῦ κλίτους (Εἰκ. 37.2). Στὸν δεόμενο ἅγιο Δημήτριο, ποὺ ἐμφανίζεται στὴν εἴσοδο τοῦ μαρμαρίνου κιβωρίου του ὁδηγεῖται ἀπὸ ἐνήλικα ἀγνώστου φύλου ἕνα παιδί.[2] Ἀπὸ δεύτερο ζευγάρι προσερχομένων, ποὺ ὑπῆρχε στὴν ἄλλη πλευρὰ τοῦ ἁγίου σώζεται μόνον τὸ ἐμπρόσθιο τμῆμα τοῦ παιδιοῦ. Οἱ μορφὲς εἶναι ἐνδεδυμένες ὁμοιόμορφα μὲ λευκὰ ἱμάτια καὶ ἐσωτερικὸ κλειστὸ χιτωνίσκο μὲ κόψιμο στὸ λαιμό. Παρόμοια ἐσωτερική ἐνδυμασία δὲν ἦταν ἀσυνήθης. Φέρει καὶ ὁ ἰατρὸς Δαμιανός, ὁ Κοσμᾶς καὶ ἄλλες μορφὲς στὰ ψηφιδωτὰ τῆς Ροτόντας. Οἱ Γ. καὶ Μ. Σωτηρίου (1952, 192) διατύπωσαν τὴν ἄποψη ὅτι θέμα τῆς παράστασης εἶναι ἡ ἀφιέρωση παιδιῶν στὸν ἅγιο Δημήτριο ἐπειδὴ ἔδωσαν βαρύνουσα σημασία στὸ ρόλο τῆς δεύτερης μορφῆς.[3] Ἡ ὁμοία ὡστόσο στάση προσερχομένων μὲ τὰ χέρια κάτω ἀπὸ τὰ ἱμάτια συναντᾶται σὲ ὅλα τὰ ψηφιδωτὰ τοῦ ναοῦ (βλ. παρακάτω), στὰ ὁποῖα ἀπεικονίζονται ἐνήλικες καὶ δὲν ἔχουν σχέση μὲ ἀφιέρωση παιδιῶν. Ἀντιθέτως ἡ στάση αὐτὴ τοῦ σώματος, καὶ σύμφωνα μὲ τὶς ἐπιγραφὲς ποὺ συνοδεύουν τὰ ψηφιδωτά (βλ. παρακάτω παράγρ. 3), προσιδιάζει σὲ ἔκφραση σεβασμοῦ καὶ εὐχαριστίας (Μπακιρτζῆς 2012, 144). Συνεπῶς θέμα τῆς συγκεκριμένης ψηφιδωτῆς παράστασης δὲν μπορεῖ νὰ εἶναι ἡ ἀφιέρωση ἢ καθοσίωση παιδιῶν στὸν ἅγιο Δημήτριο, ἀλλὰ παιδιὰ ποὺ ὁδηγοῦνται ἀπὸ τοὺς κηδεμόνες (;) τους καὶ μαζὶ εὐχαριστοῦν τὸν ἔμπροσθεν τοῦ κιβωρίου εὑρισκόμενο ἅγιο Δημήτριο λόγω κάποιας εὐεργεσίας πρὸς αὐτά, τῆς ἀποθεράπευσής των ἀπὸ ἀσθένεια ὑποστηρίζει ἡ C. Hennesy (2008, 89). Ὁ χῶρος

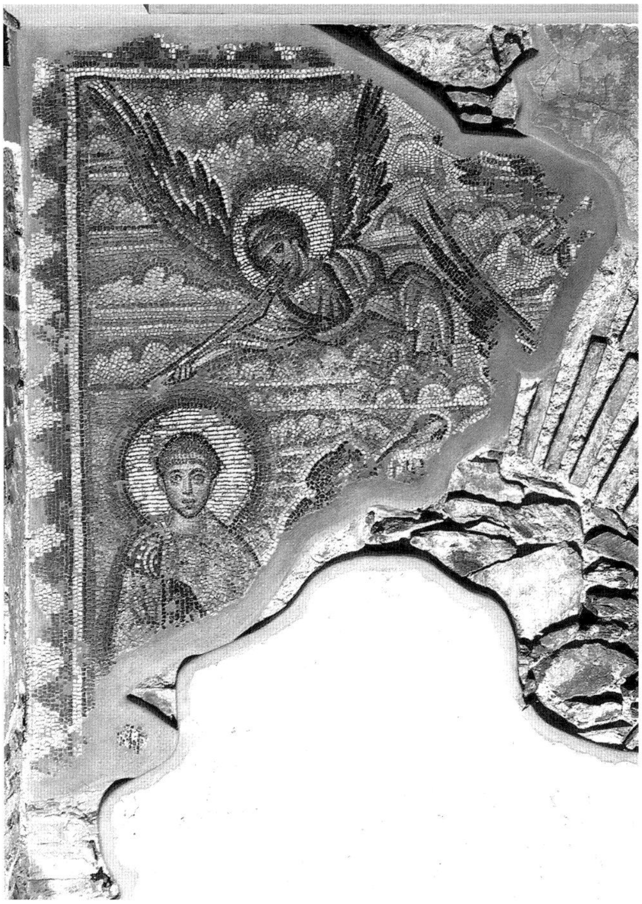

Εἰκ. 37.3. Ψηφιδωτὸ μὲ παράσταση καθιέρωσης ἁγίου Δημητρίου ὡς ἀρχιάτρου (9η Ἐφορεία Βυζαντινῶν Ἀρχαιοτήτων)

ποὺ συμβαίνει τὸ «γεγονὸς» αὐτὸ καὶ ὅπου βρίσκεται στημένο τὸ κιβώριον τοῦ ἁγίου Δημητρίου εἶναι ἕνας κῆπος (βλ. παρακάτω παράγρ. 3).

2. Τὸ δεύτερο ψηφιδωτὸ βρίσκεται ἐπάνω ἀπὸ τὴν εἴσοδο τοῦ νάρθηκα πρὸς τὸ πρῶτο βόρειο κλίτος, σὲ ἰδιαίτερα σημαίνουσα θέση: μπροστὰ στὴν εἴσοδο πρὸς τὰ δύο ΒΔ γωνιακὰ διαμερίσματα, ποὺ χρησίμευαν, ὅπως πιστεύω, ὡς θάλαμος τῶν ἀσθενῶν καὶ ὅπου ἀπὸ τὰ τέλη τοῦ 7ου αἰώνα βρίσκεται ὁ τάφος τοῦ ἁγίου Δημητρίου (Bakirtzis 2002, 188, εἰκ. 10). Σώζεται μόνον τὸ ἀριστερὸ τμῆμα του, ἤτοι τὸ 1/3 τῆς ψηφιδωτῆς παράστασης (Εἰκ. 37.3). Ἀπεικονίζεται κάτω ἀριστερὰ ὁ ἅγιος Δημήτριος – ὄχι σὲ στάση δέησης ἀλλὰ πιθανὸν σὲ στάση προσοχῆς – καὶ ἄνω ἄγγελος ποὺ κρατᾶ «σάλπιγγα» καὶ προβάλλει μέσα ἀπὸ πολύχρωμα σύννεφα. Δεξιά σώζονται φτερὰ δευτέρου ἀγγέλου δεομένου (διακρίνεται τὸ δεξί του χέρι), καὶ κάτω ἀπὸ αὐτὸν φτερὰ τρίτου ἀγγέλου. Ἀνάμεσα στὸν τρίτο ἄγγελο καὶ τὸν ἅγιο Δημήτριο ἀδιάγνωστο θέμα (βράχος;). Μετὰ τὶς πρόσφατες ἐργασίες καθαρισμοῦ τοῦ ψηφιδωτοῦ (Bakirtzis, Mastora and Pitsalidis 2005, 501–11) φαίνεται καθαρὰ ὅτι τὸ ἄκρο τῆς «σάλπιγγας», τὸ ἐπιστόμιό της, δὲν προσαρμόζεται οὔτε

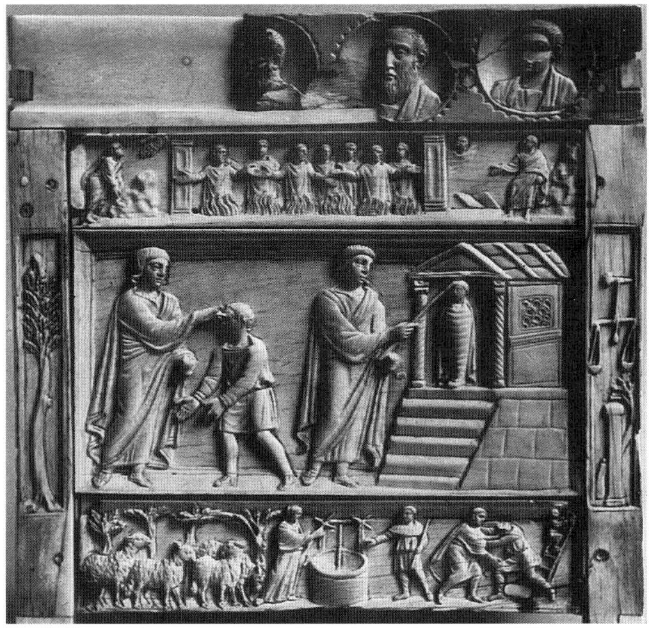

Εἰκ. 37.4. Κιβωτίδιο ἀπὸ ἐλεφαντοστὸ (περ. 360–370) μὲ παράσταση Ἀνάστασης τοῦ Λαζάρου (Fr. Abbate (ed), *Christian Art of the 4th to the 12th Centuries*, London 1972, 33)

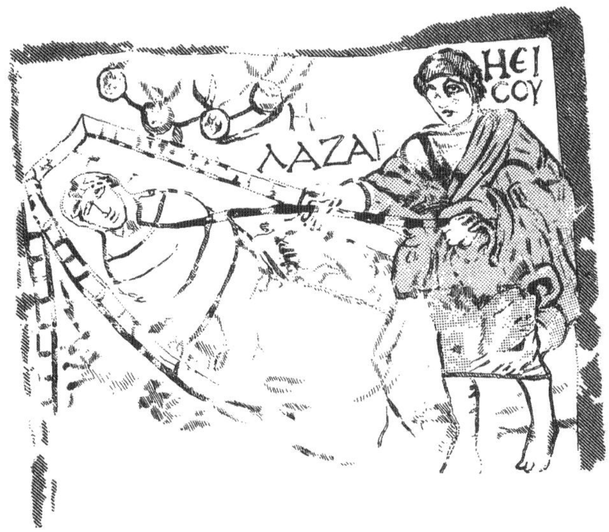

Εἰκ. 37.5. Τοιχογραφία ἀπὸ τάφο μὲ παράσταση Ἀνάστασης τοῦ Λαζάρου (Π. Μαρκῆ, *Ἡ νεκρόπολη τῆς Θεσσαλονίκης στοὺς ὑστερορωμαϊκοὺς καὶ παλαιοχριστιανικοὺς χρόνους,* σχέδιο 69)

κατευθύνεται πρὸς τὰ χείλη τοῦ ἀγγέλου ἀλλὰ στηρίζεται στὸν ὦμο του καὶ κρύβεται πίσω ἀπὸ τὸ κεφάλι του. Συνεπῶς ὁ ἄγγελος δὲν σαλπίζει ἀλλὰ φέρει μὲ τὸ δεξί του χέρι κάτι ἐπίμηκες, ἐλαφρῶς καμπύλο, πρὸς τὸν ἅγιο Δημήτριο, πρὸς τὸν ὁποῖο καὶ προσβλέπει. Τὸ πρὸς τὸν ἅγιο ἄκρο τοῦ ἀντικειμένου αὐτοῦ εἶναι πλατύτερο.[4] Στηριζόμενος στὴν

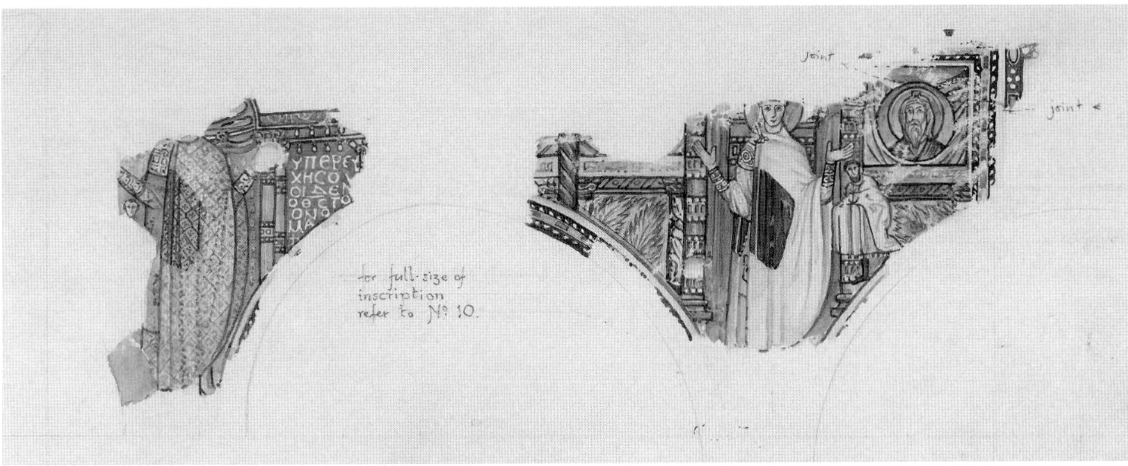
joint
joint
for full-size of
inscription
refer to Nº 10.

Εἰκ. 37.6. Ψηφιδωτὰ βόρειας μικρῆς κιονοστοιχίας: α΄ διάχωρο (ὑδατογραφία W. S. George, *Ὁ ναὸς τοῦ Ἁγίου Δημητρίου. Ὑδατογραφίες καὶ σχέδια τοῦ W. S. George*, Κατάλογος ἔκθεσης τοῦ Δήμου Θεσσαλονίκης)

ἀπόχρωση τῶν ψηφίδων ποὺ χρησιμοποιήθηκαν γιὰ τὴν ἀπόδοση τοῦ ἀντικειμένου αὐτοῦ συμπεραίνω ὅτι εἶναι ξύλινο κυκλικῆς διατομῆς μὲ ἐπένδυση φύλλου χρυσοῦ. Συνεπῶς δὲν πρόκειται γιὰ σάλπιγγα, ὅπως νομίζαμε, οὔτε στεφάνι, ὅπως ὑποστήριξε ὁ Β. Ψευτογκᾶς (2001, 55–6), ἀλλὰ ράβδος, ἡ ὁποία δὲν κρατιέται ἁπλῶς ἀλλὰ προσφέρεται ἀπὸ τὸν ἄγγελο στὸν ἅγιο Δημήτριο ἐπειδὴ τὸ πιὸ χοντρὸ ἄκρο της, ἡ λαβή της, βρίσκεται πρὸς τὴν πλευρὰ τοῦ ἁγίου (Μπακιρτζῆς 2012, 146). Παρομοίου σχήματος εἶναι οἱ ράβδοι ποὺ κρατοῦν οἱ ἰατροί, ὅπως εἰκονίζονται σὲ παραστάσεις τῆς Ἀνάστασης τοῦ Λαζάρου νὰ κρατῶνται ἀπὸ τὸν Χριστὸ-ἰατρό, π.χ. στὸ ἐλεφαντοστέινο κιβωτίδιο (περ. 360–370) στο Civico Museo Dell'Età Cristiana στη Brescia (Εἰκ. 37.4) ἢ καὶ σὲ τοιχογραφία παλαιοχριστιανικοῦ τάφου στὴ Θεσσαλονίκη (Εἰκ. 37.5). Τὴν ἰατρικὴ ράβδο λοιπὸν προσφέρει ὁ ἄγγελος στὸν ἅγιο Δημήτριο ἀπονέμοντάς του ἐκ Θεοῦ τὸ χάρισμα τοῦ θεραπεύειν. Τὸ θεῖο αὐτὸ χάρισμα ρητῶς ὁμολογεῖται ἀπὸ τὸν ἅγιο Δημήτριο στὸν ἀσθενὴ ἔπαρχο Μαριανό: *ἕτοιμος ἡ τοῦ Χριστοῦ δι᾽ἐμοῦ σοι βοήθεια*, ὅπως διασώζουν τὰ *Θαύματα* (Lemerle 1979, 66.1–2).[5] Στὸ κατεστραμμένο τμῆμα τοῦ ψηφιδωτοῦ ὑποθέτω ὅτι θὰ συμπληρωνόταν ἡ σκηνὴ τῆς καθιέρωσης τοῦ ἁγίου Δημητρίου ὡς ἀρχιάτρου μὲ κάποια ἀπεικόνιση σπουδαίας θαυματουργικῆς ἴασης, *χορεύων χαρὰν μετ᾽ ἀγγέλων* κατὰ τὴν ποιητικὴ ἔκφραση τοῦ Ὑμνογράφου Ἰωσὴφ (843 ἢ λίγο ἀργότερα) (Ἀγγελᾶτος 1985, 1396.369). Γιὰ τὴ σημασία τῆς παράστασης αὐτῆς στὸ κοινωνικὸ περιβάλλον τῆς Θεσσαλονίκης σημειώνω τὴν ἰδιαίτερα σημαντικὴ θέση ποὺ κατεῖχαν οἱ ἀρχίατροι ἀνάμεσα στοὺς λειτουργοὺς τῆς Θεσσαλονίκης καὶ ἄλλων πόλεων τῆς Μακεδονίας (Κανατσούλης 1964, 126).

3. Τὸ τρίτο ψηφιδωτὸ (βλ. σημ. 1) εἶναι μία σύνθεση τεσσάρων συνεχομένων διαχώρων στὸ νότιο μέτωπο τῆς πρώτης βόρειας κιονοστοιχίας (Cormack 1969, 17–52. Μπακιρτζῆς 2012, 148–57). Ἀναπτύσσεται δηλαδὴ κατὰ μῆκος τοῦ πρώτου βόρειου κλίτους μέσω τοῦ ὁποίου συνδεόταν ἡ αἴθουσα τῶν ἀσθενῶν μὲ τὸ ἱερὸ βῆμα καὶ τὸ βόρειο πτερύγιο τοῦ ἐγκαρσίου κλίτους τῆς βασιλικῆς. Στὰ δύο, α΄ καὶ δ΄, ἀκραῖα διάχωρα (Εἰκ. 37.6 καὶ 9), ποὺ ἔχουν ἀνεξάρτητα πλαίσια, εἰκονίζονται δεόμενοι ὁ ἅγιος Νέστωρ καὶ ὁ ἅγιος Λοῦπος στὸ α΄ διάχωρο, καὶ ὁ ἅγιος Δημήτριος στὸ δ΄ διάχωρο, ἔμπροσθεν πολυτελῶν οἰκοδομημάτων ποὺ μιμοῦνται αὐτὰ τῶν ψηφιδωτῶν τῆς Ροτόντας. Στοὺς ἁγίους προσέρχονται κατὰ τὸ πρότυπο τοῦ πρώτου ψηφιδωτοῦ πολυτελῶς ἐνδεδυμένοι ἄνδρες εὐχαριστοῦντες, καὶ ἕνα παιδὶ (;) στὸ δ΄ διάχωρο. Στὶς σκηνὲς παρίστανται ἅγιοι εἰκονιζόμενοι μέσα σὲ κυκλικὰ καὶ τετράπλευρα ἀνοίγματα στὸ ἄνω τμῆμα τῆς παράστασης. Στὸ φωτοστέφανο ἑνὸς ἀπὸ τοὺς ἁγίους αὐτούς, στὸ δ΄ διάχωρο, ὑπάρχει ἡ ἐπιγραφὴ '*Ὁ ἅγι[ος Ἀλέξα]νδρος*'. Οἱ ἀπεικονίσεις τῶν δωρητῶν συνοδεύονται ἀπὸ τὴν ἐπιγραφὴ '*Ὑπὲρ εὐχῆς οὗ οἶδεν ὁ Θεὸς τὸ ὄνομα*', ποὺ αἰωρεῖται.[6]

Στὸ β΄ διάχωρο ἀπεικονίζεται στὸ μέσον ἔνθρονη ἡ Παναγία μὲ τὸν Χριστὸ καὶ δύο ἀγγέλους (Εἰκ. 37.7). Ἀριστερὰ ἕνας ἄνδρας προσέρχεται ὁδηγούμενος ἀπὸ τὸν ἅγιο Δημήτριο καὶ δεξιὰ ἵσταται ὁ ἅγιος Θεόδωρος δεόμενος. Τὴ σκηνὴ παρακολουθοῦν μέσα ἀπὸ κυκλικὰ καὶ τετράπλευρα ἀνοίγματα δύο ἄνδρες ἅγιοι καὶ τρεῖς γυναῖκες ἁγίες, ἀπὸ τὶς ὁποῖες δύο συνοδεύονται ἀπὸ τὰ ὀνόματά τους, ἡ ἁγία Ματρώνα καὶ ἡ ἁγία Πελαγία. Στὸ δεξὶ ἄκρο τῆς παράστασης γυναικεία μορφὴ σὲ κατάσταση ἐγκυμοσύνης προσέρχεται στὴ σκηνή (Μπακιρτζῆς 2012, 151).

Στὸ γ΄ διάχωρο (Εἰκ. 37.7–9) ἀπεικονίζεται σὲ τέσσερα ἐπεισόδια ἡ ἱστορία τῆς παιδίσκης Μαρίας ἀπὸ τὴν βρεφικὴ ἕως τὴν παιδικὴ ἡλικία, ἡ ὁποία συνοδευόμενη ἀπὸ τὴ μητέρα της καὶ ἄλλες γυναικεῖες ὡς ἐπὶ τὸ πλεῖστον μορφὲς προσέρχεται στὴν Παναγία καὶ στὸν ἅγιο Δημήτριο.[7] Ὁ Χριστὸς μάλιστα στὸ 1ο ἐπεισόδιο μὲ τὴν παρουσία τῆς ἁγίας Ματρώνας ἐκδηλώνεται ὑπὲρ τῆς παιδίσκης μετὰ ἀπὸ μεσολάβηση τοῦ καθήμενου ἁγίου Δημητρίου ἔξω τοῦ

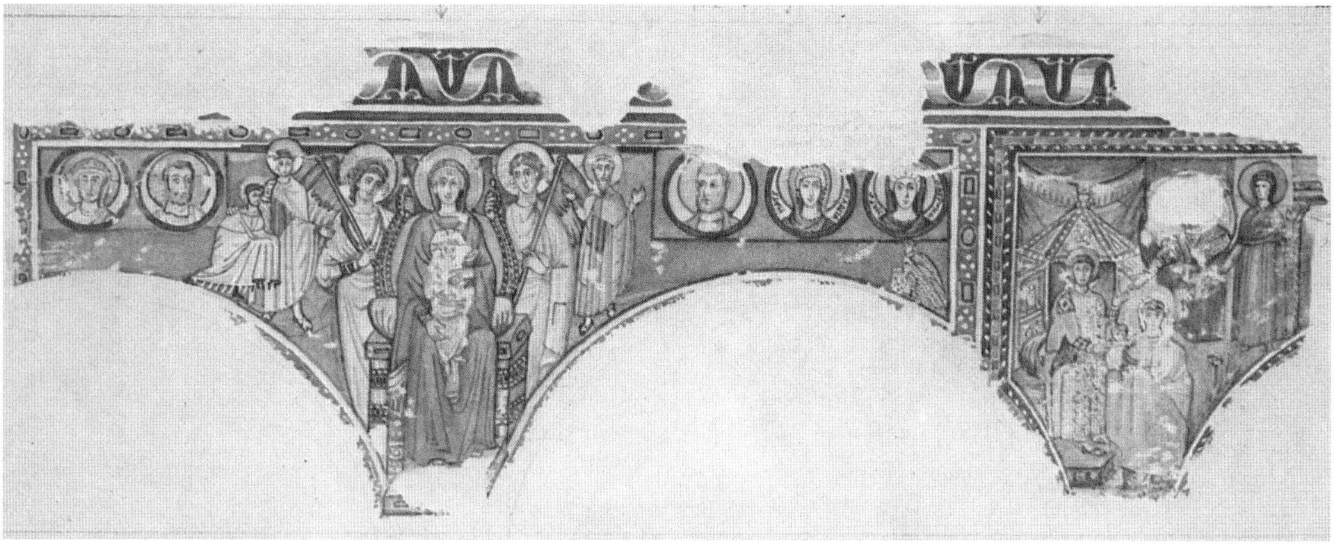

Εἰκ. 37.7. Ψηφιδωτὰ βόρειας μικρῆς κιονοστοιχίας: β´ διάχωρο, καὶ 1ο ἐπεισόδιο γ´ διαχώρου (ὑδατογραφία W. S. George, *Ὁ ναὸς τοῦ Ἁγίου Δημητρίου. Ὑδατογραφίες καὶ σχέδια τοῦ W. S. George*, Κατάλογος ἔκθεσης τοῦ Δήμου Θεσσαλονίκης)

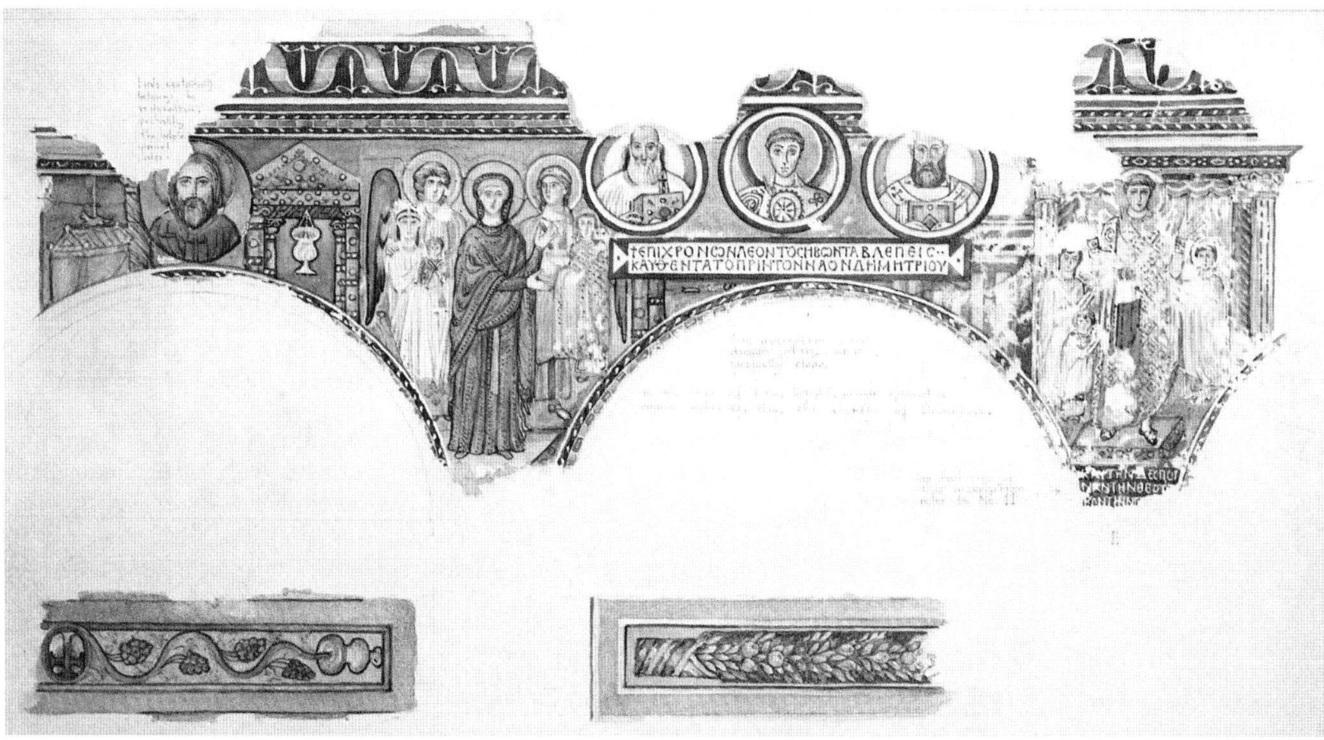

Εἰκ. 37.8. Ψηφιδωτὰ βόρειας μικρῆς κιονοστοιχίας: 2ο καὶ 3ο ἐπεισόδιο γ´ διαχώρου, καὶ μεταγενέστερη προσθήκη (ὑδατογραφία W. S. George, *Ὁ ναὸς τοῦ Ἁγίου Δημητρίου. Ὑδατογραφίες καὶ σχέδια τοῦ W. S. George*, Κατάλογος ἔκθεσης τοῦ Δήμου Θεσσαλονίκης)

κιβωρίου του. Ὁ σταυρὸς στὸ μέτωπο τῆς Μαρίας, ἡ συνεχὴς σχέση της εἰκονογραφικὰ μὲ τὸν ἅγιο Δημήτριο καὶ τὴν Παναγία, οἱ προσφορὲς καὶ οἱ εὐχαριστίες δηλώνουν ὅτι ἡ παιδίσκη Μαρία εἶχε δεχθῆ τὴ θεραπευτικὴ παρέμβαση τοῦ ἁγίου Δημητρίου. Ἡ ἐπιγραφή: *'Καὶ σὺ δέσποτα ἡμῶν, ἅγιε Δημήτρη, βοήθη ἡμῖν τοῖς δούλοις σου καὶ τῇ δούλῃ σου Μαρίᾳ ἣν ἔδωκες ἡμῖν'* βεβαιώνει ὅτι ἡ παρέμβαση τοῦ ἁγίου Δημητρίου εἶχε ἀρχίσει ἤδη ἀπὸ τὴ διαδικασία τῆς γεννήσεως τῆς παιδίσκης. Τρεῖς ἄνδρες ἅγιοι καὶ μία γυναίκα ἁγία μέσα ἀπὸ ὀμφάλια παρακολουθοῦν τὰ ἐπεισόδια. Ἡ σύμπραξη αὐτὴ ἐμφανίζεται καὶ στὴ λογοτεχνία, στὸν ὕμνο τοῦ Θεσσαλονικέως Στεφάνου Στουδίτη πρὸς τὸν ἅγιο Δημήτριο

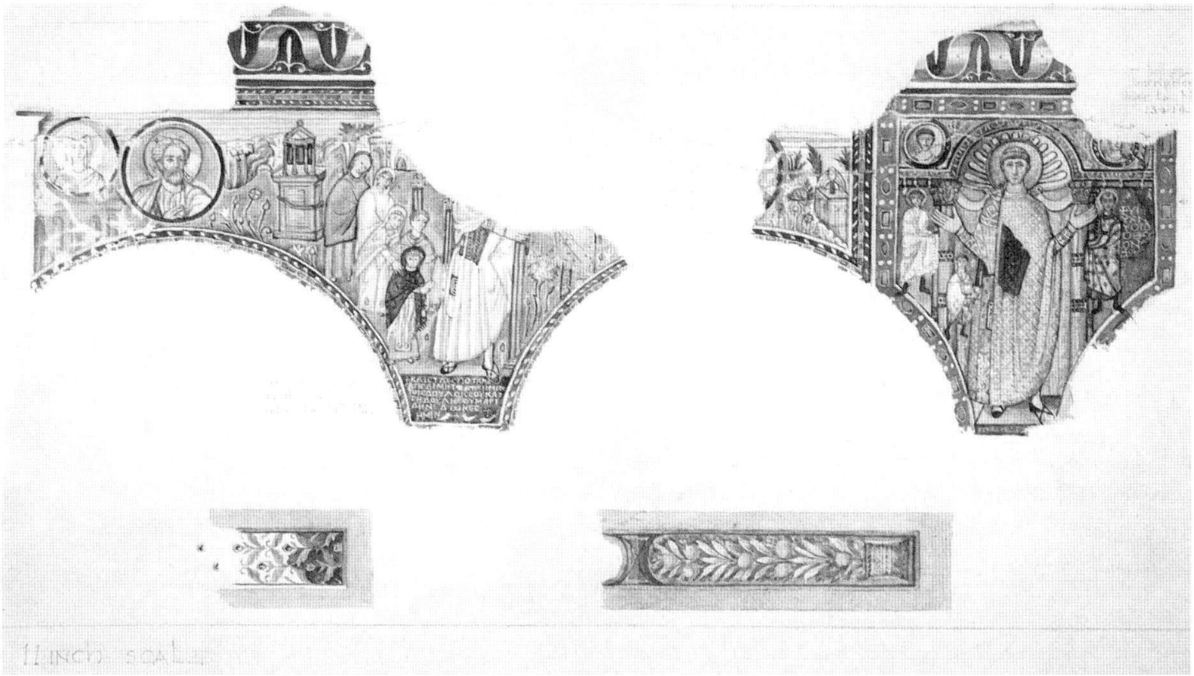

Εἰκ. 37.9. Ψηφιδωτὰ βόρειας μικρῆς κιονοστοιχίας: 4ο ἐπεισόδιο γ΄ διαχώρου, καὶ δ΄ διάχωρο (ὑδατογραφία W. S. George, *Ὁ ναὸς τοῦ Ἁγίου Δημητρίου. Ὑδατογραφίες καὶ σχέδια τοῦ W. S. George,* Κατάλογος ἔκθεσης τοῦ Δήμου Θεσσαλονίκης)

'*ῥῦσαι ἡμᾶς τοῦ σεισμοῦ τῆς ἀνάγκης, φιλάνθρωπε, πρεσβείαις τῆς Θεοτόκου, τῶν ἁγίων καὶ πάντων μαρτύρων σου*' (Δετοράκης 2001, 182). Ὁ χῶρος ποὺ συμβαίνουν τὰ 'γεγονότα' αὐτά, ὅπου τὸ ὅραμα συγχέεται μὲ τὴν πραγματικότητα, εἶναι ἕνας κῆπος. Ὁ κῆπος δὲν εἶναι μόνον ὁ Παράδεισος, ὅπως ἔχει ὑποστηριχθῆ, ἀλλὰ καὶ ὁ ναὸς τοῦ Ἁγίου Δημητρίου ἐπειδὴ ἐντὸς τοῦ κήπου ὑπάρχουν κατασκευὲς σχετιζόμενες μὲ τὴ λατρεία τοῦ ἁγίου Δημητρίου, π.χ. τὸ κιβώριον. Τὸν συσχετισμὸ αὐτὸν περιγράφει ὁ Ὑμνογράφος Ἰωσήφ: '*ἰδοὺ ὁ οἶκος σου, μάκαρ, ὡς παράδεισος θεῖος ὁρᾶται*' ἢ '*ὁ τερπνότατός σου οἶκος μέσον σε ἔχων θάλλει ὡς παράδεισος*' (Ἀγγελᾶτος 1985, 1387.139–41 καὶ 1403.550–3).

Τὰ παλαιότερα τοῦ 7ου αἰώνα ψηφιδωτὰ ἔχουν ὁρισμένα κοινὰ χαρακτηριστικά:

1. Ὅλα τὰ ψηφιδωτὰ σχετίζονται ἄμεσα ἢ ἔμμεσα μὲ τὴν ἴαση ἀσθενῶν καὶ ἔχουν πρωταγωνιστὴ τὸν ἅγιο Δημήτριο. Οἱ προσευχόμενοι δωρητὲς τῶν ψηφιδωτῶν εἶναι βέβαια συγκεκριμένα πρόσωπα, τὰ εἰκονιζόμενα ὅμως φυσιογνωμικὰ χαρακτηριστικά τους εἶναι γενικά.

2. Ἡ παρουσία τῶν παιδιῶν στὴν εἰκονογραφία τῶν ψηφιδωτῶν αὐτῶν εἶναι ἔντονη. Τὰ παιδιὰ συνοδευόμενα ἀπὸ τοὺς οἰκείους των ἀπευθύνουν, καὶ οἱ δύο μαζί, εὐχαριστίες καὶ προσφορὲς στὸν ἅγιο Δημήτριο καὶ στὴν Παναγία μὲ τὴν παρουσία καὶ ἄλλων ἁγίων, ὅπως τῶν Θεσσαλονικέων ἁγίων Ἀλεξάνδρου καὶ Ματρώνας, ἐπειδὴ ἐδέχθησαν τὴ θεραπευτικὴ βοήθεια τοῦ ἁγίου Δημητρίου τῇ μεσιτείᾳ τῆς Παναγίας ἢ ἀκόμη ἐπειδὴ τοῦ ὀφείλουν καὶ αὐτὴ τὴ γέννησή τους. Ἡ εἰκονογραφικὴ συμπαράταξη ἁγίου Δημητρίου καὶ Παναγίας καὶ ἡ ἀνεύρεση σχετικοῦ χαράγματος μαρτυροῦν τὴ συλλατρεία Παναγίας καὶ ἁγίου Δημητρίου στὴ βασιλικὴ τοῦ πολιούχου (Σωτηρίου 1952, 233–4), ποὺ εἶναι γνωστὴ ἀπὸ μεταγενέστερες πηγές καὶ γιὰ τὸν ναὸ τῆς Παναγίας Ἀχειροποιήτου στὴ Θεσσαλονίκη (Ξυγγόπουλος 1950, 22–5).

3. Ὁ ἅγιος Δημήτριος ἀπεικονίζεται μὲ ἐπίσημη ἐνδυμασία, ὅπως περιγράφεται στὰ *Θαύματα* ὅτι ἐμφανιζόταν στὰ ὁράματα: '*καὶ κατὰ νύκτα ὡς ἐν ἐκστάσει γινόμενος ἑώρα τὸν ἅγιον χλαμύδα ἠμφιεμένον καὶ εὔροδον καὶ χαρίεν τὸ πρόσωπον ἔχοντα, ὥς τινα ὕπατον παρὰ βασιλέως ἐξουσίαν λαβόντα διανεῖμαι τῷ δήμῳ τὰς χάριτας*' (Lemerle 1979, 80.19–22). Γιὰ τὸ λόγο αὐτὸ οἱ ἄνθρωποι δὲν ἀγγίζουν τὸν ἅγιο οὔτε αὐτὸς αὐτούς.

4. Ἡ ἀπόδοση εὐχαριστιῶν τελεῖται ἐντὸς κήπων, ὅπου ὑπάρχουν μεμονωμένα κτίσματα, π.χ. τὸ κιβώριον, ποὺ σχετίζονται μὲ τὴ λατρεία τοῦ ἁγίου Δημητρίου, εἰς τρόπον ὥστε καθίσταται ἡ ἐμφάνιση τοῦ ἁγίου Δημητρίου «πραγματική». Παρόμοιους συσχετισμοὺς λογοτεχνικοὺς παρουσιάζουν καὶ οἱ διηγήσεις τοῦ Α΄ Βιβλίου τῶν *Θαυμάτων*, ὅπου ὁ ἅγιος λουσμένος στὸ φῶς τοῦ ὁράματος ἔχει ἀνάγκη συνεχοῦς μαρτυρίας αὐτοπτῶν (*Ἁγίου Δημητρίου Θαύματα*, 14).

Ψηφιδωτὸ ποὺ δὲν σώζεται ἀλλὰ θὰ ἀνῆκε στὴν ἴδια ὁμάδα σχετικὸ μὲ τὴν ἴαση τοῦ ἐπάρχου Μαριανοῦ ὑπῆρχε, κατὰ τὴ μαρτυρία τῶν *Θαυμάτων*, στὸ νότιο ἐξωτερικὸ τοῖχο τῆς βασιλικῆς: '*ἱστορείτω τὴν ἐκ μουσείου συντεθειμένην ἐκεῖσε γραφὴν ἔξω τοῦ ναοῦ*' (Lemerle 1979, 67.15–16). Αὐτὸ σημαίνει ὅτι τὸ εἰκονογραφικὸ θέμα τῶν ὑπερευχομένων στὸν ἅγιο Δημήτριο ἰαθέντων ἀσθενῶν δὲν ἦταν περιορισμένο σὲ συγκεκριμένους χώρους τῆς βασιλικῆς ἀλλὰ κυρίαρχο στὴν εἰκονογράφιση τῆς βασιλικῆς μὲ ψηφιδωτά.[8] Πιστεύω ὅτι οἱ στίχοι τοῦ Ὑμνογράφου Ἰωσήφ, ποὺ ἐγκαταβίωσε στὴ Θεσσαλονίκη μία περίπου δεκαετία καὶ φημίζεται ὄχι μόνον γιὰ τὴ γλυκύτητα τοῦ ποιητικοῦ ὕφους ἀλλὰ καὶ γιὰ τὴν εἰκονιστικὴ δύναμη τῶν στίχων του, '*ὡς θαυμαστός σου ὁ οἶκος, πηγάζων θαύματα.. καὶ τὰς λαμπρότητας ἐκπέμπων τῶν θαυμάτων καὶ πάντας καταυγάζων*' (Ἀγγελᾶτος 1985, 1431.1256–61 καὶ 1458.1466), ἀντλοῦν τὴν ἔμπνευσή τους ἀπὸ τὰ ψηφιδωτὰ τῆς βασιλικῆς ἐπειδὴ θὰ μποροῦσαν νὰ συσχετισθοῦν καὶ μὲ τὰ θέματα τῶν ψηφιδωτῶν καὶ μὲ τὸ αἰσθητικὸ φῶς ποὺ ἐκπέμπουν καὶ λόγῳ ἀντανάκλασης τοῦ φυσικοῦ φωτός. Ὡς ἐκ τούτου οἱ ἐκφράσεις, ὅπως '*ὁ σὸς πανάγιος ναὸς ἰατρεῖον ἄμισθον πᾶσιν πρόκειται*' (Ἀγγελᾶτος 1985, 1395.343–5), δὲν εἶναι ὑπερβολικὲς ποιητικῇ ἀδείᾳ, ἀλλὰ πιστεύω ὅτι ἀνταποκρίνονται στὴν πραγματικότητα καὶ ὅτι ἡ κύρια λειτουργία τῆς βασιλικῆς στὴν πρώιμη βυζαντινὴ περίοδο ἦταν αὐτὴ τοῦ ξενώνα (νοσοκομείου).

Β. Τὰ ἑπόμενα τρία ψηφιδωτὰ ἀνήκουν στὴ δεύτερη ὁμάδα, χρονολογοῦνται ἀπὸ τοῦ 7ου αἰώνα καὶ ἑξῆς καὶ βρίσκονται ἐπὶ τοῦ ΒΔ πεσσοῦ τοῦ ἱεροῦ βήματος.

1. Στὸ ψηφιδωτὸ τῆς δυτικῆς πλευρᾶς εἰκονίζεται ἅγιος μὲ δύο παιδιὰ σὲ στάση σεβασμοῦ καὶ εὐχαριστίας μὲ περισσότερο ἐμφανῆ φυσιογνωμικὰ χαρακτηριστικά (Εἰκ. 37.10). Γι' αὐτὸ καὶ διατυπώθηκαν ὑποθέσεις γιὰ τὴν ταύτισή τους μὲ συγκεκριμένα πρόσωπα, οἱ ὁποῖες δὲν ἔχουν γίνει δεκτές.[9] Τὸ περιεχόμενο τῆς παράστασης μᾶς διαφεύγει ἐπειδὴ δὲν ἔχει σωθῆ ἡ ἐπιγραφὴ (*damnatio memoriae*;) στὸ κάτω τμῆμα τοῦ ψηφιδωτοῦ, ὅπου ὑπάρχει ὁ σχετικὸς χῶρος. Ἡ στάση τοῦ ἁγίου νὰ ἀγγίζει μὲ τὸ ἀριστερὸ χέρι τὸν ὦμο τοῦ μεγαλυτέρου παιδιοῦ καὶ νὰ δέεται μὲ τὸ δεξὶ δὲν ἀφήνει ἀμφιβολία ὅτι τὰ δύο παιδιὰ βρίσκονται ὑπὸ τὴν προστασία του. Ἡ C. Hennesy (2008, 90) μάλιστα διατύπωσε τὴν ἄποψη ὅτι πρόκειται γιὰ δύο παιδιὰ ποὺ θεραπεύθηκαν ἀπὸ ἀσθένεια. Μετὰ τὴν ἀνεύρεση γραπτῆς ἐπιγραφῆς ἄνω τοῦ ψηφιδωτοῦ *Ὁ ἅγιος Γεώργις*, εἴμαστε βέβαιοι ὅτι ὁ εἰκονιζόμενος φουντομάλλης καὶ κοκκινομάλλης ἅγιος δὲν εἶναι ὁ ἅγιος Δημήτριος, οὔτε ὁ ἅγιος Βάκχος, ὅπως ὑποστηρίχθηκε, ἀλλὰ ὁ ἅγιος Γεώργιος (Μπακιρτζῆς 2006, 127–34· 2012, 158). Συνεπῶς τὰ παιδιὰ δὲν ἀποτελοῦν εἰκονογραφικὴ ἀποκλειστικότητα τοῦ ἁγίου Δημητρίου, ὅπως νομίζαμε, οὔτε βεβαίως καὶ τοῦ ἁγίου Γεωργίου ἐξ ὅσων γνωρίζουμε ἀπὸ τὴν εἰκονογραφία του. Ἡ σκηνὴ λαμβάνει χώρα μπροστὰ στὰ τείχη τῆς πόλεως.

2. Στὴ νότια πλευρὰ τοῦ πεσσοῦ εἰκονίζονται μπροστὰ στὰ τείχη τῆς πόλεως δύο μορφές εἰκονογραφικὰ ἀνόμοιες (Εἰκ. 37.11). Δεξιὰ ὁ ἅγιος, ποὺ ἔχει τὰ φυσιογνωμικὰ χαρακτηριστικὰ τοῦ ἁγίου Θεοδώρου Τήρωνα-Στρατηλάτη, εἰκονίζεται κατενώπιον καὶ δεόμενος κατὰ τὸ πρότυπο τῶν παλαιῶν ἀπεικονίσεων τῶν ἁγίων. Ἀριστερὰ ἡ Παναγία εἶναι στραμμένη σὲ 3/4 καὶ τὸ σῶμα της ἀποδίδεται μὲ ἐλαφρὰ πλαστικότητα. Γι' αὐτὸ καὶ χρονολογήθηκε μετὰ τὴν Εἰκονομαχία, ὄχι πέραν τοῦ 9ου αἰώνα (Σωτηρίου 1952, 195–6).[10] Ἡ Παναγία κρατᾶ εἰλητάριο μὲ τὴν δέηση: '*Δέησις. Κύριε ὁ Θεὸς εἰσάκουσον τῆς φωνῆς, τῆς δεήσεώς μου ὅτι ὑπὲρ τοῦ κόσμου δέομαι*'. Ὁ Α. Ξυγγόπουλος στηριζόμενος στὴν ἀνώνυμη κτητορικὴ ἐπιγραφὴ τοῦ ψηφιδωτοῦ '*Πᾶσιν ἀνθρώποις ἀπελπισθεὶς παρὰ δὲ τῆς σῆς δυνάμεως ζωοποιηθεὶς εὐχαριστῶν ἀνεθέμην*' διατύπωσε τὴν ἄποψη ὅτι τὸ ψηφιδωτὸ εἶναι ἀνάθημα ἀσθενοῦς ποὺ θεραπεύθηκε ἀπὸ θαῦμα (Ξυγγόπουλος 1946, 40). Δὲν ὑπάρχει λόγος νὰ μὴν γίνει δεκτὴ ἡ ἄποψη αὐτὴ καὶ στὸ '*ἀνθρώποις*' νὰ ἐννοηθοῦν οἱ ἰατροί (Μπακιρτζῆς 2012, 162).

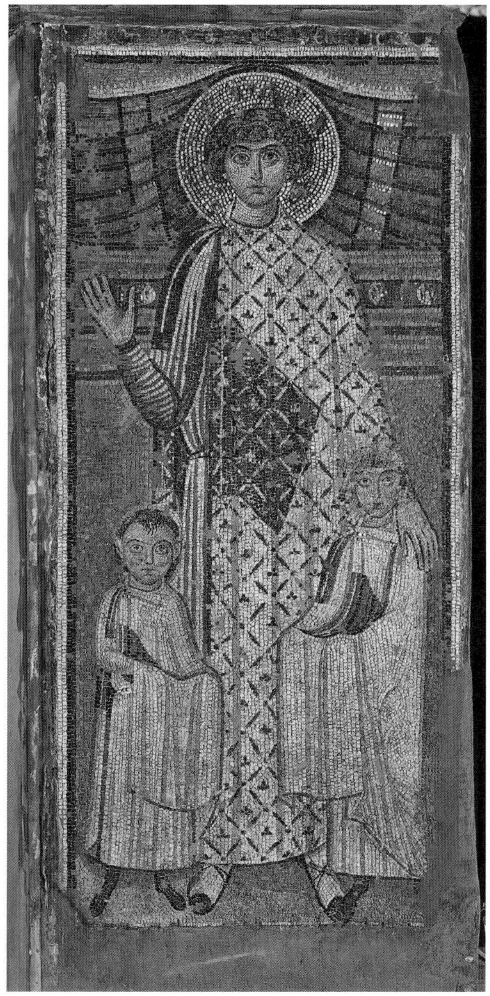

Εἰκ. 37.10. Ψηφιδωτὸ μὲ παράσταση ἁγίου Γεωργίου μὲ παιδιά (9η Ἐφορεία Βυζαντινῶν Ἀρχαιοτήτων)

Τὸ μαρμάρινο τόξο ἀπὸ τὸ κιβώριο τῆς ἁγίας τραπέζης

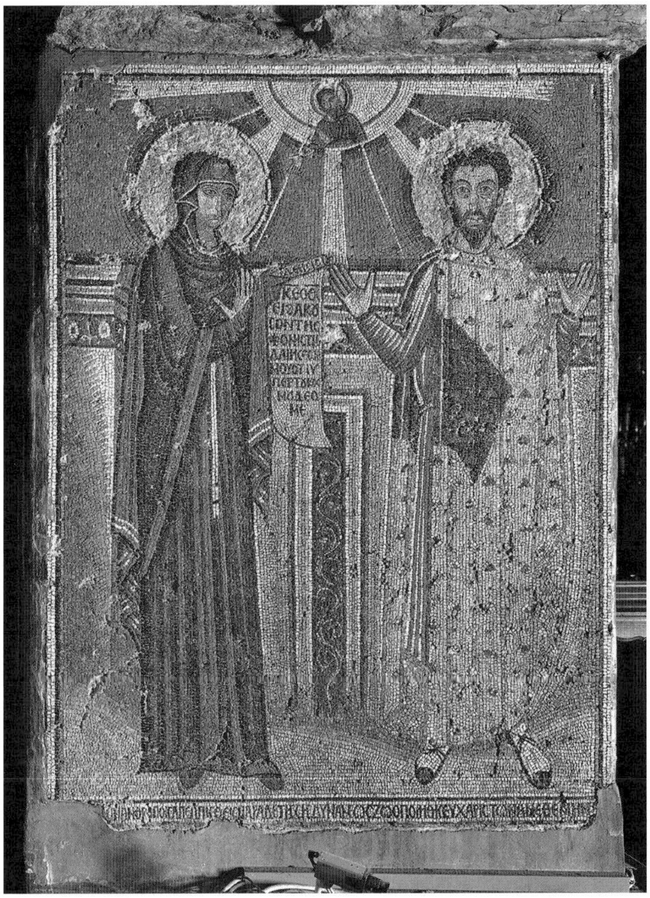

Εἰκ. 37.11. Ψηφιδωτὸ μὲ παράσταση δέησης Παναγίας καὶ ἁγίου Θεοδώρου (9η Ἐφορεία Βυζαντινῶν Ἀρχαιοτήτων)

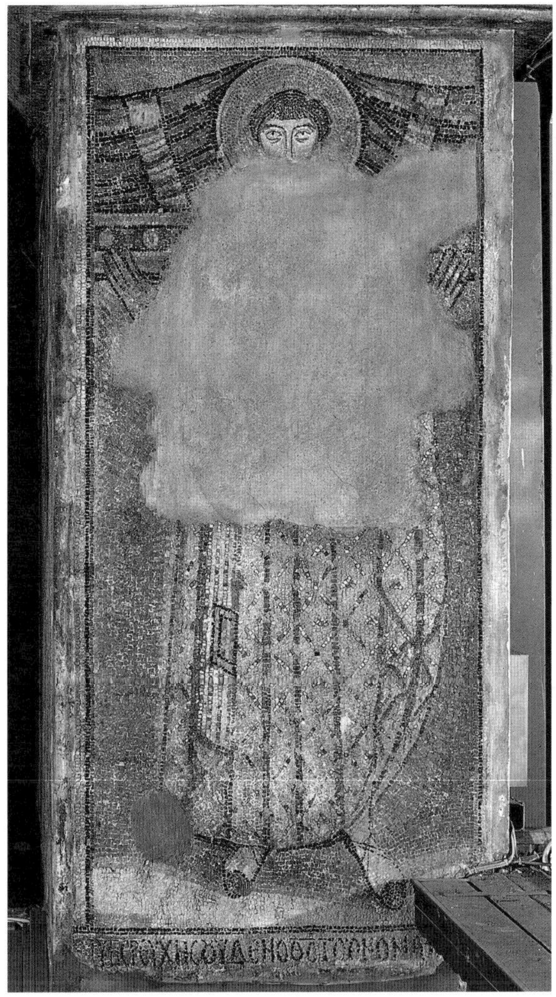

Εἰκ. 37.12. Ψηφιδωτὸ μὲ παράσταση ἁγίου Νέστορα δεομένου (9η Ἐφορεία Βυζαντινῶν Ἀρχαιοτήτων)

τῆς βασιλικῆς μὲ τὴν κτητορικὴ ἐπιγραφὴ τοῦ *παγκλεοῦς Θεοδώρου* (Σωτηρίου 1952, πίν. 57), τὸν ὁποῖο ὁ Γ. Βελένης (2005, 221–6) συσχέτισε μὲ τὸν ἀρχιεπίσκοπο Θεσσαλονίκης Θεόδωρο (866–879), θὰ μποροῦσε νὰ συσχετισθῆ μὲ τὸ ἐν λόγῳ ψηφιδωτὸ ἐπειδὴ αὐτὸ βρίσκεται ἀκριβῶς ἀπέναντι τῆς ἁγίας τραπέζης, καὶ νὰ θεωρηθοῦν καὶ τὰ δύο, κιβώριο καὶ ψηφιδωτό, ἀναθήματα τοῦ ἰδίου Θεοδώρου, ἐπειδὴ ἰάθηκε μὲ τὴ βοήθεια τῆς Παναγίας μετὰ ἀπὸ ἀποτυχημένες προσπάθειες τῶν ἰατρῶν.

3. Στὴν ἀνατολικὴ πλευρὰ τοῦ ἰδίου πεσσοῦ εἰκονίζεται μπροστὰ στὰ τείχη τῆς πόλεως ἅγιος σὲ στάση δέησης (Εἰκ. 37.12). Τὸ κεντρικὸ τμῆμα τοῦ ψηφιδωτοῦ μαζὶ μὲ μέρος τοῦ προσώπου τοῦ ἁγίου εἶναι κατεστραμμένα. Καὶ γιὰ τὴ μορφὴ αὐτὴ ἔχει διατυπωθῆ ἡ ἄποψη ὅτι πρόκειται ἐπίσης γιὰ τὸν ἅγιο Δημήτριο (Εἰκ. 37.13) (Σωτηρίου 1952, 197–8). Τὰ φυσιογνωμικὰ ὡστόσο χαρακτηριστικὰ ὁδηγοῦν σὲ ἄλλες σκέψεις ταύτισης, ποὺ γίνονται ἀκόμη πιθανότερες ἐφ᾽ὅσον στὶς ἄλλες δύο πλευρὲς τοῦ ἰδίου πεσσοῦ εἰκονίζονται ὁ ἅγιος Γεώργιος καὶ ὁ ἅγιος Θεόδωρος. Συνεπῶς ὁ ἅγιος Νέστωρ εἶναι πολὺ πιθανὸς ὑποψήφιος γιὰ τὴν ταύτιση τοῦ εἰκονιζομένου στὸ ψηφιδωτὸ ἁγίου, ἀποκλειομένου πλέον τοῦ ἁγίου Δημητρίου (Μπακιρτζῆς 2006, 133; 2012, 164). Ἡ παρουσία στρατιωτικῶν ἁγίων στὴ βασιλικὴ τοῦ Ἁγίου Δημητρίου ἑρμηνεύεται ἀπὸ τὸν συγγραφέα τῶν *Θαυμάτων τοῦ Ἁγίου Δημητρίου*, ὁ ὁποῖος διαβεβαίωνε ὅτι ὁ πολιοῦχος τῆς Θεσσαλονίκης μὲ τὴ βοήθεια καὶ ἄλλων ἁγίων, στρατιωτικῶν ἐννοεῖ, ἔσωζε τὴν πόλη: '*μετὰ καὶ ἑτέρων, ὥς φασιν, ἁγίων, τῆς πόλεως τὴν σωτηρίαν ἀπεργαζόμενος*' (Lemerle 1979, 195.6–7). Τὸ ψηφιδωτὸ ὑπογραμμίζεται ἀπὸ τὴν ἐπιγραφή: '*Ὑπὲρ εὐχῆς οὗ (ο)ἶδεν ὁ Θ(εὸ)ς τὸ ὄνομα*', ὅπως καὶ τὰ ψηφιδωτὰ τῆς βόρειας μικρῆς κιονοστοιχίας.

Τὰ τρία ψηφιδωτὰ ἔχουν ὁρισμένα κοινὰ χαρακτηριστικὰ ποὺ ἄλλα ὁμοιάζουν καὶ ἄλλα διαφέρουν ἀπὸ τὰ χαρακτηριστικὰ τῶν παλαιοτέρων τοῦ 7ου αἰώνα ψηφιδωτῶν:

1. Δὲν ἀπεικονίζουν ἐπεισόδια ἀλλὰ ἅγιες μορφὲς ἐν στάσει. Πρωταγωνιστὴς δὲν εἶναι ὁ ἅγιος Δημήτριος ἀλλὰ σύντροφοί του στρατιωτικοὶ ἅγιοι καὶ ἡ Παναγία.

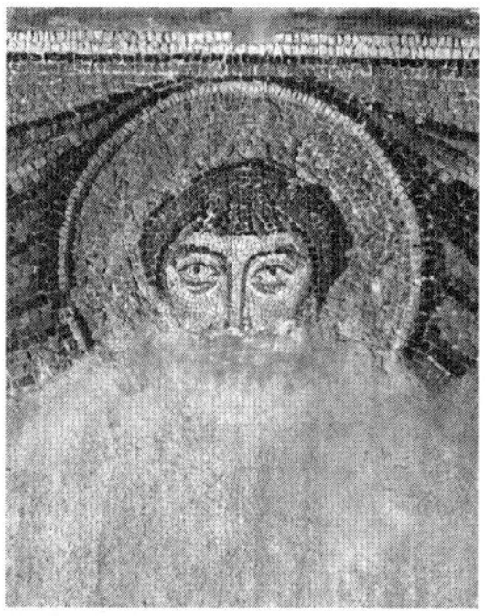

Εἰκ. 37.13. Λεπτομέρεια. Πρόσωπο ἁγίου Νέστορα (9η Ἐφορεία Βυζαντινῶν Ἀρχαιοτήτων)

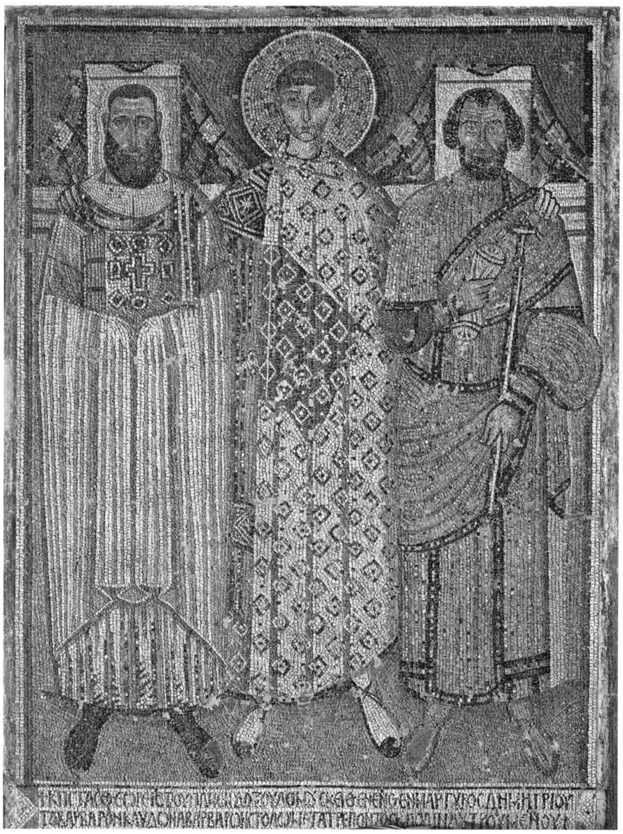

Εἰκ. 37.14. Ψηφιδωτὸ μὲ παράσταση ἁγίου Δημητρίου μὲ τοὺς *κτίστας* (ἀρχιεπίσκοπο καὶ ἔπαρχο) (9η Ἐφορεία Βυζαντινῶν Ἀρχαιοτήτων)

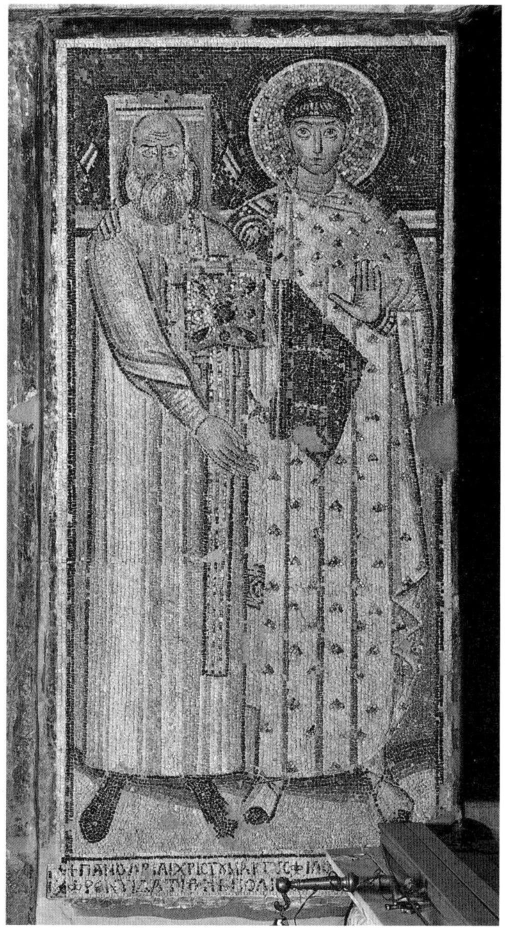

Εἰκ. 37.15. Ψηφιδωτὸ μὲ παράσταση ἁγίου Δημητρίου μὲ διάκονο (9η Ἐφορεία Βυζαντινῶν Ἀρχαιοτήτων)

2. Κατὰ τὶς διατυπωθεῖσες ἀπόψεις τὰ ψηφιδωτὰ αὐτὰ σχετίζονται ἐπίσης μὲ ἰάσεις ἀσθενῶν. Ἐὰν κρίνουμε ἀπὸ δύο ἐπιγραφὲς ποὺ σώθηκαν εἶναι ἀναθήματα δωρητῶν, τὰ ὁποῖα συμπλήρωσαν τὸ εἰκονογραφικὸ πρόγραμμα τῆς βασιλικῆς μετὰ τὴν πυρκαγιὰ *c*. 620.

3. Στὸ ἕνα ἀπὸ τὰ τρία ψηφιδωτὰ εἰκονίζονται καὶ πάλι παιδιά σὲ σχέση ὄχι μὲ τὸν ἅγιο Δημήτριο ἀλλὰ μὲ τὸν ἅγιο Γεώργιο. Ὁ ἅγιος Γεώργιος δὲν εἶναι ἀπόμακρος, ὅπως ὁ ἅγιος Δημήτριος στὰ παλαιότερα ψηφιδωτά, ἀλλὰ προστατεύει τὰ παιδιὰ ἀγγίζοντάς τα.

4. Ὁ κῆπος τῶν παλαιοτέρων ψηφιδωτῶν ἔχει ἀντικατασταθῆ μὲ ἀστικὸ χῶρο. Ὅλες οἱ ἐμφανίσεις ἁγίων προσώπων συμβαίνουν μπροστὰ στὰ τείχη τῆς Θεσσαλονίκης.

Ἐὰν τὰ ψηφιδωτὰ τοῦ βορείου πεσσοῦ, τοῦ βορείου κλίτους καὶ τοῦ δυτικοῦ τοίχου σχετίζονται μὲ τὴ σωτηρία ἀνθρώπων, τὰ ψηφιδωτὰ τοῦ νοτίου πεσσοῦ σχετίζονται μὲ τὴ σωτηρία τῆς πόλεως καὶ τῆς βασιλικῆς, καὶ μὲ τοὺς ἐκπροσώπους της (Μπακιρτζῆς 2012, 166–73). Ὁ Θ. Παπαζῶτος μάλιστα διατύπωσε τὴν ἄποψη ὅτι τὸ πρῶτο καὶ τὸ δεύτερο ψηφιδωτὸ ἀποτελοῦν μία ἑνότητα (1983, 365–76): 1) Τοὺς *κτίστας* τῆς βασιλικῆς, τὸν ἀνακαινιστὴ τῆς βασιλικῆς ἀρχιεπίσκοπο Θεσσαλονίκης καὶ βικάριο τοῦ πάπα Ρώμης, καὶ τὸν ἱδρυτὴ τῆς βασιλικῆς ἔπαρχο Λεόντιο, μὲ διακριτοὺς τοὺς ρόλους των: τὸ εὐαγγέλιο ὁ πρῶτος, τὴν ἐξουσία καὶ τὰ χρήματα ὁ δεύτερος (Εἰκ. 37.14 καὶ 37.16). 2) Τὸν ἡλικιωμένο διάκονο πού, ὡς μαρμάρινος κορμὸς κίονος, εἶναι '*εἷς ἐκ τῶν γνησίως ὑπουργούντων τὸν ἅγιον*', ὅπως πρῶτος ὑποστήριξε ὁ O. Tafrali.[11] Ἔχω διατυπώσει

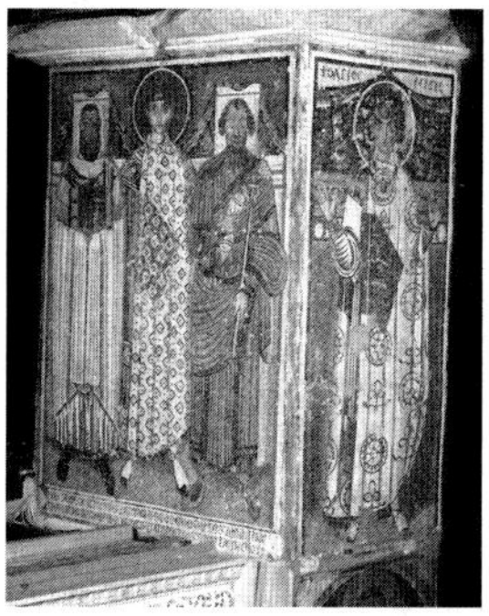

Εἰκ. 37.16. ΝΑ πεσσὸς ἱεροῦ βήματος μὲ τὸ ψηφιδωτὸ τῶν *κτιστῶν* καὶ τοῦ ἁγίου Σεργίου (9^{η} Ἐφορεία Βυζαντινῶν Ἀρχαιοτήτων)

τὴ γνώμη ὅτι ἀντὶ τοῦ εὐαγγελίου κρατᾶ τὸ βιβλίο τῶν Θαυμάτων τοῦ Ἁγίου Δημητρίου (*Ἁγίου Δημητρίου Θαύματα*, 414–5) (Εἰκ. 37.15). Ὁ ἴδιος δέεται ὁ πολιοῦχος νὰ φροντίζει καὶ τοὺς πολίτες καὶ τοὺς ξένους ποὺ στὰ τέλη τοῦ $6^{ου}$ καὶ τὸν $7^{ο}$ αἰώνα συνέρρεαν στὴν πόλη ὡς πρόσφυγες καὶ μετανάστες: '*Πανόλβιε Χριστοῦ μάρτυς φιλόπολις φροντίδα τίθη καὶ πολιτῶν καὶ ξένων*'. 3) Ἡ ἐνεπίγραφη ἀπεικόνιση τοῦ ἁγίου Σεργίου στὴ δυτικὴ πλευρὰ τοῦ ἰδίου πεσσοῦ (Εἰκ. 37.16) πιστεύω πὼς εἶναι δημόσια δήλωση τῆς Ἐκκλησίας Θεσσαλονίκης ὅτι διεκδικεῖ τὴν καταγωγὴ τοῦ στρατιώτη ἁγίου ποὺ μαρτύρησε στὴ Συρία γιὰ νὰ ἐμπλουτίσει καὶ μὲ ἄλλους στρατιωτικοὺς ἁγίους τὴ δημητριανὴ προσωπογραφία τῆς Θεσσαλονίκης (Μπακιρτζῆς 2006, 133).

Στὰ ψηφιδωτὰ τῆς δεύτερης ὁμάδας δὲν τονίζεται τὸ φωτόλουστο γεγονὸς τοῦ ὁράματος ἀλλὰ ἡ γήινη παρουσία των εἰκονιζομένων, ὅπως στὶς διηγήσεις τοῦ Β΄ βιβλίου τῶν *Θαυμάτων* τὰ ἱστορικὰ γεγονότα κατατίθενται ἁπλῶς προκειμένου νὰ ἀνατραποῦν ἀπὸ τὸν ἅγιο (*Ἁγίου Δημητρίου Θαύματα*, 14–5).

Συμπεράσματα:

1. Ἡ εἰκονογραφία τῶν ψηφιδωτῶν τῆς βασιλικῆς τοῦ Ἁγίου Δημητρίου ἔχει σχέση μὲ τὴν κύρια λειτουργία της, αὐτὴ τοῦ ξενώνα. Γιὰ τὸ λόγο αὐτὸ δικαίως ὁ ἅγιος Δημήτριος χαρακτηρίζεται ἀπὸ τὸν Ὑμνογράφο Ἰωσὴφ '*ἰατρὸς πανάριστος ὑπάρχων*', '*ἰατρὲ τῶν νοσούντων πανάριστε*', '*ἰατρὲ τῶν νοσούντων πάσας μου ἰάτρευσον τὰς νόσους δέομαι*' (Ἀγγελᾶτος 1985, 1402.517–8, 1405.598, 1435.1351–2). Μετὰ τὴν Εἰκονομαχία ὁ μυροβλύτης ἅγιος Δημήτριος εἶναι ἡ συνέχεια τοῦ ἰατροῦ ἁγίου Δημητρίου τῆς πρώιμης βυζαντινῆς περιόδου.[12]

2. Τὰ ψηφιδωτὰ εἶναι ἀναθήματα ἰαθέντων ἀσθενῶν ποὺ ἐγνώρισαν ἐντὸς τῆς βασιλικῆς τὴν χάριν τοῦ ἁγίου Δημητρίου, τῆς Παναγίας καὶ ἄλλων ἁγίων. Εὔγλωττη εἶναι ἡ ἔκφραση τοῦ πατριάρχη Κωνσταντινουπόλεως Γερμανοῦ Α΄ (715–730): '*τῶν θαυμάτων εἴληφας τὴν ἐνέργειαν ἀνθρώποις παρέχων τὰς ἰάσεις ἀφθόνως*' (Μέντζος 1994, 94). Σχετικὲς ἐκφράσεις εἶναι κοινὸς τόπος στὴν περὶ τοῦ ἁγίου Δημητρίου ὑμνολογία.

3. Τὰ εἰκονιζόμενα παιδιὰ δὲν σχετίζονται οὔτε μὲ τὸν ἅγιο Δημήτριο, οὔτε μὲ τὴν Παναγία, οὔτε μὲ τὸν ἅγιο Γεώργιο ἢ ἄλλους ἁγίους. Γιὰ τὸ λόγο αὐτὸ δὲν ἐμφανίζονται στὴν εἰκονογραφία τους ἐκτὸς τῆς βασιλικῆς τοῦ Ἁγίου Δημητρίου Θεσσαλονίκης. Πιστεύω ὅτι τὰ παιδιὰ εἶναι συστατικὸ τῆς θεραπευτικῆς διαδικασίας τοῦ ξενώνα τοῦ Ἁγίου Δημητρίου. Στηριζόμενος στὴν εἰκονογραφία τῶν ψηφιδωτῶν τῆς βασιλικῆς καὶ τὶς ἐπιγραφές τους ἔχω τὴ γνώμη ὅτι ὁ ξενὼν τοῦ Ἁγίου Δημητρίου ἦταν ἐξειδικευμένος στὰ παιδιατρικὰ καὶ μαιευτικὰ περιστατικά. Γιὰ τὸ λόγο αὐτὸ καὶ ἡ παρουσία τῶν ἁγίων γυναικῶν στὴν εἰκονογράφηση τῆς βασιλικῆς εἶναι μεγάλη καὶ ὁ ρόλος τῆς Παναγίας στὴ λατρεία τῆς βασιλικῆς σημαντικός.

4. Ἡ χωροθέτηση τῶν ψηφιδωτῶν στὴ βασιλικὴ ὑποδεικνύει τὴν προσκυνηματικὴ πορεία τῶν προσερχομένων ἀπὸ τὴν κεντρικὴ ὁδὸ ἀσθενῶν καὶ προσκυνητῶν: ἀπὸ τὸ προσκολλημένο στὸ νότιο τοῖχο τῆς βασιλικῆς προστῶο στὴν κυρία νοτία εἴσοδο, στὸ πρῶτο νότιο κλίτος, στὸν νάρθηκα, στὸ πρῶτο βόρειο κλίτος, στὸν θάλαμο τῶν ἀσθενῶν, κατὰ μῆκος τοῦ πρώτου βορείου κλίτους πρὸς τὸ ἱερὸ βῆμα καὶ τὸ βόρειο πτερύγιο τοῦ ἐγκαρσίου κλίτους.

5. Τὰ ψηφιδωτὰ τῆς βασιλικῆς τοῦ Ἁγίου Δημητρίου συγκροτοῦν ἕνα ἰατρικὸ ζωγραφικὸ σύνολο παλαιοχριστιανικῶν χρόνων, ποὺ συνεχίζει τὴν παράδοση τῆς ἀναθηματικῆς εἰκονογραφίας τῶν Ἀσκληπιείων καὶ τῶν Σαραπείων τῆς ἀρχαιότητας.

Σημειώσεις

1 Φωτογραφίες δημοσιεύθηκαν ἀπὸ τὸν Πέτρο Παπαγεωργίου 1908, 321–81 καὶ τὸν Th. Uspensky 1909, 1-61. Ὑδατογραφίες ἐξεπόνησε ὁ Βρεττανὸς Walter S. George (Cormack 1985b, Μπακιρτζῆς 2012, 148-57). Ἀντίγραφα τῶν ψηφιδωτῶν εἶχε ἐκπονήσει καὶ ὁ ζωγράφος Κωνσταντῖνος Μαλέας, ἀρχιτέκτων τοῦ Δήμου Θεσσαλονίκης (1914), τὰ ὁποῖα πιθανὸν καταστράφηκαν στὴν πυρκαγιὰ τῆς Θεσσαλονίκης τὸ 1917.

2 Ἀγένειο ἄνδρα κατὰ τὸν Cormack 1985a, 82. Οἱ προηγούμενες ἀπόψεις χαρακτήριζαν τὴ δεύτερη μορφὴ ὡς γυναίκα, μητέρα τοῦ παιδιοῦ. Γιὰ τὸ μαρμάρινο καὶ ἐν συνεχείᾳ ἀσημένιο κιβώριο τοῦ Ἁγίου Δημητρίου βλ. Bakirtzis 2002, 181.

3 Τὴν ἑρμηνεία αὐτὴ ποὺ ἀκολούθησαν καὶ ἄλλοι μελετητές (Μπακιρτζῆς 1998, 45 καὶ ἄλλοι) ἀμφισβήτησε ὁ Ψευτογκᾶς 2001, 54, ὁ ὁποῖος ὑποστήριξε ὅτι ἡ παράσταση αὐτὴ καὶ οἱ ὅμοιές της στὴ βασιλικὴ σχετίζονται μὲ τὴ διδακτικὴ δράση τοῦ ἁγίου Δημητρίου.

4 Βλ. σχέδιο τοῦ ψηφιδωτοῦ εἰς Kanonidis and Mastora, 2003, 412, εἰκ. 3.

5 Πρβλ. τὸ τροπάριο τοῦ Ἀνδρέου Κρήτης (β΄μισὸ $7^{ου}$ αἰ. ἢ ἀρχὲς $8^{ου}$ αἰ.) πρὸς τὸν ἅγιο Δημήτριο: *τὸν ... τῶν Θεσσαλονικέων προϊστάμενον...δοξάζομεν Χριστὸν τὸν Θεόν, τὸν ἐνεργοῦντα δι᾽αὐτοῦ πᾶσι τὰ ἰάματα* (Μέντζος 1994, 95).

6 Πρβλ. τοὺς στίχους τοῦ Ὑμνογράφου Ἰωσήφ: *ἰάτρευσον πάσης ἐπηρείας ταῖς προσευχαῖς σου, ἡμᾶς ἐκλυτρούμενος* (Ἀγγελᾶτος 1985, 1433.1301–1302).

7 Ἀνάμεσα στὸ δεύτερο καὶ τὸ τρίτο ἐπεισόδιο, ἔναντι τῆς εἰσόδου τοῦ κιβωρίου ποὺ ὑπῆρχε στὸ κεντρικὸ κλίτος τῆς βασιλικῆς, παρεμβάλλεται μεταγενέστερη προσθήκη ψηφιδωτοῦ ποὺ ἀνήκει στὴ δεύτερη ὁμάδα καὶ ἀπεικονίζει τὸν ἅγιο Δημήτριο μὲ ἕναν ἀρχιεπίσκοπο καὶ ἕναν διάκονο σὲ ὀμφάλια. Ἡ ἐπιγραφὴ τοῦ ψηφιδωτοῦ αὐτοῦ ἀναφέρεται σὲ ἀναστήλωση τῆς βασιλικῆς μετὰ ἀπὸ πυρκαγιά.

8 Μέρος τῶν ψηφιδωτῶν αὐτῶν θὰ κατεστράφη στὴν πυρκαγιὰ τοῦ *c*. 620.

9 Βλ. συγκεντρωτικὰ Ψευτογκᾶς 2001, 47–8.

10 Γιὰ τὴν ταύτιση τοῦ ἁγίου καὶ τὴ χρονολόγηση τοῦ ψηφιδωτοῦ στὸν 9° αἰ. βλ. Φουντούλης 1991, 175–84. Γιὰ τὶς πρωιμότερες χρονολογήσεις βλ. συγκεντρωτικά Anderson 1999, 55.

11 Βλ. συγκεντρωτικὰ Παπαζῶτος 1983, 371–2.

12 Γιὰ τὶς μεταμορφώσεις τοῦ ἁγίου Δημητρίου βλ. Μπακιρτζῆς 2007, 37–45.

Βιβλιογραφία

Ἀγγελᾶτος, Φ. 1985: 'Κανόνες ἀνέκδοτοι εἰς τὸν ἅγιον Δημήτριον', *Βυζαντινὰ* 13/2, *Δώρημα εἰς Ἰωάννη Καραγιανόπουλο*, 1371–476.

Ἁγίου Δημητρίου Θαύματα. Οἱ Συλλογὲς ἀρχιεπισκόπου Ἰωάννου καὶ Ἀνωνύμου. Ὁ βίος, τὰ θαύματα καὶ ἡ Θεσσαλονίκη τοῦ Ἁγίου Δημητρίου, εἰσαγωγή, σχόλια, ἐπιμέλεια Χ. Μπακιρτζῆς, μετάφραση Ἀ. Σιδέρη, Ἀθήνα 1997.

Anderson, J. 1999: 'A Note on the Sanctuary Mosaics of St Demetrius, Thessalonike', *Cahiers Archéologiques* 47, 55.

Bakirtzis, Ch. 2002: 'Pilgrimage to Thessalonike: The Tomb of St. Demetrios', *Dumbarton Oaks Papers* 56, 175–92.

Bakirtzis, Ch. 2010: 'Late Antiquity and Christianity in Thessalonikē: Aspects of a Transformation, 397–426 in L. Nasrallah, Ch. Bakirtzis and S. J. Friesen (eds), *From Roman to Early Christian Thessalonikē, Studies in Religion and Archaeology* (Harvard Theological Studies 64), Cambridge, MA.

Bakirtzis, Ch., Mastora, P. and Pitsalidis, N. 2005: 'Conservation, Maintenance, and Presentation of the Wall Mosaics in the Basilica of St Demetrios, Thessaloniki: Principles, Methods, and Results', 501–11 in Ch. Bakirtzis (ed.), *Proceedings of the VIIIth Conference of the International Committee for the Conservation of Mosaics (ICCM), 'Wall and Floor Mosaics: Conservation, Maintenance, Presentation, Thessaloniki 29 October – 3 November 2002* (European Centre of Byzantine and Post-Byzantine Monuments — Ephoreia of Byzantine Antiquities of Thessaloniki), Thessaloniki.

Βελένης, Γ. 2005: 'Ἡ ἐπιγραφὴ τοῦ Θεοδώρου στὸ τετράπλευρο κιβώριο τῆς βασιλικῆς τοῦ Ἁγίου Δημητρίου Θεσσαλονίκης', *Τὸ ἀρχαιολογικὸ ἔργο στὴ Μακεδονία καὶ Θράκη* 19, 221–6.

Cormack, R. 1969: 'The Mosaic Decoration of St. Demetrios, Thessaloniki: A Re-examination in the Light of the Drawings of W. S. George', *Annual of the British School at Athens* 64, 17–52.

Cormack, R. 1985a: *Writing in Gold. Byzantine Society and Its Icons*, London.

Cormack, R. 1985b: *Ὁ ναὸς τοῦ Ἁγίου Δημητρίου. Ὑδατογραφίες καὶ σχέδια τοῦ W. S. George*, Κατάλογος ἔκθεσης τοῦ Δήμου Θεσσαλονίκης, Κ΄ Δημήτρια, διοργάνωση Βρεττανικοῦ Συμβουλίου, Θεσσαλονίκη.

Dauphin, C. 1999: 'From Apollo and Asclepius to Christ. Pilgrimage and Healing at the Temple and Episcopal Basilica of Dor', *Liber Annuus* (Studium Biblicum Franciscanum, Jerusalem) 49, 419–25.

Δετοράκης, Θ. 2001: 'Ὁ ἅγιος Δημήτριος στὴν πρώιμη Βυζαντινὴ ὑμνογραφία (4ος–10ος αἰ.)', 177–88 εἰς *ΛΓ΄ Δημήτρια, Πρακτικὰ τοῦ ΙΒ΄ ἐπιστημονικοῦ συμποσίου «Χριστανικὴ Θεσσαλονίκη: Ὁ ἱερὸς ναὸς τοῦ Ἁγίου Δημητρίου Θεσσαλονίκης. Προσκύνημα Ἀνατολῆς καὶ Δύσης', Μονὴ Βλατάδων, 1–3 Ὀκτωβρίου 1999*, Θεσσαλονίκη.

Hennessy, C. 2008: *Images of Children in Byzantium*, Farnham.

Κανατσούλης, Δ. 1964: *Ἱστορία τῆς Μακεδονίας μέχρι τοῦ Μεγάλου Κωνσταντίνου*, Θεσσαλονίκη.

Kanonidis, I. and Mastora, P. 2003: 'Preservation of the Mosaics at the Rotunda of Agios Georgios, the Basilica of Agios Demetrios and the Church of Agia Sophia – Thessaloniki, 1997–1999', 403–13 in P. Blanc (ed.), *Actes de la VIIème Conférence du Comité International pour la Conservation des Mosaïques (ICCM), "Les mosaïques: Conserver pour présenter?", 22–28 novembre 1999, Musée de l'Arles antique-Arles, Musée archéologique de Saint-Romain-en-Gal*, Arles.

Koester, H. 2007: *Paul and His World. Interpreting the New Testament and Its Context*, Minneapolis.

Lemerle, P. 1979: *Les plus anciens recueils des Miracles de Saint Démétrius, I Le texte*, Paris.

Μέντζος, Α. 1994: *Τὸ προσκύνημα τοῦ Ἁγίου Δημητρίου Θεσσαλονίκης στὰ βυζαντινὰ χρόνια*, Ἀθῆναι.

Miller, T. S. 1998: *Ἡ γέννησις τοῦ νοσοκομείου στὴν βυζαντινὴ αὐτοκρατορία*, Ἀθήνα.

Μπακιρτζῆς, Χ. 1998: *Ἡ βασιλικὴ τοῦ Ἁγίου Δημητρίου*. 2η ἔκδοση, Θεσσαλονίκη.

Μπακιρτζῆς, Χ. 2006: 'Προεικονομαχικὸ ψηφιδωτὸ τοῦ ἁγίου Δημητρίου στὴ Θεσσαλονίκη', 127–34 εἰς *Δῶρον, τιμητικὸς τόμος στὸν καθηγητὴ Νίκο Νικονάνο*, Θεσσαλονίκη.

Μπακιρτζῆς, Χ. 2007: 'Οἱ μεταμορφώσεις τοῦ ἁγίου Δημητρίου', 37–45 εἰς *1700 ἔτη (305–2005) ἀπὸ τοῦ σεπτοῦ μαρτυρίου τοῦ Ἁγίου Δημητρίου, Πρακτικὰ ἡμερίδος*, Θεσσαλονίκη.

Μπακιρτζῆς, Χ. (ἐπιμ.) 2012: Χ. Μπακιρτζῆς, Ε. Κουρκουτίδου-Νικολαΐδου καὶ Χρ. Μαυροπούλου-Τσιούμη, *Ψηφιδωτὰ της Θεσσαλονίκης, 4ος–14ος αἰώνας*, Ἀθήνα / Bakirtsis, Ch. (ed.) 2012: Ch. Bakirtzis, E. Kourkoutidou-Nikolaidou and Chr. Mavropoulou-Tsioumi, *Mosaics of Thessaloniki, 4th–14th century*, Athens.

Ξυγγόπουλος, Α. 1946: *Ἡ βασιλικὴ τοῦ Ἁγίου Δημητρίου Θεσσαλονίκης*, Θεσσαλονίκη.

Ξυγγόπουλος, Α. 1950: 'Αἱ περὶ τοῦ ναοῦ τῆς Ἀχειροποιήτου Θεσσαλονίκης εἰδήσεις τοῦ Κωνσταντίνου Ἀρμενοπούλου', Ἀνάτυπον ἐκ τοῦ *Πανηγυρικοῦ τόμου ἑξηκονταετηρίδος Ἀρμενοπούλου*, Θεσσαλονίκη.

Ξυγγόπουλος, Α. 1969: *Τὰ ψηφιδωτὰ τοῦ ναοῦ τοῦ Ἁγίου Δημητρίου Θεσσαλονίκης*, Θεσσαλονίκη.

Παπαγεωργίου, Π. 1908: 'Μνημεῖα τῆς ἐν Θεσσαλονίκη λατρείας τοῦ μεγαλομάρτυρος Δημητρίου', *Byzantinische Zeitschrift* 17, 321–81.

Παπαζῶτος, Θ. 1983: 'Τὸ ψηφιδωτὸ τῶν κτητόρων τοῦ Ἁγίου Δημητρίου Θεσσαλονίκης', 365–76 εἰς *Ἀφιέρωμα στὴ μνήμη Στυλιανοῦ Πελεκανίδη*, Θεσσαλονίκη.

Σωτηρίου, Γ. καὶ Μ. 1952: *Ἡ βασιλικὴ τοῦ Ἁγίου Δημητρίου Θεσσαλονίκης*, Ἀθῆναι.

Τζαναβάρη, Κ. 2003: 'Ἡ λατρεία τῶν θεῶν καὶ τῶν ἡρώων στὴ Θεσσαλονίκη', 237–52 εἰς Δ. Β. Γραμμένος (ἐπιμ.), *Ρωμαϊκὴ Θεσσαλονίκη*, Θεσσαλονίκη.

Uspensky, Th. 1909: 'O vnov otkrytyh mozaikah v cerkvi Sv. Dimitrija v Soluni', *Izvestija Russkago Archeologičeskago Instituta v Konstantinopole* 14, 1–61.

Φουντούλης, Ι. 1991: 'Τὸ ψηφιδωτὸ τοῦ ναοῦ τοῦ Ἁγίου Δημητρίου Θεσσαλονίκης μὲ τὴν παράσταση τῆς Παναγίας καὶ τοῦ ἁγίου Θεοδώρου', 175–84 εἰς *ΚΔ' Δημήτρια, Γ' ἐπιστημονικὸ συμπόσιο 'Χριστιανικὴ Θεσσαλονίκη. Ἀπὸ τῆς ἰουστινιανείου ἐποχῆς ἕως καὶ τῆς Μακεδονικῆς δυναστείας», Μονὴ Βλατάδων, 18–20 Ὀκτωβρίου* 1989, Θεσσαλονίκη.

Ψευτογκᾶς, Β. 2001: 'Ἡ θεολογία τῶν εἰκονογραφικῶν παραστάσεων τοῦ ναοῦ τοῦ Ἁγίου Δημητρίου Θεσσαλονίκης', 39–96 εἰς *ΛΓ' Δημήτρια, Πρακτικὰ τοῦ ΙΒ' ἐπιστημονικοῦ συμποσίου 'Χριστανικὴ Θεσσαλονίκη: Ὁ ἱερὸς ναὸς τοῦ Ἁγίου Δημητρίου Θεσσαλονίκης. Προσκύνημα Ἀνατολῆς καὶ Δύσης', Μονὴ Βλατάδων, 1–3 Ὀκτωβρίου 1999,* Θεσσαλονίκη.

38. Πληροφορίες Ιατρικού Ενδιαφέροντος σε Πηγές του Κανονικού Δικαίου

Πρωτοπρεσβύτερος Βασίλειος Χρ. Τρομπούκης

Byzantine medicine continued an ancient tradition in its equal interest in the health of both body and soul. Of the various primary and secondary sources illustrating the Church's relation to medicine, the present paper examines the information that can be culled from the Orthodox Canon Law which relates to a number of topics including the role of administering holy and extreme unction, castration and abortion, as well as the practice of medicine by the clergy and the role of monasteries as nursing centres.

Κατά τη διδασκαλία της Ορθοδόξου Εκκλησίας ο άνθρωπος αποτελείται από ψυχή και σώμα. Για την Εκκλησία το φοβερό του θανάτου μυστήριο έγκειται ακριβώς στο βίαιο χωρισμό της ψυχής από το σώμα, που υπήρξε το πρώτο της υποστάσεώς του, εντός του οποίου ο Θεός ενεφύσησε τη λογική ψυχή.[1]

Εξάλλου, Αυτός που ενδιαφέρεται κυρίως για την ψυχοσωματική υγεία του ανθρώπου είναι στην ορθόδοξο πίστη ο ίδιος ο Χριστός, η ενανθρώπηση του οποίου αποτελεί μυστήριο, το μυστήριο της αγάπης και της φιλανθρωπίας με μοναδικό σκοπό να σώσει τον άνθρωπο, ως σύνολο ψυχής και σώματος. Κατά τον Μέγα Αθανάσιο «ἀλλ' ὅτι ἀσώματος ὢν τῇ φύσει καὶ Λόγος ὑπάρχων, ὅμως κατὰ φιλανθρωπίαν καὶ ἀγαθότητα τοῦ ἑαυτοῦ Πατρὸς διὰ τὴν ἡμῶν σωτηρίαν ἐν ἀνθρωπίνῳ σώματι ἡμῖν πεφανέρωται» (*PG XXV* στ. 97). Η διατύπωση του χριστολογικού δόγματος αποτελεί την τελειότερη έκφραση της ψυχοσωματικής οντότητας του ανθρώπου. Ο ίδιος ο Θεός Λόγος, το δεύτερο πρόσωπο της Αγίας Τριάδος, ενηνθρώπησε. Η υποστατική ένωση των δύο φύσεων, θεότητας και ανθρωπότητας, στην υπόσταση του Χριστού, δεν ήταν στιγμιαία ή παροδική, αλλά αιώνιος. Στην καινή κτίση ο Λόγος του Θεού είναι ενωμένος με την ανθρώπινη φύση στο πρόσωπο του Χριστού. Ο Θεός Λόγος κατά την ενανθρώπισή του προσέλαβε ολόκληρη την ανθρώπινη φύση και κατά συνέπεια ο αγιασμός και η σωτηρία αφορά στο σύνολο του ανθρώπου και όχι μόνο στην ψυχή.[2]

Η πίστη στη συναμφότερη ύπαρξη ψυχής και σώματος βρήκε απόλυτη έκφραση στη βυζαντινή ιατρική που ενδιαφερόταν ταυτοχρόνως για τη σωματική αλλά και την ψυχική υγεία (Κωνσταντέλος 1994, 150). Η συμπόρευση του ενδιαφέροντος για την υγεία ψυχής και σώματος δεν ήταν νέα αφού ήδη στην ελληνική αρχαιότητα οι μεγάλες αυθεντίες της ιατρικής επιστήμης, ο Ιπποκράτης και ο Γαληνός, πίστευαν ότι το σώμα και η ψυχή του ανθρώπου αποτελούν μια ενότητα και ότι ήταν αναγκαίο το φιλοσοφικό υπόβαθρο του ιατρού. Κατά τον Γαληνό «ὁ ἄριστος ἰατρὸς καὶ φιλόσοφος» (Marquardt, Müller et Helmreich 1884–1893, 1–8· πρβλ. Hunger 2000, 108· Κωνσταντέλος 1994, 151).

Έτσι, με την ευαγγελική επιταγή για φιλανθρωπία, την ποιμαντική των πασχόντων της χριστιανικής πίστης, ταυτίζονται και αντιλήψεις του εθνικού κόσμου. Η Εκκλησία δεν αντιστρατεύεται στην ιατρική αλλά τη στηρίζει και τη διακονεί με γνώμονες τον σεβασμό στη μοναδική και ανεπανάληπτη αξία του ανθρωπίνου προσώπου και την ανιδιοτελή αγάπη προς τον πλησίον, που συνοψίζει το νόημα του ευαγγελίου. Με την παραβολή του καλού Σαμαρείτη (Λουκά 10, 30–36) ο Χριστός δίνει το μήνυμα του Ευαγγελίου για τη θυσιαστική προσφορά στον ελάχιστο αδελφό, στηλιτεύοντας δοξασίες του Νόμου περί μιάσματος των ασθενών. Ο Μέγας Βασίλειος, ως ιατρός και επίσκοπος, είδε στην άσκηση της ιατρικής το απόλυτο διακόνημα προσφοράς.[3]

Οι πληροφορίες για θέματα που αφορούν στην άσκηση της ιατρικής στο Βυζάντιο προέρχονται από κείμενα της βυζαντινής γραμματολογίας όχι πάντα αμιγώς ιατρικού ενδιαφέροντος. Διάσπαρτες πληροφορίες απαντώνται και σε πηγές του Κανονικού Δικαίου του κλάδου εκείνου της θεολογικής και νομικής επιστήμης, που εξετάζει τους εκκλησιαστικής προελεύσεως κανόνες που διέπουν τη ζωή της Εκκλησίας. Οι πηγές αυτές διακρίνονται σε βασικές και δευτερεύουσες.[4] Στις βασικές πηγές ανήκουν η Αγία Γραφή και οι Ιεροί Κανόνες, οι ρυθμίσεις δηλαδή που αφορούν στη ζωή των μελών της Εκκλησίας και που προέρχονται από τους Αγίους Αποστόλους, τις Οικουμενικές και Τοπικές Συνόδους και Πατέρες της Εκκλησίας και που επικυρώθηκαν με τον δεύτερο κανόνα της Πενθέκτης Οικουμενικής Συνόδου. Στις δευτερεύουσες πηγές ανήκουν κανόνες άλλων τοπικών συνόδων, αποκρίσεις πατέρων, εγκύκλιοι εκκλησιαστικών αρχών, μοναστηριακά τυπικά, ερμηνευτικά κείμενα κανονολόγων και κάποιες διατάξεις πολιτειακής προέλευσης που θεσπίσθηκαν με τη συναίνεση ή την ανοχή της Εκκλησίας και που αφορούν σε θέματα εκκλησιαστικά ή σχέσεων Εκκλησίας και Πολιτείας.

Ανατρέχοντας λοιπόν στις πηγές του Κανονικού Δικαίου ανθολογούμε πληροφορίες ιατρικού ενδιαφέροντος, τις οποίες παρουσιάζουμε στη συνέχεια.

Στην Καινή Διαθήκη σημαντική είναι η αναφορά στο μυστήριο του ευχελαίου που ίδρυσε ο ίδιος ο Κύριος Ιησούς Χριστός αποστέλλοντας τους μαθητές στις πόλεις της Παλαιστίνης για να κηρύξουν και αυτοί «ἐξελθόντες ἐκήρυξαν ... καὶ ἤλειφον ἐλαίῳ πολλοὺς ἀρρώστους καὶ ἐθεράπευον» (Μάρκου 6, 13). Και ο άγιος Ιάκωβος ο Αδελφόθεος επαναλαμβάνει:

> «...ἀσθενεῖ τις ἐν ὑμῖν, προσκαλεσάσθω τοὺς πρεσβυτέρους τῆς ἐκκλησίας καὶ προσευξάσθωσαν ἐπ' αὐτὸν ἀλείψαντες (αὐτόν) ἐλαίῳ ἐν τῷ ὀνόματι τοῦ Κυρίου καὶ ἡ εὐχὴ τῆς πίστεως σώσει τὸν κάμνοντα καὶ ἐγερεῖ αὐτὸν ὁ Κύριος· κἂν ἁμαρτίας ᾖ πεποιηκὼς ἀφεθήσεται αὐτῷ...». (Ιακώβου 5, 14–15)

Το μυστήριο του ευχελαίου δηλαδή γίνεται προς θεραπεία σωματικών και ψυχικών νόσων, οι οποίες είναι συνδεδεμένες μεταξύ τους. Οι σωματικές νόσοι μπορεί να οφείλονται σε λανθάνον αμάρτημα του ασθενούς. Το μυστήριο του ευχελαίου τελείται για την πολυπόθητη υγεία η οποία επέρχεται μόνο με την αρμονική συνύπαρξη σωματικής και ψυχικής υγείας. Γι' αυτό και στην Ορθόδοξη Εκκλησία το ευχέλαιο απευθύνεται μόνο στα ζώντα μέλη της. Αντίθετα οι «καινοτομοῦντες Λατίνοι» κατά την έκφραση του αγίου Συμεών Θεσσαλονίκης τελούσαν το μυστήριο στους ετοιμοθάνατους προκειμένου να συγχωρεθούν οι αμαρτίες τους ενόψει της επερχόμενης μετάβασής τους εις τας ουρανίους μονάς (*PG* 155, στ. 516 επ.· πρβλ. περί του μυστηρίου του Ευχελαίου γενικώς και ειδικότερα από λειτουργικής επόψεως Φουντούλης 1985, 183 επ.).

Χαρακτηριστικό είναι ότι επιλέγεται και αγιάζεται από την Εκκλησία το κατεξοχήν θεραπευτικό στοιχείο της φύσεως, το έλαιον, πρωτογενές συστατικό των περισσοτέρων φαρμάκων. Στην κανδήλα του ευχελαίου κάτω από το λάδι τοποθετείται κρασί το φυσικό, και πάλι, αντισηπτικό. Η θεραπεία δεν επέρχεται με τρόπο μαγικό, όπως σε αρχαίες θρησκείες, στις οποίες ο ιερεύς ταυτίζεται με τον ιατρό–μάγο, αλλά με την επίκληση της αγιαστικής και σωστικής χάριτος του παναγίου πνεύματος «ἡ εὐχὴ τῆς πίστεως σώσει τὸν κάμνοντα» (Ιακώβου 5, 15). Η Εκκλησία δεν δέχεται τη χρήση μαγικών συμβόλων παρά μόνο τη χρίση δι' ελαίου χωρίς όμως αυτό να σημαίνει ότι απορρίπτει τη ιατρική. Αντιθέτως, προτρέπει τους πιστούς να καταφεύγουν στους γιατρούς, τους οποίους διακρίνει από τους αγύρτες. Ο ιερός Χρυσόστομος (Ομιλία 8, *PG* LXII, στ. 358) αναφέρει χαρακτηριστικώς:

> «Τὰ γὰρ περίαπτα, κἂν μυρία φιλοσοφῶσιν οἱ ἐκ τούτων χρηματιζόμενοι, λέγοντες ὅτι τὸν Θεὸν καλοῦμεν, καὶ οὐδὲν πλέον ποιοῦμεν, καὶ ὅσα τοιαῦτα καὶ Χριστιανή ἐστιν ἡ γραῦς καὶ πιστή, εἰδωλολατρεία ἐστί. Πιστὴ εἶ σφράγισον, εἰπέ. Τοῦτο ἔχω τὸ ὅπλον μόνο τοῦτο τὸ φάρμακον ἄλλο οὐκ οἶδα. Εἰπέ μοι, ἐάν προσελθὼν ἰατρός, καὶ τὰ τῆς ἰατρικῆς φάρμακα ἀφείς, ἐπάδη, τοῦτον ἰατρὸν ἐροῦμεν;».

Αν δηλαδή κάποιος ισχυρίζεται ότι είναι χριστιανός πρέπει να σφραγίζεται μόνο (δια του συμβόλου του σταυρού και δι' ελαίου) και να μην χρησιμοποιεί κανένα μαγικό. Γιατί και τον ιατρό που αφήνει τα φάρμακα της επιστήμης του και τραγουδά για να γίνει καλά ο ασθενής πώς θα μπορούσαμε να τον πούμε ιατρό (βλ. και Τρωιάνος 1997, 27–8). Ο 83ος Κανόνας του Μεγάλου Βασιλείου επιβάλλει το επιτίμιο της «ἐξαετίας» σε όσους καλούν στους οίκους τους μάγους για την ανεύρεση «φαρμακειῶν» (Ανάλογοι και οι Κανόνες 3 του Αγίου Γρηγορίου Νύσσης, 24 Αγκύρας, 36 Λαοδικείας). Ο Θεόδωρος Βαλσαμών σε ερμηνεία του στον εν λόγω κανόνα αναφέρει το παράδειγμα της συζύγου του Αλεξίου Κομνηνού Ζωής, η οποία ήταν βαριά άρρωστη και οι γιατροί είχαν αποκλείσει κάθε πιθανότητα θεραπείας της, γεγονός που εκμεταλλεύθηκαν μάγοι οι οποίοι ενεφανίσθησαν υποσχόμενοι ότι μπορούν να την θεραπεύσουν. Προκειμένου μάλιστα να γίνουν πιστευτοί έκρυψαν σε διάφορα σημεία του σπιτιού κέρινα ομοιώματα προσποιούμενοι στη συνέχεια ότι τα ανακάλυπταν, εξουδετερώνοντας έτσι τις μαγγανείες (Ράλλης και Ποτλῆς 1852–1859 [2002], τ. Δ΄, σελ. 251 επ.· πρβλ. Τρωιάνος 1997, 31). Φυσικά η αυτοκράτειρα απεβίωσε.

Άλλη σημαντική ευαγγελική ρήση, τα λόγια του Χριστού «...εἰσὶν γὰρ εὐνοῦχοι οἵτινες ἐκ κοιλίας μητρὸς ἐγεννήθησαν οὕτως, καὶ εἰσὶν εὐνοῦχοι οἵτινες εὐνουχίσθησαν ὑπὸ τῶν ἀνθρώπων, καὶ εἰσὶν εὐνοῦχοι οἵτινες εὐνούχισαν ἑαυτοὺς διὰ τὴν βασιλείαν τῶν οὐρανῶν, ὁ δυνάμενος χωρεῖν χωρείτω» (Ματθαίου 19, 12) έμελλε να παρερμηνευθεί και να αναγκάσει Εκκλησία και Πολιτεία στο Βυζάντιο να θεσπίσουν αυστηρούς κανόνες και νόμους για την απαγόρευση του ευνουχισμού.

Ο ευνουχισμός χρησιμοποιήθηκε στον αρχαίο ανατολικό κυρίως κόσμο για την δημιουργία φυλάκων των γυναικωνιτών. Οι ευνούχοι διακρίνονταν σε τρεις κατηγορίες, σύμφωνα με αναφορά του Θεόδωρου Βαλσαμώνος, τους εκτομίους ή καστράτους των οποίων τα γεννητικά όργανα είχαν αφαιρεθεί πλήρως δια χειρουργικής επεμβάσεως, τους θλιβίας οι οποίοι κατέστρεψαν τα γεννητικά τους όργανα δι' εκθλίψεως και τους σπάδωνας οι οποίοι κατεστάθησαν ανίκανοι προς παιδοποιΐα λόγω ψύξεως ή παθήσεως των όρχεων ή γιατί εγεννήθησαν χωρίς όρχεις (Ράλλης και Ποτλής 1852, τ. Β΄, 30). Οι κανόνες αναφέρονται στις περιπτώσεις κατά τις οποίες επιδιώκεται ο ευνουχισμός ως μορφή ακραίου ασκητισμού από πιστούς που ερμηνεύουν κατά γράμμα την ευαγγελική ρήση. Ο Χριστός αναφέρεται στην κατά "Χριστόν παρθενία", δηλαδή εκούσια αποχή από τη γεννετήσιο λειτουργία, που επιτυγχάνεται με τη χάρη του παναγίου πνεύματος και όχι στον αυτοακρωτηριασμό. Χαρακτηριστική είναι η περίπτωση του Ωριγένους ο οποίος ευνουχίσθηκε σε νεαρή ηλικία για λόγους πίστεως και στη συνέχεια χειροτονήθηκε κληρικός. Η χειροτονία του χαρακτηρίσθηκε αντικανονική διότι κατά τους κανόνες ο θεληματικός ευνουχισμός αποτελεί κώλυμα ιερωσύνης. Ενδεικτικώς αναφέρουμε τους Κανόνες 22, 23 και 24 των Αγίων Αποστόλων:

> «Ὁ ἀκρωτηριάσας ἑαυτὸν μὴ γινέσθω κληρικός· αὐτοφονευτὴς γάρ ἐστι ἑαυτοῦ, καὶ τῆς Θεοῦ δημιουργίας ἐχθρός», «Εἴ τις κληρικὸς ὤν, ἑαυτὸν ἀκρωτηριάσοι, καθαιρείσθω φονεὺς γάρ ἐστι ἑαυτοῦ» και «Λαϊκὸς ἑαυτὸν ἀκρωτηριάσας, ἀφοριζέσθω ἔτη τρία· ἐπίβουλος γάρ ἐστι τῆς ἑαυτοῦ ζωῆς».

Αντιθέτως, κατά τον Κανόνα 21 των Αγίων Αποστόλων ο ευνουχισθείς δια νόσον ή εξ επηρείας ανθρώπων σε διωγμό και ο γεννηθείς έτσι, αν κατά τα λοιπά είναι άξιος μπορεί να γίνει κληρικός.

Αυστηρή όμως παρουσιάζεται και η αυτοκρατορική νομοθεσία για τους ευνουχίσαντες, τους ιατρούς δηλαδή ή όποιους άλλους συγκατατιθέμενοι στο αίτημα κάποιου προβαίνουν στον ευνουχισμό του. Κατά τη Νεαρά 142 του Ιουστινιανού οι ευνουχίσαντες τιμωρούνται με ταυτοπάθεια (ευνουχίζονται δηλαδή κι αυτοί βιαίως), δήμευση της περιουσία τους και εξορία για το υπόλοιπο της ζωής τους.

Τίθενται έτσι με κανόνες και νόμους περιορισμοί στην άσκηση της ιατρικής· ένα είδος ιατρικής δεοντολογίας στην οποία προέχει ο σεβασμός στη ζωή ως δώρο Θεού και έπεται ο αυτεξουσιασμός και η αυτοδιάθεση του σώματος. Ο πρώτος Κανόνας της Α΄ Οικουμενικής Συνόδου αναφέρει «Εἴ τις ἐν νόσῳ ὑπὸ ἰατρῶν ἐχειρουργήθη ... οὗτος μενέτω ἐν τῷ κλήρῳ». Ο ιατρός στο Βυζάντιο, όπως και σήμερα, με την ίδια επέμβαση μπορούσε να σώσει ζωή ή να προβεί σε πράξη αντίθετη στην περί ηθικής αντίληψη της εποχής του, ερχόμενος αντιμέτωπος με την εκκλησιαστική και την ποινική δικαιοσύνη.

Ανάλογες κανονικές απαγορεύσεις υπάρχουν για την άμβλωση. Ενδιαφέρον παρουσιάζουν οι αναφορές σε «αμβλωθρίδια», ειδικά δηλαδή σκευάσματα που χορηγούνταν από ειδικούς με σκοπό την άμβλωση. Στο Νομοκάνονα του Φωτίου αναφέρεται:

> «ὁ πόμα δεδωκὼς πρὸς ἀμβλωθρίδιον, εὐτελὴς μὲν ὢν μεταλλίζεται, τίμιος δὲ ἐξορίζεται μετὰ μερικῆς δημεύσεως ἐσχάτη δὲ τιμωρία ἐπάγεται, ἐάν τις ἀπέθανεν ἐκ τούτου· ταῦτα κἂν χωρὶς δόλου τὸ ἀμβλωθρίδιον δέδωκε» (Νομοκάνων Φωτίου, τίτλος ΙΓ΄, κεφ. Ι΄: Ράλλης και Ποτλής 1852–1859, τ. Α΄, 312).

Ο Μέγας Βασίλειος περισσότερο επιστημονικός και ακριβής τονίζει ότι η γυναίκα που φθείρει το έμβρυό της «κατ' ἐπιτήδευσιν, φόνου δίκην ὑπέχει» (Κανόνας 2, Μεγάλου Βασιλείου). Δεν υπάρχει ελαφρυντικό στην περίπτωση που το έμβρυο ήταν «ἀνεξεικόνιστον», δεν διακρινόταν δηλαδή ακόμη τα ανθρώπινα χαρακτηριστικά, γιατί δεν τιμωρείται μόνο η φθορά του εμβρύου αλλά και η επιβουλή της μητρός, διότι «ὡς ἐπὶ τὸ πολὺ ἀποθνήσκουσι ταῖς τοιαύταις ἐπιχειρήσεσιν αἱ γυναῖκες». Ερνηνεύοντας τον κανόνα κατά τον 11ο αιώνα ο Ιωάννης Ζωναράς επεκτείνεται σε περιγραφή της ανάπτυξης του εμβρύου «τὸ γὰρ σπέρμα τῇ μήτρᾳ καταβαλλόμενον, πρότερον μὲν ἐξαιματοῦται, εἶτα εἰς σάρκα πήγνυται ἀμόρφωτον, εἶτα ἐξεικονίζεται καὶ διατυποῦται εἰς μέλη καὶ μόρια» (Ράλλης και Ποτλής 1852–1859, τ. Δ΄, 96). Χαρακτηριστικό είναι ότι η αντίστοιχη κανονική ρύθμιση του Κανόνα 91 της Πενθέκτης Οικουμενικής Συνόδου «τὰς τὰ ἀμβλωθρίδια διδούσας φάρμακα» και του Κανόνα 8 του Μεγάλου Βασιλείου «αἱ τοίνυν τὰ ἀμβλωθρίδια διδοῦσαι φάρμακα φονεύτριαι εἰσὶ καὶ αὐταί» αφορά σε γυναίκες που χορηγούν τα σκευάσματα για την έκτρωση. Είναι βέβαιο ότι στο Βυζάντιο οι γυναίκες ασκούσαν το επάγγελμα του ιατρού και περιοριζόταν συνήθως στην μαιευτική και τη γυναικολογία, αντικείμενα με τα οποία δεν μπορούσαν να ασχοληθούν οι άνδρες ιατροί (βλ. Μπουρδάρα 1989 και γενικώς περί της ασκήσεως της ιατρικής επιστήμης στο Βυζάντιο Ευτυχιάδης 1983). Εξάλλου και αυτός ο όρος που απαντάται στις πηγές «ἰάτρινα» σήμαινε τη μαία, αν και από έμμεσες πληροφορίες καταδεικνύεται η ενασχόληση των γυναικών και με τη γενική ιατρική και τη συγγραφή ιατρικών συγγραμμάτων. Για τους όρους που αποδίδουν τη γυναίκα ιατρό στο Βυζάντιο βλ. αντί άλλων Μέντζου-Μεϊμάρη 1982α. Σε κάθε περίπτωση όμως οι γυναίκες ιατροί ασχολούνταν με την περίθαλψη των γυναικών ασθενών (βλ. προχείρως Νικολάου 2007, όπου και η παλαιότερη βιβλιογραφία). Σε ειδικές μάλιστα περιπτώσεις μόνο γυναίκες ιατροί καλούνταν ως μάρτυρες σε δίκες έπειτα από αυτοψία επί γυναικών. Χαρακτηριστική η αναφορά στη Νεαρά 48 του Λέοντος ΣΤ΄ Σοφού: «ἐν πράγμασι δὲ γυναιξὶν ἰδιάζουσιν, οὗ μὴ θεμιστὸν ἐντυγχάνειν ἀνδράσιν φημὶ δὲ ἐπί τε ὠδίνων καὶ ἤ τι ἕτερον ὅ μόνη θῆλυς ὄψις ὁρᾷ τὰ οἰκεῖα καὶ ἀρρένων ὀφθαλμοῖς ἀθέατα μαρτυρείτωσαν».

Ανάλογοι περιορισμοί στην άσκηση του ιατρικού επαγγέλματος υπήρχαν για τους κληρικούς (βλ. Χριστοφιλόπουλος 1957, 83–4 και Κωνσταντέλος 1994, 152 για αναφορές σε κληρικούς ιατρούς). Με διάταξη της πατριαρχικής συνόδου της Κωνσταντινουπόλεως επί πατριαρχείας Λουκά Χρυσοβέργη, τον 12ο αιώνα, απαγορεύθηκε οι κληρικοί να ασκούν την ιατρική διότι «ἀνένδεκτον εἶναι τοὺς μετὰ φαινολίων καὶ στιχαρίων τὰ ἅγια μεταχειριζομένους κοσμικὰς στολὰς ἐνδιδύσκεσθαι καὶ μετὰ λαϊκῶν ἀνδρῶν, τῶν ἰατρῶν δηλαδή, προπομπεύειν» (βλ. Γεδεών 1889, 19. Πρβλ. «Βαλσαμῶνος, ἑρμηνεία στὸν καν. 16 Καρθαγένης», Ράλλης και Ποτλής 1852–1859, τ. Γ΄, 344 επ.). Και ο Βαλσαμών σε ερώτηση για τα επαγγέλματα που μπορεί να ασκεί ο κληρικός, αποκρίνεται ότι η τέχνη των ιατρών αν και παρά των σοφών ορίζεται ότι είναι περιποιητική της υγείας, εντούτοις αφορά σε επινοήσεις των ανθρώπων που ενδέχεται να είναι λανθασμένες· γιατί λοιπόν να απέχει ο κληρικός από την άμεμπτο και ασφαλή διακονία που του απονεμήθηκε και να ασχολείται με την αμφίβολο και συχνά επικίνδυνη (Ράλλης και Ποτλής 1852, τ. Δ,΄ 469–70);

Παρά ταύτα δεν είναι λίγες οι μαρτυρίες περί κληρικών ιατρών (Χριστοφιλόπουλος 1957, 83–4 και Κωνσταντέλος 1994, 152), ενώ είναι αναμφίβολη η οργανωμένη παροχή τόσο κοινωνικών εν γένει όσο και νοσηλευτικών ειδικότερα υπηρεσιών από την Εκκλησία. Ο Ζωναράς σε ερμηνεία του στον όγδοο κανόνα της Δ΄ Οικουμενικής Συνόδου αναφέρει «πτωχεία δέ εἰσι τὰ εἰς πτωχῶν ἀφωρισμένα πρόνοιαν καὶ διοίκησιν, τὰ γηροκομεῖα δηλονότι, καὶ ὀρφανοτροφεῖα, καὶ τὰ τοιαῦτα, ἐν οἷς καταπαθεῖς ἀνάκεινται καὶ τρέφονται» (Ράλλης και Ποτλής 1852–1859, τ. Β΄, 234–35). Η Εκκλησία επίσημα περιθάλπει τους ασθενείς (βλ. ενδεικτικώς Γρηγορίου Νύσσης, Περὶ φιλοπτωχίας, *PG* LXLVI, στ. 472 επ.). Ο Μέγας Βασίλειος είχε ιδρύσει λεπροκομείο το οποίο περιγράφει ο άγιος Γρηγόριος ο Θεολόγος σε επιτάφιο λόγο του προς τον Μεγάλο Βασίλειο (*PG* 36, στ. 577 επ.). Η αναφορά του Γρηγορίου επεκτείνεται σε λεπτομέρειες για την αντιμετώπιση των χρονίως πασχόντων από την κοινωνία, την απομόνωση και εγκατάλειψή τους που δεν αρμόζει σε εικόνες Χριστού, και την παρηγορία και περιποίηση που έβρισκαν στα εκκλησιαστικά ιδρύματα. Χαρακτηριστικότερο όλων είναι το νοσοκομείο που λειτουργούσε εντός της μονής Παντοκράτορος στην Κωνσταντινούπολη, γνωστό ως «ξενὼν τοῦ Παντοκράτορος», περιθάλποντας τους ασθενείς της Πόλης. Οι πληροφορίες που αντλούμε από το λεπτομερές τυπικό της μονής (Gautier 1974) μας οδηγούν αβίαστα στο συμπέρασμα ότι επρόκειτο για πλήρως οργανωμένο νοσηλευτικό ίδρυμα που παρείχε ολοκληρωμένες ιατρικές υπηρεσίες. (Για τα μοναστηριακά τυπικά εν γένει, βλ. αντί άλλων Μανάφης 1970, και από νομικής επόψεως Κονιδάρης 2003. Για τα νοσηλευτικά ιδρύματα στο Βυζάντιο βλ. μεταξύ άλλων Miller 1998, Μέντζου-Μεϊμάρη 1982β, Χαριζάνης 2004–2005).

Από τα ανωτέρω γίνεται κατ' αρχάς σαφής η αλληλένδετη σχέση ψυχικής και σωματικής υγείας, πίστη κοινή στον αρχαίο-εθνικό και βυζαντινό-χριστιανικό κόσμο. Καταδεικνύεται ο εναγκαλισμός της ιατρικής με την χριστιανική πίστη. Η Εκκλησία στηλιτεύει τις δεισιδαιμονικές δοξασίες και πρακτικές και στηρίζει την ιατρική τέχνη ενώ παραλλήλως ευθύνεται για τη διαμόρφωση της ιατρικής δεοντολογίας. Χρησιμοποιεί τέλος την ιατρική στα υπό την εποπτεία της ιδρύματα ως την προσφορότερη επιστήμη για την υλοποίηση την ευαγγελικής προτροπής προσφοράς στον πάσχοντα αδελφό.

Σημειώσεις

1 Γεν. 2, 4-8. Τον χωρισμό ψυχής και σώματος περιγράφει χαρακτηριστικώς ο άγιος Ιωάννης ο Δαμασκηνός (*Μικρόν Ευχολόγιον* 1996, 243) σε ιδιόμελο της εξοδίου ακολουθίας: «ὄντως φοβερώτατον τὸ τοῦ θανάτου μυστήριον, πῶς ψυχὴ ἐκ τοῦ σώματος βιαίως χωρίζεται ἐκ τῆς ἁρμονίας καὶ τῆς συμφυΐας ὁ φυσικώτατος δεσμὸς θείῳ βουλήματι ἀποτέμνεται ...»· (σημειωτέον ότι το ανωτέρω ιδιόμελο δεν περιλαμβάνεται στις εκδόσεις του Μεγάλου Ευχολογίου αν και σε κάθε περίπτωση απηχεί ακριφνώς την ορθόδοξη διδασκαλία περί θανάτου· πρβλ. Φουντούλης 1985, 462 επ.).

2 «Ὁμολογοῦμεν τοιγαροῦν τὸν Κύριον ἡμῶν Ἰησοῦν Χριστόν, τὸν Υἱὸν τοῦ Θεοῦ τὸν Μονογενῆ, Θεὸν τέλειον καὶ ἄνθρωπον τέλειον ἐκ ψυχῆς λογικῆς καὶ σώματος, πρὸ αἰώνων μὲν ἐκ τοῦ Πατρὸς γεννηθέντα κατὰ τὴν θεότητα, ἐπ' ἐσχάτων δὲ τῶν ἡμερῶν τὸν αὐτόν, δι' ἡμᾶς καὶ διὰ τὴν ἡμετέραν σωτηρίαν, ἐκ Μαρίας τῆς Παρθένου κατὰ τὴν ἀνθρωπότητα, ὁμοούσιον τῷ Πατρὶ τὸν αὐτὸν κατὰ τὴν θεότητα καὶ ὁμοούσιον ἡμῖν κατὰ τὴν ἀνθρωπότητα. Δύο γὰρ φύσεων ἕνωσις γέγονε, διὸ ἕνα Χριστόν, ἕνα Υἱόν, ἕνα Κύριον ὁμολογοῦμεν», Ὅρος τῶν Διαλλαγῶν (433), *PG* 77, στ. 172–6· βλ. αντί πολλών Ανδρούτσος 2005, 173 και Φειδάς 2004, 617–8.

3 Γενικότερα για τη σχέση του Μεγάλου Βασιλείου με την ιατρική, βλ. προχείρως Μουρατίδης 1968, 33–60· Κέκης 1959, 13–7· Παλαιός 1978, 179–85.

4 Βλ. ενδεικτικώς για τη διάκριση αυτή και εν γένει για τις πηγές του Κανονικού Δικαίου, Μίλας 1906, 49 επ.· Ροδόπουλος 1988, 39 επ.· Κονιδάρης 2000, 35 επ.· Μπούμης [3]2008, 32 επ.

Βιβλιογραφια

Ἀθανάσιος Ἀρχιεπίσκοπος Ἀλεξανδρείας, *Λόγος περὶ τῆς ἐνανθρωπήσεως τοῦ Λόγου, καὶ τῆς διὰ σώματος πρὸς ἡμᾶς ἐπιφανείας αὐτοῦ*, *PG* XXV στ. 95–200.

Ανδρούτσος, Χρ. 2005: *Δογματική της Ορθοδόξου Ανατολικής Εκκλησίας*, Αθήναι.

Γεδεών, Μ. Ί. 1889: *Κανονικαὶ διατάξεις*, τ. Β΄, Κωνσταντινούπολη.

Γρηγόριος ὁ Νύσσης, *Περὶ φιλοπτωχίας*, *PG* XLVI, στ. 472 επ.

Ευτυχιάδης, Α. 1983: *Η άσκησις της βυζαντινής ιατρικής επιστήμης και κοινωνικαί εφαρμογαί αυτής κατά σχετικάς διατάξεις*, Αθήναι.

Ζωναρᾶς, *Ἑρμηνεία στὸν Κανόνα 2 Μεγάλου Βασιλείου*: Ράλλης και Ποτλής 1852–1859 (2002), τόμ. Δ΄.

Gautier, P. 1974: 'Le typikon du Christ Sauveur Pantocrator', *Revue des Etudes Bibliques* 32, 1–145.

Hunger, H. 2000: *Βυζαντινή Λογοτεχνία, Η λόγια κοσμική γραμματεία των Βυζαντινών*, τ. Γ΄ (μετάφρ. κεφαλαίου «Ιατρική», Ιωάννα Οικονόμου-Αγοραστού), Αθήνα.

Θεόδωρος Βαλσαμών, *Ἑρμηνεία στὸν κανόνα 21 τῶν Ἁγίων Ἀποστόλων*: Ράλλης και Ποτλής 1852–1859 (2002), τόμ. Β΄.

Ἰωάννης ὁ Δαμασκηνός, *Μικρὸν Εὐχολόγιον*, Αθήνα: εκδ. Αποστολικής Διακονίας της Εκκλησίας της Ελλάδος, 1996.

Κέκης, Β. 1959: «Ο Μέγας Βασίλειος και η ιατρική», *Ακτίνες* 22, 13–7.

Κονιδάρης, Ι. Μ. 2000: *Εγχειρίδιο Εκκλησιαστικού Δικαίου*, Αθήνα-Κομοτηνή.
Κονιδάρης, Ι. Μ. 2003: *Νομική θεώρηση των Μοναστηριακών τυπικών*, Αθήνα-Κομοτηνή.
Κωνσταντέλος, Δ. Ι. 1994: *Πενία, κοινωνία και φιλανθρωπία, στον Μεταγενέστερο Μεσαιωνικό, Ελληνικό Κόσμο* (μετάφρ. εκ της αγγλικής Αθανασίας Κοντογιαννακοπούλου), Θεσσαλονίκη.
Μανάφης, Κ. Α. 1970: *Μοναστηριακά Τυπικά-Διαθήκαι, Μελέτη φιλολογική* («Αθηνά». Σειρά διατριβών και μελετημάτων 7), Αθήναι.
Marquardt, J., Müller, I. von and Helmreich, G. (eds.) 1884–1893: *Claudii Galeni Pergameni scripta minora* II, Leipzig.
Μέντζου-Μεϊμάρη, Κ. 1982α: «Η παρουσία της γυναίκας στις ελληνικές επιγραφές από τον Δ΄ μέχρι τον Ι΄ μ.Χ. αιώνα», *Jahrbuch der Österreichischen Byzantinistik* 32/2, 433–43
Μέντζου-Μεϊμάρη, Κ. 1982β: «Επαρχιακά ευαγή νοσηλευτικά ιδρύματα μέχρι τού τέλους της Εικονομαχίας», *Βυζαντινά* 11, 243–308.
Μίλας, Ν. 1906: *Τὸ ἐκκλησιαστικὸν δίκαιον τῆς Ὀρθοδόξου Ἀνατολικῆς Ἐκκλησίας* (μετάφραση Μελετίου Αποστολοπούλου), Αθήναι (φωτοτυπική ανατύπωσις: Αθήναι 1970).
Miller, T. 1998: *Ἡ γέννησις τοῦ Νοσοκομείου στήν Βυζαντινή Αὐτοκρατορία*, ἀπόδοσις στά ἑλληνικά Ν. Κελερμένος, Ἀθήνα 1998.
Μουρατίδης, Κ. Δ. 1968: «Η ιατρική του σώματος τύπος της κατά ψυχήν θεραπείας κατά την διδασκαλία του Μεγάλου Βασιλείου», *Θεολογία* 39, 33–60.
Μπούμης, Π. Ι. 2008: *Κανονικόν Δίκαιον*, Αθήνα.
Μπουρδάρα, Κ. Α. 1989: «Η άσκηση του ιατρικού επαγγέλματος από τη γυναίκα στο Βυζάντιο και η νομική της κατοχύρωση», 121–34 εις *Πρακτικά Α΄ Διεθνούς Συμποσίου «Η καθημερινή ζωή στο Βυζάντιο»*, Κέντρο Βυζαντινών Ερευνών / Ε.Ι.Ε., Αθήνα.
Νικολάου, Κ. 2007: «Ασθένειες και θεραπεία των γυναικών στο Βυζάντιο», *Αρχαιολογία* 103, 28–33.
Παλαιός, Κ. 1978: *Ο Μέγας Βασίλειος και η ιατρική*, (Ριζάρειος Εκκλησιαστική Παιδεία 1), Αθήναι.
PG: J.-P. Migne, *Patrologia Graeca,* Paris 1857–1858.
Ράλλης, Γ. καὶ Ποτλῆς, Μ. 1852–1859: *Σύνταγμα θείων καὶ ἱερῶν κανόνων*, τ. Α΄–ΣΤ΄, Αθήναι (ανατύπωση Θεσσαλονίκη 2002).
Ροδόπουλος, Π. 1988: *Μητροπολίτου Τυρολόης και Σερεντίου, Επιτομή Κανονικού Δικαίου*, Θεσσαλονίκη.
Συμεών, Ἀρχιεπίσκοπος Θεσσαλονίκης, *Περί τῆς ἱερᾶς τελετῆς τοῦ εὐχελαίου*, *PG* CLV, στ. 516 επ.
Τρωιάνος, Σ. Ν. 1997: *Μαγεία και Δίκαιο στο Βυζάντιο*, Αθήναι.
Φειδάς, Β. Ι. 2004: *Εκκλησιαστική Ιστορία*, τ. Α΄, Αθήναι.
Φουντούλης, Ι. Μ. 1985: *Θέματα Ευχολογίου* (Κείμενα Λειτουργικής, τεύχ. Β΄), Θεσσαλονίκη.
Χαριζάνης, Γ. 2004–2005: «Παροχή νοσοκομειακής περίθαλψης από τις βυζαντινές μονές, κατά τον 10ο –12ο αιώνα», *Βυζαντινός Δόμος* 14, 171–82.
Χριστοφιλόπουλος,, Α. 1957: *Θέματα Βυζαντινού Εκκλησιαστικού Δικαίου*, Αθήναι.
Ἰωάννης Χρυσόστομος, *Ὑπόμνημα είς τὴν πρὸς Κολοσσαεῖς Ἐπιστολήν, Ὁμιλία 8*, *PG* LXII, στ. 358.

39. Ασθένειες όπως Περιγράφονται σε Βίους Ιαματικών Αγίων και Τρόποι Θεραπείας Αυτών

Δήμητρα Παπαϊωάννου

This paper examines diseases as described in the Lives of (male and female) saints; both medical and non-medical saints are included. The first aim is to catalogue and describe diseases and their symptoms and the second to examine the ways of treatment by medical and non-medical saints. Emphasis is given to scientific medical treatment, but miraculous treatment associated with belief in God is also addressed. At the same time, Byzantine and Post-Byzantine icons and frescoes depicting the medical miracles of Saints Cosmas and Damian are briefly presented.

Τα ιάματα που μελετηθήκαν από τους βίους των ιατρών αγίων Κοσμά και Δαμιανού, Κύρου και Ιωάννου, Παντελεήμονα και Σαμψών του Ξενοδόχου διαχωρίστηκαν αρχικά σε δύο κατηγορίες: σε αυτά που πραγματοποιήθηκαν κατά τη διάρκεια της ζωής τους και σε αυτά που έγιναν μετά θάνατον, κατά την εγκοίμηση των ασθενών είτε στους ναούς όπου λατρεύονταν οι άγιοι Κοσμάς και Δαμιανός, Κύρος και Ιωάννης είτε στον ξενώνα του Σαμψών του Ξενοδόχου. Κατά τη διάρκεια της νύχτας και ενώ οι ασθενείς κοιμόνταν εντός του ναού ή του ξενώνα, οι άγιοι εμφανίζονταν σε όνειρο ή σε όραμα και αποκάλυπταν στους ασθενείς τον τρόπο της θεραπείας, την πραγματοποιούσαν είτε με θαυματουργικό τρόπο είτε με ιατρική επέμβαση είτε συνιστούσαν τη λήψη συγκεκριμένης διατροφής.[1]

Στα ιάματα των Κοσμά και Δαμιανού καθώς και του Σαμψών του Ξενοδόχου πραγματοποιήθηκαν και χειρουργικές επεμβάσεις, αναίμακτες ή μη, ενώ στα ιάματα των Κύρου και Ιωάννου και του Παντελεήμονα ουδέποτε παρατηρούμε χειρουργικές επεμβάσεις παρά μόνο αναίμακτους χειρισμούς, καθώς και υποδείξεις για τη λήψη διαφόρων ουσιών, όπως πόση εκχυλίσματος μυρσίνης με οίνο ή επάλειψη με πηλό ή πλύσιμο με χυλό μπιζελιών. Την κυριότερη ωστόσο κατηγορία των θεραπειών τους αποτελούν τα θαύματα, τα οποία στοχεύουν στη διάδοση του Χριστιανισμού, καθώς και στην εκτέλεση ευσεβών πράξεων.

Ιάματα Αγίων Αναργύρων

Τα ιάματα των Κοσμά και Δαμιανού ανήκουν στη δυάδα των εκ Μικράς Ασίας Αναργύρων και περιγράφονται στον κώδικα Edfu του Βρετανικού Μουσείου, με αριθμό 37534P7944 (Rupprecht 1935). Με τα ονόματα Κοσμάς και Δαμιανός, υπάρχουν τρεις συζυγίες Αγίων Αναργύρων, σύμφωνα με το Μέγα Συναξαριστή και την Ερμηνεία του Διονυσίου Εκ Φουρνά[2], οι οποίοι παριστάνονται ως «νέοι οξυγένειοι» οι Ρωμαίοι, «μελανοί αρχιγένειοι, έχοντες εις τα κεφάλια μανδήλα τυλιγμένα» οι Άραβες και «νέοι αρχιγένειοι» οι Ασιάτες (Νικόδημος Αγιορείτης, Τ. 1, 137–8).

Η πρώτη δυάδα των αδελφών Κοσμά και Δαμιανού, γεννήθηκε και έζησε επί αυτοκράτορα Καρίνου στη Ρώμη. Ήταν σπουδαίοι γιατροί και γιάτρευαν όχι μόνο ανθρώπους αλλά και ζώα χωρίς να λαμβάνουν αμοιβή παρά μόνο ζητούσαν από όσους γιάτρευαν να πιστέψουν στον Χριστό. Ο διδάσκαλός τους στην ιατρική και άλλοι συνάδελφοί τους, λόγω φθόνου, τους ανέβασαν σε ένα βουνό δήθεν για να μαζέψουν βότανα και εκεί τους λιθοβόλησαν το 284. Εορτάζουν την 1 Ιουλίου (Νικόδημος Αγιορείτης, Τ. 1, 138).

Η δεύτερη δυάδα των Αγίων Αναργύρων Κοσμά και Δαμιανού καταγόταν από την Αραβία. Μαζί με τα τρία αδέλφια τους, Άνθιμο, Ευπρέπιο και Λεόντιο, επισκέπτονταν πόλεις και χωριά, θεράπευαν αρρώστους και κήρυτταν την

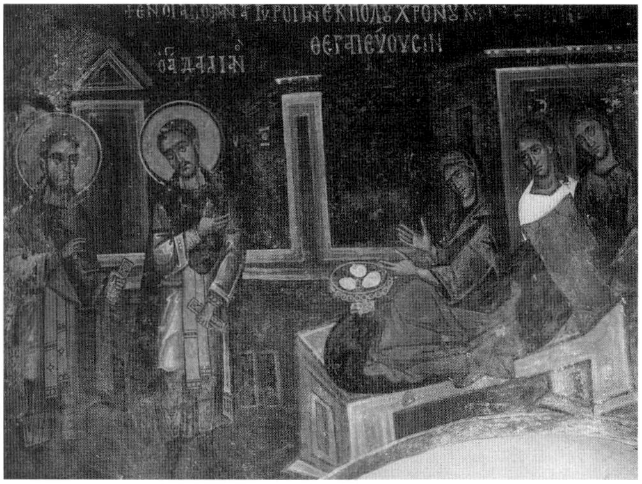

Εικ. 39.1. Μυστράς, Μητρόπολη Αγίου Δημητρίου. Διακονικό. Η θεραπεία της Παλλαδίας (Χατζηδάκης 1977–79, πίν. 40β)

πίστη του Χριστού. Μετά από βασανιστήρια αποκεφαλιστήκαν και τα πέντε αδέλφια μαζί το 292 επί Διοκλητιανού, στην πόλη Αιγαίς της Λυκίας. Εορτάζουν στις 17 Οκτωβρίου (Νικόδημος Αγιορείτης, Τ. 1, 138).

Η τρίτη δυάδα γεννήθηκε στη Μικρά Ασία. Μητέρα τους ήταν η Θεοδότη. Πέθαναν εν ειρήνη, πρώτα ο νεότερος αδελφός Δαμιανός και λίγες μέρες αργότερα ακολούθησε και ο Κοσμάς. Τάφηκαν και οι δύο στην πόλη Φερεμάν της Ασίας. Μετά τον θάνατό τους συνέχισαν να γίνονται πολλά θαύματα στον ανεγερθέντα στη μνήμη τους ναό. Εορτάζουν την 1η Νοεμβρίου (Νικόδημος Αγιορείτης, Τ. 1, 137–8, 180).

Από ιατρικής πλευράς ενδιαφέρον παρουσιάζουν τα ιάματα στα οποία συστήθηκε από τους αγίους διαιτητική ή φαρμακευτική θεραπεία ή έστω και εικονική επέμβαση (Τούλ 1975–1976, 265). Δύο είναι τα ιάματα των αγίων εν ζωή. Τα υπόλοιπα πραγματοποιούνταν στο ναό τους ή στον τάφο τους έπειτα από όραμα ή όνειρο κατά την εγκοίμηση των ασθενών.

Ιάματα στα οποία δεν αναφέρεται ο τρόπος θεραπείας

Στην κατηγορία αυτή ανήκει η θεραπεία της Παλλαδίας η οποία υπέφερε από ημιτριταίο (ο επανερχόμενος κάθε 2 ημέρες και μισή πυρετός). Το θαύμα αυτό έγινε εν ζωή των δύο Αγίων χωρίς ωστόσο να περιγράφεται ο τρόπος θεραπείας (Rupprecht 1935, 6–7) .

Εικονίζεται στον κύκλο θαυμάτων των αγίων Κοσμά και Δαμιανού στο διακονικό της Μητρόπολης του Αγίου Δημητρίου στο Μυστρά (Εικ. 39.1). Στην τοιχογραφία που χρονολογείται στα 1272–1288[3] απεικονίζεται η στιγμή που η θεραπευμένη Παλλαδία προσφέρει σε ένδειξη ευγνωμοσύνης και ως ελάχιστο δώρο για τη θεραπεία της τρία ωά (αυγά) στον νεότερο αδελφό Δαμιανό.[4] Η αποδοχή των αυγών, προκάλεσε ρήξη ανάμεσα στα δύο αδέλφια διότι, κατά τον μεγαλύτερο αδελφό Κοσμά, ο Δαμιανός υπέπεσε στο μεγάλο αμάρτημα της φιλαργυρίας, πολύ δε περισσότερο γιατί παρέβη τη ρητή συμφωνία τους να μη λαμβάνουν ποτέ δώρα για τη θεραπεία ασθενών.

Το ίδιο θαύμα απεικονίζεται και στο φύλλο 197^{α} στο τέταρτο διάχωρο της ολοσέλιδης μικρογραφίας του ευαγγελισταρίου της μονής Παντελεήμονος στο Άγιον Όρος (Εικ. 39.2). Η ολοσέλιδη μικρογραφία χωρίζεται με ταινίες σε τέσσερα διάχωρα, στο καθένα εικονίζεται μία σκηνή από τον κύκλο θαυμάτων των αγίων Αναργύρων. Ο κώδικας είναι από περγαμηνή. Χρονολογείται στον 12° αιώνα και είναι από τα πιο αξιόλογα ευαγγελιστάρια του Αγίου Όρους (Πελεκανίδης κ. ά., 1975, 349–51, εικ. 278).

Η ίδια σκηνή παριστάνεται στο τελευταίο διάχωρο στα δεξιά, στην αμφιπρόσωπη εικόνα των αγίων Αναργύρων στο Βυζαντινό Μουσείο της Καστοριάς, η οποία χρονολογείται στο τέλος του $12^{ου}$ – αρχές του $13^{ου}$ αιώνα (Τσιγαρίδας 2002, 6, εικ. 3· Κακαβάς 1996, 6). Παρόλη την κακή κατάσταση διατήρησης της εικόνας στην κύρια όψη εικονίζονται οι θεραπευτές άγιοι με δώδεκα σκηνές του βίου τους. Η εικόνα ήταν λατρευτική του βυζαντινού ναού των Αγίων Αναργύρων.

Το δεύτερο θαύμα έγινε εν ζωή ενός εκ των δύο αγίων και συγκεκριμένα του Κοσμά. Αφορά στην ίαση του κατάγματος της ομιλούσης καμήλου χωρίς να αναφέρεται αν έγινε εκ θαύματος ή εφαρμογής ιατρικών μεθόδων (Rupprecht 1935, 9). Στην εικόνα της Καστοριάς η ίαση της καμήλου (η οποία είπε ότι είναι θέλημα θεού να ταφούν στο ίδιο μέρος τα δύο αδέλφια, στον τόπο που καλείται Φερεμάν) απεικονίζεται στο κάτω διάχωρο αριστερά (Τσιγαρίδας 2002, 6, εικ. 3· Κακαβάς 1996, 6).

Ασθένειες στις οποίες συστήθηκε ως θεραπεία διαιτητική αγωγή

Σε δύο αιμοπτύσεις (στο 9° και 29° θαύμα) οι άγιοι συνέστησαν σε όνειρο στον μεν πρώτο ασθενή να σταματήσει να τρώει όρνιθες και να κάνει δίαιτα με λάχανα και ψωμί και να τηρεί τις νηστείες (Rupprecht 1935, 25–6), ενώ στον δεύτερο, που ήταν και ο ίδιος ιατρός και παρόλο που είχε εφαρμόσει τις μεθόδους του Γαληνού και του Ιπποκράτη δεν είχε θεραπευτεί, του συνέστησαν να φάει χονδροκοπανισμένο σιτάρι και να κάνει εντριβές στο στήθος με θερμό λάδι (Rupprecht 1935, 49–50). Στο 42° θαύμα, όπου η πάθηση αναγράφεται ως σπληνική, προς ανακούφιση των συμπτωμάτων της ασθένειας, δηλαδή των γαστρικών πόνων και της δύσπνοιας, οι άγιοι συνέστησαν εντριβές με θυμίαμα και αποχή από τα όσπρια (Rupprecht 1935, 68–70).

Ασθένειες που θεραπεύτηκαν με χειρουργικές επεμβάσεις

Το 5° θαύμα του βίου τους αναφέρεται στη θεραπεία του υδρωπικού. Ο ασθενής αφού ανέμενε στο ναό μάταια για καιρό την εμφάνιση των αγίων αποφάσισε να επιστρέψει σπίτι του και μεταφέρθηκε με φορείο στην παραλία όπου ανέμενε το πλοίο. Οι άγιοι εμφανίστηκαν υπό τη μορφή διαβατών και αφού τον επέπληξαν για την ολιγοπιστία του, τον έπεισαν να επιστρέψει στο ναό, όπου οι ίδιοι τον μετέφεραν με φορείο. Τη νύχτα εμφανίστηκαν ξανά και πραγματοποίησαν βαθιά τομή στην κοιλιά του αρρώστου, απ' όπου έτρεξε πολύ δυσώδες υγρό, ενώ την επόμενη μέρα έφεραν κηρωτή για την επούλωση του τραύματος (Rupprecht 1935, 17–20). Το θαύμα εικονίζεται στην εικόνα της Καστοριάς στη ζώνη αριστερά (Τσιγαρίδας 2002, 6, εικ. 3· Κακαβάς 1996, 6), καθώς και στην ολοσέλιδη μικρογραφία, στο διάχωρο πάνω δεξιά, του ευαγγελισταρίου της μονής Παντελεήμονος (Πελεκανίδης κ. ά, 1975, 351, εικ. 278) (Εικ. 39.2).

Στο 37° θαύμα η ασθενής έπασχε από απόστημα στο μαστό. Ο γιατρός που την επισκέφθηκε συνέστησε διάνοιξη, η ίδια όμως επειδή φοβήθηκε την επέμβαση κατέφυγε στο ναό των αγίων. Σε όραμα οι άγιοι εμφανίστηκαν ταυτόχρονα και στην ασθενή και στον γιατρό. Στην πρώτη περιχάραξαν με το δάκτυλο το απόστημα και έκαναν το σημείο του σταυρού, ενώ στον γιατρό υπέδειξαν ποιο φάρμακο να επιθέσει. Ο γιατρός την επόμενη μέρα, αφού γύμνωσε το μαστό, είδε την τομή που έκαναν οι άγιοι και επέθεσε το φάρμακο που του είχαν υποδείξει (Rupprecht 1935, 61–2).

Στο 34° θαύμα, σε γυναίκα που είχε απόστημα στη γνάθο οι άγιοι, αφού εμφανιστήκαν στο όνειρό της, τη διέταξαν να ανοίξει το στόμα και με τα δάκτυλα πέτυχαν να σπάσουν το απόστημα. Την επόμενη νύχτα εμφανίστηκαν ξανά και επέθεσαν στην κλίνη της κηρωτή για να επουλωθεί η πληγή (Rupprecht 1935, 57–9).

Στο 23° θαύμα ο ασθενής μετά από πτώση από άλογο έσπασε το πόδι στην κνήμη. Οι γιατροί που κλήθηκαν να τον θεραπεύσουν έδεσαν το πόδι του με καλάμια και του έδωσαν ως φάρμακο κηρωτή έπειτα από επιθυμία του ασθενούς. Τη νύχτα φάνηκαν οι άγιοι στον ύπνο του, έλυσαν εν μέρει την επίδεση με τα καλάμια και του ανήγγειλαν ότι θα επανέλθουν μετά από τρεις μέρες. Οι γιατροί που τον παρακολουθούσαν αποσύρθηκαν μετά την ανάμειξη των αγίων. Μετά την πάροδο τριών ημερών οι άγιοι επανήλθαν, τον βοήθησαν να σηκωθεί και με τον τρόπο αυτό θεραπεύτηκε (Rupprecht 1935, 34–6).

Κηρωτή

Σε πολλά ιάματα οι άγιοι χορηγούσαν ως θεραπεία την κηρωτή, που όπως συνάγουμε από την περιγραφή της, ήταν είδος εμπλάστρου που κατασκευάζονταν από τα αναμμένα

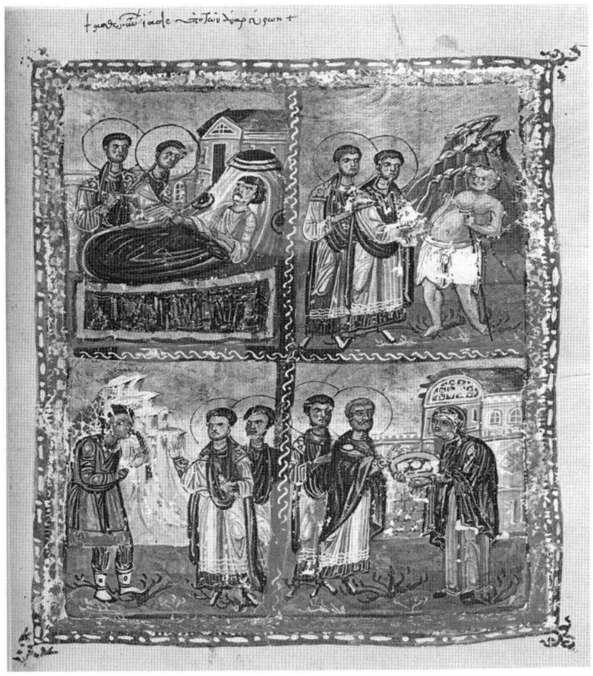

Εικ. 39.2. Άγιο Όρος. Μονή Παντελεήμονος: Ευαγγελιστάριο 12^{ου} αι., Φύλλο 197^{α} (Πελεκανίδης, Χρήστου, Μαυροπούλου-Τσιούμη και Καδά 1975, εικ. 278)

κεριά του ναού. Η εν λόγω αγωγή δόθηκε στη θεραπεία οφθαλμολογικών παθήσεων, στη θεραπεία χειρουργικών τομών, σε αποστήματα γνάθου, σε κατάγματα κνήμης.

Ιάματα που έγιναν με θαυματουργικό τρόπο

Στη θεραπεία της υδρωπικής στο 24° θαύμα οι άγιοι βγήκαν από την εικόνα στην οποία απεικονίζονταν και τη θεράπευσαν αγγίζοντας την κοιλιά της (Rupprecht 1935, 37–40).

Στο θαύμα του γεωργού που κατά τη διάρκεια του θερισμού κοιμήθηκε τις μεσημβρινές ώρες στη σκιά δέντρου και χωρίς να το αντιληφθεί όφις εισήλθε στο στόμα του κατά τη διάρκεια του ύπνου. Το φίδι άρχισε να μετακινείται στο στομάχι του και να τον σπαράζει. Ο γεωργός κατέφυγε στο ναό των αγίων, όπου οι άγιοι εμφανίστηκαν σε όραμα το ίδιο βράδυ και διέταξαν το φίδι να εξέλθει από το στομάχι του γεωργού (Rupprecht 1935, 10–2). Το εν λόγω θαύμα εικονίζεται στον κύκλο θαυμάτων των αγίων Κοσμά και Δαμιανού στο διακονικό της Μητρόπολης του Αγίου Δημητρίου στο Μυστρά (Rupprecht 1935, υποσημείωση 9) (Εικ. 39.3), καθώς και στο τρίτο διάχωρο της ολοδέλιδης μικρογραφίας του ευαγγελισταρίου της μονής Παντελεήμονος (Πελεκανίδης κ. ά., 1975, 351, εικ. 278) (Εικ. 39.2).

Στο θαύμα που επιγράφεται ως «Περί του ξηρά έχοντος την χείρα» και το οποίο εικονίζεται στο πρώτο διάχωρο της μικρογραφίας του ευαγγελισταρίου (εικ. 39.2), η θεραπεία

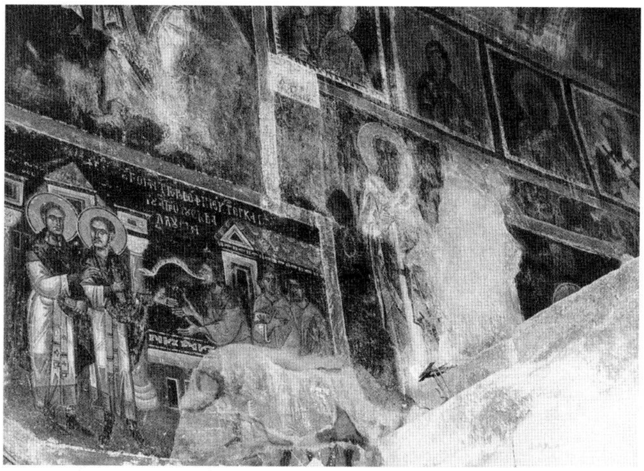

Εικ. 39.3. Μυστράς, Μητρόπολη Αγίου Δημητρίου. Διακονικό. Η θεραπεία του γεωργού (Μαρίνου 2002, πίν. 13α, 63β)

εικονίζεται να πραγματοποιείται από τους ίδιους τους αγίους ενώ στον κώδικα η θεραπεία πραγματοποιείται από ζώο και συγκεκριμένα ελάφι (Rupprecht 1935, 24), ίσως κατά αντιστοιχία ή σε ανάμνηση των θεραπειών υπό των ιερών ζώων του Ασκληπιού.

Ιάματα Κύρου και Ιωάννη

Για την καταγραφή των θαυμάτων βασιστήκαμε στην περιγραφή του βίου τους από τον Σωφρώνιο. Ο Σωφρόνιος γεννήθηκε στη Δαμασκό περί το 550 και ήταν μοναχός. Επισκέφθηκε την Αίγυπτο επί πατριάρχου Ιωάννου του Ελεήμονος, όπου και πιθανόν έγραψε τα ιάματα των αγίων περί το 615. Συνολικά περιγράφει 70 ιάσεις.

Σε όλα τα ιάματα που περιγράφει ο Σωφρόνιος δεν παραλείπει να τονίσει την αποτυχία των γιατρών και να εξάρει τα θεαματικά αποτελέσματα των θαυματουργικών ιαμάτων των αγίων ενώ συγχρόνως τονίζει ότι προϋπόθεση για κάθε θεραπεία αποτελεί η πίστη του ασθενούς. Η έλλειψη αυτής τιμωρείται από τους θεραπευτές αγίους, όπως στο θαύμα 29, όπου οι άγιοι έστειλαν στη δυσπιστούσα Αλεξανδρινή τον τιμωρό ψύλλο (Σωφρόνιος Μοναχός, *PG* CXIV, στ. 3512).

Ο Κύρος ήταν ιατρός στο επάγγελμα και καταγόταν από την Αλεξάνδρεια (Σωφρόνιος Μοναχός, *PG* CXIV, στ. 1232), ενώ ο Ιωάννης ήταν στρατιωτικός και καταγόταν από την Έδεσσα της Μεσοποταμίας (Σωφρόνιος Μοναχός, *PG* CXIV, στ. 1240). Ο Κύρος θεράπευε ανιδιοτελώς τους αρρώστους και είχε μεγάλη φήμη. Κατά τους διωγμούς του Διοκλητιανού κατέφυγε σε μοναστήρι στον Αραβικό κόλπο. Ακούγοντας για το σπουδαίο έργο του ο Ιωάννης εγκατέλειψε τη στρατιωτική σταδιοδρομία, έγινε στενός συνεργάτης του και τον βοηθούσε στο ιατρικό και φιλανθρωπικό του έργο. Βασανίστηκαν και οι δύο και αποκεφαλίστηκαν όταν θέλησαν να συνδράμουν στη φυλακή την Αγία Αθανασία και τις τρεις κόρες της (Νικόδημος Αγιορείτης, Τ. 1, 434 και Τ. 2, 229· Σωφρόνιος Μοναχός, *PG* CXIV, στ. 1240–5), επί Διοκλητιανού περί το 292. Η μνήμη τους εορτάζεται στις 31 Ιανουαρίου.

Θαύματα στα οποία η θεραπεία συνίστατο σε καταπλάσματα

Στο 1° θαύμα του βίου ο νεαρός Αμμώνιος έπασχε από χοιράδες στον τράχηλο (εξογκώματα και σκλήρυνση των αδένων του τραχήλου). Προσέπεσε στο μνήμα των αγίων, οι οποίοι του συνέστησαν με όραμα να επιθέσει στον τράχηλο κατάπλασμα από κηρωτή αναμεμειγμένο με άρτο. Μετά από λίγες ημέρες οι χοιράδες κατέπεσαν μπροστά στο μνήμα των αγίων (Σωφρόνιος Μοναχός, *PG* CXIV, στ. 3424–5).

Στο 6° θαύμα ο Γεδδαίος έπασχε από συρίγγιον στους βουβώνες. Προσήλθε στο ναό και σε όραμα άκουσε από τους αγίους τη θεραπεία που έπρεπε να ακολουθήσει: να φτιάξει κατάπλασμα από σουσάμι, μέλι και άρτο. Μετά την εφαρμογή της θεραπείας η σύριγξ ανεπήδησε (Σωφρόνιος Μοναχός, *PG* CXIV, στ. 3433–6).

Στο 13° θαύμα στον πάσχοντα από λέπρα Ηλία δόθηκε με όνειρο η εντολή από τους αγίους να επαλείψει ολόκληρο το σώμα του με κοπριά από τη τέταρτη καμήλα ενός καραβανιού. Ο ασθενής ακολούθησε την εντολή αλλά παρέλειψε λόγω απέχθειας να αλείψει το πρόσωπό του. Η λέπρα θεραπεύτηκε αλλά παρέμειναν τα στίγματα στο πρόσωπό του (Σωφρόνιος Μοναχός, *PG* CXIV, στ. 3461–5).

Μητρορραγία

Στο 25° θαύμα στην άρρωστη συστήθηκε από τους αγίους με όραμα ως θεραπεία η πόση εκχυλίσματος μυρσίνης με οίνο (Σωφρόνιος Μοναχός, *PG* CXIV, στ. 3496).

Θεραπεία υδρωπικών (συλλογή υγρού στην κοιλιά)

Ο Σωφρόνιος απέδιδε την αρρώστια σε υπερβολική υδατοποσία. Στο 42° θαύμα η θεραπεία του αρρώστου επήλθε σε όραμα με απλό άγγιγμα της κοιλιάς από τους αγίους. Την επομένη αισθάνθηκε την ανάγκη να αφοδεύσει και απέβαλε τα υγρά (Σωφρόνιος Μοναχός, *PG* CXIV, στ. 3584–5).

Στο 20° θαύμα στην ασθενή που είχε πρηστεί σε όλο της το σώμα και δεν εύρισκε γιατρειά από τους άλλους γιατρούς, οι άγιοι σε όνειρο της αποκάλυψαν τον τρόπο θεραπεία της:

να αλειφθεί σε όλο της το σώμα με νερό από την πηγή κοντά στο ναό και στη συνέχεια να καλυφθεί με παξιμάδι. Το κατάπλασμα με το παξιμάδι αφού ξεράθηκε τράβηξε τα υγρά από το σώμα της και με τον τρόπο αυτό γιατρεύτηκε η πάσχουσα (Σωφρόνιος Μοναχός, *PG* CXIV, στ. 3480–1).

Στον υδρωπικό ασθενή του 66° θαύματος οι άγιοι συνέστησαν ως θεραπεία την κάλυψη ολόκληρου του σώματος με άμμο (Σωφρόνιος Μοναχός, *PG* CXIV, στ. 3649–52).

Θεραπεία τραυμάτων

Στο 9° ίαμα η ασθενής μετά από πτώση στα λουτρά τραυματίστηκε στον αγκώνα. Οι άγιοι μέσα από όραμα συνέστησαν να επιθέσει σ' αυτό κρέας από λαυράκι και οίνο (Σωφρόνιος Μοναχός, *PG* CXIV, στ. 3444–8).

Στο 3° ίαμα σε τραύμα που προήλθε από κάταγμα της κνήμης ύστερα από πτώση από κλίμακα, οι άγιοι συνέστησαν ως θεραπεία την αλοιφή του ποδιού με λάδι από την κανδήλα του ναού (Σωφρόνιος Μοναχός, *PG* CXIV, στ. 3429).

Στο 67° θαύμα ο νυχτοκόρακας έδρασε ως απεσταλμένος του διαβόλου. Φώλιασε στη στοά όπου διανυκτέρευε ο πάσχων και τον ρύπαινε με ακαθαρσίες. Αν και ο ασθενής μετέφερε πολλές φορές σε άλλα σημεία την κλίνη του, ο νυχτοκόρακας τον ακολουθούσε και απελπισμένος ο ασθενής αυτοσφαγιάσθηκε. Οι άγιοι εμφανίστηκαν και μαστίγωσαν τον υπηρέτη επειδή προσέφυγε σε βοήθεια γιατρού για να συρράψει το τραύμα, και τον θεράπευσαν με επαλείψεις ελαίου και οίνου ενώ εσωτερικά του τραύματος έθεσαν αλόη (Σωφρόνιος Μοναχός, *PG* CXIV, στ. 3652–6·, Τούλ 1975–1976, 282 κ. ε.).

Θεραπεία δαιμόνων

Στον μανιακό που είχε καταληφθεί από δαιμόνια στο 57° θαύμα οι άγιοι συνέστησαν ως θεραπεία την επάλειψη με κονιορτοποιημένο ψητό κρέας μόσχου αναμεμειγμένο με οίνο προς εντριβή του πάσχοντα (Σωφρόνιος Μοναχός, *PG* CXIV, στ. 3628–9), ενώ στο 54° θαύμα σε επιληπτικό δαιμονιόπληκτο παιδί συνέστησαν στη μητέρα του με όραμα να το επαλείψει με χοιρινό λίπος (Σωφρόνιος Μοναχός, *PG* CXIV, στ. 3621–5).

Θεραπεία Μαγείας

Το 35° θαύμα αφορά σε ειδική περίπτωση μαγείας, τον κατάδεσμο, και ο ασθενής είχε παραλύσει και στα τέσσερα άκρα. Μετά από επίκληση των αγίων στο ναό τους του φανέρωσαν με όραμα να μισθώσει έναν ψαρά. Ο ασθενής το έκανε και ο ψαράς έπιασε στα δίχτυα ένα κιβώτιο, το οποίο άνοιξε ο οικονόμος του ναού. Εντός του βρήκε χάλκινο αγαλμάτιο με καθηλωμένα τα τέσσερα άκρα. Όταν ο οικονόμος αφαίρεσε από το άγαλμα τα καρφιά ο ασθενής θεραπεύτηκε (Σωφρόνιος Μοναχός, *PG* CXIV, στ. 3541–5).

Σκώληκες

Ο Σωφρόνιος αποδίδει πολλά νοσήματα σε σκώληκες οι οποίοι εισχωρούν στο σώμα, στο στομάχι, στα έντερα, στο κεφάλι, και οι οποίοι αποστέλλονται από το διάβολο προς βασανισμό των ανθρώπων.

Στο 18° ίαμα ο ασθενής έπασχε από κεφαλαλγίες και εμβοές. Οι άγιοι με όραμα τον διέταξαν να πάει στο δημόσιο δρόμο και να ραπίσει τον πρώτο διερχόμενο. Πράγματι το έκανε, αλλά αυτός ήταν στρατιώτης και χτύπησε τον ασθενή στο κεφάλι με ραβδί. Από το τραύμα εξήλθε πλήθος σκωλήκων και με τον τρόπο αυτό γιατρεύτηκε (Σωφρόνιος Μοναχός, *PG* CXIV, στ. 3476–7).

Στο 4° θαύμα η αιτία των αιμοπτύσεων αποδίδεται σε σκώληκα ο οποίος κατέτρωγε τον πνεύμονα του ασθενούς. Αφού έφαγε κίτρο κατ' εντολή των αγίων απέβαλε με εμετό το σκουλήκι και θεραπεύτηκε (Σωφρόνιος Μοναχός, *PG* CXIV, στ. 3432).

Σε γυναίκα που υπέφερε από κοιλιακούς πόνους εμφανίστηκαν οι άγιοι στον ύπνο της, άνοιξαν το στόμα της και φύσηξαν εντός της τρεις φορές. Την επόμενη ημέρα η άρρωστη αισθάνθηκε την ανάγκη εκκένωσης, κατά την οποία απέβαλε τον σκώληκα και θεραπεύτηκε (Σωφρόνιος Μοναχός, *PG* CXIV στ. 3481–4).

Ιάματα Αγίου Παντελεήμονα

Ο άγιος Παντελεήμων καταγόταν από τη Νικομήδεια. Το αρχικό του όνομα ήταν Παντολέων και μετονομάστηκε λόγω της φιλανθρωπικής του δράσης σε Παντελεήμονα (Συμεών Λογοθέτης, *PG* CXV, στ. 476). Σπούδασε ιατρική κοντά στο γιατρό Ευφρόσυνο και διδάχθηκε τον χριστιανισμό από τον ιερέα Ερμόλαο (Νικόδημος Αγιορείτης, Τ. 2, 284). Μοίρασε την περιουσία του σε φτωχούς και φυλακισμένους, απελευθέρωσε τους δούλους του και γιάτρευε αρρώστους δωρεάν. Λόγω της φήμης του και της θεραπείας τυφλού προκάλεσε το φθόνο των συναδέλφων του, οι οποίοι τον συκοφάντησαν στον αυτοκράτορα Μαξιμιανό. Επειδή δεν απαρνήθηκε την πίστη του, βασανίστηκε και αποκεφαλίστηκε το 306 μαζί με τους δασκάλους του αγίους Ερμόλαο, Έρμιππο και Ερμοκράτη (Νικόδημος Αγιορείτης, Τ. 2, 277). Από αυτούς ο Ερμόλαος, αν και ιερέας, λογίζεται στους αγίους Αναργύρους. Ο Παντελεήμων συγκαταλέγεται ανάμεσα στους σπουδαιότερους ιαματικούς αγίους του Βυζαντίου. Η μνήμη του εορτάζεται στις 27 Ιουλίου.

Στο βίο του αγίου Παντελεήμονα από τον Συμεών το Μεταφραστή περιγράφονται τρεις ιάσεις εν ζωή του αγίου, οι οποίες και πραγματοποιήθηκαν με θαυματουργικό τρόπο μετά από επίκληση του Χριστού. Η πρώτη αφορά στην ανάσταση του νεκρού παιδιού που το είχε τσιμπήσει έχιδνα.

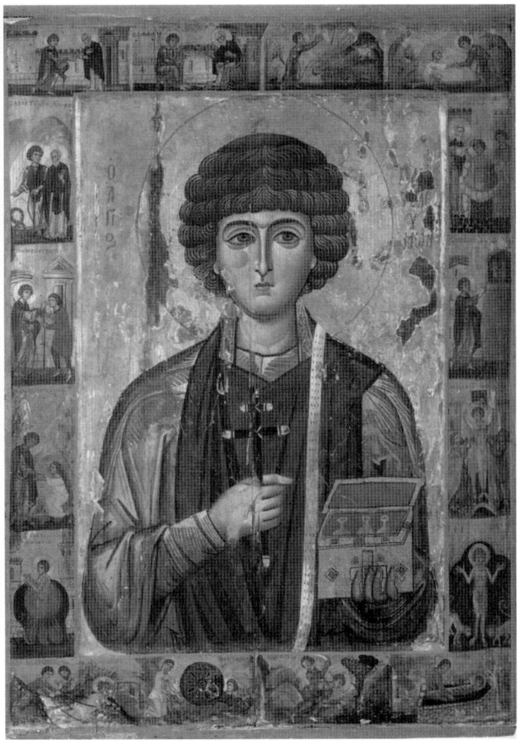

Εικ. 39.4. Σινά. Φορητή εικόνα του αγίου Παντελεήμονα με σκηνές του βίου του (αρχές 13ου αι.) (Thomas 1997, 378, fig. 249)

Ο Παντελεήμων προσευχήθηκε στο Χριστό και το παιδί αναστήθηκε ενώ το φίδι χάθηκε. Το δε θαύμα αυτό αποτέλεσε και την αιτία για να ασπαστεί τον χριστιανισμό που του δίδασκε ο δάσκαλός του Ερμόλαος (Συμεών Λογοθέτης, *PG* CXV, στ. 452· Συμεών Μεταφραστής 1805, 305). Το δεύτερο θαύμα αναφέρεται στη θεραπεία του τυφλού, τον οποίον δεν μπόρεσε να θεραπεύσει ούτε ο διδάσκαλος του στην ιατρική Ευφρόσυνος. Ο Παντελεήμων τον θεράπευσε ακουμπώντας το δεξί του χέρι στους οφθαλμούς του σχηματίζοντας το σημείο του σταυρού (Συμεών Λογοθέτης, *PG* CXV, στ. 456· Συμεών Μεταφραστής 1805, 306). Το τρίτο θαύμα αναφέρεται στην ίαση του παραλυτικού τον οποίο γιάτρεψε ο Παντελεήμων μετά από επίκληση στο Θεό μπροστά στο βασιλιά Μαξιμιανό (Συμεών Λογοθέτης, *PG* CXV, στ. 461· Συμεών Μεταφραστής 1805, 309).

Και τα τρία θαύματα απεικονίζονται στη φορητή εικόνα από το Σινά, που χρονολογείται στις αρχές του 13ου αιώνα (Εικ. 39.4). Στο κέντρο απεικονίζεται μετωπικός- στηθαίος ο άγιος Παντελεήμονας, ενώ την κεντρική παράσταση του αγίου περιβάλλουν 16 σκηνές του βίου του. Μεταξύ αυτών η ανάσταση του νεκρού παιδιού απεικονίζεται σε δύο σκηνές στην άνω ζώνη, ενώ η θεραπεία του τυφλού και του παραλυτικού απεικονίζονται σε δύο διάχωρα στη ζώνη στην αριστερή πλευρά της εικόνας (Thomas 1997, 379, fig. 249).

Ιάματα Σαμψών

Ο Σαμψών έζησε επί εποχής Ιουστινιανού Α΄ (527–565). Ήταν Ρωμαίος ευγενής που είχε σπουδάσει την ιατρική και την ασκούσε δωρεάν (Συμεών Λογοθέτης *PG* CXV, στ. 280–1). Τον 6° αιώνα πήγε στην Κωνσταντινούπολη όπου χειροτονήθηκε ιερέας. Ανεπαύθη εν ειρήνη σε μεγάλη ηλικία και η μνήμη του εορτάζεται στις 27 Ιουνίου.

Στον βίο του από τον Συμεών τον Μεταφραστή περιγράφεται η ίαση του αυτοκράτορα Ιουστινιανού στα πρώτα χρόνια της βασιλείας του, με terminus ante quem τις εργασίες ανοικοδόμησης της Αγίας Σοφίας (Συμεών Λογοθέτης *PG* CXV, στ. 289). Ο Σαμψών θεράπευσε τον αυτοκράτορα από ασθένεια στο υπογάστριο, που του είχε προκαλέσει πρήξιμο στην κοιλιά και στα αιδοία (Συμεών Λογοθέτης *PG* CXV, στ. 284), με απλό άγγιγμα και για να αποφύγει τον έπαινο ότι αυτός ήταν η αιτία της θεραπείας επάλειψε την περιοχή με αλοιφή από βότανα. Ο Ιουστινιανός για να τον ευχαριστήσει ανέγειρε μεγάλο ξενώνα, το ξενοδοχείο του Σαμψών, από τα πρώτα γνωστά νοσοκομεία, όπου περιέθαλπτε δωρεάν τους αρρώστους του (Συμεών Λογοθέτης *PG* CXV, στ. 289).

Οι υπόλοιπες ιάσεις που περιγράφονται στον βίο του πραγματοποιήθηκαν μετά θάνατον κατά την εγκοίμηση των ασθενών στο ναό ή στο ξενοδοχείο. Ο Θεοδώρητος, ο οποίος έσπασε το πόδι του μετά από πτώση από σκάλα, θεραπεύτηκε σε όραμα με απλό άγγιγμα του ποδιού από τον άγιο (Συμεών Λογοθέτης *PG* CXV, στ. 293–7). Η υδρωπική Ειρήνη, που υπηρετούσε στον ξενώνα, θεραπεύτηκε μετά από όραμα, στο οποίο εμφανίστηκαν οι άγιοι Ανάργυροι Κοσμάς και Δαμιανός και ο Σαμψών. Ο τελευταίος διέταξε τον ένα εκ των δύο να πραγματοποιήσουν τομή με ξυράφι, από την οποία βγήκε πολύ υγρό (Συμεών Λογοθέτης *PG* CXV, στ. 305–7).

Σε όλα τα ιάματα–θεραπείες, που πραγματοποιήθηκαν μετά θάνατον των αγίων, παρατηρήσαμε το κοινό στοιχείο της εγκοίμησης και την ίαση των ασθενών με την εμφάνιση των αγίων σε όραμα ή σε όνειρο και την αποκάλυψη του τρόπου θεραπείας τους ή την πραγματοποίησή της με θαυματουργικό τρόπο. Εγκοίμηση συνδέει τις ιάσεις-θαύματα των θεραπευτών αγίων με τον Ασκληπιό και την εγκοίμηση στα Ασκληπιεία.

Ενδεικτικά αναφέρουμε το Ασκληπιείο της Επιδαύρου – έδρα του θεού ιατρού της αρχαιότητας – το σημαντικότερο θεραπευτικό κέντρο όλου του ελληνικού και ρωμαϊκού κόσμου. Το ιερό του Ασκληπιού ήταν οργανωμένο γύρω από το ιερό φρέαρ (το οποίο αργότερα ενσωματώθηκε στη στοά του αβάτου και τον χώρο του κτηρίου Ε), όπου υπήρχε ο πρώτος βωμός τέφρας και ο χώρος των τελετουργικών γευμάτων. Το φρέαρ ήταν βασικό στοιχείο της ίασης που επιτυγχανόταν με τη διαδικασία της κάθαρσης.[5]

Στη σύνθετη στοά του αβάτου επιτυγχανόταν η ίαση του ασθενούς μέσω της εγκοίμησης και κατά συνέπεια μέσω της επαφής του με το θείο. Ο ασθενής αφού είχε εξαγνιστεί με νερό από το ιερό πηγάδι κοιμόταν στο έδαφος, σε επαφή με τη χθόνια κατοικία του θεού και ο θεός ο ίδιος ή τα ιερά ζώα του εμφανιζόταν στον ύπνο του και τον θεράπευαν ή του υποδείκνυαν τον τρόπο της θεραπείας του.[6]

Στο ιερό του Ασκληπιού στη νότια κλιτύ της Ακρόπολης, η μεγάλη στοά στο ανατολικό τμήμα του ιερού λειτουργούσε ως «εγκοιμητήριον», χώρο δηλαδή για την εγκοίμηση και τη θαυματουργική ίαση των ασθενών. Μετά την καταστροφή του στα τέλη του 5ου ή στις αρχές του 6ου αι. μ.Χ., ανεγέρθηκε στα ερείπιά του μία τρίκλιτη βασιλική αφιερωμένη στους αγίους Αναργύρους, τους αγίους θεραπευτές του χριστιανισμού[7], οι οποίοι πήραν τη θέση του Ασκληπιού.

Σημειώσεις

1 Ευχαριστώ θερμά τον καθηγητή κ. Στέφανο Γερουλάνο για τις χρήσιμες υποδείξεις του και τις γόνιμες παρατηρήσεις του.

2 Διονύσιος εκ Φουρνά 161, 270, 283. Για το θέμα των τριών συζυγιών των Αγίων Αναργύρων καθώς και την εικονογραφική τους απόδοση παράβαλε Ξυγγόπουλος 1965, 84 και εξής.

3 Millet 1910, pl. 74, 2· Dufrenne 1970, 60, pl. 7, 8· Χατζηδάκης 1977–1979, 144, 158· Χατζηδάκης 2000, 35· Μαρίνου 2002, 95–6, όπου υποστηρίζεται ότι ο χώρος του διακονικού δεν κατείχε αυτή τη θέση, αλλά ενός παρεκκλησίου αφιερωμένου στη λατρεία των θεραπευτών αγίων, καθώς και στη δέηση για τη θεραπεία των ασθενούντων. Η λειτουργία αυτή άλλωστε σχετίζεται με τον ρόλο των μητροπόλεων και των επισκοπών ως κέντρων περίθαλψης των πιστών.

4 Τα αυγά που προσέφερε η Παλλαδία σχετίζονται κατά τη γνώμη μας, όχι μόνο με τον συμβολισμό του αυγού ως αναγέννηση της γης, του εύθραυστου κόσμου, της ζωής, αλλά και την αναγέννηση του ανθρώπου, και συγκεκριμένα την αναγέννηση της ιδίας της Παλλαδίας, μετά από θεραπεία της ασθένειάς της από τους αγίους Αναργύρους.

5 Το νερό ως στοιχείο της ίασης απαντά και στα θαύματα των Κύρου και Ιωάννου όπως λ.χ., στη θεραπεία της υδρωπικής στο 20° θαύμα. Στην Κύπρο μία από τις πιο σημαντικές πηγές με ιαματικό νερό βρίσκεται στην Πάφο, στο μοναστήρι των αγίων Αναργύρων Κοσμά και Δαμιανού, ενώ σύμφωνα με την τοπική παράδοση οι δύο άγιοι έζησαν και έδρασαν στην περιοχή αυτή, βλ. Egoumenidou και Michaelides 2008, 146–9.

6 Ψυχογιού Όλγα, 'Αρχαιολογικός Χώρος Ασκληπιείου Επιδαύρου', βλ. http/Υπουργείο Πολιτισμού/ Οδυσσέας/ Αρχαιολογικός Χώρος Ασκληπιείου Επιδαύρου, όπως στις 22/8/2008.

7 Πλάτων 1964, 21–37· Travlos 1971, 127–37· Aleshire 1989· Κασαπόγλου Έφη, 'Ασκληπιείο', βλ. http/Υπουργείο Πολιτισμού/Οδυσσέας/ Ασκληπιείο, όπως στις 22/8/2008.

Βιβλιογραφία

Aleshire, S. B. 1989: *The Athenian Asklepieion*, Amsterdam.

Διονύσιος ὁ ἐκ Φουρνᾶ, *Ἑρμηνεία τῆς ζωγραφικῆς τέχνης καὶ αἱ κύριαι αὐτῆς πηγαί, Ἐκδιδομένη μετὰ προλόγου νῦν τὸ πρῶτον πλήρης κατὰ τὸ πρωτότυπον αὐτῆς κείμενον ὑπὸ* Ἀ. Παπαδοπούλου-Κεραμέως, ἐν Πετρουπόλει, 1909.

Dufrenne, S. 1970: *Les Programmes iconographiques des Églises Byzantines de Mistra*, Paris.

Egoumenidou, E. and Michaelides, D. 2008: 'The exploitation of mineral springs in Cyprus during British rule (1879–1960): dreams unfulfilled', 133–56 in P. Lysaght (ed.), *Sanitas per Aquas, Spas, Lifistyles and Foodways, Proceedings of the 16th Conference of the International Commission for Ethnological Food Research, Innsbruck, Austria, and Meran(o), Italy, 25 September–1 October 2006*, Innsbruck.

Κακαβάς, Γ. 1996: *Βυζαντινό Μουσείο Καστοριάς*, Αθήνα.

Μαρίνου, Γ. 2002: *Άγιος Δημήτριος. Η Μητρόπολη του Μυστρά*, Αθήνα.

Millet, G. 1910: *Monuments byzantins de Mistra*, Paris.

Νικοδήμου Αγιορείτου, *Συναξαριστής των Δώδεκα μηνών του ενιαυτού*, Τόμος Α΄ και Β΄. Ανετυπώθη υπό του Εκδοτικού Οίκου Κων. Χ. Σπανού, Αθήνησι (χ.χ.).

Ξυγγόπουλος, Α. 1965: «Το ανάγλυφον των αγίων Αναργύρων εις τον Άγιον Μάρκον της Βενετίας», *Αρχαιολογικόν Δελτίον* 20, 84–95.

Πελεκανίδης, Στ., Χρήστου, Π., Μαυροπούλου-Τσιούμη, Χρ. και Καδά, Σ. (επιμ.) 1975: *Οι θησαυροί του Αγίου Όρους*, Τόμος Β΄, Αθήνα.

PG: J.-P. Migne, *Patrologia Graeca,* Paris 1857–1858.

Πλάτων, Ν. 1964: «ΙΙ. Εργασίαι διαμορφώσεως και τακτοποιήσεως του αρχαιολογικού χώρου Ακροπόλεως», *Αρχαιολογικόν Δελτίον* 12, B_1 *Χρονικά*, 21–37.

Rupprecht, E. (ed.) 1935: *Cosmae et Damiani sanctorum medicorum, vitam et miracula e codice Londinesi* (Neue Deutsche Forschungen 20), Berlin.

Συμεὼν ὁ Μεταφραστής, *Ἐκλόγιον, τουτέστιν οἱ ὡραιότεροι βίοι τῶν ἁγίων*, Βενετία 1805.

Thomas, T. 1997: 'Christians in the Islamic East', 364–401 in H. C. Evans and W. D. Wixom (eds), *The Glory of Byzantium, Art and Culture of the Middle Byzantine Era, A.D. 843–1261*, New York.

Τουλ, Χ. 1975–76: «Τα ιάματα των Αγίων Αναργύρων», *Επετηρίς Εταιρείας Βυζαντινών Σπουδών*, ΜΒ΄, 253–97.

Travlos, I. 1971: *Pictorial Dictionary of Ancient Athens*, London.

Τσιγαρίδας, Ε. 2002: *Βυζαντινό Μουσείο Καστοριάς. Βυζαντινές και μεταβυζαντινές εικόνες*, Αθήνα.

Χατζηδάκης, Μ. 1977–1979: «Νεώτερα για την ιστορία και την τέχνη της Μητρόπολης του Μυστρά», *Δελτίον της Χριστιανικής Αρχαιολογικής Εταιρείας Θ΄*, 143–75.

Χατζηδάκης, Μ. 2000: *Μυστράς. Η μεσαιωνική πολιτεία και το κάστρο*, Αθήνα.

Part IX

Byzantine, Arab and Medieval Sources

40. The Role of the Egyptian Sea and Land Routes in the Justinian Plague: the Case of Pelusium

Costas Tsiamis, Effie Poulakou-Rebelakou and George Androutsos

The aim of our study is to present the sea and land commercial routes of Byzantine Egypt and their role in the dissemination of the plague bacterium Yersinia pestis *from the Red Sea to the Mediterranean ports. Independently of the fact that the Mediterranean port of Pelusium was the starting point of the first plague pandemic, according to the historical, archaeological and epidemiological data, the port of Clysma in the Red Sea can be assumed as a possible entrance gate of* Yersinia pestis.

Introduction

The narration of the Justinian plague (6th century AD) by contemporary Byzantine historians and chronicle writers highlights an important historical and epidemiological question: *where was the real gateway of the plague to Europe during the 6th century AD?* According to Procopius (*De Bellis* 249–59), the epidemic started from the city of Pelusium. But, *was Pelusium the real gateway of the plague?*

At that time, Justinian's empire was at its greatest strength, with the Mediterranean Sea becoming a Byzantine *'mare nostrum'*. No historical source mentions anything about the existence of such a disease in other Mediterranean cities before the start of the known epidemic. It seems impossible that the disease was transferred to Pelusium from any other Mediterranean port and it is logically concluded that the disease must have reached Pelusium from inland Egypt.

The position of Pelusium is identified near to the current site of *Tell el-Farama*, on the eastern branch of the Nile delta (the Roman *Ostium Pelusiacum*), 30 km from the entrance of the Suez Canal at Port Said. Pelusium was about 4 km from the shores of the Mediterranean and only small boats could approach it, through the canals that crossed the marshes and swamplands that surrounded the city (Procopius *De Aedificiis* 171–2). The port of Pelusium was overshadowed by the great Alexandria, from where ships left for the capital of the empire, Constantinople. Pelusium mainly served the maritime and land transport of goods such as salted food, oil and textiles to Palestine and Syria (Milani 1977, 216). The two major Egyptian ports in the Mediterranean, Alexandria and Pelusium, communicated with the Nile through a network of canals. According to the descriptions of Procopius in his work *On Constructions* (*De Aedificiis* 171–2), which described all public works of the Justinianic era, the bulk of the Nile reached the small town of Chaereus which was linked to Alexandria through a canal. In the eastern Delta, Pelusium was linked to the Nile through the city Bubastis (Redmount 1995, 127–36).

In the late Roman era, the eastern delta of the Nile hosted the channel of the Emperor Trajan (*Amnis Traianus*), which crossed the Bitter Lakes of the Sinai Peninsula and ended in the Red Sea (Sijpesteijn 1963). Trajan's canal was not a new construction, but an improvement to the old 'canal of the Pharaohs', starting from the city of Pithom in Sinai and ending in Babylon, on the Nile. Claudius Ptolemeus (*Geographica* IV, 5, 54) indicates that in his days the canal flowed between Heroopolis of Sinai and Babylon. With the improvements to the old canal, Trajan's river, as it was often referred to, apart from Babylon, also connected the Bitter Lakes with the town of Bubastis (Redmount 1995, 127–36; Uphill 1968, 291–315).

The commercial importance of the Red Sea

In the 6th century AD, the Red Sea was the setting of a peculiar struggle between the Persians and the Byzantines. The Byzantines exercised political influence on the kingdom of the Axumites (current Ethiopia) and the Persians on the Jewish kingdom of Homerites (current Yemen). In the east, the Persians controlled the trade in the Persian Gulf, part of the trade in the Indian Ocean and land routes of the Silk Road. But the sea was not completely under their control, so the Axumites and the Christian Homerites (on behalf of the Byzantine traders) reached Ceylon (Byzantine Taprovani) and southern India, as testified by the findings of Byzantine coins there (Laiou 2006, 346). Since the 4th century AD, thanks to the commercial agreements of Emperor Constantius, the kingdom of Axum operated as an alternative commercial solution (Laiou 2006, 346; Bidez and Winkelman 1972, 32–3).

The Axum kingdom played the role of the retail commercial hub of Central Africa and India. The merchant ships transferred herbs, spices, precious and semi-precious stones, ivory and silk fabrics from India (Casson 1989, 17–8). A journey from Africa or Arabia to India had many stopovers which were used in the following centuries by the Arabs. According to the descriptions of the Arab geographers Ibn Hawqal and Muqaddasi (10th century AD), a journey from Aden (Yemen) to India would take place along the coast of the Arabian Peninsula and beyond the Persian Gulf with stops at the ports of Baçra, Chatt ar-Arab, Siraf, Çuhar and Dayboul (Miquel 1977, 131–45). The Byzantine ships received the goods of the Axumites and headed to the Red Sea ports. Through the old Roman road, Via Hadriana, which joined the major ports of Berenike and Myos Hormos with the cities of the Nile Antinoopolis, Apollonopolis Magna and Coptos, the goods reached the commercial stations of the river (Sidebotham 1997, 385–93, Sidebotham and Wendrich 2002, 31–44). Myos Hormos was essentially the last accessible port, since beyond this navigation was very difficult (Young 2001, 75–8).

The role of the ports of the Sinai Peninsula

According to Procopios' narration, from Pelusium the disease spread west to Alexandria and gradually affected the rest of Egypt, and east to Palestine (Procopius *De Bellis* 249–59). The disease probably arrived in Alexandria in mid-September 541 (Stathakopoulos 2004, 277–80). In the east, through the trade routes of Gaza, the disease affected Ashkelon and the towns in the region of the Negev Desert, about one month after Pelusium, in the middle of August (Kislinger and Stathakopoulos 1999, 76–98). The information that the epidemic started from Pelusium limits the possible port portals of the plague to those in Sinai.

The Sinai Peninsula had two ports, Ailana (current Aqaba) and Arsinoe (Sidebotham 1991, 78). From Ailana, the goods left for Palestine and Syria through the Via Nova Traiana, while Arsinoe served the movement of goods to the Nile. Arsinoe, however, was abandoned due to the region's strong north-eastern winds. This resulted in the creation of a new port (about five kilometres to the west), to the side of the current Suez Canal, the old port of Clysma (Sidebotham 1991, 78). Of course, Clysma faced the same problem of strong winds but a series of historical events rendered it perhaps the most important Red Sea port.

Clysma was located in Sinus Hieroopoliticus (Gulf of Suez) and was a known port in ancient times, but was abandoned because of its shallow waters. The population of the city is unknown but we do have information on their water supply problems as residents brought water from the oasis of Ayum Musa, about 2 km to the southeast (Mayerson 1996, 119–26). Between the 2nd and 4th centuries AD, the surrounding area was uninhabited. In AD 383, we have a testimony of the pilgrim Egeria, surviving in the 11th century work by Petros Diakonus '*Liber de locis sancti*' (Geyer 1965, 93–103). From Egeria's description, the city was more of a frontier fortress than a busy port. Following dredging works, Clysma developed into a port with great commercial activity (Ward 2007, 161–71). The choice of Clysma was far from random, as it was essentially the entrance to the canal of Trajan, which, like all other canals, was logically highly dependent on the level of the Nile.

The role of the River Nile

The Nile is the largest river in Africa. The climatic conditions in Central Africa play an important role, as it has been observed that the level fluctuations are linked not only with the quantity of water but also with the humid or dry tropical climate of equatorial Africa (Mikhailova 2001; Fraedrich and Bantzer 1991). Hydrological and paleo-climatology research shows a relationship between the fluctuations of the Nile and other 'climatic events' with a periodicity of about 25 years (Mikhailova 2001). The highest and lowest level fluctuations occur in a timeframe of about a century (80–170 years) (Mikhailova 2001). The lowest level of the river is from March to May. As of June, the level begins to rise rapidly to reach its peak in mid-September (Eltahir 1996, 131–7). No matter how strange it may seem, in antiquity, the Nile presented many difficulties in navigation, and journeying in the river was a slow process. Since the time of the Pharaohs, ships travelled there only during the day, while in some places the Nile was not navigable and the ships had to be towed from the banks using animals. It is estimated that a boat on the Nile could travel a distance of 40–70 km a day (Collin 2007, 17–46). The journey – 1,545 km – from Sudan to the Mediterranean would take 28 days. The shipment of goods from Axum to Clysma and from there to Pelusium or Palestine took almost half of that time. Even the first border trading Byzantine station in the Nile, Elephantine (Aswan), was thirty days by land from Axum (Procopius, *De Bellis* 104).

It has been argued that the canal of Trajan did not operate for centuries and that just a section was still used to carry fresh water from the Bitter Lakes to Clysma (Mayerson 1996, 119–26). The theory is apparently strengthened by the evaluation of French engineers of the mid-19th century, who believed that during the late Roman era the trade of the Red Sea stopped during the summer months due to lack of water in the channels of the Nile (*Travaux 1847*, 99). However, in his monumental work *Historia Francorum*, Gregory of Tours (6th century AD), trying to explain the Biblical Exodus, quotes a remarkable fact. Referring to testimonies by travellers of his time, he describes the existence of constructions from Babylon on the Nile to the Bitter Lakes in Sinai (Krusch 1937, 11). He also notes that Clysma was built not because the area was fertile but because that was where Trajan's river ended and that the port was used to transport products to Egypt, which then made their way to India (Krusch 1937, 11). The time of the works in Clysma also manifests the importance of the canal, as this was used to bring supplies to workers and equip the ships anchored in the port (Collin 2007, 17–46). Also, according to Gregory, these constructions took water from the Nile and the flow of water was from the west (Egypt) to the east (Sinai) (Kruch 1937, 11). This fact reinforces the view that the operation of the canal was inextricably linked with the fluctuations of the Nile. Given that the epidemic broke out in Pelusium in mid-July and in Alexandria in mid-September and taking into account the level of the Nile, we could create a geographical-historical link of the course of the disease, from Clysma to Pelusium and Alexandria, through the canal network.

Clysma as a possible gateway

The suggestion that the port of Clysma, and no other port of the Red Sea, could have acted as the gateway of the plague is supported by a series of historical events. In the 6th century, the ports of Myos Chormos and Berenike had been abandoned, while the Via Hadriana had been destroyed (Sidebotham 1997; Sidebotham and Zitterkopf 1997, 221–37). The archaeological and anthropological findings in the region of the eastern desert of Egypt show a gradual aggregation of nomads from the 3rd century, who foraged the ports of the Red Sea and the Nile, while, in AD 524–525, we identify the last report on the operation of Berenike (Ward 2007, 161–7). The upgrading of Clysma was reinforced by another historical event. Clysma protected an important commercial station in the Red Sea, the small island Iotabe. It is suggested that Iotabe is the island of Tiran located where the Gulf of Aqaba flows into the Red Sea, but archaeologists have not found any remains there. The Saracens had occupied the island and threatened Byzantine trade. In AD 498, the Duke Romanos took it back but the Saracens returned and a new campaign by Duke Aratios was required, in AD 534, for the Byzantines to re-occupy it (Ward 2007, 161–7). Clysma, therefore, represented a guarantee for the safety of the island, offering ships ready for war in an emergency. In the same period, Clysma flourished and was the seat of the *agens in rebus* (*logothetes*), a high rank official who visited the kingdom of Axum once a year as ambassador of the Byzantine emperor (Mayerson 1996, 119–26).

The mass abandonment of many ports on the coast of the Red Sea and the Nile shows the fear of the attacking nomads. It is likely that this fact contributed to the choice of this trade route from Axum to Clysma. The case of a direct link of Clysma with Pelusium along the Bitter Lakes must be considered as something of a problem. The main reason for this is the geography of the region with its scalding sun and lack of wells, which made travellers describe it as a 'terrible desert' (Collin 2007, 17–46). However, the risk of attacks on the caravans by the Saracens of the Peninsula was very real and frequent. The findings also suggest the state's failure to protect the land roads of Sinai from the Saracens. The archaeological discoveries show numerous defence walls in the settlements of the peninsula, a fact obviously linked to the government's abandonment of the region of Sinai and the effort of the residents to protect themselves (Ward 2007). The gradual rise of the Saracens from the 3rd century AD may be linked with the movement of the Legio X Fretensis to Ailana in order to guard the valuable road, the Via Nova Traiana leading to Syria, leaving Sinai unprotected (Parker 2002).

Conclusions

Some of the trade routes in the area were estimated, with the help of historical and archaeological sources. The above suggest a vast commercial traffic in the Red Sea and the importance Clysma acquired during the 6th century AD. For historical reasons, it is believed that Clysma is most likely to have been the gateway of *Yersinia pestis* in Byzantine Egypt when the epidemic broke out. The month of the epidemic's occurrence in Pelusium, Clysma's geographic position and their close trade relationship, strengthen this theory. The use of the canal of Trajan at the time of the epidemic is under question, without, however, its operation being precluded. In concluding we would like to mention that we believe that the multidisciplinary collaboration of different scientific fields, often completely unconnected at first glance, always helps to find answers to medico-historical questions.

Bibliography

Bidez, J. and F. Winkelman (eds) 1972: *Philostorgius. Kirchengeschichte*, Berlin.

Casson, L. 1989: *The Periplus Maris Erythraei: text, translation and commentary*, Princeton.

Collin, A. 2007: *Land Transport in Roman Egypt. A Study of Economics and Administration in a Roman Province*, Oxford.

Eltahir, E. 1996: 'El Niño and the natural variability in the flow of the Nile River', *Water Resources Research* 32, 131–7.

Fraedrich, K. and Bantzer, C. 1991: 'A note to fluctuations of the Nile river flood levels (715–1470)', *Theoretical and Applied Climatology* 44, 167–71.

Geyer, P. 1965: 'Peter the Deacon. *Liber de locis sancti. Appendix ad Itineriarium Egeriae II*', 93–103 in P. Geyer and O. Cuntz (eds), *Itineraria et alia Geographica*, Turnhout.

Kislinger, E. and Stathakopoulos D. 1999: 'Pest und Perserkriege bei Prokop. Chronologische Überlegungen zum Geschenen 540–545', *Byzantion* 69, 76–98.

Krusch, B. 1937: *Gregorii episcopi Historiarum Libri X* (*Historia Francorum*), Hannover.

Laiou, A. 2006: *The Economic History of Byzantium*, Athens.

Mayerson, P. 1996: 'The port of Clysma (Suez) in transition from Roman to Arab Rule', *Journal of Near Eastern Studies* 55, 119–26.

Mikhailova, M. 2001: 'Hydrological regime of the Nile delta and dynamics of its coastline', *Water Resources* 28, 526–39.

Milani, C. 1977: *Itinerarium Antonini Placentini: Un viaggio in terra Santa del 560–570 d.C*, Rome.

Miquel, A. 1977: *L'Islam et sa civilization VIIe–XXe siècle*, Paris.

Parker, S. 2002: 'The Roman frontier in Jordan: an overview', 77–82 in P. Freeman (ed.), *Limes XVII: Proceedings of the XVIIIth International Congress of Roman Frontier Studies*, Amman.

Procopii Caesariensis: *Opera Omnia, De Bellis. Libri I–II*, edited by J. Haury and G. Wirth, Leipzig 1905.

Procopii Caesariensis: *Opera Omnia VI, De aedificiis*, edited by J. Haury, Leipzig 1964.

Redmount, C. 1995: 'The Wadi-Tumilat and the canal of Pharaohs', *Journal of Near Eastern Studies* 54, 127–36.

Sidebotham, S. 1991:'Ports of the Red Sea and the Arabia-India trade', 78 in V. Begley and R. De Puma, *Rome and India: The Ancient Sea Trade,* Madison.

Sidebotham, S. 1997: 'Caravans across the Eastern Desert of Egypt: recent discoveries on the Berenike-Apollonopolis Magna-Koptos road', 385–93 in A. Avanzini (ed.), *Profumi d'Arabia: Atti del convegno*, Rome.

Sidebotham, S. and Wendrich, W. 2002: 'Berenike: Archaeological fieldwork at a Ptolemaic-Roman port on the Red Sea coast of Egypt 1999–2000', *Sahara* 13, 31–44.

Sidebotham, S. and Zitterkopf, R. 1997: 'Survey of the Via Hadriana: the 1996 season', *Bulletin de l' Institut français d'Archéologie orientale* 2, 221–37.

Sijpesteijn, P. 1963: 'Der ΠΟΤΑΜΟΣ ΤΡΑΙΑΝΟΣ', *Aegyptus* 43, 70–83.

Stathakopoulos, D. 2004: *Famine and pestilence in the Late Roman and Early Byzantine Empire: A systematic survey of subsistence crises and epidemics*, London.

Travaux de la Brigade française: *Rapport de l'ingénieur*, Société d'études historiques et géographiques de l'isthme de Suez, Nîmes, 1847.

Uphill, E. 1968: 'Pithom and Ramses: their location and significance', *Journal of Near Eastern Studies* 27, 291–315.

Ward, W. 2007: 'Aila and Clysma: the rise of northern ports in the Red Sea in Late Antiquity', 161–71 in J. Starkey *et al.*, *Natural Resources and Cultural Connections of the Red Sea* (British Archaeological Report International Series 1661), Oxford.

Young, G. 2001: *Rome's Eastern Trade: International Commerce and Imperial Policy 31 B.C.–305 A.D.*, London.

41. Du Diagnostic différentiel aux Thérapies prudentes : *Le traité de la rougeole et de la variole* de Râzî

Mehrnaz Katouzian-Safadi and Jean-Marc Bonmatin

One of the major interpreters of Galen in Arabic is revealed to be Abû Bakr Mohammed Zakarîya al-Râzî (865-925). A work of great originality, 'al-Djudarî wa al-hasba' *or* Smallpox and Measles *reveals a detailed scientific and medical reading of Galen by Râzî, and critical remarks on the absence of precise descriptions of these diseases by Galen. This work has marked the history of medicine as far as differential diagnosis, and different ways of translating are concerned. Indeed, it would be translated from Arabic into Greek, Latin and several European languages. The Greek translation seems to have been commissioned by an emperor of Constantinople. The work was known in Europe by the Greek translations, translated into Latin. A Latin edition was made in Venice in 1556 entitled* De pestilentia. *Later, in the 18th century, the first translation from Arabic to Latin was made by Mead in 1747. Other translations followed.*

We examine the passages which lead to Râzî's personal observations, and to his discoveries. Râzî suggests observing every little change in the patient's condition. The care and treatment of disease need permanent attention and Râzî calls for caution. In general, treatments by specific nutrition predominate over powerful drugs. We compare this major work with other books where the author treated the same diseases. Thus, we were able to clarify which treatments are essential for him when the patient is in mortal danger. At the same time, we can also learn about Râzî's methods of healing and collecting information.

I. Introduction

Râzî se situe à une période essentielle des sciences écrites, médiévales et arabes, période où des œuvres et des créations scientifiques inédites sont réalisées. Après les traductions effectuées par Hunayn Ibn Ishâq (809–877) et ses collaborateurs, les œuvres des grands médecins grecs furent accessibles en langue arabe aux médecins et aux étudiants (Gutas 2005, 197–203). Hunayn Ibn Ishâq donne lui-même la liste des œuvres qu'il a traduites (Muhaqeq 2001). Ces traductions ont conduit à la formation d'un vocabulaire médical unifié. Dès le début de cette période, des œuvres originales apparaissent dans le domaine de la médecine (Pormann et Savage-Smith, 2007) et de la pharmacie (Hamarneh 1973 ; Katouzian-Safadi 2004a, 870–4). Les Livres de Râzî sont des témoignages de cette époque riche en créativité (Ullmann 1970, 141–4). Le traitement des maladies comme la variole et la rougeole est un des exemples historiques démontrant ces nouveautés médicales et thérapeutiques. En effet, pour ces nouvelles délimitations de maladies, il est fort pertinent de voir comment l'auteur puise ses pratiques thérapeutiques dans les vastes usages déjà existants et qui sont inscrits dans les textes ou présents dans les pratiques courantes. L'examen de quatre œuvres de Râzî, adressées à des publics ayant des niveaux de connaissances et de besoins différents, permet de mieux comprendre la méthode de travail de l'auteur.

II. Examen des œuvres

II.1. *Œuvres majeures de Râzî sur la variole et la rougeole*

L'auteur décrit ces deux maladies dans plusieurs œuvres

rédigées au cours de sa vie. Nous examinons uniquement les quatre plus importantes ici :

a) L'ouvrage *Kitâb al-Mansûrî fî al-tibb* a été commandé par Mansûr, homme politique du 10e siècle, au service de la dynastie des bouyides. Le livre est formé de dix chapitres et est destiné aux médecins s'intéressant à la théorie et à la pratique. Il aborde l'essentiel de l'enseignement théorique et pratique de la médecine médiévale, c'est à dire toutes les maladies de la tête aux pieds ainsi que les médicaments simples et composés. Le chapitre 10 est consacré aux fièvres ou '*fî al-humîyyât*', aux signes ou '*al- 'alâmât*', aux périodes critiques ou '*al-buhrân*', aux urines ou '*al-bowl*' et aux pouls ou '*al-nabd*'. Au sein de la partie consacrée aux fièvres, dix-huit catégories de fièvres fortes sont décrites. Elles sont nommés par le mot 'fièvre' suivi d'un 'qualificatif' ; on peut citer les dernières : sur les fièvres des inflammations,'*fî al-huma al-haditha 'an al-awrâm*', sur les fièvres épidémiques ou '*fî al-huma al-wabâiyya*', sur les fièvres composées ou '*fî al-huma al-murakkaba*' et enfin le dernier cas, le dix-huitième est mentionné par les termes, 'sur la variole et la rougeole' ou '*fî al-djudarî wa al-hisba*'. Il faut souligner que ces derniers cas sont bien classés dans le chapitre des fièvres mais sans la mention '*fièvres de …*' qui aurait signifié une catégorie supplémentaire de fièvre. Ces dernières atteintes avec *forte fièvre* sont définies comme des maladies spécifiques avec une terminologie précise. Ce court passage est formé approximativement de 570 mots (pour l'arabe voir, al-Siddîqî 1987 ; *Mansûrî*, 489–91 et pour l'anglais voir Greenhill 1848a). Ce livre a précédé les trois autres textes décrits ci-dessous. Nous le nommerons *Mansûrî* par la suite.

b) *Le livre de la division et de l'arborisation, Kitâb al-taqsîm wa al-tashdjîr* est un abrégé des travaux médicaux (Hamâmî 1992 ; traduction anglaise Grennhill 1848b). Dans son introduction, l'auteur précise qu'il s'agit d'un livre qui réunit les maladies, leurs divisions, leurs symptômes et la façon de les traiter. Il ajoute qu'il le met à la disposition des praticiens ou de simples personnes averties en absence d'un médecin confirmé. Il le qualifie de compendium en matière de diagnostic de traitements et de remèdes. L'auteur y décrit les premiers soins vitaux à apporter aux malades. Ce livre est donc destiné à un public moins averti que le précédent. L'auteur dira pour commencer et clore ce livre (Hamâmî 1992, 706–7 ; la traduction est modifiée par nos soins) 'C'est un livre qui contient ce qui est nécessaire au médecin '*al-tabîb*', au praticien '*al-mutitabib*' et à celui qui n'a pas de médecin auprès de lui '*man la yadaruhu tabîb*'.

Le texte est divisé en cent cinquante entrées '*bâb*', abordant toutes les maladies classées de la tête au pied selon la tradition admise de l'Antiquité à la période médiévale. Les dix dernières entrées sont consacrées aux diverses fièvres qui affectent l'ensemble du corps. Comme dans le *Mansûrî*, la dernière concerne les deux maladies de la variole et de la rougeole citées par leur noms et non simplement comme des fièvres avec des qualifications (Greenhill 1848b, et Hamâmî 1992, 697–707). Ce court passage est formé approximativement de 200 mots. Ce livre est rédigé après *Mansûrî* car l'auteur y fait référence. Par exemple au chapitre 34, pour les abcès lacrymaux et fistules, l'auteur renvoie le lecteur à *Mansûrî* (al-Siddîqî 1987, 135) et pour les tumeurs chaudes il écrit '*tous ces sujets sont traités dans al-Mansûrî et nous n'avons rien à leur ajouter*' (Hamâmî 1992, 575–6). Nous nommerons ce livre *Division* dans la suite de l'article.

Souvent, les ouvrages sur l'histoire de la médecine affirment que les fièvres représentaient dans la période médiévale un simple symptôme et non pas une catégorie de maladie déterminée (voir par exemple, Pormann et Savage-Smith 2007, 57–8). Le cas de ces deux maladies nous enseigne qu'il faudrait prendre quelques précautions avant de généraliser cette affirmation. Ici plusieurs symptômes sont clairement définis, ces maladies *accompagnées de très forte fièvre sont diagnostiquées et portent deux noms distincts et spécifiques ; dans ces deux cas la fièvre est un symptôme parmi d'autres pour des états de maladies, celles-ci bien différenciées et répertoriées comme telles.*

c) L'œuvre la plus aboutie et la plus complète de Râzî consacrée uniquement et spécifiquement à ces deux maladies fulgurantes et dangereuses est *Le Livre sur la Variole et la Rougeole*, ou en arabe '*al-Djudari wa al-hasba*'. Ce livre est rédigé après *Mansûrî* car l'auteur y fait référence. Par exemple le chapitre 14 sur 'les signes dangereux des varioles et des rougeoles mortelles et bénignes', évoque le livre de *Mansûrî* (Nadjmâbâdî 1992, 27 ; Greenhill 1848c, 71 ; Leclerc et Lenoir 1866, 44). C'est notre référence principale pour l'analyse comparative des écrits de Râzî sur ces deux maladies. Il est composé de 7600 mots et est organisé en 14 chapitres ; dans cet article, nous le mentionnons par *La Variole et la Rougeole* ou *la V et R*.

d) Les notes personnelles de Râzî, nommées *Kitâb al-Hâwî fî al-tibb*, ont été rassemblées, au 10e siècle, après sa mort par ses étudiants à la demande d'Ibn Amîd, homme politique sous la dynastie des Bouyides ; une personnalité politique importante de la ville de Ray, ville natale du médecin (ville située en Iran près de la ville de Téhéran d'aujourd'hui). La publication sans édition critique de l'ensemble de ces notes en 25 volumes a été réalisée après presque vingt années de travail (Abdu'l Mu 'id Khan 1955–1973). *Al-Hâwî* rassemble des réflexions, des notes de lecture, des considérations et des pratiques médicales personnelles et expérimentées par Râzî (Iskandar 1959, 73–92). La lecture de cet ouvrage demande beaucoup d'attention pour reconnaître les citations précises des médecins antérieurs à Râzî et les réflexions personnelles de l'auteur (Brysson 2000, 6, 22). Ces notes personnelles n'ont pas l'organisation d'une œuvre rédigée et destinée vers un public spécifique. Dans les manuscrits nous trouvons cet ouvrage organisé en de nombreux volumes. Dans cette œuvre immense nous considérons deux fragments. Le premier se trouve au volume 7, nommé '*fî al-djudarî wa al-hasba*' ou 'sur la variole et la rougeole', composé de 5000 mots, et le second est un paragraphe d'une dizaine de lignes (200 mots) consacré à l'étude d'un cas particulier d'une jeune femme atteinte de la variole (Greenhill 1848d, 97–132). Nous nous référerons à cette œuvre en l'appelant les notes de Râzî ou *Hâwî*.

Nous comparons ces quatre livres, pour mieux comprendre l'approche médicale de la variole et de la rougeole, sa méthode de travail lors de la collecte d'informations qui se fait par lectures des livres de grands médecins, par les échanges oraux avec son entourage et par observations personnelles au chevet de malades. Le Tableau 41.1 rassemble des descriptions brèves sur ces quatre œuvres analysées.

II.1.1. Histoire d'un difficile diagnostic différentiel

Selon Grmek, la rougeole et la variole n'ont pas été décrites dans l'antiquité et lorsqu'un corps était couvert de boutons des termes comme *exanthema*, *boubon* ou *loimos* étaient usités (Grmek 1994, 222–3, note 56). Cette absence de diagnostic de la variole a été expliquée par la multiplicité des symptômes de diverses épidémies. Biraben (1995) écrit à propos des épidémies en cours au second siècle et de la peste d'Antonin :

> 'pour les années 167 à 172 de notre ère : Cette fois les descriptions médicales de l'épidémie sont abondantes, peut-être même un peu trop pour que le tableau soit clair. Galien, qui est témoin de cette épidémie et fuit Rome pour y échapper, en parle à sept reprises dans son œuvre. Il la nomme "grande pestilence" (*megas loimos*) et déclare qu'elle est semblable à la "peste d'Athènes" décrite par Thucydide'.

Pour cette époque certains diagnostics rétrospectifs ont été faits par Littman et Littman (1973, 243–55) qui trouvent des cas de variole dans leurs études approfondies des œuvres de Galien. Il semble que l'œuvre de Râzî est celle qui décrit aussi bien la maladie, les symptômes et propose des traitements (Grmek 1994, 243–55). Selon G. Strohmaier (1995, 123–49), Râzî différencie la rougeole et la variole en proposant un tableau clinique claire et rigoureux.

II.1.2. Transmission : traductions des œuvres en grec, latin et langues vernaculaires

Le livre, *al-Mansûrî fi al-tibb*, destiné à un public de médecins demandant la théorie et la pratique médicale a été traduit en latin par le grand traducteur Gérard de Crémone (1114–1187) sous le nom *Liber ad Almansorem*. La traduction anglaise du fragment issu de ce livre et concernant la variole et la rougeole est faite par Greenhill d'après le manuscrit arabe de la bibliothèque de Bodleian à Oxford (*March*, 248) ; selon l'auteur la version latine est conforme à la version originale arabe étudiée (Greenhill 1848a).

Le livre *Des divisions des maladies* ou *Kitâb al-Taqsîm wa al-tashdjîr* a été également traduit en latin par Gérard de Crémone sous le nom de *Divisio Morborum* ou *Liber Divisionum*. La traduction anglaise de Greenhill (1848b) est faite d'après le texte latin, sans être comparée à la version arabe du manuscrit de la bibliothèque de Venise (catalogue collection Naniana, vol. ii, 238). Nous avons comparé la traduction anglaise de Greenhill à l'édition arabe de *Mansûrî* pour notre analyse.

Les notes et les remarques personnelles de Râzî, *Hâwî*, rassemblés par ses élèves n'ont pas été sélectionnées pour la traduction latine par Gérard de Crémone au 12e siècle ; certes s'agissant des notes personnelles, l'usage pratique et médical a été jugé moins aisé. Cet ensemble de notes a été traduit en latin en 1279 sous le nom *Continens,* pour Charles d'Anjou, le roi de Naples (Richter-Bernburg 2003). Le traducteur est un médecin de Sicile, Faradj Ibn Sâlim (parfois nommé Faragut). Nous avons comparé l'édition anglaise et arabe pour ce travail (Greenhill 1848d).

Le traité de *La rougeole et de la variole*, écrit en langue arabe, a marqué l'histoire de la médecine par son apport au diagnostic différentiel et par ses multiples voies de traductions qui ne sont pas encore toutes élucidées. Congourdeau (1996, 99–111) montre que la thèse d'une première traduction en syriaque est fausse et que la traduction a été faite directement de l'arabe en grec ; de nombreux manuscrits sont conservés dans les bibliothèques européennes (Greenhill 1848c, 4, note 3). L'Europe découvre cette œuvre dans la langue grecque. Le titre des premières traductions latines est *De Pestilentia* ; ce terme est probablement une trace du titre de la traduction grecque où un terme unique générique, exprimant une forte fièvre et une diffusion rapide de la maladie, est usité au lieu des deux termes arabes pour deux maladies distinctes que sont la variole et la rougeole.

L'histoire des voies de traductions latines n'est pas encore totalement établie. *De Pestilentia* a été édité treize fois entre 1498 et 1586 (Sezgin 2001, vol. III, 386–7 ; voir également Greenhill 1848c, 5–9). A partir du 18e siècle diverses traductions de l'arabe sont réalisées en latin par Channing (1766), en anglais par Greenhill (Greenhill 1848c), en français par Leclerc et Lenoir (1866) et en persan par Nadjmâbâdî (1992). Steinschneider (1956, no. 178) décrit une version allemande que nous n'avons pas examiné pour nos travaux. Si l'histoire de la transmission du texte a fait l'objet d'études multiples, le contenu thérapeutique exige encore des examens et des analyses.

II.2. Les thérapies de ces nouvelles entités nosologiques

Il est légitime de se demander à quels registres thérapeutiques fait appel Râzî, pour traiter ces deux maladies dont il définit le diagnostic différentiel. Dans toutes les maladies aiguës, Râzî opte pour un traitement rafraîchissant, comme il le précise dans ses aphorismes (aphorisme n° 337, Iskandar 1980 et Moubachir 1996). Râzî sélectionne avec grande précaution, les traitements usuels pour les fièvres fortes et

Tableau 41.1. Comparaison des conditions de rédaction des œuvres majeures de Râzî traitant de la rougeole et de la variole.

Œuvres	***Kitâb al-Mansûrî*** ***Le Livre de Mansûrî***	***Kitâb al- Taqsîm wa al- tashdjîr*** ***Le livre des divisions des maladies***	***K al Djudarî wa al-Hisba*** ***La Rougeole et la Variole***	/ / / / / / /	***Kitâb al-Hâwî fî al-tibb*** ***Le livre d'al-Hâwî***
Abréviation dans notre article	*Mansûrî*	*Division*	*V et R*	/ / /	*Hâwî*
Ordre chronologique de rédaction	1er	2ème Après *Mansûrî*	2ème ou 3ème o- Après *Mansûrî* o- Avant ou après *Taqsîm* ?	/ / / /	Lors de l'exercice de la médecine au cours de sa vie
Diffusion de l'œuvre	De son vivant	De son vivant	De son vivant	/ /	Posthume
Nombre mots consacrés à la variole et à la rougeole	570	500	7600	/	5000 + 200 (1 cas de malade)
%	8	7	100	/	66
Commande par un mécène	Oui	Non indiqué	Oui	/ / /	- Non car notes personnelle - Sur commande rassemblé à titre posthume
Lecteurs Destinataires Contenus	Médecins débutants ou confirmés Théories et pratiques	Praticiens grand public ou en absence de médecin Pratiques	Médecins confirmés Théories et Pratiques	/ / / / /	Notes personnelles pas destinées à un grand public Théories et Pratiques

ainsi des remèdes très ordinaires interviennent pour des maux fort dangereux, effrayants pour le malade et le médecin (Katouzian-Safadi 2012, 23–51).

Traitement de l'ensemble du corps – Au sein du traité de la *V et R*, les conseils sur l'alimentation sont présents dans toutes les étapes de l'évolution de la maladie (prévention, crise et convalescence). Au chapitre 5 de ce traité, Râzî réserve une grande place aux repas de la personne malade (Nadjmâbâdî 1992, 8, et Leclerc et Lenoir 1866, 19). Il propose des aliments qui 'éteignent le feu' ou '*al-mutfîyât*' : les lentilles jaunes décortiquées cuites '*tafshîla*' avec verjus '*hasramîya*', des bouillons '*sikbâj*' avec peu de graisse, du francolin, du chevreau '*al-judâ'* ', de l'agneau '*al-hilmân*' et des poules domestiques '*al-dadjadj*'.

Dans les quatre œuvres examinées, la viande de poussin '*al-faradj*' est fortement déconseillée aux fiévreux (par exemple voir Abdu'l Mu 'id Khan 1955–73, vol. 17, 10). En effet dans un autre livre sur *Les qualités et les méfaits des aliments*, il décrit la chair du poussin comme étant chaude (Râzî 1984, 105–6) ; cette chair crée des inflammations et sa graisse (*al-shuhum*) a une chaleur apparente et évidente. Elle ne convient donc pas aux fiévreux et Râzî la déconseille dans les traités concernant la fièvre.

L'eau est une matière essentielle du traitement : pour boire, pour s'y baigner et pour humidifier l'espace environnant. Comme dans le cas des fièvres aiguës, l'espace est rafraîchi en permanence par des vaporisations d'eau, associées ou non à des arômes comme le santal et le camphre (Katouzian-Safadi et Ben Ghachem 2012). Le malade doit se laver vers le milieu du jour dans de l'eau froide en s'y plongeant tout entier (Katouzian-Safadi et Bensaad 2013, à paraître). L'eau froide apaise, humidifie, adoucit les effets de la fièvre. L'eau chaude peut accélérer l'éruption des pustules sur la paume de la main ou la plante du pied. Les jus de fruits et de légumes sont administrés fréquemment pour ces maladies : jus de prune, de grenade, de pastèque, de concombre, de courge. L'eau d'orge est un aliment-médicament essentiel. Comme médicament simple, le mucilage des graines de psyllium est employé. Pour les deux maladies et dans toutes les œuvres examinées le médecin évite fortement la diarrhée, c'est pour cela la grenade est utilisée avec sa chair, écrasée et associée à son jus.

Traitement des parties du corps – Dans ces quatre œuvres, Râzî rappelle que la rougeole est plus dangereuse que la variole, mais pour les yeux, c'est la variole qui est à craindre. Les yeux sont traités avec l'eau de rose simple ou trempée avec du sumak lorsqu'un début de marque apparaît dans l'œil (Greenhill 1848b, 92 et Hamâmî 1992, 700, 701). La gorge est protégée par des gargarismes à l'eau de rose et l'oreille par du glaucium '*mamithâ*' au vinaigre associé aux extraits de plantes qui apaisent la chaleur (Greenhill 1848c ; Nadjmâbâdî 1992, ch. 7). S'il y a des picotements dans les extrémités (la plante du pied ou la paume de la main), l'éruption des boutons est favorisée modérément en les trempant dans l'eau tiède. Les argiles sont des remèdes bien connues par Râzî pour leurs qualités fort variées (Rautureau *et al.* 2010, 23–5). Une argile spécifique est appliquée pour protéger les articulations (Greenhill 1848c, 54 ; Nadjmâbâdî 1992, 18) et pour lutter contre le relâchement du ventre (Greenhill 1848c ; Nadjmâbâdî 1992, ch. 13).

Les cas particuliers de malades – Dans *Hâwî* ou ses notes personnelles, Râzî livre le cas d'une femme atteinte de la variole (Greenhill 1848d, 130 ; Meyerhof 1935, 321–72, cas n°11). Il s'agit d'une patiente déjà connue du médecin. Elle vient consulter Râzî accompagnée par une autre femme. Râzî commence à prendre soin des yeux de la patiente pour éviter la cécité ; c'est grâce à ces premiers soins attentifs que Râzî arrive à gagner la confiance de l'accompagnatrice craintive. D'autres cas sont cités dans *Hâwî* (Greenhill 1848d) où note des pratiques de traitements de pustules où une femme emploie les feuilles d'iris pour assécher les pustules (Greenhill 1848d, 111–2). Il cite le cas fatal d'une femme variolique (Greenhill 1848d, 113) ; il expérimente un médicament pour permettre l'éruption des pustules (Greenhill 1848d, 113) ; il note son expérience sur les difficultés de respiration et de suffocation (Greenhill 1848d, 117). Il donne des indications sur ses observations sur l'effet bénéfique des saignements du nez (Greenhill 1848d, 117) ; il décrit le cas particulier d'une longue fièvre avec angoisse, révélant la rougeole (Greenhill 1848d, 119) ; il rappelle le cas fatal d'un variolique, avec perte d'une jambe par amputation (Greenhill 1848d, 122) ; il cite le cas des personnes ayant très mal à la jambe lors des atteintes de la variole (Greenhill 1848d, 121). Suite à son enseignement, ses élèves rapportent dans un autre livre les histoires de dix-huit cas de personnes atteintes de la variole et de la rougeole (Harbî 2006, 294–7). Les nombreux cas particuliers, cités dans plusieurs livres, indiquent que Râzî avait observé de nombreuses personnes atteintes de la variole et de la rougeole ; ainsi ses recherches et ses prescriptions sont le fruit de ses lectures et de ses observations personnellement collectées. La narration de cas particuliers de malades constitue un genre littéraire au sein des écrits médicaux en langues arabe ou persane (Alvares Milan 2010). Chez Râzî, ces récits de cas particuliers, ne sont pas uniquement un compte-rendu d'observations mais ils font partie intégrante de sa pratique médicale. Les descriptions et les observations des comportements de patients forment la base de sa médecine, de sa thérapie et probablement de son enseignement.

Tous les traitements administrés pour ces maladies graves et dangereuses sont des remèdes fort courants et facilement disponibles (Katouzian-Safadi et Ben Ghachem 2012) ; les aliments–médicaments, comme le jus d'orge, sont fréquents ; les rares médicaments composés contiennent peu d'ingrédients ; Râzî qui a contribué à l'usage de nouveaux médicaments provenant du monde de l'alchimie (McVaugh 2003, 55–76) n'en propose pratiquement pas l'usage dans ces textes consacrés au traitement de la variole et de la rougeole. Les médicaments puissants comme l'opium sont rares ; l'auteur l'utilise rarement, par exemple lorsque la diarrhée et l'insomnie persistent et deviennent un danger pour le malade (Nadjmâbâdî 1992, 24 ; Greenhill 1848c, 64).

Dans le livre de la *Division*, nous pouvons retrouver le plus petit dénominateur commun pour la thérapie présente dans les quatre œuvres ; des traitements semblables sont appliqués pour d'autres atteintes ayant les mêmes symptômes, par exemple : les fièvres fortes et 'les fièvres de deuxième catégorie' (Hamâmî 1992, 661–8) et surtout 'la fièvre continue' ou '*al-huma al mutbiqa*' (Hamâmî 1992, 669–74) et les tumeurs chaudes (Hamâmî 1992, 570–3) ; Râzî donne le qualificatif de fièvre 'continue' à celle présente dans la variole et la rougeole.

II.2.1. La mort et les séquelles destructrices et effrayantes

Le taux élevé de la mortalité par ces deux maladies était une des causes majeures de crainte des médecins. La fièvre élevée conduisait à des délires, les atteintes aux yeux présentaient un risque important de cécité et les ravages de la variole sur le visage effrayaient médecins et malades. Au Proche-Orient, le savant et écrivain des 8–9e siècles, al-Djahiz, révèle les peurs que de nombreuses maladies de peau provoquaient auprès de la population ; les séquelles sur la peau pouvaient créer des réactions de rejets de l'entourage, même après la maladie ; al-Djahiz appelle ses contemporains à plus de compassion pour ces malades ; il souligne que ces ravages corporelles n'influencent pas la réussite sociale de ces individus s'ils s'acharnent à l'apprentissage des arts et des connaissances (Katouzian-Safadi 2013).

Il faut rappeler ici la mort terrible de Louis XV en France (Darmon 1989, 111–6 ; Katouzian-Safadi 2012). Dans la période médiévale en Europe, nous avons des récits mémorables de mariages princiers défaits par la défiguration des mariés après contractions de la variole. Jusqu'à des époques récentes, ce sont les souffrances et la mortalité causées par ces maladies qui imposaient l'intérêt pour les traitements et donc la traduction des ouvrages. Ce n'est que très récemment avec les campagnes de vaccination que la variole a disparu comme maladie courante et que la fréquence de la rougeole a baissé (Glynn 2004).

Râzî qui a rencontré lui-même des cas de malades victimes de ces maladies, consacre les dernières lignes de ses œuvres aux signes bénins ou mortels des maladies. Il considère que la rougeole est plus dangereuse que la variole ; la variole risque cependant de provoquer la cécité (Hamâmî 1992, 700–1). Les symptômes graves sont décrits dans les quatre livres de Râzî : pour les deux maladies si l'éruption des boutons est trop lente et que l'anxiété et la fièvre persistent la maladie est fatale ; les boutons verts, violets ou noirs, avec palpitations et syncope sont considérés comme des mauvais présages. Pour la variole si après l'apparition des boutons, l'état de la personne ne s'améliore pas et si la fièvre augmente, l'affection risque d'être fatale.

II.2.2. Comparaison des symptômes dans les quatre œuvres de Râzî

C'est dans la *Division* que Râzî donne la plus courte description des symptômes (Hamâmî 1992, 696–7) : une fièvre chaude continue (ou rémittente), *huma hara mutbiqa*, dorsalgie, le prurit du nez (sensation de démangeaisons) et des rêves effrayants. La tristesse et l'oppression se révèlent plus fortes dans le cas de la rougeole. Râzî appelle les signes indiqués dans la *Division* comme 'les signes caractéristiques' des deux maladies. Les symptômes sont plus nombreux dans *Mansûrî* où l'auteur ajoute : sommeil, lourdeur de tête, rougeur aux yeux. Dans *V et R*, Râzî multiplie ces signes enrichit le tableau des symptômes : rougeur des pommettes, pléthore, douleur de la gorge et de la poitrine accompagnée de dyspnée, de toux, la sécheresse de la bouche, l'épaississement de la salive, la raucité de la voix, la céphalalgie, la pesanteur dans la tête, l'inquiétude, le trouble, la lipothymie, l'anxiété, avec une plus grande anxiété dans la rougeole que dans la variole ; la douleur dorsale et les rougeurs de tout le corps et surtout de la gencive qui sont plus spécifiques à la variole. Dans *Hâwî*, on peut retrouver ces signes rassemblés dans la *V et R* sous forme plus restreinte et dans des paragraphes épars.

Quelques descriptions physiognomoniques sont données dans *Hâwî* et dans le traité de la *V et R* (Leclerc et Lenoir 1866, 16) pour décrire les corps qui attirent plus facilement ces deux maladies :

> '…les corps humide, blancs, à chaires abondantes, riche de couleur, rouges ; les corps bruns pareillement quand ils sont chargés de chairs ; ceux qui sont fréquemment et promptement atteint de la fièvre chaude et continue (*mubtaqa*), d'hémorragie nasale, d'ophtalmie, de pustules …'

De telles indications n'ont pas été précisées dans des textes courts et utilitaires comme *Mansûrî* ou *Division*.

II.2.3. Etiologie de la maladie

Râzî rappelle dans ses œuvres que ces deux maladies se diffusent très rapidement au sein de la population (*wâfid*). Certaines saisons et certaines conditions atmosphériques sont propices à ces maladies (Katouzian-Safadi 2012, 31). Dans le traité de la *V et R* au premier chapitre, Râzî souligne que les enfants sont beaucoup plus sensibles à ces maladies que les adultes. Pour proposer une étiologie de ces maladies, Râzî fait appel à deux registres différents, la théorie médicale humorale et l'alchimie.

Afin d'illustrer la grande fragilité des enfants, fragilité qui baisse avec l'âge, Râzî propose une métaphore. Cette image riche en capacité heuristique est celle de la succession des états du liquide lors de la fermentation du jus de fruit : le sang des nouveau-nés et des enfants rappelle le jus de fruit (*usara*). Sa cuisson (*al-tabkh*), son bouillonnement (*nashîsh*) et son ébullition (*ghalayân*) conduit à la maturation (*al-nadzǧ* ou *qawâm*), à la putréfaction (*'ufûnat*) du liquide qui se transforme en vin qui rappelle le sang de l'adulte ; ce vin évolue vers le vinaigre qui ressemble au sang de la personne âgée (Katouzian-Safadi 2012). La transformation du jus de fruit en vinaigre nourrit l'imagination scientifique de Râzî pour expliquer ainsi deux points : a) la rapidité fulgurante du cours de la maladie, difficilement contrôlable, comme l'ébullition du jus de fruit par la fermentation, et b) la grande vulnérabilité des enfants par rapport au plus vieux, constatée lors des examens des cas de malades. Le Tableau 41.2 donne un résumé simple du déroulement de la maladie, mis en parallèle avec l'évolution du jus de fruit.

Tableau 41.2. Termes transposées de l'alchimie vers la médecine. Etiologie de la rougeole et de la variole par Râzî.

Domaine médical : théorie des humeurs en fonction de l'âge	*Notions de l'alchimie transférées vers la théorie médicale des humeurs : Notions communes aux deux domaines*
Assèchement du corps	la putréfaction (*'ufûnat*) la cuisson (*tabkh*)
Perte de chaleur	l'ébullition (*ghalayân*)
Digestion	le bouillonnement (*nashîsh*) la maturation (*nadzdj ou qawâm*)
Résultat	la transformation (*inqilâb*)
Comparaisons des matières liquides permettant le rapprochement et l'étiologie	
sang des enfants	jus de fruit *(usara)*, **qualité : immature**
sang des jeunes	vin (*sharâb*), **qualité : plus stable**
sang des vieux	ressemble au vinaigre après le vin (*yashbahu sharâb*), **qualité : totalement stable**

II.3.1. Sagesse et prudence face à la variole et à la rougeole

Dans le traité principal sur la *V et R*, le médecin suit pas-à-pas l'évolution du malade selon le schéma de l'étiologie décrite comme un chimiste contrôlant une ébullition dangereuse et une fermentation non maîtrisée. Il met en garde les médecins contre toute tentative hâtive de traitement. Dans le chapitre cinq '*Pour éviter la variole avant son apparition et limiter sa propagation*', Râzî use de diverses thérapies pour refroidir progressivement le sang et ralentir 'l'ébullition'. Le médecin se trouve devant un dilemme : s'il persiste dans ce traitement de refroidissement, il pourrait dépasser le niveau nécessaire et s'il ne le préconise pas, le danger guette le malade et l'évolution serait fatale. Râzî sermonne le médecin en l'appelant à agir sereinement et rappelle que certains médecins ne veulent pas évoquer ces problèmes par ignorance de l'art médical (*bakhlan minhu bi-sanâ'a*), par stupidité (*djahl*), ou par égoïsme (*istibdâd*). Il emploie ces qualificatifs outrageants, rares chez Râzî, pour éviter des erreurs fatales et demande au médecin de ne pas se précipiter sur des prescriptions de médicament injustifié (Katouzian-Safadi et Bensaad 2013).

Râzî recommande au médecin et philosophe de conserver un esprit critique sur les propositions des autres médecins et sur ses propres pratiques ; son livre, *Les doutes sur Galien* (Mohaghegh 1993 et Labib Abdul-Ghani 2005) témoigne d'une lecture admirative mais critique de Galien (Katouzian-Safadi 2004b, 377–90). La réflexion et la prudence doivent guider le médecin tout au long du processus rapide et incertain de ces maladies fulgurantes.

II.3.2. Justifications et références bibliographiques dans le traité de V et R

L'introduction du *Livre sur la rougeole et la variole* montre la connaissance profonde des œuvres de Galien par Râzî. Dans ce passage, Râzî cite et indique les chapitres des traités du médecin de Pergame discutant des maladies semblables à la variole. Il s'agit de : 1– *Qâtâdjânis* ou *De compositione medicamentorum secundum locos* (Kühn, 1821–33, Tome XIII, 361) ; 2– *De pulsibus ad tirones* (Kühn, Tome VIII, 462) ; 3– *Kitâb al-manâfi' al-'aada'* ou *De usu partium corporis humani* (Kühn, Tome VIII, livre I–XI, Tome IX, livre XII–XVII) ; et 4– *Kitâb al-Tîmawûs ou De iis quae medice scripta sunt in Platonis Timaeo* (non traduit par Kühn). Ce dernier a été traduit par Daremberg (1848) ; Kühn ne l'a pas intégré à son édition et son attribution à Galien a été débattue par Nickel (2002, 73–78). Toutes ces œuvres ont été traduites à l'époque de Hunayn Ibn Ishâq, le grand et prestigieux traducteur du 9e siècle (Balty-Guesdon 1992 ; 2008). Hunayn a rédigé lui-même la liste de ses traductions des œuvres médicales (Bergsträsser1925 ; Muhaqeq 2001). Râzî donne le contenu médical précis de chaque œuvre citée. Dans le premier livre sur *Les médicaments composés selon les lieux*, Galien indique une pommade pour la maladie. Dans les trois œuvres suivantes, Galien préconise une étiologie de la maladie qui proviendrait des aliments et de leurs superfluités, non transformés en sang ou en bile. Ces informations étant insuffisantes, Râzî signale qu'il a également consulté en vain ses collègues connaissant le grec ou le syriaque à la recherche d'éventuels ouvrages pas encore traduits en arabe (voir Tableau 41.3). Cette introduction et ces expositions critiques des œuvres de Galien sont présentes uniquement sous cette forme dans la *V et R*. Cette présentation révèle la méthode de travail de Râzî qui entreprend la rédaction d'un nouveau traité après l'examen des livres disponibles ; il associe la lecture des livres à sa pratique médicale au chevet du malade. Il informe les médecins et les lecteurs, sur sa méthode de travail, et justifie ainsi la nécessité de la rédaction de son traité.

Mansûrî et *Le traité de la Rougeole et de la Variole* sont tous les deux des traités commandés par un mécène. Les passages de *Mansûrî* et de *Division* qui sont destinés à la pratique médicale sont dépourvus de ces argumentations bibliographiques qui faisaient partie de la méthode d'enseignement de Râzî et qui intéressaient surtout le public des médecins avertis à qui *Le traité de la Rougeole et de la variole* est adressé.

III. Conclusion sur la méthode de recherches et de thérapie médicamenteuse

C'est la jeunesse de la population atteinte, la rapidité de l'évolution de la maladie et l'excès de fièvre qui permettent la formulation du schéma étiologique du traité de la *V et la R*. Après l'examen des ces quatre œuvres nous remarquons que Râzî sélectionne les thérapies dans les livres, d'après les pratiques et les propos rapportés dans son entourage et il y associe ses expériences personnelles citées minutieusement.

Avec ces traitements, Râzî réussit à baisser la mortalité et les séquelles profondes de la peau et des yeux. Dans les œuvres examinées, les substances thérapeutiques sont des matières accessibles, au quotidien au plus grand nombre de soignants comme : l'eau chaude et froide, les lentilles, le verjus, le jus de grenade, le vinaigre, la grenade pilée et souvent l'eau d'orge (*ma'al-sha'îr*). A part les saignées à pratiquer avant l'apparition des symptômes, l'ensemble des traitements pour ces deux maladies graves et dangereuses est à base d'arômes (Katouzian-Safadi et Ben Ghachem 2012), d'aliments ou de médicaments qui sont faciles à trouver sur les marchés et dans les boîtes de pharmacie les plus rudimentaires (Katouzian-Safadi et Bensaad 2013).

Le choix de ces substances pourrait se justifier car ainsi Râzî facilite l'accessibilité de traitements à tous les thérapeutes pour ces maladies fulgurantes. Mais surtout, par principe, la prudence encourage l'auteur à ne pas intervenir avec violence dans le cours de ces maladies. En effet, face à ces maladies graves et souvent fatales, l'auteur suggère diverses voies qui révèlent une grande prudence d'intervention ; très souvent une alimentation spécifique l'emporte sur une thérapie médicamenteuse intensive. La comparaison de ces quatre œuvres (voir Tableau 41.4), le

Tableau 41.3. Introduction du *Traité sur la rougeole et la variole*. Examen des quatre citations par Rāzī de Galien.

Ordre des citations par Râzî	*Titres des livres de Galien cités par Râzî*	*Lettre ou Risala de Hunayn (Bergsträsser1925 ; Muhaqeq 2001)*	*Sezgin 2001*	*Kühn ref.*
1ère	في المقالة الثانية *من قاطاجانس*... *Qâtâdjânis* *De compositione medicamentorum secundum locos* (VII-X) *De compositione medicamentorum per genera* in *al-Hawî* plus de141 citation de *Mayâmîr* in *al-Hâwî*, plus de 30 citations de *Qâtâdjânis* in *al-Shukûk*, 1 citation, critique d'une pommade (*marham*) – voir Sezgin, 2001	p. 44 n° 79	p.172 n° 63	Tome XIII, p. 361
2ème	في اول المقالة الرابعة عشرة *من النبض*... *Kitâb al-nabd* اصناف النبض –تَعَرّف النبض –اسباب النبض –تقدمه المعرفة من النبض *De pulsibus ad tirones* *De pulsuum differentia* *De diagnoscendis pulsibus* *De causis pulsuum* *De praesagitione ex pulsibue* *Synopsis Librorum Suorum de pulsibus* *al-Hâwī* : plus de 33 citations Râzî a écrit un résumé et un commentaire sur les livres de Galien sur le pouls. *ikhtisâr k. al-nabd al-Kabîr* ***إختصار كتاب النبض الكبير لجالينوس***	p. 15 n° 16 Voir note a	p. 137 n° 16	T VIII p. 493–765 ; 766–961 T IX p.1–204 ; 205–430 ; 431–549
3ème	**و قال في التاسعة من *منافع الأعضاء*...** *Kitâb fī al-manâfio al-'adâ'* *De usu partium corporis humani* in *al-Hâwî* plus de 24 citations in *al-shukûk* , 7 citations	p. 32 n° 49 Voir note b	p. 156 n° 40	Tome VIII Book I–XI Tome IX Book XII–XVII
4ème	**و قال في الرابعة من *كتاب طيماوس*...** *Kitâb al-Tîmâwûs* *De iis quae medice scripta sunt in Platonis Timaeo (Timaeus)* in *al-shukûk* : 1 citation	p. 61 n° 122 Voir note c	p. 183 n° 90	Daremberg 1848 Nickel 2002

Notes Tableau 41.3 :

(a) Traduction partielle par Serdjius de Reshayna (7 chapitres) ; les 7 autres chapitres ont été traduits par Ayyûb Rahâwî pour Gibraïl Ibn Bakhtîshû. Le premier chapitre a été traduit par Hunayn en arabe. Les autres chapitres ont été traduits en arabe par Hubaysh. Mais, une traduction complète pour Ibn Massawayh a été faite par Hunayn en 16 chapitres et 4 parties. Car, Hunayn, comme maître de traduction a critiqué la version de Hubaysh pour sa rapidité et son impatience.

(b) Hunayn : livre à 17 chapitres. Hunayn a traduit 4 chapitres en syriaque pour Salmawayh, et le premier chapitre en arabe, après la mauvaise traduction Serdjiûs.

(c) Cela peut être lu dans la lettre ou *Risâla* de Hunayn (Muhaqeq 2001) à propos des livres de Galien :

كتابه فيما ذكره افلاطون في كتابه المعروف بطيماوس من علم الطّب

'son livre sur ce que Platon a écrit dans son livre connu sous le nom de *Timawûs* sur la science médicale'. Hunayn a traduit 4 chapitres en syriaque, et seulement le premier en arabe. Ishâq Ibn Hunayn a traduit les trois derniers chapitres en arabe. Un tableau moins élaboré avait été présenté par Katouzian-Safadi (2007).

Tableau 41.4. Comparaison des œuvres majeures traitant de la rougeole et de la variole chez Râzî.

Livres	*V et R*	*Mansûrî*	*Division*	*Hâwî*
Thèmes				
Commande	oui	oui	non déclaré	notes personnelles
Récits bibliographiques	oui	non	non	non
Citations d'auteurs	oui	-	-	oui
Distinction rougeole et variole	Oui, nombreuses symptômes différenciés	Pas de symptômes différenciés	Rougeole plus oppressante	oui : multiples paragraphes
Descriptions des symptômes	Chap. II	oui : 2 lignes précisant plus chez enfants et jeunes	oui : 2 lignes sans donner d'âge	oui : multiples paragraphes épars
Etiologie	Longue description image : digestion et Alchimie	non	non	oui : multiples paragraphes
Prévention	Chap. V	oui	oui	oui
Prédisposition				
âge	Chap. II	oui	non	oui
Physiognomonie	Chap. IV : 3 types de corps	non	non	oui
saison	oui	non	non	oui
Soins curatifs yeux	Chap. VII	quelques lignes	quelques lignes	multiples paragraphes épars
Pustules à accélérer	Chap. VI			
Maturation pustules	Chap. VIII			
Assèchement pustules	Chap. X	Quelques mots	Quelques mots	multiples paragraphes épars
Escarre pustules	Chap. X	-	-	-
Convalescence séquelles Yeux	Chap. XI	quelques lignes	quelques lignes	multiples paragraphes épars
Alimentation	Chap. XII			
Évacuation intestinale	Chap. XII			
Distinction maladie curable ou incurable	A la fin, Chap. XIV	en fin du texte	en fin du texte	multiples paragraphes épars

récit des cas graves ou mortels, les doutes sur l'évolution du cours de la maladie, nous permettent d'élucider comment Râzî applique cette grande prudence. Nous remarquons que l'auteur aborde les traitements de ces deux maladies principalement comme les 'fièvres continues' et les 'tumeurs provenant de l'excès de chaleur', c'est-à-dire d'autres états maladifs avec des symptômes similaires.

Râzî agit avec la prudence d'un médecin et philosophe averti. Les multiples mis en garde et les appels à la prudence sont clairs, nombreux et insistants dans la *V et R*. Le médecin et philosophe Râzî était influencé par l'éthique médicale qu'il exprime dans de nombreuses œuvres philosophiques et médicales. Un autre médecin et philosophe, Averroès (m. 1198) prônait les vertus des médicaments composés dans son livre *Les généralités sur la médecine* '*al-Kullîyyat fî al-tibb*' ; cependant, il rappelait au médecin de rester prudent car toutes les *qualités* d'un médicament composé n'étaient pas prévisibles (Katouzian-Safadi 2011, 135–45). La conscience des effets incertains engendre le doute chez le médecin. La prudence thérapeutique au cours des maladies, rapproche ces deux philosophes et médecins, pourtant éloignés par le temps et par leur pratique ; en effet contrairement à Râzî, l'activité principale d'Averroès n'était probablement pas la médecine. Malgré des parcours et des formations distincts, des philosophies différentes ou parfois opposées, on retrouve une filiation méthodologique sur l'usage de la prudence lors de l'administration médicamenteuse.

Le livre de la *V et R* de Râzî est un exemple où la reconnaissance des doutes du philosophe, influence l'éthique médical et guide le médecin à choisir entre une intervention excessive et une attente observatrice et angoissante. Le médecin philosophe, doit modestement rassembler et connaître les œuvres écrites des autres médecins, être au chevet du malade pour observer et noter les cas particuliers dans un cahier personnel. Ensuite, il intervient d'abord par les aliments, puis par les médicaments simples et bien connus, et ensuite par des médicaments composés (Iskandar 1980 et Moubachir 1996, chapitre 'De la composition des médicaments', Aphorismes n° 174 et 5).

La *Division* et *Mansûrî* sont dépourvus de la bibliographie détaillée des œuvres de Galien ; ils ne contiennent pas non plus la longue description étiologique de la maladie. La description des symptômes est courte. Mais, les signes indiquant l'issue fatale des maladies sont décrits dans les quatre traités analysés. Ces derniers semblent être indispensables à toute personne soignante pour reconnaître les circonstances où le médecin doit cesser ses interventions. Lors de la rédaction de la *Division*, écrit après *Mansûrî*, Râzî connaissait un grand nombre de cas particuliers de malades, de multiples symptômes et la population fragile et susceptible de contracter ces maladies.

Or, Râzî sélectionne et restreint le tableau clinique en fonction des publics destinataires de ses œuvres : des médecins avisés (*al-tabîb*), des médecins praticiens (*al-mutitabib*) et des lettrés non médecin, 'n'ayant pas à leur proximité un médecin'. Dans un passage intitulé 'La séparation de la médecine et de la pharmacie' ('Kitâb al-saydala fî al-tibb', in M. Abdu'l Mu 'id Khan, 1955–1973, vol. XXII [1971], 1–4), l'auteur écrit que la pratique thérapeutique médicamenteuse est beaucoup plus complète et complexe dans les grandes cités urbaines qu'à la campagne (Katouzian-Safadi 2002, 217–22.). La *Division*, adressée à 'ceux qui ne disposent pas de médecin', pourrait être fort utile dans ces espaces loin des grandes cités urbaines arabo-musulmanes. Loin de ces centres, la pratique, le diagnostic, la thérapie et les remèdes doivent être simplifiés et c'est ainsi que procède ce médecin et philosophe Râzî.

En fonction des publics et dans un souci de faciliter la transmission des savoirs Razi adapte son savoir médical écrit. Cela montre que la démarche du médecin philosophe est double ; il a à la fois le souci de soigner la maladie mais également celui de permettre la discussion qui modifie l'état des savoirs. Il présente cette position audacieuse dans l'introduction de son livre *Les doutes sur Galien* (Mohaghegh 1993, Labib Abdul-Ghani 2005) où il décrit les conditions de travail et l'éthique du médecin philosophe qui veut tendre vers une avancée ou vers un progrès dans le domaine des sciences de la nature.

Remerciements

Ce travail a été réalisé avec les soutiens du Ministère français de l'Agriculture et de l'Environnement et de la Commission Européenne (EC 1221/97 & 917/2004 programs). Nous remercions le Dr Michael Chase pour les lectures des textes grecs et le Dr D. Bacalexi pour les discussions scientifiques. Nous avons bénéficié lors de nos recherches des conseils du Professeur R. Rashed pour associer en permanence les recherches historiques et les connaissances scientifiques contemporaines.

Translitération simplifiée adoptée Arabe et persan

Arabe	Translittération simplifiée dans cet article	Translittération internationale	*Encyclopé-die de l'Islam*
أ	'	'	'
ا	â	ā	ā
ث	th	c	th
ج	dj	ğ	dj
ح	h	h	h
خ	kh	k	kh
ذ	dh	x	dh
ش	sh	š	sh
ص	s	s	s
ض	d	d	d
ط	t	t	t
ظ	z	z	z
ع	'	o	o
غ	gh	r	gh
ق	q	q	k point dessous
و	û w	ū	ū
ي	î– y	ī	ī

Codes de la translittération simplifiée pour l'arabe et le persan. Graphie arabe	Translittération simplifiée dans cet ouvrage	Translittération internationale
أ	**'**	'
ع		O
د	**d**	d
ض		d
ه	**h**	h
ح		h
ت	**t**	z
ط		t
ز	**z**	z
ظ		z

Nous avons adopté un système simplifié proche de celui de certaines parutions (Cheddadi et Abdesselam, *Les Arabes et l'appropriation de l'histoire*, Sindbad, Actes Sud, Paris, 2004). Nous avons translittéré les deux lettres *hamza* et *ayn* en utilisant pour les deux l'apostrophe droite. Nous ne marquons pas les signes désignant les emphatiques et les vélaires. Ainsi, les arabophones sauront retrouver la transcription conventionnelle et les non arabophones disposeront d'une lecture plus aisée.

Bibliographie

Abdu'l Mu 'id Khan, M. 1955–1973 : *Kitâb al-Hâwî fî al-tibb* [Rhazes' *Liber Continens* – éd. arabe], 25 volumes, Hydarâbâd.

al-Siddîqî, H. B. (éd.) 1987 : *al-Mansûrî fî al-tibb* [*Le livre de Mansûrî*], *Manshûrât ma'had al-makhtûtât al-'arabîyya*, Kuwait.

Álvarez Millán C. 2010 : 'The case history in Medieval Islamic medical literature : *Tajârib* and *Mujarrabât* as Source', *Medical History*, 54(2), 195–214.

Balty-Guesdon, M.-G. 1991 : 'Le Bayt al-Hikma de Baghdad', *Arabica*, 39/2, 131–50.

Balty-Guesdon, M.-G. 2008 : 'La maison de la sagesse : une institution hors de l'histoire ? ', 85–98 dans M. Leibowicz (éd), *L'islam médiéval en terres chrétiennes, science et idéologie*, Villeneuve d'Asq.

Bergsträsser, G. (ed.) 1925 : *Hunain Ibn Ishâq. Über die syrischen und arabischen Galen-Übersetzungen zum ersten Mal herausgegeben und übersetzt*, in *Abhandlungen für die Kunde des Morgenlandes*, Band XVII, N° 2.

Biraben, J.-N. 1995 : 'Les maladies en Europe : équilibres et ruptures de la pathocénose', in M. Grmek (org.), *Histoire de la pensée médicale en Occident*, Paris, 283–310.

Brysson, J. S. 2000 : *The kitâb al-Hawî of Râzî (ca. 900 A.D.), Book One of the Hāwī on Brain, Nerve, and Mental Disorder : studies in the transmission of medical texts from Greek into Arabic into Latin*, Ph.D. dissertation, Yale University, UMI Number 9991125.

Channing, I. J. 1766 : *Rhazes, De variolis et morbilis*, London (éd. arabe et trad. Latine).

Congourdeau, M.-H. 1996 : 'Le traducteur grec du traité de Rhazès sur la variole', 99–111 dans A. Garzya et J. Jouanna (éds), *Storia e ecdotica dei testi medici greci, Atti del II Convegno Internazionale, Parigi, 24–26 maggio 1994*, Napoli.

Daremberg, C. 1848 : *Fragments du Commentaire de Galien sur le Timée de Platon*, Paris.

Darmon, P. 1989 : *La variole, les nobles et les princes, la petite vérole mortelle de Louis* XV, Bruxelles.

Glynn, I. and J. 2004 : *The Life and Death of Smallpox*, Cambridge.

Greenhill, W. A. (trans.) 1848a : '*Liber ad Almansorem*' (Lib. X, cap. 18), 74–86, dans *A treatise on the Small-Pox and Measles, by Abú Becr Mohammed ibn Zacaríyá ar-Rází (commonly called Rhazes)*, London. Site : http://books.google.fr/books?id=LC0IAAAAIAAJ&pg=PA7&dq=GREENHILL

Greenhill, W. A. (trans.) 1848b : '*Divisio morborum*' [fragment du *Kitâb al-Taqsîm wa al-tashdjîr, Livre de la division et de l'arborisation*], 87–98 dans *A treatise on the Small-Pox ...*

Greenhill, W. A. (trans.) 1848c : 'A Treatise on the Smallpox and Measles' [trad. anglaise de la version arabe *Kitâb al-djudarî wa al-hasba*], 1–74 dans *A treatise on the Small-Pox ...*

Greenhill, W. A. (trans.) 1848d : '*Liber continens*' [fragment du chapitre d'*al-Hâwî fî al-tibb*], 97–132 dans *A treatise on the Small-Pox ...*

Grmek, M. 1994 : *Les maladies à l'aube de la civilisation occidentale*, Paris (1ère éd. 1983).

Gutas, D. 2005 : *Pensée grecque, culture arabe. Le mouvement de traduction gréco-arabe à Bagdad et la société abbasside primitive (11-IV/VIII-X siècles)*, trad. de l'anglais par A. Cheddadi, Paris.

Hamâmî, S. M. (éd.) 1992 : *Kitâb al-taqsîm wa al-tashdjîr* [*Le livre de la division et de l'arborisation* – édition arabe et traduction française], Alep.

Hamarneh, S. 1973 : 'Origins of Pharmacy and Therapy in the Near East', The Naito Foundation, English Publications, Series 1, No. 2, Tokyo.

Harbî K. (éd.) 2006 : *Kitâb al-tadjârib* [*Le livre des expériences*] Alexandrie.

Iskandar, A. Z. 1959 : *A study of ar-Râzî's medical writings with selected texts and English translations*, Ph.D. thesis, Oxford University.

Iskandar, A. Z. (éd.) 1980 : *Kitâb al-murshid aw al-fusûl* [*Les aphorismes de Râzî*, éd. Arabe], *Madjallât ma had al-maktûtât al- 'arabiyya*, vol. 7, fasc. 1, Le Caire.

Katouzian-Safadi, M. 2002 : 'Séparation de la médecine et de la pharmacie : Plaidoyer d'Al-Rāzī', 217–22 dans S. M. Razaullah Ansari (éd.), *Science and Technology in the Islamic World*, Turnhout.

Katouzian-Safadi, M. 2004a : 'La pharmacie arabe', 870–74 dans D. Lecourt (dir.), *Dictionnaire d'histoire et philosophie de la médicine*, Paris.

Katouzian-Safadi, M. 2004b : 'La cornue et l'alambic, instrument d'analyse et de preuve dans *Les doutes sur Galien* de Râzî', 377–90 dans R. Morelon et A. Hasnawi (éds), *De Zénon d'Elée à Poincarré, Recueil d'études en hommage à Roshdi Rasehed*, Louvain et Paris.

Katouzian-Safadi, M. 2011 : 'Lois de la composition des médicaments : propriétés prévisibles et imprévisibles selon Averroès', 135–45 dans A. Hasnawi (éd.), *La lumière de l'intellect. La pensée scientifique et philosophique d'Averroès dans son temps. Actes du IVe Colloque International de la SIHSPAI (Société Internationale d'Histoire des Sciences et de la Philosophie Arabes et Islamiques), Cordoue, 1998*, Leuven.

Katouzian-Safadi, M. 2012: « *Une histoire des soins dans le monde arabe médiéval. La variole, la lèpre, la mélancolie, Le médecin face aux déséquilibres* », 23-50 dans V. Adam et L. Revol-Marzouk (éds), *La contamination : lieux symboliques et espaces imaginaires*, Paris.

Katouzian-Safadi, M. à paraître : 'Histoire de quelques infirmités visibles, les maladies de la peau : la lèpre, la variole, la rougeole', *Actes du colloque International sur Jâhiz, Tetouan, Maroc, novembre 2011*, dans A. Aarab (dir.), éd. faculté des lettres et sciences humaine de Tétouan, Université Abdelmalek Essaadi.

Katouzian-Safadi, M. à paraître : 'The Treatise on *Smallpox and measles, al-djudari wa al-hasba* of al-Râzî (865–925) : a history of innovation, transmission and teaching', *Fourth international conference of Translated Manuscripts, 29 May–1 June, 2007, Alexandrie.*

Katouzian-Safadi, M et Ben Ghachem, A. 2012 : '*Les arômes et les parfums au sein d'un faisceau de traitements. Examen de quelques traités médicaux médiévaux*', *Symposium international d'aromathérapie, Grasse*. Site : http://www.aromatherapie.ville-grasse.fr/ (Log-in: conferencier, Mot de passe: symparoma).

Katouzian-Safadi, M. et Bensaad, M. à paraître : 'Une nouvelle définition de la rougeole et de la variole chez le savant médiéval Râzî (865 – 925)', *Actes du colloque, Les crises sanitaires en Méditerranée antique et médiévale, novembre 2010, Poitiers*, éd. CRHIA–CESCM.

Kühn, C. G. (éd.) 1821–33 : *Claudii Galeni Opera Omnia*, Leipzig (reprint Hildesheim 1964–65).

Labib Abdul-Ghani, M. (éd.) 2005 : *Kitâb al-Shukûk 'alâ Jâlînûs* [*Les doutes sur Galien*], Le Caire.

Leclerc, J. et Lenoir, A. 1866 : *Traité de la variole et de la rougeole de Razès* [traduction française de la version arabe *Kitâb al-djudarî wa al-hasba*], Paris.

Littman, R. J. and Littman, M. L. 1973 : 'Galen and the Antonine Plague', *American Journal of Philology*, 94.

McVaugh, M. R. 2003 : 'Alchemy in the *Chirurgia* of Teodorico Borgognoni', 55–76 dans Ch. Crisciani e A. Paravicini Bagliani (éds), *Alchimia e medicina nel Medioevo*, Florence.

Meyerhof, M., 1935 : 'Thirty-three clinical observations by Rhazes (ca 900 A.D.)', *Isis* 23 :2, 321–72.

Mohaghegh, M. (éd.) 1993 : *Kitâb al-Shukûk 'alâ Jâlînûs* [*Les doutes sur Galien*], International Institute of Islamic Thought & Civilisation (ISTAC), Malaysia and Institute of Islamic Studies, Tehran University, Tehran.

Moubachir, E.-A. (éd.) 1996 : *Râzî, Guide du médecin nomade* [traduction française]. Paris.

Muhaqeq, M. (éd.) 2001 : *Risalâ Hunayn Ibn Ishâq* (*La Lettre de Hunayn Ibn Ishâq*) [éd. arabe, trad. Persane], Tehéran et Montréal.

Nadjmâbâdî, M. 1992 : *Kitâb al-djudarî wa al-hasba* [*Le livre de la rougeole et de la variole*, éd. arabe et traduction persane], 3ème éd. Téhéran.

Nickel, D. 2002 : 'On the authenticity of an "excerpt" from Galen's *Commentary on the Timaeus*', 73–8 in V. Nutton (ed.), *The unknown Galen*, London.

Pormann, P. and Savage-Smith, E. 2007 : *Medieval Islamic Medicine*, Edinburgh.

Rautureau, M., Liewig, N., Gomes, C. et Katouzian-Safadi, M. 2010 : *Argiles et Santé – Propriétés, usages thérapeutiques*, Paris.

Râzî 1984 : *Manafi' al-adwîya wa daf' madârrihâ* [*Les bienfaits et les méfaits des aliments* -éd. Arabe), Dâr Ihyâ'al-'ulûm, Beyrouth.

Richter-Bernburg, L. 2003 : '*Hâwî, Al-*', *Encyclopédie Iranica*, site : http://www.iranicaonline.org/articles/hawi-medical-book

Sezgin, F. (éd.) 2001/1380 H : *Tarikhe negâresh-hâye 'arabi*, vol. III, Téhéran. Traduction persane de l'allemand : F. Sezgin, 1970 : *Geschichte des arabischen Schrifttums*, Band III : Medizin, Pharmazie, Zoologie, Tierheilkunde bis ca 430 H, Leiden.

Steinschneider, M. 1956 : *Die europäischen Übersetzungen aus dem Arabischen bis Mitte des 17. Jahrhunderts*, Graz.

Strohmaier, G. 1995 : 'La médecine dans le monde byzantine et Arabe', 123–14 in Grmek, M. (dir.), *Histoire de la pensée médicale en Occident. Vol.1. Antiquité et Moyen Age*, Paris.

Ullmann, M. 1970 : *Die Medizin im Islam*, Handbuch der Orientalistik, I Abteilung, Ergänzungsband VI, 1 Abschnitt, Leiden-Köln.

42. The Ancient Background of Witelo's Theory of Vision

Maria-Magdalena Weker

Erazmus Ciolek, known as Witelo, Vitello Thuringopolonis, born c. *1230 and died before 1310, was a Polish theologian and a scientist: physicist, natural philosopher and mathematician. Witelo defined vision as a special kind of contact. The* pyramis radialis *stimulates the* organum viritus visivae. *The* cella aranea *collects the images from the crystal humour and the* spiritus visibilis *transports them to the brain. Witelo's concept of vision was an example of the combination of eye anatomy and geometric knowledge. Connections to the ancient theories of vision are clearly visible in the aspects of eye anatomy and function characteristics. Witelo's major surviving work on optics* Peri optikes *was one of the most influential works until the 17th century.*

Vision is the ability to perceive the visible external world. The primary task of the theory of vision is to explain how useful information about the external world is recovered from the changing retinal image. Theorists of vision have proposed various explanations of the nature of the processing responsible for our perception of size, shape and distance. Ancient philosophers and physicians explained vision in terms of *pneuma* theories of elementary cognition. Arab optic theorists created geometric models of vision and construed visual processing as a type of mathematical calculation.

The views of ancient scholars spread to the science of the Middle Ages and had a significant impact on the creation of the scientific image of the world. In numerous cases, they determined the ideas and theories created by the scholars of the Middle Ages. Clear references to the scientific theories created by those scholars may be found in the theories describing the functioning of man, in particular those concerning the cognitive processes. Those references are so clearly visible in some cases that they raise questions about the originality of a given theory. Witelo's theory is an example of such a theory, since it was considered a compilation of the views of ancient and Arab scholars and its originality was questioned. The aim of this article is to point to several clear references to the ancient theories of vision which, nevertheless, do not devalue the theory of Witelo.

Witelo: Life

Witelo, also known as Vitellio, Vitello, Vitello Thuringopolonis, Vitulon was in fact Erazm Ciołek. The appellation Witelo is almost certainly a Latinised form of the original Polish family name (*vitellus*, *vitellum* – a calf; *ciołek* – a young bull calf, a calf). The form Vitellio or Vitello used at first was transformed into Witelo in the 19th century (Bukowska 2006).

His date of birth is unknown. He was probably born around 1230 and died around 1300. Scholars give different dates of Witelo's birth and death. According to C. Baeumker, he lived between 1230 and 1270; according to A. Birkenmajer between1230 and 1314; while J. Burchardt believes that Witelo was born before 1237 and died after 1281 (Birkenmajer 1936; Bieganowski *et al.* 1991).

Witelo was educated at colleges in Wrocław, Legnica, Paris and Padua, and studied at the University of Paris in 1250. Around 1262, he began his studies at the academy in Padua. He studied theology, philosophy, mathematics, medicine and Canon law. In 1268, Witelo went to Viterbo and then moved to Rome where he worked at the Pope's court. It was there that he met Wilhelm von Moerbeke (William of Moerbeke, Guillelmus Morbeka), who became his tutor; and thanks to Moerbeke's translations from Greek to Latin, Witelo could study the dissertations of ancient philosophers.

Around 1275, Witelo returned to Poland and worked as

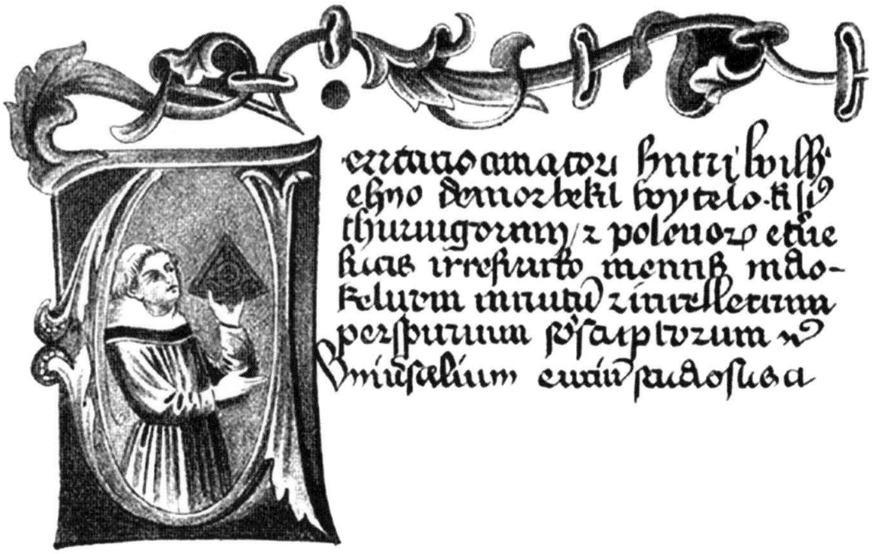

Fig. 42.1. Page from a manuscript of *De Perspectiva* by Witelo with a miniature showing the author, end of 13th century (http://monika.univ.gda.pl/~literat/grafika/optyk.htm)

a lecturer in the academies in Wrocław and Legnica. Then he was a diplomat at the Czech King Ottokar's diplomatic service and later at the court of the German Emperor Rudolf. Around 1281, he entered a monastic order in Vicogne in France. The place where he died is unknown but most probably it was Vicogne or Wrocław in Poland.

Witelo: Research

Witelo carried out research on many philosophical, scientific and natural phenomena. He wrote a number of treatises on such topics as meteorological and psychological phenomena, and metaphysical and theological issues. His most important research concerned eye anatomy and physiology of vision, as well as psychological, psychiatric and psychopathological knowledge. He also analysed the issue of light propagation, reflection, dispersion, refraction, as well as meteorological phenomena related to light and the psychological aspect of perception. In order to better understand and analyse the light, Witelo studied the treatises on mathematics and optics by, *inter alios*, Archimedes, Eutokios, Euclid, Ptolemy, Aristotle, Avicenna, Alhazen, Robert Grosseteste and Roger Bacon.

Witelo presented the results of his research along with the summary of the then knowledge on vision in his major work known as Περὶ ὀπτικῆς (*Peri optikes*, that is *On Perspective*), which was written between 1270 and 1278 (Fig. 42.1). It was first printed in 1535 with the title *Vitellionis mathematici doctissimi de optica, id est de natura, ratione et proiectione radiorum visum, luminum, colorum atque formarum, quam vulgo Perspectivam vocant, libri X.* There were no editorial changes in that edition or the next one, of 1551. The third edition was printed in 1572, together with Alhazen's dissertation on optics, as one book titled *Opticae thesaurus Alhazeni Arabis libri septem, nunc primum editi Eiusdem liber De Crepusculis et nubium ascensionibus, Item Vitellonis Thuringopoloni libri X.* Witelo's part was titled *Vitellonis Thuringopoloni opticae libri decem. Instaurati, figuris novis illustrati ataque aucti infinitisque erroribus, quibus antea scatebant, expurgati, a Federico Risnero*. Risnero, in fact, made many corrections and supplements to Witelo's original dissertation.

Peri optikes means perspective

The treatise contains a description of the works of Euclid, Ptolemy, Archimedes, Heron and Alhazen on geometry, optics, physiology and structure of the eye. Witelo analysed the information from the works of ancient scholars and Arab researchers, organised it and combined it into one coherent whole (Tejszerska 2004).

Peri optikes consists of ten books, each of which begins with a summary and compilation of the definitions and theses used therein. The first book includes the information related to geometry. It contains some definitions, including the definition of the pole, convex line, concave line, convex and concave surface intersecting circles, equal spheres, parallel spheres and circles, tangent and intersecting spheres, plane tangent to a sphere, denominator of proportion and compound proportions. The second book presents the research on the propagation of light. Witelo discusses light rays, the straight line through which light goes. Another

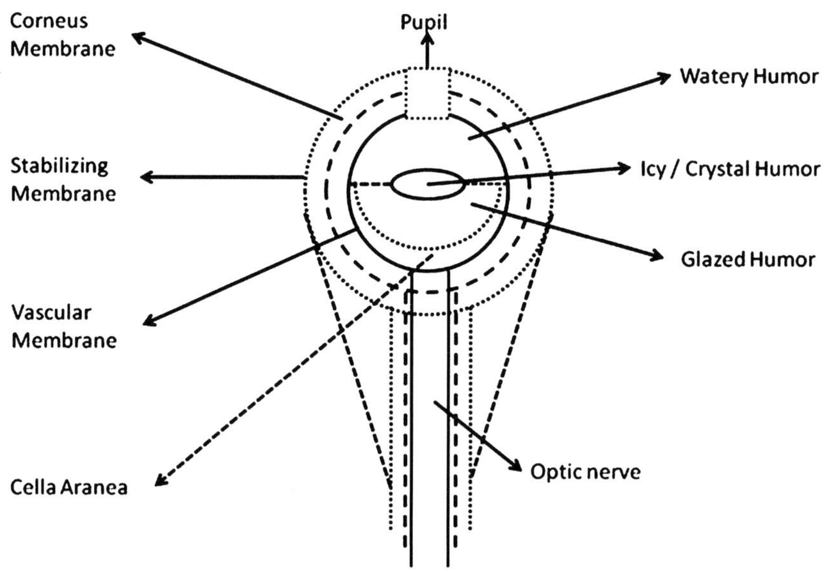

Fig. 42.2. Drawing of the eye according to Witelo (M.-M. Weker based on an illustration of the eye in Witelo's *Peri optikes* (1535 and 1572)).

topic discussed concerns the shadow, its creation, shape, size and relation to the light. The third book describes the eye anatomy and the seeing process. The next book is about the conditions and principles of vision. Book number five deals with the issues related to the reflection in flat mirrors. The sixth to ninth books deal with the reflections in spherical, concave, cylindrical and conical mirrors. The last book is devoted to the refraction of light and meteorological phenomena (Bieganowski *et al.* 1991; Bieganowski, Bielski and Wróblewski 1994; Bielski and Wróblewski 2003). *Peri optikes* was an important work for its time and until the 17th century it remained one of the major treatises on light, optical phenomena and vision.

Theory of vision

Witelo developed an original theory of vision which included the issues related to eye anatomy and physiology, the process of seeing and the conditions for seeing.

Eye anatomy

As regards eye anatomy, Witelo referred to the theory of Galen. Such references may be traced in the description of eye structure and eye functions. Witelo wrote about both eyes seeing in the same way as Galen. The similarity is also visible in the description of the movements of the eyeball and the characteristics of eye muscles.

According to Witelo, the eye is a sphere consisting of three membranes: the corneous, the stabilising and the vascular membrane. The corneous membrane is located at the front, the stabilising on the sides, while the vascular membrane is inside the eye. In the front of the eye there is an opening, i.e. a pupil. The inside of the sphere is filled with three transparent fluids called humours, namely the watery, the icy and the glazed humour. The watery humour is located at the front, the icy (crystal) humour in between, while the glazed humour is at the back (Fig. 42.2).

Witelo used the term icy/crystal humour to refer to the pupil. The crystal humour was small, spherical, with a structure similar to that of crystal or ice. Its moistness was the same as the moistness of the seen objects (wetter for a living being and less wet for rock or sand). According to Witelo, the characteristic of the crystal humour was the vision.

The glazed humour is a transparent liquid, which he placed in the centre of the eyeball. Its task is to provide nutrition to the eye. It is separated from the crystal humour by a web membrane (*cella aranea*). There is an optic nerve at the back of the sphere. It consists of an external and an internal membrane and has the shape of a funnel. Inside the nerve there is an empty channel. The spirit of vision (*spiritus visibilis*) created in the front part of the brain moves within the optic nerve. The interior of the channel is covered with a special membrane, the *cella aranea,* which covers also the back of the eyeball and the icy/crystal humour, that is the pupil (*organum viritus visivae*), which is the organ which directly senses the light. According to Witelo, the so-called 'light pyramid' *(pyramis radialis)* plays an important role in the process of vision. Its base is on the seen object and its top is in the eye/pupil. Only objects within the limits of the pyramid can be seen.

Table 42.1. Elements of Witelo's theory that match the ancient conceptions of vision

WITELO theory	*ANCIENT scholars*
Moistness	Democritus
Spiritus visibilis	Galen, Aristotle
Pyramis radialis	Euclid, Ptolemaeus Claudius
Organum viritus visivae/icy humour	Galen
Anatomy	Galen

Table 42.2. Elements of Witelo's theory that match the Arabic conceptions of vision

WITELO theory	*ARABIC scholars*
Spiritus visibilis	Hunayn Ibn Ishaq
Pyramis radialis	Qusta Ibn Luqa, Al-Kindi
Organum viritus visivae/icy humour	Avicenna
Cella aranea	Averroes
Anatomy	Alhazen

The vision process

According to Witelo, vision occurs as a result of the contact of the sight with the seen item and there is no vision without this contact. There are several stages in the process of vision. At the beginning, the light pyramid connects the eye with an object and the beams from the light pyramid fall on the pupil. Next, they create the picture on the pupil and it is caught by the *cella aranea.* Finally, they are sent to the brain by the *spiritus visibilis.* The process of seeing is a result of light being reflected from an object. Alhazen wrote that light goes from seen objects to the eye and, in accordance with Aristotle, he considered it was not a source of light. Witelo proves that light rays are drawn to the eye surface from each point of the seen object but only the orthogonal one passes through. All these orthogonal lines create a cone surface with a vertex being the centre of the eye and the pupil being the base.

Ancient references

References to the ancient theories of vision may be found in several places in the works of Witelo. His description of the eye anatomy contains an element which seems to be inspired by ancient philosophers (Table 42.1).

The moistness of the eye, which determines the seeing, may be found in the theory of vision developed by Democritus. The *spiritus visibilis* seems to be the part of Aristotle's conception of soul and mind. We can also find the same kind of *spiritus* in Galen's theory of eye anatomy and his theory of vision. The light pyramid is taken from the conceptions developed by Euclid and Claudius Ptolemaeus. The most important references concern the anatomy of the eye, where there are many connections to Galen's anatomy of the eye and the structure of the eyeball.

Some of the references result from Witelo's knowledge of Arabic treatises (Table 42.2). The *spiritus visibilis* kind of mental fluids may be found in Arabic dissertations, written by Hunayn Ibn Ishaq. The links concerning *pyramis radialis* are obvious if we compare the dissertations of Witelo and Qusta Ibn Luqa or Al-Kindi. The conceptions of the *organum viritus visivae*, that is the icy-crystal humour, may be found in Avicenna's theory; and, according to Averroes, the *cella aranea* is the most important element of the eye. Moreover, there are many connections to Alhazen's anatomy of the eye and the structure of the eyeball.

Some other aspects of vision

Witelo formulated a number of principles and rules of vision. The most important and most interesting include the following:

- We do not see any object in whole but only in parts.
- The distance of the seen object from the eyes is not measured by seeing itself but by the way of thought (analysis in thought) on the acuteness of seeing and the distinction from the background; there may be certain mistakes in the estimation of the size of the object due to the incorrect assessment of the surroundings of the seen object.
- The impression of beauty is created by images easy to see and comprehend, pleasant for the soul, or consisting of many elements with appropriate proportions.
- The impression of ugliness is created by images and figures which, alone and combined, do not correspond to the concept of beauty.
- The blackness of things which is not black may occur as a result of the lack of sight.

In his main work on optics, as well as in his earlier treatise *Tractatus de primaria causa poenitentiae et de natura daemonum* of 1268, Witelo argued that visual illusions are the result of observations, imagination and the method of thinking, and wrote, e.g., 'the eye does not receive any other information apart from light, colour and angle measure' and it is the brain which processes the impressions with the use of images taken from experience.

Conclusion

Witelo's concept of vision was an example of the combination of eye anatomy and geometric knowledge. The references to the ancient theories of vision are clearly visible in the aspects of eye anatomy and function characteristics. The originality of Witelo's theory lies in the combination of the discoveries of the ancient and Arab scholars with the knowledge of the Middle Ages, which was available to him. The combination of these elements resulted in the theory which, up to the 17th century was the most famous conception, and recognised as the best theory. It was studied by Leonardo da Vinci and Nicolaus Copernicus; and the work of Witelo and Alhazen, published as *Thesaurus opticus*, was the canon of optic knowledge until the 17th century. In 1604, Johannes Kepler published his own treatise on optics entitled *Ad Vitellonem Paralipomena*, that is Supplements to Witelo.

Bibliography

Bieganowski, L., Bielski, A. and Wróblewski, W 1994: *Witelona Perspektywy Księga IV. Przekład na język polski ze wstępem i komentarzami* (Studia Copernicana XXXIII), Warszawa.

Bieganowski, L., Bielski, A., Dygdała, R. S. and Wróblewski, W. 1991: *Witelona Perspektywy Księga II i III. Przekład na język polski ze wstępem i komentarzami* (Studia Copernicana XXIX), Wrocław.

Bielski, A. and Wróblewski, W. 2003: *Witelona Perspektywy Księga V, VI, VII. Przekład na język polski ze wstępem i komentarzami. Wstęp, opracowanie przekładu i komentarz* (Studia Copernicana XL), Toruń.

Birkenmajer, A. 1936: *Witelo najdawniejszy śląski uczony,* Katowice.

Bukowska D. 2006: 'Witelo. Życie i twórczość polskiego przyrodnika, zagubionego w zakamarkach przeszłości', *Foton* 95, 43–9.

Tejszerska, A. 2004: 'Witelo and Alhazen the most prominent perspective scientists of the middle ages', available from <http://ogigi.polsl.pl/biuletyny/zeszyt_9/z9_8.pdf> [Accessed May 2008].